Fitness for Life

SEVENTH EDITION

Charles B. Corbin
Arizona State University

Darla M. Castelli
The University of Texas at Austin

Benjamin A. Sibley
Appalachian State University

Guy C. Le Masurier
Vancouver Island University

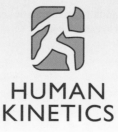

**HUMAN
KINETICS**

Library of Congress Cataloging-in-Publication Data

Names: Corbin, Charles B., author. | Castelli, Darla M., 1967- author. | Sibley, Benjamin A., author. | Le Masurier, Guy C., author.

Title: Fitness for life / Charles B. Corbin, Arizona State University, Darla M. Castelli, The University of Texas at Austin, Benjamin A. Sibley, Appalachian State University, Guy C. Le Masurier, Vancouver Island University.

Description: Seventh edition. | Champaign, IL : Human Kinetics, [2022] | Includes index.

Identifiers: LCCN 2020045984 (print) | LCCN 2020045985 (ebook) | ISBN 9781492591511 (hardback) | ISBN 9781718200623 (paperback) | ISBN 9781492591528 (epub)

Subjects: LCSH: Physical fitness.

Classification: LCC RA781 .C584 2022 (print) | LCC RA781 (ebook) | DDC 613.7--dc23

LC record available at https://lccn.loc.gov/2020045984

LC ebook record available at https://lccn.loc.gov/2020045985

ISBN: 978-1-4925-9151-1 (hardback)
ISBN: 978-1-7182-0062-3 (paperback)

Acquisitions Editor: Scott Wikgren; **Developmental Editor:** Melissa Feld; **Managing Editor:** Derek Campbell; **Copyeditor:** Heather Hutches; **Indexer:** Beth Nauman-Montana; **Permissions Manager:** Dalene Reeder; **Senior Graphic Designer:** Nancy Rasmus; **Cover Designer:** Keri Evans; **Cover Design Specialist:** Susan Rothermel Allen; **Photograph (front cover):** PeopleImages/Getty Images; **Photographs (back cover):** Getty Images/FatCamera (left), © Human Kinetics (middle), Marc Dufresne/E+/Getty Images (right); **Photographs (interior):** © Human Kinetics, unless otherwise noted; **Photo Asset Manager:** Laura Fitch; **Photo Production Manager:** Jason Allen; **Senior Art Manager:** Kelly Hendren; **Illustrations:** © Human Kinetics, unless otherwise noted; **Printer:** Walsworth

Printed in the United States of America   1 2 3 4 5 6 7 8 9 10   WPC   25 24 23 22 21

The paper in this book was manufactured using responsible forestry methods.

Human Kinetics
1607 N. Market Street
Champaign, IL 61820
USA

United States and International
Website: **US.HumanKinetics.com**
Email: info@hkusa.com
Phone: 1-800-747-4457

Canada
Website: **Canada.HumanKinetics.com**
Email: info@hkcanada.com

E7818 (hardback) /
E8195 (paperback)

Tell us what you think!
Human Kinetics would love to hear what we can do to improve the customer experience. Use this QR code to take our brief survey.

Contents

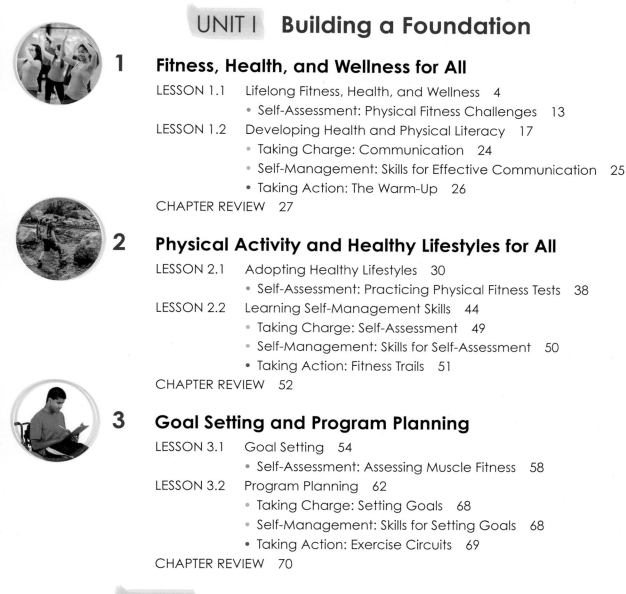

UNIT I   Building a Foundation

UNIT II   Safe and Smart Health-Enhancing Physical Activity

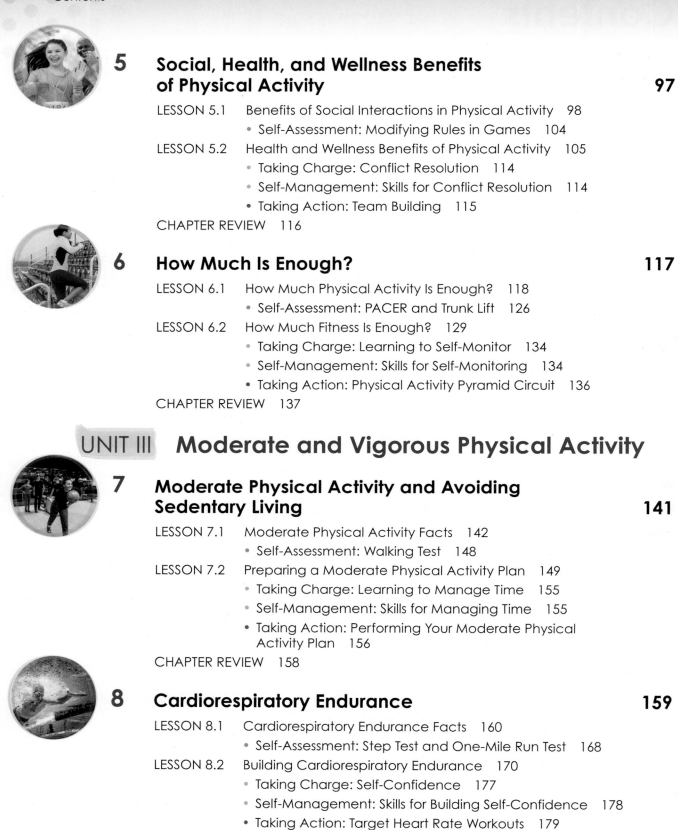

UNIT III   Moderate and Vigorous Physical Activity

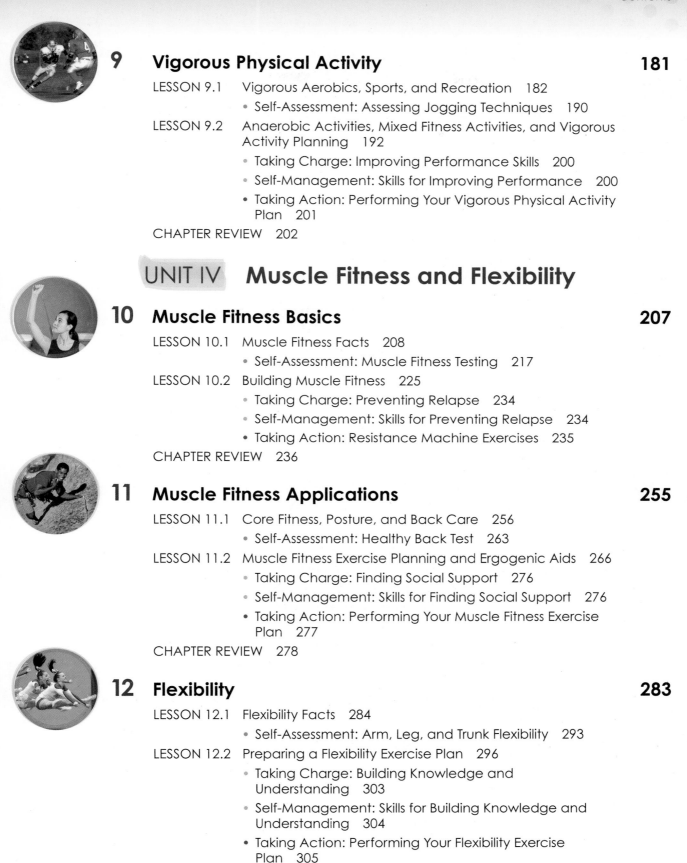

UNIT VII   Moving Through Life

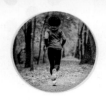

Touring *Fitness for Life*

Do you want to be healthy and fit? Do you want to look your best and feel good?

Fitness for Life is based on the proven HELP philosophy: **H**ealth for **E**veryone for a **L**ifetime in a very **P**ersonal way.

H = Health

E = Everyone

L = Lifetime

P = Personal

The HELP philosophy allows you to take personal control of your future fitness, health, and wellness.

Fitness for Life helps you become a physically literate person so that you can

- understand and apply important concepts and principles of fitness, health, and wellness;
- understand and use self-management skills that promote healthy lifestyles for a lifetime;
- be an informed consumer and critical user of fitness, health, and wellness information; and
- adopt healthy lifestyles now and later in life.

Fitness for Life is the winner of the Texty Award for textbook excellence.

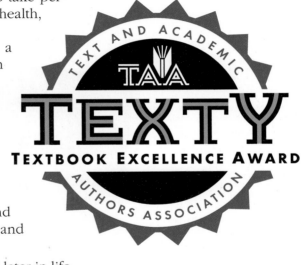

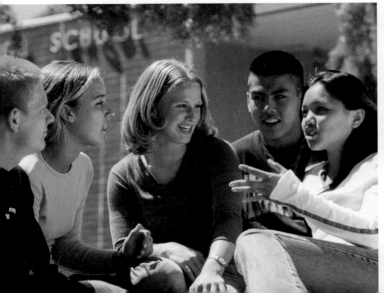

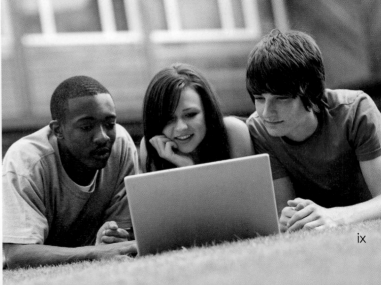

Fitness for Life will help you meet your fitness and physical activity goals. Take this guided tour to learn about all of the features of this textbook.

Two lessons are included in each chapter to help you learn key concepts relating to fitness, health, and wellness.

Unit Opener: Provides a brief overview of the content in each unit.

Healthy People 2030 Goals and Objectives: Lists national health goals and objectives covered in each unit.

Chapter Opener: Provides a brief overview of the content of the chapter.

UNIT III

Moderate and Vigorous Physical Activity

CHAPTER 7   **Moderate Physical Activity and Avoiding Sedentary Living**
CHAPTER 8   **Cardiorespiratory Endurance**
CHAPTER 9   **Vigorous Physical Activity**

Healthy People 2030 Goals and Objectives
Overarching Goals
- Attain healthy, thriving lives and well-being, free of preventable disease, disability, injury, and premature death.
- Eliminate health disparities, achieve health equity, and attain health literacy to improve the health and well-being of all.

Objectives
- Reduce the proportion of people who do no physical activity in their free time.
- Increase the proportion of adolescents and adults who do enough aerobic physical activity for health benefits.
- Increase the proportion of teens who participate in daily school physical education.
- Increase the proportion of teens who play sports.
- Increase the proportion of teens who walk or
- Increase the proportion of teens who limit scre
- Improve cardiovascular health and reduce th blood pressure, high blood lipids, heart attack
- Reduce unintentional injuries including brain i

Self-Assessment Features in This Unit
- Walking Test
- Step Test and One-Mile Run Test
- Assessing Jogging Techniques

Taking Charge and Self-Management Featur
- Learning to Manage Time
- Self-Confidence
- Improving Performance Skills

Taking Action Features in This Unit
- Performing Your Moderate Physical Activity Plan
- Target Heart Rate Workouts
- Performing Your Vigorous Physical Activity Plan

Features: Lists the Self-Assessment, Taking Charge and Self-Management, and Taking Action features in each unit.

In This Chapter: Lists the main elements of each chapter.

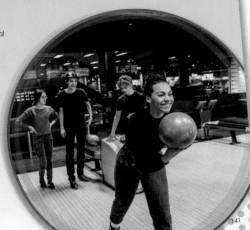

7

Moderate Physical Activity and Avoiding Sedentary Living

In This Chapter

LESSON 7.1
Moderate Physical Activity Facts

SELF-ASSESSMENT
Walking Test

LESSON 7.2
Preparing a Moderate Physical Activity Plan

TAKING CHARGE
Learning to Manage Time

SELF-MANAGEMENT
Skills for Managing Time

TAKING ACTION
Performing Your Moderate Physical Activity Plan

141

Lesson Objectives: Describes what you will learn in each lesson.

Lesson Vocabulary: Lists key terms in each lesson, which are defined in the glossary and on the student website.

Web Icon: Reminds you that additional information is available on the web resource for each lesson.

LESSON 1.1
Lifelong Fitness, Health, and Wellness

Lesson Objectives

After reading this lesson, you should be able to

1. define *health* and *wellness* and describe how they are interrelated;
2. define *physical fitness* and describe the six parts of health-related fitness and the five parts of skill-related fitness;
3. define *functional fitness* and explain why it is important; and
4. describe the warm-up, the workout, and the cool-down and explain why each is important.

Lesson Vocabulary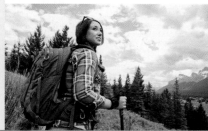

agility
balance
body composition
body fat level
calisthenics
cardiorespiratory endurance
cool-down
coordination
dynamic warm-up
flexibility
functional fitness
general warm-up
health
health-related physical fitness
hypokinetic condition
muscular endurance
physical fitness
power
quality of life
reaction time
skill-related physical fitness
skill warm-up
speed
state of being
strength
stretching warm-up
warm-up
wellness
workout

4

If you were granted one wish, what would it be? Some people might wish for material things, such as money, a new car, or a new house. But after some consideration, most people would wish for good health for themselves and their families. With health, fitness, and wellness, you can enjoy life to its fullest. Without them, no amount of money will allow you to do everything you would like to do. More than 90 percent of all people, including teens, agree that good health is important because it helps you feel good, look good, and enjoy life with the people you care about most.

As you read this book, you'll learn more about good lifestyle choices that can help you be fit, healthy, and well. You'll learn how to prepare a healthy personal lifestyle plan and how to use self-management skills to stick with your plan. The goal of this book is to help you become an informed consumer who makes effective decisions about your lifelong fitness, health, and wellness.

Before you can start developing a plan, you need some basic information. In this lesson, you'll learn definitions for some key words used throughout this course. You'll better understand the meaning of the words *fitness*, *health*, and *wellness*, and you'll learn about each of their components.

I took good health for granted until my dad had a heart attack. Then health became very important to me.

Jamis Abernathy

Teen Quotes: Statements from teens about fitness, physical activity, and healthy lifestyles.

SCIENCE IN ACTION: The Warm-Up

Experts have studied the warm-up for nearly 100 years, and over that time, ideas about what constitutes a good warm-up have changed. For many years a stretching warm-up was the preferred method of getting ready for a workout, but the current evidence suggests that the type of warm-up you use depends on the type of activity you plan to perform (see tables 1.1 and 1.2).

STUDENT ACTIVITY

List the three activities that you most commonly do as part of your workout, then use the information in this section to choose the best type of warm-up for each activity.

The cool-down usually consists of slow to moderate activity, such as walking or slow jogging, to allow the muscles to gradually recover and heart rate and blood pressure to return to normal. This also helps prevent dizziness and fainting. If you suddenly stop running, for example, the blood can pool in your legs, leaving your heart with less blood to pump to your brain. But if you continue moving after a hard run, your muscles will squeeze the veins of your legs, helping the blood continue to circulate. The following list provides some more cool-down guidelines.

- Do not sit or lie down immediately after vigorous activity.
- Gradually reduce the intensity of activity during the cool-down (for example, if you were running, slow to a jog, then a walk, and then consider gentle stretching).
- Walk or do other moderate total body movements.
- You may choose to do some of the stretching exercises presented in chapter 12, Flexibility, after your general cool-down while your muscles are still warm.

Lesson Review: Helps you review and remember the information you learned in the lesson.

LESSON REVIEW

1. How are health and wellness defined, and how are the two interrelated?
2. How do you define physical fitness, the six parts of health-related fitness, and the five parts of skill-related fitness?
3. How do you define functional fitness, and why is it important?
4. What are the warm-up, the workout, and the cool-down, and why each is important?

Fit Fact: Offers interesting information about key topics.

Tech Trends: Helps you become aware of new technological information related to fitness, health, and wellness and helps you try out and use new technology.

FIT FACT
On average, Americans of all ages take about 5,000 steps per day. This is considerably less than the averages in some other countries—for example, 9,000 or more in Australia and Switzerland and 7,000 or more in Japan—where obesity rates are much lower. Children (ages 5-12) average 12,500 steps per day.

progression. Instead of starting with a high goal such as 10,000 steps per day, which some experts recommend for adults, increase your step count gradually. Monitor your activity for a full week and then determine your average daily step count. Each week add 500 to 1,000 steps to your daily step count. The average teen takes about 10,000 steps a day (11,000 for boys and 9,000 for girls), and those involved in sports activities often accumulate 12,000 to 15,000 steps per day. Experts indicate that 12,000 steps per day is a reasonable long-term step goal for teens.

Tracking Energy Expended

Another way to determine whether you perform enough moderate activity is to track the energy you expend in activity. Some activity trackers estimate the calories you expend during physical activity. To allow the counters to estimate calories, you enter personal data such as your age and weight. The counter then uses this information as well as the time and intensity of your activity to estimate the calories expended during the day. During 60 minutes of moderate activity, such as brisk

TECH TRENDS: Pedometers and Activity Trackers (Accelerometers)

As described in chapter 6, a **pedometer** is a small, battery-powered device that counts each step you take and displays the running count on a meter. You simply open the face of the pedometer or push a button to see how many steps you've taken. If you choose a pedometer to monitor physical activity, additional information can be useful. Some pedometers allow you to enter the length of your step (your stride length) and your body weight so that the computer can estimate the distance you walk and the number of calories you expend. More expensive pedometers can also track the total time you spend in activity during the day. Less expensive pedometers must be reset at the end of the day, but some more expensive ones can store steps for several days. Pedometers are good for counting steps when walking but are not as good for tracking other forms of activity.

Activity trackers such as the Fitbit and the Apple Watch contain an **accelerometer**, which tracks body movements (forward and backward, up and down, and side to side). The accelerometer uses a formula determine how

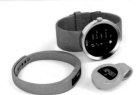

A pedometer counts steps and is a good way to self-monitor moderate activity.

much you move each day. Activity trackers are similar to pedometers but measure physical activity in more detail, including the intensity of your movements (METs) and the amount of time you spend at different intensities. With these measurements, most activity trackers can estimate the energy you expend in many types of activity. Accelerometers are now available in watches, phones, and devices worn on your belt or carried in your pocket.

USING TECHNOLOGY
Check your pedometer for accuracy (you may also use a smartphone app or fitness monitor). Set the counter to zero, count as you take 100 steps, and check the pedometer to see how many steps it counted. If it is within 3 steps (97-103) it is counting well. Next, estimate the number of steps you take on a typical weekday and a typical weekend day. Then wear a pedometer to see how many steps you actually take on these days. See if you're as active as you think you are!

Servings and Serving Sizes

A healthy eating pattern includes appropriate amounts of macro- and micronutrients from the various food groups. The FDA requires that food labels contain the size of a serving and the number of servings in a food package. Size of servings are shown in common measurements (e.g., cup, tablespoon, piece, slice). The size of serving on a food container is not a recommendation of how much to eat or drink. Rather, a serving size is based on the amount of food people typically consume rather than how much they *should* consume. The size of serving is provided so that you know the nutrition value of food in a serving of the size noted on the package.

Consumer Corner: Provides information to help you become a good consumer and avoid quackery.

CONSUMER CORNER: MyPlate

The Dietary Guidelines for Americans 2020–2025 provide easy-to-use information about eating for good health. Earlier you learned about the food groups from which you can choose to eat well (see figure 16.3). The guidelines also recommend the use of MyPlate (see figure 16.4) to encourage you to fill your plate with a variety of foods at each meal. As noted earlier, oils do not constitute a separate food group, so they are not included in MyPlate.

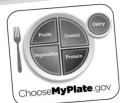

Figure 16.4 MyPlate: A USDA food graphic.
FROM USDHHS and USDA.

STUDENT ACTIVITY
Explore the MyPlate website to learn more about the different food choices that contribute to healthy eating patterns.

Science in Action:
Helps you understand how new information is generated using the scientific method.

SCIENCE IN ACTION: Optimal Challenge

Scientists in many fields have collaborated to find ways to help people stay active, eat well, and stick with other healthy lifestyle behaviors. They have discovered that in order to be successful, you must set goals that provide optimal challenge. If a challenge is too easy, there's no need to try hard—it's not really a challenge. On the other hand, if a goal is too hard, we fail, which may lead us to give up because our effort seems hopeless (see figure 3.2).

An optimal challenge requires reasonable effort. Meeting an optimal challenge allows us to experience success and makes us want to try again. In fact, optimal challenge is one reason that video games are so popular. They challenge you by making the task more difficult as you improve, which makes you want to play again and again. You can use optimal challenge when setting your own goals to help you succeed.

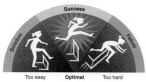

Figure 3.2 Some challenges can lead to boredom or failure, but optimal challenges can lead to success.

STUDENT ACTIVITY

Imagine that you want to help a friend learn a skill—for example, hitting a tennis ball. How could you use optimal challenge to help your friend learn the skill?

Fitness Quotes:
Provide quotes from famous people about fitness, health, and wellness.

If you want to live a happy life, tie it to a goal, not to people or things.

Albert Einstein, Nobel Prize–winning physicist

appropriate long-term goals because it may take you a fair amount of work and time to reach them.

The Taking Charge and Self-Management features in this chapter focus on setting goals for nutrition and fitness. Elsewhere in the book, you'll get the chance to set long-term goals for making healthy lifestyle changes (product goals). You'll also get the chance to set short-term goals (process goals) that help you move toward achieving your long-term goals.

LESSON REVIEW

Academic Connection:
Relates concepts from other academic subject areas to fitness, health, and wellness.

ACADEMIC CONNECTION: Mnemonics and Acronyms

A **mnemonic** (pronounced ni-mon'-ik) is a tool that helps you remember something. There are many types of mnemonics. Examples include rhymes, songs, and patterns of letters. For example, a rhyme is commonly used as a mnemonic to remember how many days there are in each month ("Thirty days hath September, April, June, and November") and the alphabet song is a mnemonic that helps children learn their ABCs. An **acronym** is a type of mnemonic that uses the first letter of several words to form a new word. Two examples used in this book are SMART and FIT. SMART helps you remember the characteristics of goal setting and FIT helps you remember the *frequency, intensity,* and *time* of physical activity (when the type of activity is already established).

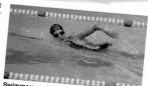

Swimmers on this team used the acronym TEAM (Together Everyone Achieves More) to help them achieve their goals.

STUDENT ACTIVITY

Create a mnemonic or an acronym related to your study in *Fitness for Life*. Briefly describe the mnemonic or acronym and explain how it might be useful.

new goal of continuing to work for five hours a week for the next eight weeks. Over the next eight weeks, Anna met her goal and was able to save $240. At this point she had saved $340 and felt confident about setting a long-term goal of saving $100 per month over the next nine months if she sticks to her schedule. If Anna meets her long-term goal, she will have saved at least $1,240 for the year ($340 + $900), more than half of what she needs for college. Now let's see whether this would be a SMART long-term goal for Anna.

Specific. Saving $100 a month for nine months is a very specific long-term goal.

Measurable. The goal of saving $100 a month is measurable. Anna can count her money every month to see how close she is to reaching the long-term goal.

Attainable. Anna set short-term goals and met them twice, so the long-term goal is likely to be attained.

Realistic. For someone else, the goal of $100 a month might not be realistic, but for Anna it is not unreasonable. She has saved at least $100 a month for three months, and if she continues to save at that rate she will meet the long-term goal as scheduled.

Timely. The goal of saving $100 a month for nine months ($900 total) has a specific and workable time line, fits her schedule, and over two years will provide the funds that she will need for college.

Product and Process Goals

Process goals involve performing a behavior, such as working a certain number of hours to earn money. *Process* refers to what you do rather than to the product resulting from what you do. Examples of process goals for fitness, health, and wellness include exercising for 60 minutes and eating five servings of fruits and vegetables every day (figure 3.1a). Process goals make good short-term goals because you can easily monitor your progress. In contrast, product goals do not make especially good short-term goals, because they typically take a while to achieve and can be discouraging, especially for a person who is just beginning to change. For example, if you chose a product goal of being able to perform 25 push-ups, it might (depending on your current fitness level) take you so long to meet the goal that you would give up. But a short-term process goal—such as performing 5 to 10 push-ups each day for two weeks—would be possible for you

56

EXERCISE CHART 3: **Elastic Band Exercises**

Choose an exercise band that offers enough resistance so that you are fatigued after the last repetition in the last set. Band length should be adjusted to allow the exercise to be performed as described. Check your bands regularly for wear and tear. If a band breaks while you are exercising it can cause injury.

Arm Press

This exercise is best performed with a tube-type band with handles. The band length should be adjusted to allow the exercise to be performed as described.

1. Anchor the band at shoulder height or higher using a secure hook (avoid hooks that may damage the band). Stand close to the anchor so that the band is not tight.
2. Face away from the anchor. Hold a handle in each hand, palm facing down. With your hands and grips in front of your shoulders, walk forward until the band is tight. Stand with one foot about two feet in front of the other.
3. Press straight forward with your hands and arms until your arms are extended. Return slowly to the starting position.

   Caution: Keep the core muscles tight and limit movement to your arms.

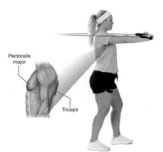

This exercise uses the muscles at the top of your shoulders, between your shoulder blades, and on the back of your arms.

Biceps Curl

This exercise is best performed with a tube-type band with handles.

1. Stand with both feet on the band with feet shoulder-width apart. Grab the handles with the arms extended and the palms facing up.
2. Flex the elbow until the handles are at shoulder level. Lower to the starting position.
3. You can also perform this exercise with your palms down.

   Caution: Do not move other joints, especially in your back.

Exercise Chart:
Provides instructions and pictures to teach you correct technique for exercises.

SELF-ASSESSMENT: **Walking Test**

Many of the self-assessments you perform in this course require very intense physical activity. If you're active and fit, the mile run or PACER may be the best way to estimate your cardiorespiratory endurance, but the walking test is especially good for beginners, those who haven't done a lot of recent activity, or those who are regular walkers but do not regularly get more vigorous activity. The walking test is also good for older people and for those who cannot do running tests due to joint or muscle problems. As directed by your teacher, record your scores and fitness ratings for the walking test. You can then use the information in preparing your personal physical activity plan. If you're working with a partner, remember that self-assessment information is confidential and shouldn't be shared without the permission of the person being tested.

1. Walk a mile at a fast pace (as fast as you can go while keeping approximately the same pace for the entire walk).
2. Immediately after the walk, count your heartbeats for 15 seconds. (For information about counting heart rate, see chapter 8.) Multiply the result by four to calculate your one-minute heart rate.
3. Use the appropriate chart to determine your walking rating.

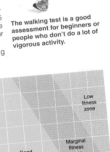

The walking test is a good assessment for beginners or people who don't do a lot of vigorous activity.

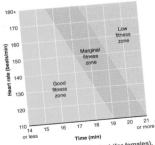

Rating chart for the walking test (for females).
Adapted from the *One Mile Walk Test* with permission of author James M. Rippe, M.D.

Rating chart for the walking test (for males).
Adapted from the *One Mile Walk Test* with permission of author James M. Rippe, M.D.

Self-Assessment:
Helps you learn more about your fitness and behaviors that affect your health and wellness and helps you prepare a personal plan for improvement.

Taking Charge and Self-Management: Provide guidelines for learning self-management skills that help you adopt healthy behaviors.

For Discussion: Helps you take charge by making good decisions.

TAKING CHARGE: Setting Goals

You probably know people who are sedentary or who eat a lot of unhealthy food. They may have tried to make lifestyle changes but been ineffective because they failed to set good goals. This feature highlights SMART goals for nutrition.

Ms. Booker, a physical education teacher, noticed that Kevin seemed a bit listless in class. She stopped by his desk and asked, "Are you all right, Kevin? You seem a bit tired."

Kevin said, "I'm okay. I was in a hurry this morning so I missed breakfast."

Later, as she passed through the cafeteria, Ms. Booker couldn't help noticing that Kevin was eating food from a vending machine for lunch. They were sitting by themself at an isolated table.

Ms. Booker walked over, sat down, and asked, "Are you feeling better now?"

Kevin replied, "Yes, but I know I need to eat better."

Ms. Booker said, "Maybe you need to make a plan to eat better. Do you remember the SMART formula we learned in class? Maybe you could use the formula to set some goals." Kevin agreed that this was a good idea.

FOR DISCUSSION

How could Kevin use the SMART formula to set good nutrition goals? What might be some good long-term goals for them? What might be some good short-term goals? What kinds of advice do you think Ms. Booker gave Kevin about goal setting? What advice would you have for Kevin? Consider the guidelines in the following Self-Management feature as you answer these discussion questions.

SELF-MANAGEMENT: Skills for Setting Goals

Now that you know more about different types of goal setting, you can begin developing some goals of your own. Use the following guidelines to help you as you identify and develop your personal goals.

- *Know your reasons for setting your goals.* People who set goals for reasons other than their own personal improvement often fail. Ask yourself, *Why is this goal important to me?* Make sure you're setting goals based on your own needs and interests.

- *Choose a few goals at a time.* As you work your way through this book, you'll establish goals for fitness, physical activity, food choices, weight management, stress management, and other healthy lifestyle behaviors. But rather than focusing on all of them at once, you'll choose a few goals at a time. Trying to do too much often leads to failure.

- *Use the SMART formula.* The SMART formula helps you to set goals that are

specific, measurable, attainable, realistic, and timely.

- *Set long-term and short-term goals.* The SMART formula helps you establish both long-term and short-term goals. When setting short-term goals, focus on process goals—that is, focus on making good lifestyle changes, not on results.

- *Put your goals in writing.* Writing down a goal represents a personal commitment and increases your chances of success. You'll get the opportunity to write down your goals as you do the activities in this book.

- *Self-assess and keep logs.* Doing self-assessments helps you set your goals and determine whether you've met them. Focus on improvement by working toward goals that are slightly beyond your current results.

- *Reward yourself.* Achieving a personal goal is rewarding. Allow yourself to feel

68

be afraid to revise it. It's better to revise your goal than to quit.

- *Consider maintenance goals.* Improvement is not always necessary. Once you reach the highest level of change, setting

continue to improve in fitness forever, and following a regular workout schedule to maintain good fitness is a reasonable goal. Likewise, once you achieve the goal of eating well, maintaining your healthy eating pattern is a worthwhile goal.

Taking Action: Lets you try out activities that can help you become fit and active for a lifetime.

Taking Action: Exercise Circuits

An exercise circuit consists of several stations, each of which features a different exercise. Typically, you move from one station to the next without resting. They also have the advantage of not requiring a lot of equipment, though you might enjoy bringing some music to listen to while working out. Exercise circuits are popular because the variety of exercises helps make the workout interesting. Circuits can be designed to focus on either health-related or skill-related fitness components, and they can be performed in a variety of places—indoors or outdoors, at home or elsewhere. **Take action** to create an exercise circuit using the following tips:

- Before starting the circuit, perform a dynamic warm-up.
- Plan stations that address all parts of your body: lower, middle, and upper.
- Avoid having two stations in a row that challenge the same body part.
- Pace yourself so that you can move continuously through the stations without stopping.
- Use correct technique at each station; if your technique fails due to fatigue, take a break.
- After doing the circuit, perform a cool-down.

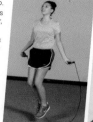

Exercise circuits use a variety of exercises at several stations.

Chapter Review: Helps you reinforce what you've learned in the chapter's two lessons.

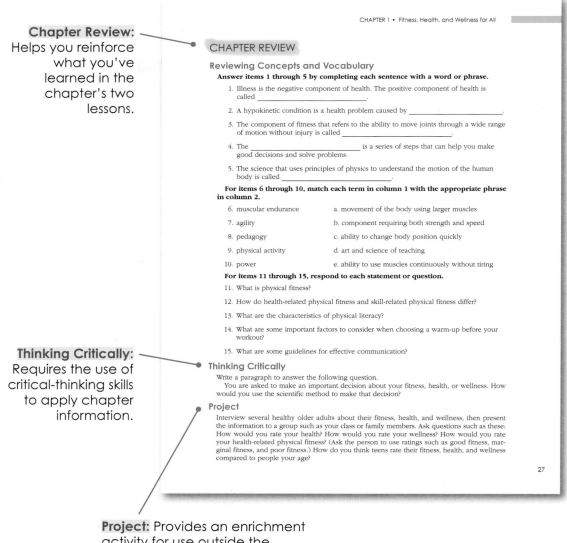

CHAPTER 1 • Fitness, Health, and Wellness for All

CHAPTER REVIEW

Reviewing Concepts and Vocabulary

Answer items 1 through 5 by completing each sentence with a word or phrase.

1. Illness is the negative component of health. The positive component of health is called _____.

2. A hypokinetic condition is a health problem caused by _____.

3. The component of fitness that refers to the ability to move joints through a wide range of motion without injury is called _____.

4. The _____ is a series of steps that can help you make good decisions and solve problems.

5. The science that uses principles of physics to understand the motion of the human body is called _____.

For items 6 through 10, match each term in column 1 with the appropriate phrase in column 2.

6. muscular endurance   a. movement of the body using larger muscles

7. agility   b. component requiring both strength and speed

8. pedagogy   c. ability to change body position quickly

9. physical activity   d. art and science of teaching

10. power   e. ability to use muscles continuously without tiring

For items 11 through 15, respond to each statement or question.

11. What is physical fitness?

12. How do health-related physical fitness and skill-related physical fitness differ?

13. What are the characteristics of physical literacy?

14. What are some important factors to consider when choosing a warm-up before your workout?

15. What are some guidelines for effective communication?

Thinking Critically

Write a paragraph to answer the following question.

You are asked to make an important decision about your fitness, health, or wellness. How would you use the scientific method to make that decision?

Project

Interview several healthy older adults about their fitness, health, and wellness, then present the information to a group such as your class or family members. Ask questions such as these: How would you rate your health? How would you rate your wellness? How would you rate your health-related physical fitness? (Ask the person to use ratings such as good fitness, marginal fitness, and poor fitness.) How do you think teens rate their fitness, health, and wellness compared to people your age?

27

Thinking Critically: Requires the use of critical-thinking skills to apply chapter information.

Project: Provides an enrichment activity for use outside the classroom.

In addition to all the textbook features, the *Fitness for Life* program includes several other components:

- **Student Web Resource:** You have access to a variety of resources in the *Fitness for Life, Seventh Edition, Web Resource*. These resources will aid your understanding of the textbook content and include video clips that demonstrate how to do the self-assessment exercises in each chapter and the exercises in chapters 10, 11, and 12, chapter reviews, and vocabulary terms with English and Spanish definitions and audio pronunciations.

- **Teacher Resources:** Your teacher has access to lessons and activities that you can do to better learn and understand the information in this textbook.

Now read on, and enjoy *Fitness for Life*!

Editorial Board

UNIT I

Building a Foundation

CHAPTER 1   **Fitness, Health, and Wellness for All**
CHAPTER 2   **Physical Activity and Healthy Lifestyles for All**
CHAPTER 3   **Goal Setting and Program Planning**

What Is Healthy People 2030?

Healthy People 2030 is a document that outlines health and wellness goals and objectives for our nation. The goals and objectives are established by hundreds of health experts, with input from the public.

Why 2030?

The first goals and objectives were initiated in 1979 with the hope that they would be met by the year 1990. Every 10 years, new health and wellness goals for the nation are established. Through personal and community action, the current national goals and objectives are meant to be attained by the year 2030.

What Are the Main Goals of Healthy People 2030?

The overarching goals of Healthy People 2030 are the following:

- Attain healthy, thriving lives and well-being, free of preventable disease, disability, injury, and premature death.
- Eliminate health disparities, achieve health equity, and attain health literacy to improve the health and well-being of all.
- Create social, physical, and economic environments that promote attaining full potential for health and well-being for all.
- Promote healthy development, healthy behaviors, and well-being across all life stages.
- Engage leadership, key constituents, and the public across multiple sectors to take action and design policies that improve the health and well-being of all.

What Are the Objectives of Healthy People 2030?

To meet the main goals of Healthy People 2030, specific objectives have been written in 41 categories. The opening page of each unit of this book provides a list of Healthy People 2030 objectives relevant to the chapters in that unit. You can find more information about other objectives at https://health.gov/healthypeople.

Why Are Healthy People 2030 Goals and Objectives Important to Me?

The overarching goals and objectives of *Fitness for Life* are consistent with those of Healthy People 2030. Since the first Healthy People initiative was started more than 40 years ago, much progress has been made, including reducing major causes of death such as heart disease and cancer and improving health behaviors that promote health and wellness. By adopting personal healthy lifestyles as outlined in Healthy People 2030, and encouraging these lifestyles among others, you contribute to the continued improvement of our nation's health and wellness.

Healthy People 2030 Goals and Objectives

Overarching Goals

- Attain healthy, thriving lives and well-being, free of preventable disease, disability, injury, and premature death.
- Eliminate health disparities, achieve health equity, and attain health literacy to improve the health and well-being of all.

Objectives

- Increase health literacy of the population.
- Increase the proportion of people who can access electronic health information.
- Reduce the proportion of people who do no physical activity in their free time.
- Increase the proportion of adolescents and adults who do enough aerobic and muscle building physical activity for health benefits.
- Create social, physical, and economic environments that promote attaining full potential for health and well-being for all.
- Promote healthy development, healthy behaviors, and well-being across all life stages.

Self-Assessment Features in This Unit

- Physical Fitness Challenges
- Practicing Physical Fitness Tests
- Assessing Muscle Fitness

Taking Charge and Self-Management Features in This Unit

- Communication
- Self-Assessment
- Setting Goals

Taking Action Features in This Unit

- The Warm-Up
- Fitness Trails
- Exercise Circuits

Fitness, Health, and Wellness for All

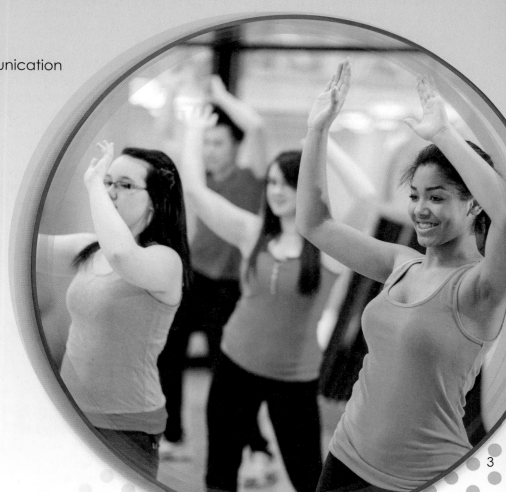

Lifelong Fitness, Health, and Wellness

Lesson Objectives

After reading this lesson, you should be able to

1. define *health* and *wellness* and describe how they are interrelated;
2. define *physical fitness* and describe the six parts of health-related fitness and the five parts of skill-related fitness;
3. define *functional fitness* and explain why it is important; and
4. describe the warm-up, the workout, and the cool-down and explain why each is important.

Lesson Vocabulary

agility
balance
body composition
body fat level
calisthenics
cardiorespiratory endurance
cool-down
coordination
dynamic warm-up
flexibility
functional fitness
general warm-up
health
health-related physical fitness
hypokinetic condition
muscular endurance
physical fitness
power
quality of life
reaction time
skill-related physical fitness
skill warm-up
speed
state of being
strength
stretching warm-up
warm-up
wellness
workout

If you were granted one wish, what would it be? Some people might wish for material things, such as money, a new car, or a new house. But after some consideration, most people would wish for good health for themselves and their families. With health, fitness, and wellness, you can enjoy life to its fullest. Without them, no amount of money will allow you to do everything you would like to do. More than 90 percent of all people, including teens, agree that good health is important because it helps you feel good, look good, and enjoy life with the people you care about most.

As you read this book, you'll learn more about good lifestyle choices that can help you be fit, healthy, and well. You'll learn how to prepare a healthy personal lifestyle plan and how to use self-management skills to stick with your plan. The goal of this book is to help you become an informed consumer who makes effective decisions about your lifelong fitness, health, and wellness.

Before you can start developing a plan, you need some basic information. In this lesson, you'll learn definitions for some key words used throughout this course. You'll better understand the meaning of the words *fitness*, *health*, and *wellness*, and you'll learn about each of their components.

> I took good health for granted until my dad had a heart attack. Then health became very important to me.
>
> *Jamis Abernathy*

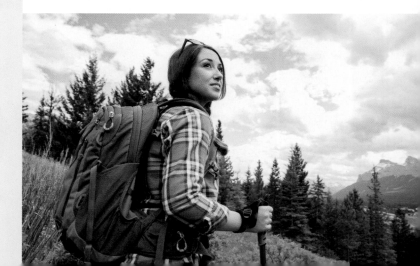

What Is Health? What Is Wellness?

The first wealth is health.

Ralph Waldo Emerson, poet

Early definitions of **health** focused on illness. The first medical doctors focused on helping sick people overcome their health problems; in other words, their main job was treating people who were ill.

But in 1947, the World Health Organization (WHO), which has representatives from 194 countries, issued a statement indicating that health meant more than freedom from disease or illness. This recognition led to a more comprehensive definition of health, which now includes wellness. According to the WHO statement, simply not being sick doesn't mean you are well. **Wellness** is the positive component of health that includes having a positive sense of personal well-being and **quality of life** (i.e., satisfaction with your current life status).

Figure 1.1 shows that a healthy person is not ill (the blue circle) and also has a strong wellness component (the green circle). Illness is the negative component of health that we want to treat or prevent, whereas wellness is the positive component of health that we want to promote.

Health and wellness have many linked components, often represented by a chain (figure 1.2). For a chain to be strong, each link must be strong. This can be accomplished by promoting the positive while avoiding the negative in each link. If you have this combination, you possess wellness and your risk of illness is reduced. The bottom line is this: Health is freedom from disease and debilitating conditions as well as optimal wellness in all five components (physical, emotional–mental, social, intellectual, and spiritual).

Each of us is interested in our own personal health and wellness. This is commonly referred to as *personal health*. To ensure our health and wellness, we should also be interested in promoting community health. *Community health* refers to the health and wellness of a group rather than an individual—small groups such as families and networks of friends, larger groups such as towns and cities, and very large groups such as states and countries. Just as each person

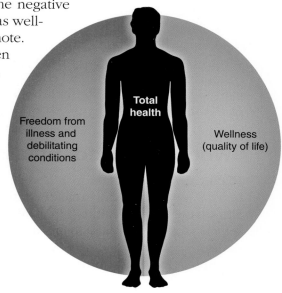

Figure 1.1 Being healthy means having wellness in addition to not being ill.

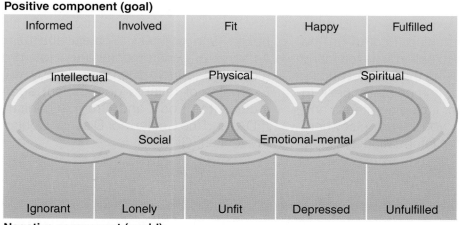

Figure 1.2 The total health and wellness chain.

sets health goals, communities do as well. Many schools, for example, have a coordinated school health program (CSHP) or comprehensive school physical activity program (CSPAP). CSHPs and CSPAPs have many components, including physical education, health education, wellness programs, and other programs designed to improve the personal health of students and the health of the school community.

One example of an ongoing large-scale community health program is the Healthy People 2030 project, in which the U.S. Department of Health and Human Services has set national health goals to be accomplished by the year 2030. Every 10 years, health experts from every state as well as federal and private agencies work together to develop health goals for the nation. Many of the Healthy People 2030 objectives are described on the unit opening pages of this book.

What Is Physical Fitness?

Physical fitness refers to the ability of your body systems to work together efficiently to allow you to be healthy, effectively perform activities of normal daily living, and effectively perform more demanding activities of life. For example, over and above the tasks of daily living, a fit person has the ability to respond to emergency situations, participate in sports and leisure activities, and perform demanding work-related activities.

Physical fitness is made up of 11 different parts. **Body composition**, **cardiorespiratory endurance**, **flexibility**, **muscular endurance**, **power**, and **strength** are the six parts of **health-related physical fitness**. They get this name because these traits reduce your risk of chronic disease and promote good health and wellness. **Agility**, **balance**, **coordination**, **reaction time**, and **speed** are the five skill-related parts of fitness. As the name implies, **skill-related physical fitness** helps you perform well in sports and other activities that require motor skills.

Health-Related Physical Fitness

Does a runner have good health-related fitness? They can probably run a long distance without tiring; thus they have good fitness in the area of endurance. However, being a runner doesn't guarantee fitness in all health-related areas. Like the runner, you may be more fit in some areas than in others. The following table describes and gives an example of each of the six parts of health-related fitness. As you read about each part, consider how fit you are in that area.

TECH TRENDS: The Internet and the World Wide Web

The Internet is a network that connects computers throughout the world. The World Wide Web consists of information located on the Internet at websites (also called links) on many different computers. Using the Internet and its websites, you can get immediate access to all kinds of information, including fitness and health information. As you'll learn elsewhere in this book, some of the information available on the web is good. However, much of it is inaccurate, especially when it comes to fitness, health, and wellness. Some websites, such as those of governmental agencies, provide more reliable information than just any website. Examples of reliable government agencies include the Food and Drug Administration (FDA) and the Centers for Disease Control and Prevention (CDC).

USING TECHNOLOGY

Search for the FDA website. Once at the site, click the search button. You can then enter words such as **health fraud** and **food supplements** or other health-related terms. Now search for the CDC website. At the site, search for topics such as health or physical activity. Your instructor may ask you to report about what you learned in your search.

The Six Parts of Health-Related Fitness

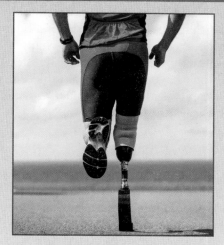

Cardiorespiratory Endurance

Cardiorespiratory endurance is the ability to exercise your entire body for a long time without stopping. It requires a strong heart, healthy lungs, and clear blood vessels to supply your large muscles with oxygen. Examples of activities that require good cardiorespiratory endurance are distance running, swimming, and cross-country skiing.

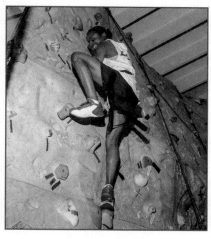

Muscular Endurance

Muscular endurance is the ability to use your muscles many times without tiring—for example, doing many push-ups or curl-ups (crunches) or climbing a rock wall.

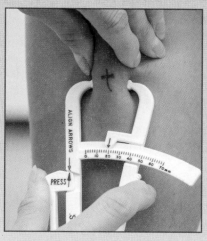

Body Composition

Body composition refers to the proportion of different types of tissues that make up your body, including fat, muscle, bone, and organs. Your level of body fat is often used to assess the component of body composition related to health. Body composition measures commonly used in schools include body mass index (based on height and weight), skinfold measures (which estimate body fatness), and waist and hip circumferences.

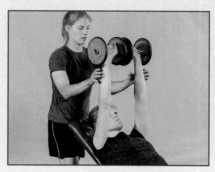

Strength

Strength is the amount of force your muscles can produce. It is often measured by how much weight you can lift or how much resistance you can overcome. Examples of activities that require good strength are lifting a heavy weight and pushing a heavy box.

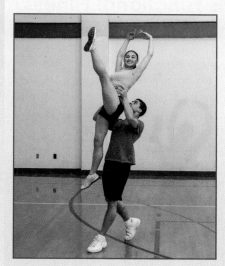

Flexibility

Flexibility is the ability to fully use your joints through a wide range of motion without injury. You are flexible when your muscles are long enough and your joints are free enough to allow adequate movement. Examples of people with good flexibility include dancers, gymnasts, and kickers in soccer or football.

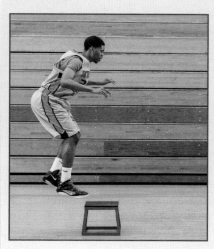

Power

Power is the ability to use strength quickly; it is sometimes referred to as *explosive strength*. People with good power can, for example, jump far or high or speed swim.

Physical fitness is not only one of the most important keys to a healthy body; it is the basis of dynamic and creative intellectual activity.

John F. Kennedy, U.S. President

FIT FACT

Cardiorespiratory endurance is also referred to as *cardiovascular fitness* or *aerobic fitness*. A national committee of experts from the National Academy of Medicine chose the name *cardiorespiratory endurance* especially for use with youth, because this type of fitness requires the cardiovascular and respiratory systems to work well together (cardiorespiratory) to allow your entire body to function for a long time without fatigue (endurance).

FIT FACT

Power, formerly classified as a skill-related part of fitness, is now classified as health related. The change is based on a report prepared by fitness experts concluding that power is important for healthy bones and muscles and is associated with wellness, higher quality of life, and reduced risk of chronic disease.

How do you think you rate in each of the six health-related fitness parts? Totally fit people are less likely to develop a health problem caused partly by lack of physical activity, known as a **hypokinetic condition**. These conditions include heart disease, some cancers, high blood pressure, diabetes, osteoporosis, or a high **body fat level**. (You'll learn more about hypokinetic conditions in other chapters of this book.) People who are physically fit also enjoy better wellness. They feel better, look better, and have more energy. You don't have to be a great athlete in order to enjoy good health and wellness and be physically fit. Regular physical activity can improve anyone's health-related physical fitness.

Skill-Related Physical Fitness

All sports, recreational activities, and activities of daily living require some level of skill-related fitness, but different activities require different parts of fitness. For example, a figure skater must have agility and balance, but this activity does not require the level of reaction time necessary for a sprinter. The following table describes and gives an example of each of the five parts of skill-related fitness.

How do you think you rate in each of the five skill-related parts of fitness? If you are like most people, you will score better on some parts than others. Learning about your own skill-related fitness will help you choose activities that best suit your abilities. Also, learning about your fitness in all 11 areas will help you determine in which areas you need improvement.

What Is Functional Fitness?

Functional fitness is the ability to function effectively in daily life, and it requires all parts of physical fitness. You have functional fitness if you can do your schoolwork and perform other daily tasks safely (for example, driving a car or doing yardwork). Having good health-related fitness not only helps you stay healthy but also helps you avoid undue fatigue. Having good skill-related fitness helps you perform daily tasks efficiently, such as when you need to stop quickly while driving a car.

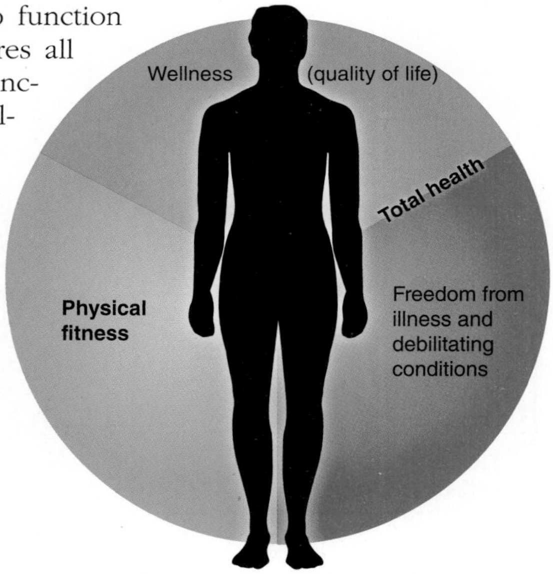

Fitness, health, and wellness are all **states of being** that can be maximized by practicing healthy lifestyles. The circle in figure 1.3 illustrates how they are interrelated. For example, if you're active on a regular

Figure 1.3 Interrelationship of fitness, health, and wellness.

basis, your fitness improves. This reduces your risk of disease, which improves your health. Your wellness is also improved because you feel better and can better enjoy the activities of daily life. Together they contribute to your functional fitness.

The Five Parts of Skill-Related Fitness

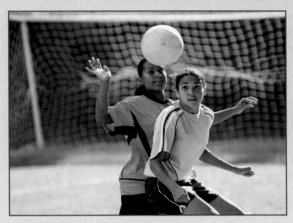

Agility

Agility is the ability to change the position of your body quickly and control your body's movements. People with good agility are likely to be good at wrestling, diving, soccer, and ice skating.

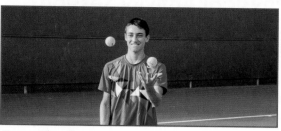

Coordination

Coordination is the ability to use your senses together with your body parts or to use two or more body parts together. People with good eye–hand or eye–foot coordination are good at juggling and at hitting and kicking games, such as soccer, baseball, volleyball, tennis, and golf.

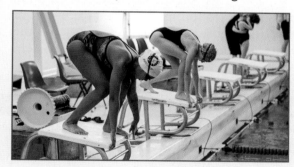

Reaction Time

Reaction time is the amount of time it takes you to move once you recognize the need to act. People with good reaction time can make fast starts in track and swimming and can dodge fast attacks in fencing and karate.

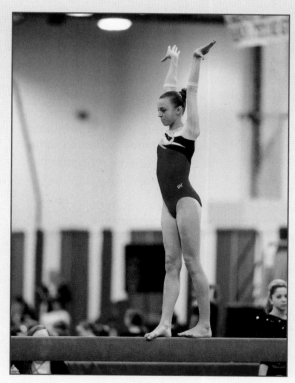

Balance

Balance is the ability to keep an upright posture while standing still or moving. People with good balance are likely to be good at gymnastics and ice skating.

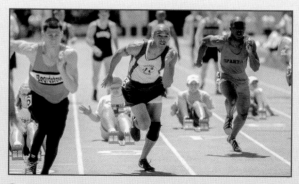

Speed

Speed is the ability to perform a movement or cover a distance in a short time. People with good speed can run fast. For example, people with good leg speed can run fast, and people with good arm speed can throw fast or hit a ball that is thrown fast.

9

What Are the Parts of a Physical Activity Session?

There are many different healthy lifestyles that contribute to good fitness, health, and wellness. Being physically active is considered to be a priority healthy lifestyle because it provides many benefits that are available to everyone regardless of age, sex, or current fitness level. The time you spend doing physical activity each day is your physical activity session. The activity session has three parts: warm-up, workout, and cool-down.

The **warm-up** is the activity you perform before your workout in order to get ready for it. The **workout** (sometimes referred to as the *conditioning phase*) is the main part of an activity session. This can involve exercise to build fitness, participation in a competitive event, or activity done just for fun. The **cool-down** is the activity you perform after your workout to help you recover. Because you will begin performing different types of physical activity early in this class, information about warming up and cooling down is presented now so that you will be ready to try each type of activity.

The Warm-Up

There are four types of warm-up that are commonly used to prepare for different types of physical activity: the **general warm-up**, the **dynamic warm-up**, the **skill warm-up**, and the **stretching warm-up** (see table 1.1).

As shown in table 1.2, the type of warm-up you choose depends on the activity you plan to perform. A light to moderate workout does not require a warm-up because the warm-up is of similar intensity to the workout. For vigorous activities, a general or dynamic warm-up is recommended. The best choices for different types of activities are shown in table 1.2.

TABLE 1.1   **Warm-Up Types and Benefits**

Type of warm-up	Description	Benefits
General warm-up Recommended by the American College of Sports Medicine (ACSM) prior to vigorous physical activity.	Consists of at least 5–10 minutes of light to moderate intensity aerobic (e.g., jogging) and body weight exercises (e.g., **calisthenics**).	• Allows the body to gradually adjust from rest to more intense physical activity • Prepares the heart and cardiorespiratory system • Prepares muscles • Prepares energy systems
Dynamic warm-up Recommended by the National Strength and Conditioning Association (NSCA) prior to activities requiring strength, power, and speed. Can be performed before any type of activity as a substitute for, or in addition to, a general warm-up.	Consists of 5–10 minutes of dynamic exercises prior to vigorous physical activity, especially activities that require strength, speed, and power. Examples of dynamic exercises include skipping, hopping, jumping, and calisthenics using the muscles to be used in the workout.	• Similar benefits to the general warm-up • Enhanced performance in activities requiring strength, power, and speed
Skill warm-up Can be used prior to sports and recreational activities.	Consists of performing the skills to be used in an activity, such as doing a layup drill in basketball. If done for 5–10 minutes at light to moderate intensity, it can substitute for a general warm-up. A less intense skill warm-up (e.g., swinging a golf club or baseball bat) does not have the benefits of a general warm-up.	• May aid performance by rehearsing movement patterns and adapting to environmental conditions • May aid mental preparation (e.g., focus on task at hand)

Type of warm-up	Description	Benefits
Stretching warm-up Can be performed prior to most activities but is most important to include before activities requiring flexibility (e.g., gymnastics, dance). Should be performed after a general warm-up. Not recommended for activities requiring strength, power, and speed.	Consists of slow static stretching of muscles beyond their normal length. The stretches should be held for 15–30 seconds and should include all muscle groups involved in the activity.	• Improves range of motion • May reduce risk of injury • May enhance performances that require flexibility, such as gymnastics and dance

TABLE 1.2   **Which Warm-Up Is Best?**

Type of physical activity	Recommended warm-up
Light to moderate physical activity such as walking, moderate jogging, and moderate biking	**No warm-up is required** because the activity is similar to a general warm-up. If desired, a stretching warm-up (see table 1.1) can be performed after 5–10 minutes of light to moderate activity.
Nonvigorous sports such as golf and bowling	**No general warm-up is required,** but a skill warm-up has some benefits (see table 1.1).
Vigorous aerobic activities such as running and mountain biking	**A general or dynamic warm-up should be performed** (see table 1.1). If desired, a stretching warm-up can be performed after the general or dynamic warm-up.
Noncompetitive vigorous sports and recreation activities such as tennis with friends or skiing for recreation	**A general or dynamic warm-up should be performed** (see table 1.1). If desired, a stretching warm-up can be performed after the general or dynamic warm-up.
Competitive vigorous sports and recreation requiring high levels of strength, power, and speed, such as sprinting, rock climbing, or shot put	**A dynamic warm-up should be performed** (see table 1.1). If it lasts for 5–10 minutes, it can double as a general warm-up. A stretching warm-up is not recommended prior to performance.
Muscle fitness exercise such as weight and interval training or activities requiring strength, power, and speed	**A dynamic warm-up should be performed** (see table 1.1). If it lasts for 5–10 minutes, it can double as a general warm-up. A stretching warm-up is not recommended prior to performance.
Flexibility exercise or activities requiring flexibility, such as gymnastics or dance	**A stretching warm-up should be performed after a general or dynamic warm-up.**

The Workout

There are many different ways to work out. You can work out as a way of training for a sports team or to prepare for an event such as a 5K race. You can also work out to improve your personal fitness and health. When you play a sport or go for a jog just for fun, you are working out. Throughout this book, you will learn about the many different ways of working out depending on your personal goals and interests.

The Cool-Down

After a workout, your body needs to recover from the demands of physical activity. To aid this process, ACSM recommends a cool-down of 5 to 10 minutes after a vigorous workout.

SCIENCE IN ACTION: **The Warm-Up**

Experts have studied the warm-up for nearly 100 years, and over that time, ideas about what constitutes a good warm-up have changed. For many years a stretching warm-up was the preferred method of getting ready for a workout, but the current evidence suggests that the type of warm-up you use depends on the type of activity you plan to perform (see tables 1.1 and 1.2).

STUDENT ACTIVITY

List the three activities that you most commonly do as part of your workout, then use the information in this section to choose the best type of warm-up for each activity.

The cool-down usually consists of slow to moderate activity, such as walking or slow jogging, to allow the muscles to gradually recover and heart rate and blood pressure to return to normal. This also helps prevent dizziness and fainting. If you suddenly stop running, for example, the blood can pool in your legs, leaving your heart with less blood to pump to your brain. But if you continue moving after a hard run, your muscles will squeeze the veins of your legs, helping the blood continue to circulate. The following list provides some more cool-down guidelines.

- Do not sit or lie down immediately after vigorous activity.
- Gradually reduce the intensity of activity during the cool-down (for example, if you were running, slow to a jog, then a walk, and then consider gentle stretching).
- Walk or do other moderate total body movements.
- You may choose to do some of the stretching exercises presented in chapter 12, Flexibility, after your general cool-down while your muscles are still warm.

LESSON REVIEW

1. How are health and wellness defined, and how are the two interrelated?
2. How do you define physical fitness, the six parts of health-related fitness, and the five parts of skill-related fitness?
3. How do you define functional fitness, and why is it important?
4. What are the warm-up, the workout, and the cool-down, and why each is important?

SELF-ASSESSMENT: **Physical Fitness Challenges**

Each chapter of this book includes a Self-Assessment feature. In most chapters, the self-assessment is designed to help you determine your personal fitness level. In this self-assessment, you'll try 11 challenges. They're called *challenges* rather than tests because they are not meant to be tests of fitness, nor are they meant to be exercises that you do to get fit. Instead, trying these challenges is a fun way to better understand the differences among the various parts of physical fitness. Please do not draw conclusions about your fitness based on your performance in these challenges. As you work your way through this book, you'll learn many self-assessments to help you determine your true fitness level.

The cardiorespiratory endurance and flexibility challenges will help you warm up before performing the other challenges. You may also want to consider additional warm-up exercises recommended by your teacher.

PART 1: Health-Related Physical Fitness Challenges

RUNNING IN PLACE (cardiorespiratory endurance)

1. Determine your resting heart rate. To do this, use your fingers to feel your pulse at your wrist or neck, then count your heartbeats for one minute.

2. Run 120 steps in place for one minute. Count one step every time a foot hits the floor.

3. Rest for 30 seconds, then again count your pulse for one minute. People with good cardiorespiratory endurance recover quickly after exercise. Is your heart rate after this exercise within 15 beats per minute of your resting heart rate before running in place?

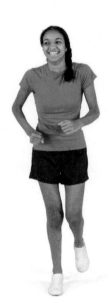

This challenge focuses on cardiorespiratory endurance.

TWO-HAND ANKLE GRIP (flexibility)

1. Squat with your heels together. Lean the upper body forward and reach with your hands between your legs and behind your ankles.

2. Clasp your hands in front of your ankles, interlocking your fingers.

3. Keep your feet still.

4. Hold the position for five seconds.

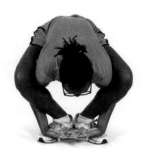

This challenge focuses on flexibility.

SINGLE-LEG RAISE (muscular endurance)

1. Bend forward at your waist so that your upper body rests on a table and your feet are on the floor.

2. Raise one leg so that it is extended straight out behind you. Complete several raises with each leg. Performing 8 or more repetitions requires muscular endurance.

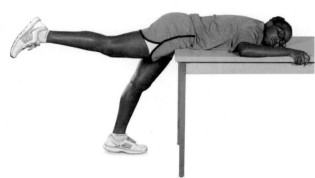

This challenge focuses on muscular endurance.

ARM SKINFOLD (body composition)

1. Let your right arm hang relaxed at your side. Have a partner gently pinch the skin and the fat under the skin on the back of your arm halfway between your elbow and shoulder. Together the skin and fat under the skin is called a *skinfold*.

2. Several skinfolds in different body locations can be used to determine the total amount of fat in the body. At this point there is no need to measure the skinfold. The skinfold on the arm is used only to illustrate the concept of body composition.

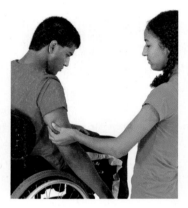

This challenge focuses on body composition.

90-DEGREE PUSH-UP (strength)

1. Lie facedown on a mat or carpet with your hands under your shoulders, your fingers spread, and your legs straight. Your legs should be slightly apart and your toes should be tucked under.

2. Push up until your arms are straight. Keep your legs and back straight—your body should form a straight line.

3. Lower your body by bending your elbows until your upper arms are parallel to the floor (elbows at a 90-degree angle), then push up until your arms are fully extended. Do one push-up every three seconds. You may want to have a partner say "up, down" every three seconds to help you. Performing five push-ups or more requires muscular strength.

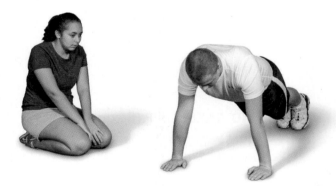

This challenge focuses on strength.

KNEES-TO-FEET (power)

1. Use a mat to kneel on your shins and knees, with your toes pointing back. Hold your arms back.
2. Without curling your toes under you or rocking your body backward, swing your arms upward and spring to your feet.
3. Hold your position for three seconds after you land.

This challenge focuses on power.

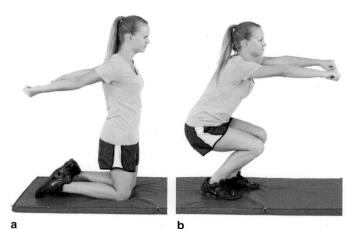

a   b

PART 2: Skill-Related Physical Fitness Challenges

LINE JUMP (agility)

1. Balance on your right foot on a line on the floor.
2. Leap onto your left foot so that it lands to the right of the line.
3. Leap across the line onto your right foot, landing to the left of the line.
4. Leap onto your left foot, landing on the line.

This challenge focuses on agility.

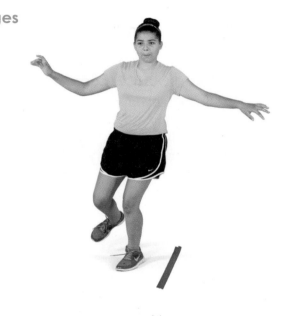

DOUBLE HEEL CLICK (speed)

1. Jump into the air and click your heels together twice before you land.
2. Your feet should be at least three inches (eight centimeters) apart when you land.

This challenge focuses on speed.

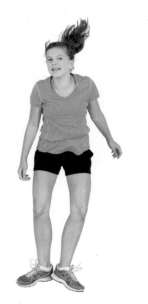

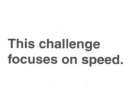

BACKWARD HOP (balance)

1. With your eyes closed, hop backward on one foot five times.
2. After the last hop, hold your balance for three seconds.

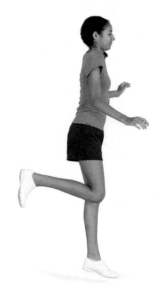

This challenge focuses on balance.

DOUBLE BALL BOUNCE (coordination)

1. Hold a volleyball in each hand. Beginning at the same time with each hand, bounce both balls simultaneously, at least knee high.
2. Bounce both balls three times in a row without losing control of them.

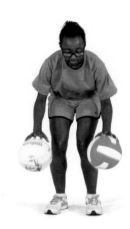

This challenge focuses on coordination.

COIN CATCH (reaction time)

1. Bend your arm and point your right elbow outward in front of you. Your right hand, palm up, should be beside your right ear. (If you're left-handed, do this activity with your left hand.)
2. Place a coin on your arm, as close to your elbow as possible.
3. Quickly lower your elbow and grab the coin in the air with the hand of the same arm.

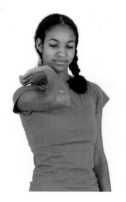

This challenge focuses on reaction time.

Developing Health and Physical Literacy

Lesson Objectives

After reading this lesson, you should be able to

1. describe the characteristics of physical literacy and health literacy;
2. describe the scientific method;
3. define and explain the importance of kinesiology and the many types of sciences within kinesiology; and
4. define and explain the importance of medical science, health science, and nutrition science.

Lesson Vocabulary

biomechanics
dietitian
exercise anatomy
exercise physiology
exercise psychology
exercise sociology
health literacy
health science
kinesiology
medical science
motor learning
motor skill
nutrition science
physical literacy
sport pedagogy

In the first lesson of this chapter, you were provided information about fitness, health, and wellness and why they are important. But how did we learn about them? Who makes decisions about how fitness, health, and wellness are defined and why they are important? In this lesson, you will learn about the sciences that provide the basis for the study of fitness, health, and wellness and the process that scientists use when studying them. You will also learn about health and physical literacy.

What Is Physical Literacy? What Is Health Literacy?

Literacy refers to being educated or cultured. Early definitions of literacy referred only to the ability to read and write, but the concept has been expanded to include other types of literacy, such as quantitative literacy (i.e., math literacy), computer and technical literacy, health literacy, and physical literacy.

> I love sports and being active. I lose track of time when I am playing. Nothing is more fun than playing a game.
>
> *Gena Gemma*

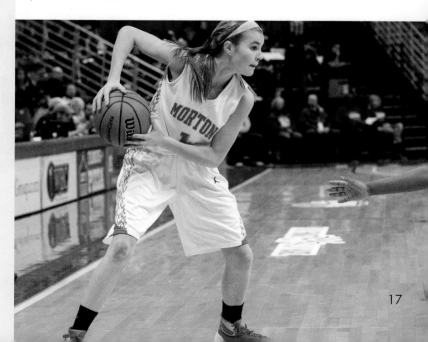

Physical Literacy

Achieving physical literacy is an important goal of physical education. People with **physical literacy** have the knowledge, skills, and fitness necessary to be active throughout life. The characteristics of physical literacy, identified by the Society of Health and Physical Educators (SHAPE America), are shown in figure 1.4.

As shown in figure 1.4, a physically literate person has the skills, knowledge, confidence, and motivation to be active and fit; values activity; and exhibits responsible personal and social behavior in physical activity and everyday life. Through your study of *Fitness for Life*, you will develop the characteristics necessary to achieve physical literacy.

Health Literacy

Just as physical literacy is important to lifelong fitness, health, and wellness, so is health literacy. **Health literacy** refers to the capacity to make sound health decisions that lead to adopting healthy lifestyles now and later in life. The characteristics of health literacy are shown in figure 1.5.

Health literacy works hand in hand with physical literacy to help you adopt healthy lifestyles. A person with health literacy knows how to obtain, process, and understand health information from reliable sources in order to make good decisions and plan healthy lifestyles, such as eating well and managing stress. In

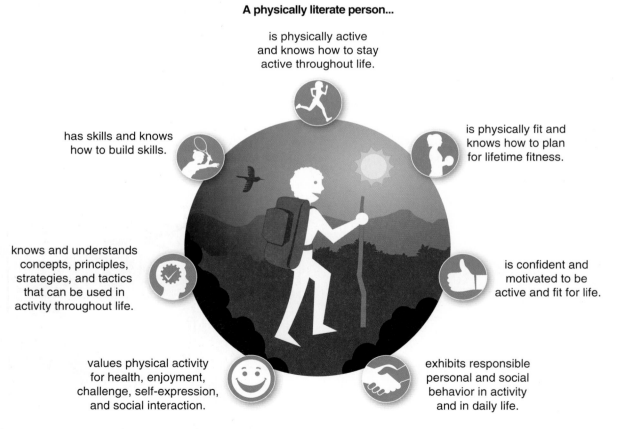

A physically literate person...

is physically active and knows how to stay active throughout life.

is physically fit and knows how to plan for lifetime fitness.

has skills and knows how to build skills.

is confident and motivated to be active and fit for life.

knows and understands concepts, principles, strategies, and tactics that can be used in activity throughout life.

exhibits responsible personal and social behavior in activity and in daily life.

values physical activity for health, enjoyment, challenge, self-expression, and social interaction.

Figure 1.4   The characteristics of physical literacy.

Adapted from SHAPE America.

addition, a person with health literacy adopts sound personal health habits (e.g., oral care, adequate sleep), avoids destructive habits (e.g., tobacco use, drug abuse), uses good safety practices (e.g., bike and auto), and seeks and uses health services. This textbook and the class that you are taking are both designed to help you develop physical and health literacy.

What Is the Scientific Method?

To achieve physical and health literacy, it is important to have scientific evidence to support what you learn. Science is the study of knowledge based on observation and experimentation. In school, you study various sciences, such as natural science (e.g., biology, chemistry, physics), social science (e.g., psychology, sociology, history), and mathematics (e.g., algebra, geometry, calculus).

Scientists of all types use the scientific method to discover new knowledge and establish principles that help us make good decisions and solve problems. A simplified form of the scientific method is presented in figure 1.6. An example issue (use of a dietary supplement) is used to illustrate the steps: identifying a problem, establishing a hypothesis, obtaining and processing information, and understanding and using information.

The information presented in this book is based on studies that use the scientific method. In addition, a special feature called Science in Action helps you see how research in kinesiology (exercise science), health and medical science, and nutrition science can help us achieve physical and health literacy. In the following section you will learn about several areas of science that provide the evidence for developing health and physical literacy.

A person with health literacy can

Process health information

Obtain health information

Understand health information

Identify and choose health services

Make appropriate health decisions

Figure 1.5 The characteristics of health literacy.
Adapted from CDC.

FIT FACT
Many of the names of sciences end with *ology*, which means "the study of."

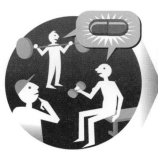
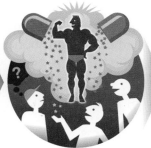
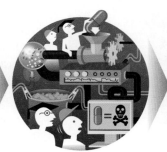
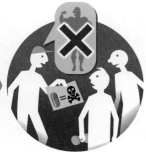

Identify the problem
Friends are considering taking a dietary supplement. Should I take one?

Establish a hypothesis
They think a supplement might help them get fit faster.

Obtain and process information
Conduct a search for information about benefits and risks associated with the supplement.

Understand and use information
Analysis and conclusion: the risks are greater than the benefits. Don't take the supplement.

Figure 1.6 A simplified form of the scientific method.

What Is Kinesiology?

Kinesiology is the study of human movement. There are, of course, many types of human movement. Some involve small muscle movements, such as the movement of your eyes when reading, the movement of your fingers when typing, and the movement of your hands when playing a musical instrument. Kinesiology specifically focuses on large muscle physical activity—in fact, the phrase "physical activity" is a general term for large muscle movement. There are many types of physical activity, including moderate activities such as walking, vigorous activities such as aerobics, sport and recreational activities, and exercise for muscle fitness and flexibility.

Within kinesiology there are many different specialties, including exercise physiology, exercise anatomy, biomechanics, exercise psychology, exercise sociology, motor learning, and sport pedagogy. These sciences provide the foundation for physical literacy and for our current understanding of the health benefits of physical activity and exercise. Exercise professionals, including physical education teachers, study all of the sciences in kinesiology as part of their training. You don't need to know as much about kinesiology as your teachers, but a basic understanding will help you understand the information in this book and help you achieve both physical and health literacy.

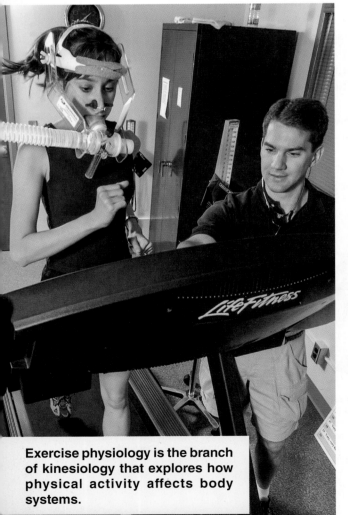

Exercise physiology is the branch of kinesiology that explores how physical activity affects body systems.

Exercise Physiology

Physiology is a branch of biology focused on the study of body systems. More specifically, **exercise physiology** is a branch of kinesiology that explores how physical activity affects the body systems (e.g., cardiovascular, respiratory, skeletal, muscular). Understanding the basic principles of exercise physiology is essential for planning physical activity programs that promote lifelong fitness, health, and wellness.

Exercise Anatomy

Scientists who study human anatomy focus on the tissues that make up the body (muscle, bone, tendon, ligament, skin, organ). Those who study **exercise anatomy** are especially interested in understanding how we use our muscles together with our bones, ligaments, and tendons to produce movement. Understanding exercise anatomy can help you choose good exercises for building your personal fitness program.

Biomechanics

The human body is like a machine. It uses a complex system of levers (bones) that are moved by the force produced when you contract your muscles. **Biomechanics** is the branch of kinesiology that seeks to understand how the human machine moves through the principles of physics. Knowing the basic principles of biomechanics can help you move efficiently and avoid injury.

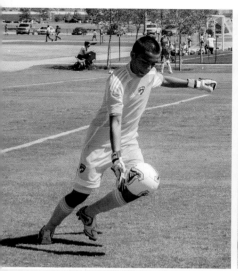
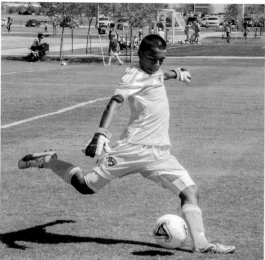
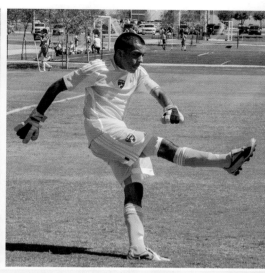

Biomechanics is the branch of kinesiology that seeks to understand the human body in motion through the principles of physics.

Exercise Psychology

Psychology is commonly referred to as the science of mind and behavior. More specifically, **exercise psychology** (also referred to as *sport psychology*) focuses on the study of human thoughts and behavior about all types of physical activity, including sport and exercise for fitness. Exercise psychology can help motivate people to be active, set realistic goals, and perform better in sports.

Exercise Sociology

Sociology is the study of society and social relationships. Within this broad field, **exercise sociology** (also referred to as *sport sociology*) focuses on social relationships and interactions in physical activity, including sports. Exercise sociology has helped people understand teamwork and cooperation, social responsibility, and cultural and ethnic differences in physical activity. Understanding key principles of exercise

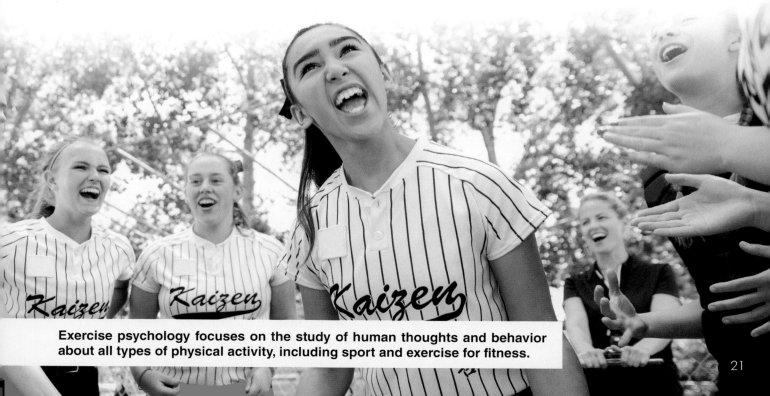

Exercise psychology focuses on the study of human thoughts and behavior about all types of physical activity, including sport and exercise for fitness.

sociology will help you experience positive social interactions in your physical activity.

Motor Learning

When you see the word *motor*, you may think of an automobile engine, but the term **motor learning** in his book refers to skill learning. When you perform a movement skill (also called a **motor skill**), your brain sends a signal through a nerve that tells the relevant muscles to contract. Nerves and muscle fibers that work together to produce movement are called *motor units*. Performing a motor skill, such as throwing a ball, requires action by many motor units (nerves and muscles). In this book, you'll learn the best ways to develop and practice the skills used in a variety of activities.

Sport Pedagogy

Pedagogy is the art and science of teaching. **Sport pedagogy** is the study of teaching and learning in physical activity settings, including school physical education, sports teams, and fitness clubs. The word *sport* is used broadly to include more than just traditional American sports. In other regions of the world, sport is used similarly to the term *physical activity* and includes activities such as riding a bike, hiking, and performing muscle fitness exercises as well

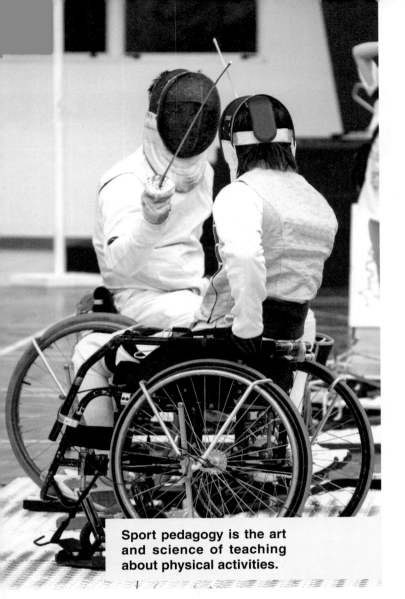

Sport pedagogy is the art and science of teaching about physical activities.

SCIENCE IN ACTION: Life Expectancy

For more than a century, the life expectancy of the average American increased with each generation. In 1900, people lived an average of 47 years. Life expectancy has now reached a high of nearly 79 years. One of the primary reasons for the increase is improved treatment for infectious diseases. As a result, diseases such as typhoid fever and smallpox, which used to be among the leading causes of death, have been conquered. COVID-19, a viral infection that plagued the nation beginning in 2020, is an exception. Before 1900, fewer than 100 medicines were available to doctors. Now there are more than 10,000, and in the United States

they must be tested before the government's Food and Drug Administration (FDA) approves them for widespread use.

Today the main causes of early death are related to unhealthy lifestyles such as lack of physical activity, poor nutrition, and unhealthy behaviors such as drug use and smoking, which lead to heart disease, cancer, diabetes, obesity, and other chronic diseases. The good news is that practicing the healthy lifestyles described in this book can greatly reduce the risk of chronic disease and help us live long and healthy lives.

STUDENT ACTIVITY

Aside from having more medicines, what do you think are the reasons for increased life expectancy?

as performing traditional sports such as basketball, volleyball, or tennis. People who study pedagogy focus on developing the best approaches to teaching, as well as understanding the many factors that influence learning.

The Medical, Health, and Nutrition Sciences

The medical, health, and nutrition sciences provide the basis to help you plan and adopt healthy lifestyles. A brief description of each of the sciences is provided here.

Medical Science

Medicine is the art and science of healing. Historically, the practice of medicine focused on diagnosing and treating disease. As early as 2000 BC, Egyptians performed surgery and began to build a scientific base for medicine. **Medical science** provides medical practitioners with the research evidence that is required before medical procedures and medicines are approved.

Health Science

Health science focuses on preventing disease and promoting wellness and high quality of life. Some health scientists study personal health issues in order to help individuals prevent disease and promote wellness. Public health scientists, sometimes called *epidemiologists*, study patterns of health and illness among populations in order to help prevent epidemics. Health psychologists investigate ways of helping people change their behaviors to enhance health and wellness.

Nutrition Science

Nutrition science is the study of nutrients (carbohydrate, protein, fat, vitamins, and minerals) and how they contribute to healthy growth and development. Food science is the study of the chemical makeup of food, whereas food technology focuses on food processing, packaging, preservation, and safety. **Dietitians** are experts who help apply the principles of nutrition in daily life.

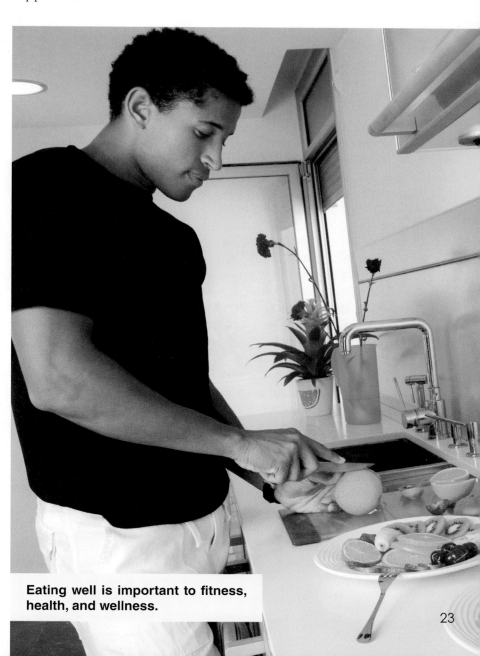

Eating well is important to fitness, health, and wellness.

LESSON REVIEW

1. How do you define physical literacy and health literacy?
2. What are the steps of the scientific method?
3. What are the types of sciences within kinesiology, and how are they important to your fitness, health, and wellness?
4. How would you describe medical science, health science, and nutrition science, and how are they important to your fitness, health, and wellness?

TAKING CHARGE: **Communication**

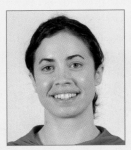 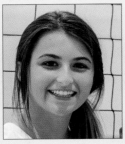 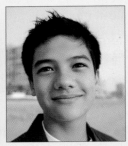

Communication refers to sharing and receiving information, ideas, and feelings with others. We communicate to learn, to be socially involved, to express our needs, to learn about the needs of others, and for a variety of other reasons. Communication can be face-to-face (in person) or from a distance (e.g., over the phone or through social media), but there are several types of communication that are typically used no matter the form. Examples include verbal (spoken), written, graphic (pictures), and nonverbal (body language).

Teagen and Josh usually walked to school together. Early this morning, Teagen got a text from her friend Piper. *WUP? Want a ride?*

Teagen remembered that she needed to meet the guidance counselor before school, so she texted back, *Ya, 7:30?* Piper texted, *K.* Because she was running late, Teagen forgot to text Josh to let him know that she was hitching a ride to school. At 7:40, Josh was getting irritated because Teagen was not at their normal meeting location. So he texted, *WRU?* Teagen had shut off her phone while she was meeting with Mr. Wolford, so she missed Josh's message. As he walked to school alone, Josh texted Teagen again, *WTH?* When he got to school Josh texted Teagen again, *PCM.* But he got no return message. So he texted Piper, *Seen Teag?* Piper replied, *OTP.* Because Piper was

on the phone, she did not answer Josh. Piper's text was the last communication Josh received before he had to go to class. Teagen texted later in the day, but Josh was upset and ignored her message.

FOR DISCUSSION

What are some things that could have been done to avoid the communication gap between Josh and Teagen? Now that things have gone wrong, what could the friends do to prevent future problems?

Communication skills, like any skills, can be improved with practice. Consider the guidelines in the following Self-Management feature as you answer these discussion questions.

SELF-MANAGEMENT: **Skills for Effective Communication**

The following guidelines will help you improve your communication skills.

General Communication Guidelines

- *Think first.* Engage your brain before speaking, typing, or posting a picture. Have a purpose to what you say and consider who you are communicating with and how will it be received.

- *Think ahead.* Try to anticipate when you might have a problem with another person. Communicate to let people know what is going on; don't assume.

- *Be respectful.* Consider the thoughts and feelings of others when you speak, write, or post.

- *Keep your message simple.* Use clear language.

- *Avoid quick or angry reactions.* Avoid raising your voice or texting angry comments. Use stress management techniques to relax before responding. Stay calm and avoid escalation.

- *Apologize when appropriate.* We all make mistakes. It's okay to say "I'm sorry."

Face-to-Face Communication Guidelines

- *Listen!* Communication is a two-way street. Ask questions to get an idea of what other people are thinking.

- *Give others your full attention.* Look at the person and avoid interrupting.

- *Take your time.* Speak slowly. Don't rush, especially when you are upset.

- *Be aware of your body language.* Make eye contact and nod to show interest. Avoid invading the personal space of others, negative facial expressions, looking down, and slouching.

Distance Communication Guidelines

- *Avoid quick responses.* Take the time to think about your response.

- *Ask yourself: Would you say this in person?* Don't say anything in a written message that you wouldn't say to the person's face.

- *Be sure that texting abbreviations are clear and understandable.* Not all abbreviations are known to everyone. Be sure you are on the same page with those you communicate with.

- *Be careful what you share.* When you use social media you are often communicating with more people than you think. Ask yourself: How will others react to your communication? Would you care if everyone could see what you shared? Remember, what goes on social media often stays on social media.

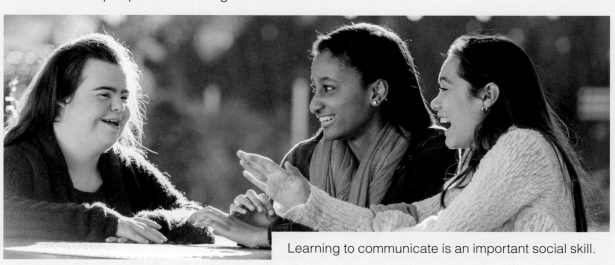

Learning to communicate is an important social skill.

Taking Action: **The Warm-Up**

Because *Fitness for Life* includes many types of activity, the type of warm-up you perform will vary as well. You will **take action** here by trying each of the different types of warm-up: general, dynamic, skill, and stretching. After you've tried them, you can work with your teacher and use the information in tables 1.1 and 1.2 to create warm-up activities for each type of workout you're planning to do.

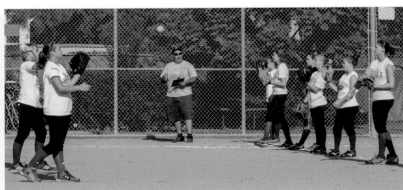

The skill warm-up.

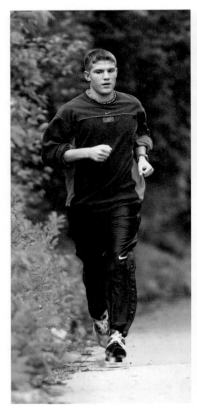

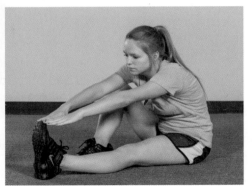

The general warm-up.   **The stretching warm-up.**

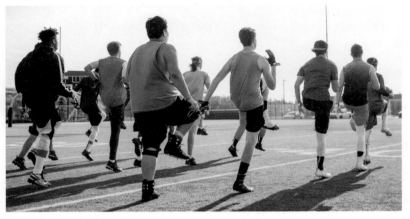

The dynamic warm-up.

CHAPTER REVIEW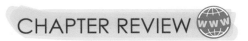

Reviewing Concepts and Vocabulary

Answer items 1 through 5 by completing each sentence with a word or phrase.

1. Illness is the negative component of health. The positive component of health is called _____.

2. A hypokinetic condition is a health problem caused by _____.

3. The component of fitness that refers to the ability to move joints through a wide range of motion without injury is called _____.

4. The _____ is a series of steps that can help you make good decisions and solve problems.

5. The science that uses principles of physics to understand the motion of the human body is called _____.

For items 6 through 10, match each term in column 1 with the appropriate phrase in column 2.

6. muscular endurance   a. movement of the body using larger muscles

7. agility   b. component requiring both strength and speed

8. pedagogy   c. ability to change body position quickly

9. physical activity   d. art and science of teaching

10. power   e. ability to use muscles continuously without tiring

For items 11 through 15, respond to each statement or question.

11. What is physical fitness?

12. How do health-related physical fitness and skill-related physical fitness differ?

13. What are the characteristics of physical literacy?

14. What are some important factors to consider when choosing a warm-up before your workout?

15. What are some guidelines for effective communication?

Thinking Critically

Write a paragraph to answer the following question.

You are asked to make an important decision about your fitness, health, or wellness. How would you use the scientific method to make that decision?

Project

Interview several healthy older adults about their fitness, health, and wellness, then present the information to a group such as your class or family members. Ask questions such as these: How would you rate your health? How would you rate your wellness? How would you rate your health-related physical fitness? (Ask the person to use ratings such as good fitness, marginal fitness, and poor fitness.) How do you think teens rate their fitness, health, and wellness compared to people your age?

Physical Activity and Healthy Lifestyles for All

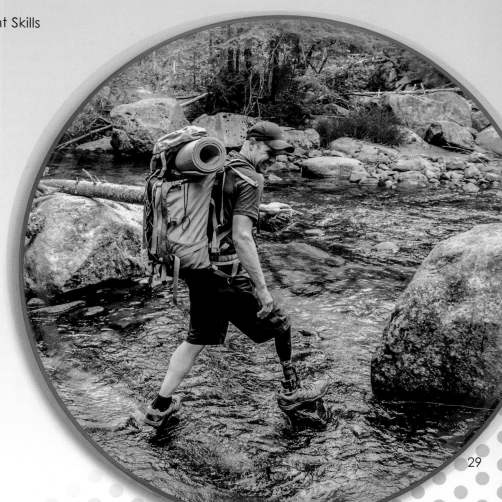

Adopting Healthy Lifestyles

Lesson Objectives

After reading this lesson, you should be able to

1. describe several examples of personal and environmental determinants of fitness, health, and wellness;

2. describe several examples of health care and social determinants of fitness, health, and wellness;

3. describe several examples of healthy lifestyle choices and the five benefits of making healthy lifestyle choices;

4. explain the Stairway to Lifetime Fitness, Health, and Wellness and how it can be used.

Lesson Vocabulary

autonomy
competence
dependence
determinant
independence
priority health lifestyle choice
self-management skills

As discussed in chapter 1, fitness, health, and wellness are interrelated, meaning that if you do something to change one, you affect the others. Your fitness, health, and wellness are also affected by many other factors. Medical and scientific experts refer to these factors as **determinants**, and the U.S. Department of Health and Human Services Healthy People 2030 project suggests that all people learn about them in order to stay fit, healthy, and well.

Personal and Environmental Determinants

As shown in figure 2.1, your fitness, health, and wellness are affected by five types of determinants: personal, environmental, health care, social, and lifestyle choices. Some determinants are more within your control than others. Figure 2.1 shows the determinant types in varying shades of orange—the lighter the color, the less control you have; the darker the color, the more control. Personal and environmental determinants, shown with light shading, are less in your control than those with darker shading.

> I know I can't control everything that happens to me. But I also know that how I live can make a difference in my fitness and health. It also makes a difference in how I perform. If I am going to make the cross-country team, I have to put in the effort—that's up to me.
>
> *Weimo Chen*

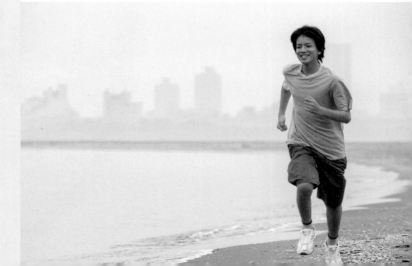

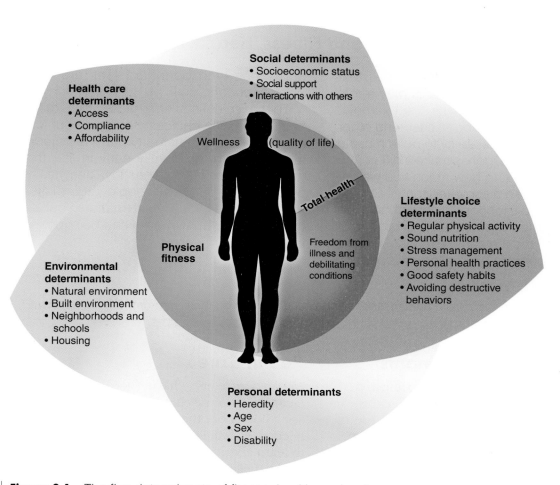

Figure 2.1   The five determinants of fitness, health, and wellness.

Adapted from C.B. Corbin et al., *Concepts of Fitness and Wellness: A Comprehensive Lifestyle Approach,* 12th ed. (St. Louis, MO: McGraw-Hill, 2019).

Personal Determinants

You have little or no control over personal determinants, which include heredity, age, sex, race or ethnicity, and disability; thus, they are shaded in light orange in the figure. Nonetheless, these factors can greatly affect your fitness, health, and wellness. For example, a person might inherit genes that cause a higher or lower than normal risk for certain diseases. Sex is also a factor—for example, males tend to have more muscle than females do, especially after the teen years. Females also have a longer life expectancy than males. Research evidence also indicates that certain chronic health conditions are more prevalent among particular racial or ethnic groups than others, so race and ethnicity can affect a person's health. Another potential factor is disability, which can affect a person's capacity to perform certain tasks. Disease risk also increases with age.

You'll learn more about personal determinants and their effects on fitness, health, and wellness in other chapters of this book. Although you cannot control personal determinants, you can be aware of them, which can help you decide to alter the determinants over which you do have control.

FIT FACT

A disability is an objective condition (impairment), whereas a handicap is the inability to do something you would like to do. A person who is disabled is not necessarily handicapped. We are all physically different, and various personal determinants affect what you can and cannot do. Understanding your own strengths and limitations helps you be the best you can be and allows you to help others be the best they can be.

SCIENCE IN ACTION: Heredity and Fitness, Health, and Wellness

Exercise physiologists have determined that genes we inherit from our parents play a role in fitness, health, and wellness. For example, some genes affect risks for disease and other genes affect a person's ability to build muscle mass. And, of course, genes make a difference in how tall you are and how much you weigh. Scientists have also discovered that, because of genetics, people respond differently to exercise. They learned this by studying groups of people who all did the same exercise. People who got big benefits are called *responders*, and those who benefited less are called *nonresponders*.

These scientists emphasize that making healthy lifestyle choices can help counteract heredity. Although heredity plays a major role in your health, especially early in life, those who practice lifelong healthy lifestyles are among the healthiest people regardless of heredity. What you inherit matters, but over the long haul, what you do can be even more important.

STUDENT ACTIVITY

Choose a component of health-related fitness and describe how you think your heredity influences it.

Environmental Determinants

Fitness, health, and wellness are also affected by many different environmental determinants. In figure 2.1, they are colored in a light shade of orange because you have limited control over them. For example, teens do not typically choose where they live and go to school. Socioeconomic factors affect housing, access to healthy food, and access to parks and green spaces. On the other hand, you can recycle, avoid use of plastics that pollute waterways and neighborhoods, and advocate for protecting the environment. As an adult, if you have the resources, you can choose to live or work in locations that are healthier than others. Every year the American College of Sports Medicine (ACSM) publishes the American Fitness Index that ranks cities based on various fitness, health, and wellness determinants.

Health Care and Social Determinants

In figure 2.1, health care and social determinants are shown in a darker orange than personal and environmental determinants. You have somewhat more control over these types of determinants than those shaded in a lighter color, but as discussed in the sections that follow, there are limits concerning the control you have over them.

Health Care

Health care refers to having access to health care facilities and medicine and having the ability to see a doctor or other health care professional as needed. Health care also includes opportunities to learn about prevention of illness and promotion of wellness. People who receive good health care live longer and have higher-quality lives compared to those who don't. This factor is in a darker shade of orange in figure 2.1 because you have some control over it; however, it is not totally under your control. People with low income have less access than those with higher income, so health care is limited for many. However, seeking health care when needed and complying with health care recommendations are things that you can control and are important to your health and wellness.

Social Determinants

There are many social factors that influence fitness, health, and wellness—too many to describe here. However, three important social determinants are socioeconomic status, social support, and interactions with other people. This factor is in a darker shade of orange in figure 2.1 because you have some control over it, particularly in terms of your social support and interactions with other people. However, socioeconomic status is not typically in the control of teens. Socioeconomic status is typically determined by income, education, and job status. People with low income have a higher than normal risk of health problems and often lack access to health insurance and health care. People of color and people with low income are more likely to be exposed to negative environmental factors (e.g., poor water and poor living conditions) and have less access to factors that lead to healthy lifestyles.

Having the support of others is important, especially to emotional and mental health. Family, community, and friends provide social support. You do have some control over social support. For example, you choose your friends and make decisions about how you interact with them. Teens who choose friends who avoid destructive habits and practice healthy ones are likely to be fit, healthy, and well themselves.

Healthy Lifestyle Choices

By far the most important determinants of your fitness, health, and wellness are your lifestyle choices. A healthy lifestyle is made up of behaviors that improve your fitness, health, and wellness. A list of several healthy lifestyle behaviors is

FIT FACT

A wellness program in the Boise, Idaho, school district helped teachers and other employees eat better, sleep better, reduce smoking, and be more physically active. Changing these behaviors reduced health care costs and improved productivity.

ACADEMIC CONNECTION: Accurate Use of Words

English language arts is an area of academic study that focuses on preparing students who are college and career ready in reading, writing, speaking, listening, and language. Learning to use words accurately and knowing how similar words differ are important in the study of the English language and in achieving literacy (being educated). In this book you learned that one of the personal determinants of fitness, health, and wellness is your sex. The American Psychological Association (APA) defines *sex* as one's sex assignment at birth. It defines *gender* as "the attitudes, feelings, and behaviors that a given culture associates with a person's biological sex" and *gender identity* as "the component of gender that describes a person's psychological sense of their gender."

In this book we use the words male and female to describe a person's sex assignment at birth. However, not all people identify with their sex assignment at birth or the terms male or female. They often use other terms to identify themselves (gender identity). The APA indicates that it is important that people be free to use the terms of their choice to describe themselves.

Throughout the book, you will be asked to determine health-related fitness ratings based on your fitness self-assessment scores, your age, and sex assignment at birth (male or female). The reason for using sex assigned at birth for fitness ratings is because scientists have determined health-risk for different rating categories based on biological characteristics associated with sex assigned at birth. Although sex assignment at birth is used for making fitness ratings, consistent with APA recommendations, students should feel free to use their own terms for their gender identity.

The APA also indicates that care should be taken when using pronouns. He, him, his, she, her, and hers are the most commonly used pronouns. However, the APA indicates that "self-identified pronouns" should be used for non-gender conforming people. When referring to individuals whose identified pronouns are not known, the terms they, them, and their are appropriate as are other self-identified pronouns.

included in figure 2.1. The first three healthy lifestyle choices are performing regular physical activity, eating well, and managing stress. They are considered to be **priority health lifestyle choices** and are emphasized in this book. Your personal health habits, safety habits (e.g., seatbelts, protective biking gear), and avoidance of destructive habits (e.g., smoking, vaping) also are lifestyle choices that influence your fitness, health, and wellness. Because you generally have a lot of control over lifestyle choices, they are colored in dark orange in figure 2.1.

A healthy lifestyle not only helps you later in life but also lets you enjoy many benefits now. Examples include looking and feeling good, learning better, enjoying daily life, and effectively handling emergencies.

Looking Good

Do you care about how you look? Experts agree that regular physical activity, proper nutrition, and good posture can help you look your best.

Feeling Good

People who do regular physical activity also feel better. If you're active, you can resist fatigue, avoid injury, and work more efficiently. National surveys indicate that active people sleep better, do better in school, and experience less depression than people who are less active. Research indicates that regular activity can increase brain chemicals called *endorphins* that give you a sensation of feeling great after exercise. You can also help yourself feel your best by eating well and managing stress wisely.

Learning Better

In recent years, scientists have found that you learn better if you are active, eat well, get enough sleep, and manage stress effectively. More specifically, studies show that teens who are active and fit score better on tests and are less likely to be absent from school. In addition, active teens who eat regular healthy meals, especially breakfast, are more alert at school and less likely to be tired in the classroom. Recent studies also show that regular exercise and good fitness are associated with high function in the parts of the brain that promote learning.

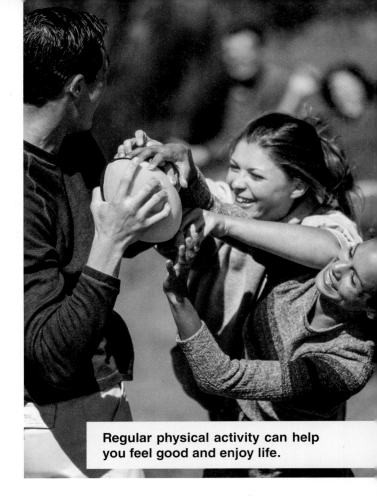

Regular physical activity can help you feel good and enjoy life.

Enjoying Life

Everyone wants to enjoy life. But what if you're too tired to participate in the activities you really like? Regular physical activity increases your physical fitness, which is the key to being able to do more of the things you want to do. People who are fit, healthy, and well are able to enjoy life to the fullest.

Meeting Emergencies

Challenging situations can arise suddenly, but you can prepare yourself for them by engaging in regular physical activity and making other healthy lifestyle choices. For example, if you're physically fit and active, you'll be able to run for help, change a flat tire, and offer assistance to others as needed.

Stairway to Lifetime Fitness, Health, and Wellness

Do you live a healthy lifestyle? Do you eat well? Are you physically active? Many teens are active and eat well, but will you continue to do so when you're older and on your own? Will you do the same kinds of activity you do now? If you answered no to any of these questions, you need to begin developing a lifetime plan for practicing a healthy lifestyle. One way to accomplish this goal is to climb the Stairway to Lifetime Fitness, Health, and Wellness. As you can see in figure 2.2, when you climb this stairway, you move from **dependence** (having others make decisions for you) to **independence** (making good decisions on your own).

> One who has health has hope; and one who has hope has everything.
>
> *Ancient proverb*

Step 1: Practicing Healthy Lifestyles (Directed by Others)

Think about the way you eat, your physical activities, and your other lifestyle practices. When you were a kid, you were dependent on other people to make these decisions for you (see step 1, figure 2.2). As you've grown older, you've started making more decisions for yourself. As an adult, you'll be almost totally responsible for making your own decisions. Living out the healthy lifestyle choices made or facilitated for you by other people is a good first step, but it's up to you to keep climbing the stairway.

Step 2: Achieving Fitness, Health, and Wellness (Directed by Others)

If you stick with the healthy living practices in step 1, you will improve your fitness, health, and wellness (step 2), but the result is still dependent on others. For example, if you get fit because of exercise prescribed by coaches and physical education teachers, your fitness is dependent on their guidance. You may also eat well because a parent buys food and prepares most or all of your meals. It's good that

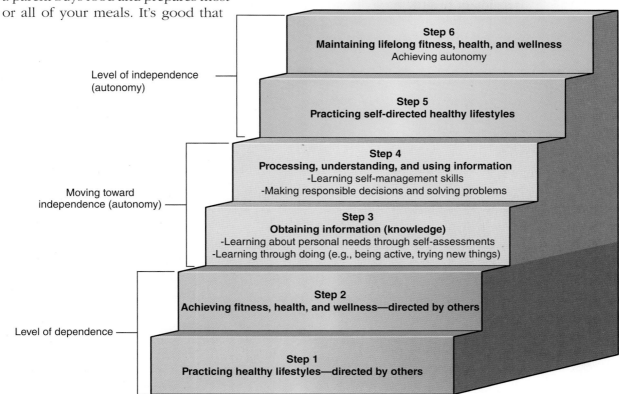

Figure 2.2 The Stairway to Lifetime Fitness, Health, and Wellness.

others help you adopt healthy lifestyles (step 1) that lead to fitness, health, and wellness (step 2). But it's not until you move to the third step in the stairway that you begin to make your own decisions and become more independent.

Step 3: Obtaining Information

An important part of the scientific method is obtaining information (see chapter 1). Reading the text and having discussions in class are ways of obtaining information. You also learn by interacting with others through family, extracurricular activities, and in the community. Performing self-assessments also helps you learn about your personal needs and interests (e.g., fitness, current eating patterns, posture and back health). Knowledge helps you as you begin to move toward **autonomy**, or the freedom to make your own well-informed decisions.

Step 4: Processing, Understanding, and Using Information

Obtaining information (step 3) is important, but just having information is not enough—now you must examine and organize it so that you can better understand it. You can use the modified scientific method to help you determine if your information is accurate and reliable. Learning and practicing **self-management skills** can also help you process and understand information. These important skills are fully described in lesson 2.2 of this chapter.

Step 5: Practicing Self-Directed Healthy Lifestyles

At stage 5 you have learned how to obtain, process, understand, and use information. You have learned and practiced the self-management skills to plan, adopt, and maintain healthy lifestyles and healthy relationships. In a way, this step is much like the first step, but now you have transitioned from being dependent on others to making your own decisions and solving your own problems.

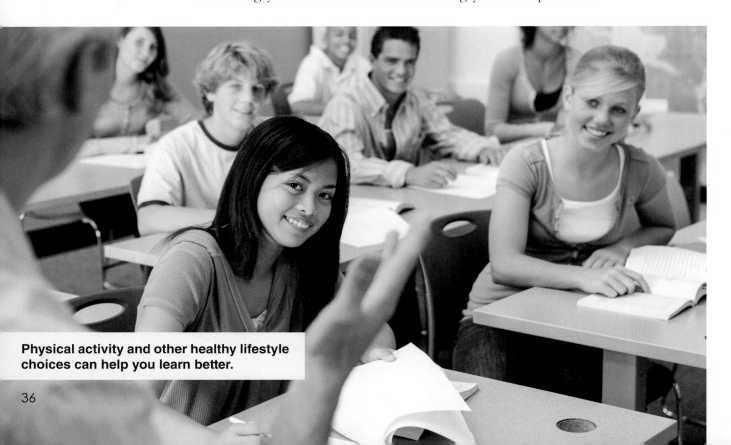

Physical activity and other healthy lifestyle choices can help you learn better.

TECH TRENDS: **FitnessGram**

FitnessGram is a fitness assessment program developed by a group of science advisors at the Cooper Institute in Dallas, Texas. It provides instructions for self-assessing your fitness using a variety of health-related test items. It also includes software that allows you to build your own personal fitness report. You'll learn how to perform and practice the items in the FitnessGram test battery in this chapter's Self-Assessment feature. Other chapters in this book provide more information about each test item and how to determine fitness ratings using FitnessGram.

USING TECHNOLOGY

Practice each of the health-related fitness tests in FitnessGram using the directions in this chapter's Self-Assessment feature. Later you will perform each test in FitnessGram. Sometimes you will test yourself (self-assessment), and sometimes you will test with the help of a partner. Your instructor may ask you to enter your results on the computer to give you access to a FitnessGram report (see figure 2.3).

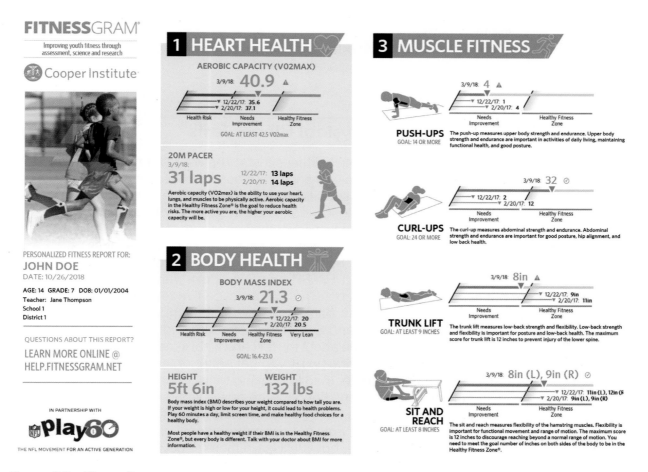

Figure 2.3   FitnessGram report.

Reprinted by permission from *FitnessGram*.

Step 6: Achieving and Maintaining Lifelong Fitness, Health, and Wellness

When you reach the top step of the stairway, you have achieved full autonomy and **competence** in using self-management, decision-making, and problem-solving skills. You have taken responsibility for your own lifetime fitness, health, and wellness, as well as for your own personal and social behavior. You'll be well on your way to achieving and maintaining the benefits of healthy lifestyle behaviors as a result of your well-informed choices.

LESSON REVIEW

1. What are some examples of personal and environmental determinants of fitness, health, and wellness?
2. What are some examples of health care and social determinants of fitness, health, and wellness?
3. What are some examples of healthy lifestyle choices, and what are the five benefits of practicing healthy lifestyles?
4. What are the steps in the Stairway to Lifetime Fitness, Health, and Wellness, and how can they help you make informed personal decisions?

SELF-ASSESSMENT: Practicing Physical Fitness Tests

In this book, you'll read about many physical fitness tests. The overall goal is to be able to select appropriate self-assessments to use now and throughout your life. Several groups have developed physical fitness assessments specifically for young people. One of these, called FitnessGram (see Tech Trends), is the most widely used test battery in the United States. This battery is a group of items designed to test several components of health-related fitness.

There are other test batteries that also assess health-related physical fitness, such as the ALPHA-FIT and Eurofit test batteries. They were developed in Europe and, like Fitness-Gram, are used throughout the world. ALPHA-FIT and Eurofit use many of the same items as FitnessGram but also some different ones. You will practice five tests from Fitnessgram (PACER, 90-degree push-up, curl-up, the back-saver sit-and-reach, and the trunk lift) as well as two tests included in ALPHA-FIT and Eurofit (grip strength and standing long jump).

Before using a physical fitness test, learn about the test and what it measures, then practice each test item that you plan to use. Practice helps you get better at taking the test properly so that you're truly measuring fitness rather than test-taking skills. For best results, give your best effort when doing the self-assessment. For now, the goal is not to determine a score or rating on the test items but to practice the tests so that you know how to perform them properly. Because body composition assessments are not performance tests, they don't require practice and thus are not described here, but you'll learn more about them later.

Remember that self-assessment information is personal and is considered confidential. It should not be shared with others without the permission of the person being tested. Record your results as directed by your teacher.

TEST OF CARDIORESPIRATORY ENDURANCE

PACER (Progressive Aerobic Cardiovascular Endurance Run, or 20-meter shuttle run)

This test is included in FitnessGram, ALPHA-FIT, and Eurofit. The test objective is to run back and forth across a 20-meter (almost 22-yard) distance as many times as you can at a predetermined pace (pacing is based on signals from a special audio recording provided by your instructor).

1. Start at a line located 20 meters from a second line. When you hear the beep from the audio track, run across the 20-meter area and touch the second line with your foot before the audio track beeps again. Turn around and get ready to run back.

2. At the sound of the next beep, run back to the line where you began. Touch the line with your foot. Again, make sure to wait for the beep before running back.

3. Practice running back and forth from one line to the other, touching the line each time. The beeps will come faster and faster, causing you to run faster and faster. When performing the actual test, you are finished when you twice fail to reach the opposite side before the beep.

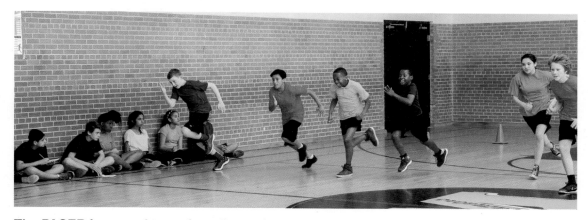

The PACER is a good test of cardiorespiratory endurance.

Practice Tips

- Practice running at the correct pace so that you arrive just before the beep that signals you to change directions.
- Practice adjusting your pace as the beeps come faster and faster.

TESTS OF MUSCLE FITNESS

CURL-UP (abdominal muscle strength and muscular endurance)

This test is included in FitnessGram.

1. Lie on your back on a mat or carpet. Bend your knees approximately 140 degrees. Your feet should be slightly apart and as far as possible from your buttocks while still allowing your feet to be flat on the floor. (The closer your feet are to your buttocks, the more difficult the movement is.) Your arms should be straight and parallel to your trunk with your palms resting on the mat.

2. Place your head on a piece of paper. The paper will help your partner judge whether your head touches down on each repetition. Place a strip of cardboard (may also substitute rubber, plastic, or tape) 4.5 inches (about 11.5 centimeters) wide and 3 feet (about 1 meter) long under your knees so that the fingers of both hands just touch the near edge of the strip. You can tape the strip down or have a partner stand on it to keep it stationary.

3. Keeping your heels on the floor, curl your shoulders up slowly and slide your arms forward so that your fingers move across the cardboard strip. Curl up until your fingertips reach the far side of the strip.

4. Slowly lower your back until your head rests on the piece of paper.

5. Practice doing one curl-up every three seconds. A partner can help you by saying "up, down" every three seconds. When performing the actual test, you are finished when you can't do another curl-up or when you fail to keep up with the three-second count.

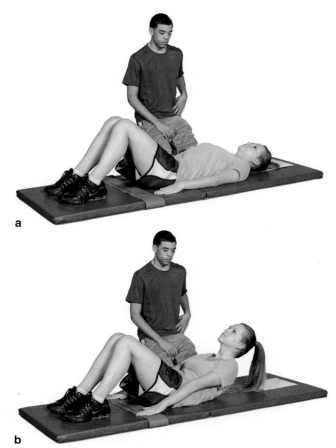

a

b

When properly performed, the curl-up is a good measure of muscle fitness of the abdominal muscles.

Practice Tips

- Practice keeping your buttocks and heels stationary as you do repetitions.
- Practice doing one repetition (up, down) every three seconds.
- Practice reaching to the end of the strip for each repetition.
- Practice lowering your head to the mat on each repetition.
- Practice as many repetitions as you can (up to 15). Have a partner check your form to make sure you are performing each curl-up correctly.

90-DEGREE PUSH-UP (upper body strength and muscular endurance)
This test is included in FitnessGram.

1. Lie facedown on a mat or carpet with your hands (palm down) under your shoulders, your fingers spread, and your legs straight. Your legs should be slightly apart and your toes tucked under.

2. Push up until your arms are straight. Keep your legs and back straight. Your body should form a straight line from your head to your heels.

3. Lower your body by bending your elbows until your upper arms are parallel to the floor (elbows at a 90-degree angle), then push up until your arms are fully extended.

4. Practice doing one push-up every three seconds. You may want to have a partner say "up, down" every three seconds to help you. When performing the actual test, you are finished when you are unable to complete a push-up with proper form for the second time or are unable to keep the pace for a second time.

Practice Tips

- Practice lowering until your elbows are bent at 90 degrees. You may want to have a partner hold a yardstick parallel to the floor (at the elbow) to help you determine when your elbows are properly bent.

- Practice pushing up all the way so that your arms are at full extension at the top of each push-up.

- Practice doing one repetition (up, down) every three seconds.

- Practice as many repetitions as you can (up to 15). Have a partner check your form to make sure you are performing each push-up correctly.

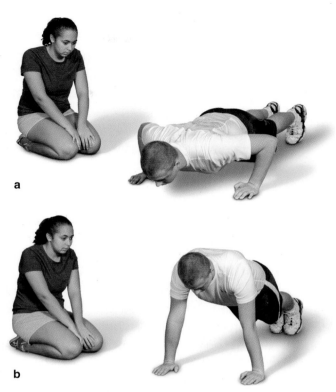

The push-up is a measure of muscle fitness of the upper body.

HANDGRIP STRENGTH (isometric hand and arm strength)

This test uses a dynamometer to measure isometric strength. It is included in ALPHA-FIT.

1. Adjust the dynamometer to fit your hand size.

2. With your arm extended and your elbow nearly straight, squeeze as hard as possible for two to five seconds. Do not touch your body with your arm or hand.

3. Practice with each hand. Alternate hands to allow a rest between each attempt.

4. Results are most often reported in kilograms (a kilogram equals about 2.2 pounds). When performing the actual test, you report your score in pounds. If the dynamometer that you use measures in kilograms, multiply your score in kilograms by 2.2. Add your best right-hand score to your best left-hand score, then divide the total by two to get your average score.

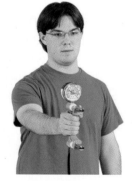

The handgrip strength test measures muscle fitness; scores are related to total body strength.

Practice Tips

- Try the grip at different settings to see which enables you to perform the best.

- Try bending your knees a bit as you squeeze to help maintain good balance, which may help your score.

STANDING LONG JUMP (leg power or explosive strength)

This test is included in ALPHA-FIT and Eurofit.

1. Mark a line on the floor with masking tape.

2. Stand with your feet shoulder-width apart behind the line. Bend your knees and hold your arms straight out in front of you.

3. Swing your arms backward, then jump forward as far as possible while vigorously swinging your arms forward and extending your legs.

4. Land on both feet and try to maintain your balance on landing. Do not run or hop before jumping.

5. When performing the actual test, measure the distance of your jump in inches as described later in the text.

Practice Tips

- For best performance, lean forward just before you jump. Practice to get the best timing of the lean followed by the forward arm swing just before you jump.

- Try the test several times so that you can land without losing your balance. Keep your arms extended in front of you and bend your knees when you land to help you absorb the shock of landing.

- Try bending your knees more or less before different jumps to see which amount of knee bend gives you the best jump.

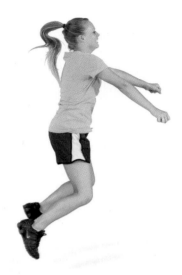

The standing long jump is a test of power (explosive strength).

TEST OF MUSCLE FITNESS AND FLEXIBILITY

TRUNK LIFT (back muscle fitness and back and trunk muscle flexibility)

This test is included in FitnessGram.

1. Lie facedown with your arms at your sides and your hands under or just beside your thighs.

2. Practice lifting the upper part of your body very slowly so that your chin, chest, and shoulders come off the floor. Lift your trunk as high as possible, to a maximum of 12 inches (30 centimeters). Hold this position for three seconds while a partner measures how far your chin is from the floor. Your partner should hold the ruler at least 1 inch (2.5 centimeters) in front of your chin. Look straight ahead so that your chin is not tipped abnormally upward.

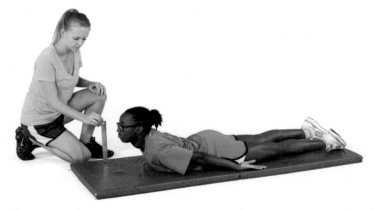

The trunk lift measures fitness and flexibility of the back and trunk muscles.

Caution: The ruler should not be placed directly under your chin, in case you have to lower your trunk unexpectedly.

Practice Tips

- Practice lifting your trunk three to five times to see if you are able to hold the lift for the required three seconds.
- Practice looking straight ahead so that your chin is not tipped up.

TEST OF FLEXIBILITY

BACK-SAVER SIT-AND-REACH (flexibility of the hip)

This test is included in FitnessGram.

1. Place a yardstick or meter stick on top of a box that is 12 inches (30 centimeters) high, with the stick extending 9 inches (23 centimeters) over the box and the lower numbers toward you. You may also use a flexibility testing box if one is available.

2. To measure the flexibility of your right leg, fully extend it and place your right foot flat against the box. Bend your left leg, with the knee turned out and your left foot 2 to 3 inches (5 to 8 centimeters) to the side of your straight right leg.

3. Extend your arms forward over the measuring stick. Place your hands on the stick, one on top of the other, with your palms facing down. Your middle fingers should be together with the tip of one finger exactly on top of the other.

4. Lean forward slowly; do not bounce. Reach forward, then slowly return to the starting position. Repeat four times. On the fourth reach, hold the position for three seconds and observe the measurement on the stick below your fingertips.

5. Repeat with your left leg.

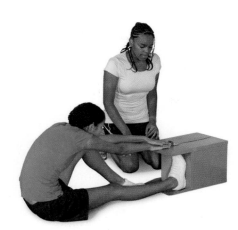

The back-saver sit-and-reach measures flexibility (range of motion) of the hip.

Practice Tips

- Do the PACER practice or another general warm-up before practicing this test.
- Practice keeping your extended leg straight (a very slight bend is okay).
- Practice keeping your other leg bent and the foot of that leg about 2 to 3 inches (5 to 8 centimeters) from your straight leg.
- Practice keeping one middle finger on top of the other.
- Practice holding your stretch for three seconds.
- Practice three to five times with each leg.

Learning Self-Management Skills

Lesson Objectives

After reading this lesson, you should be able to

1. describe the stages of change in adopting a healthy lifestyle;

2. describe the three types of self-management skills and give examples of each type;

3. describes some benefits of using self-management skills to change behavior; and

4. describe three components of social–emotional learning and give examples of each.

Lesson Vocabulary

exercise
physical activity
self-management skills
social–emotional learning

In the first lesson of this chapter, you learned about what it means to live a healthy lifestyle, as well as the many determinants of health, fitness, and wellness. In this lesson, you'll learn the self-management skills to make the lifestyle changes to enhance your fitness, health, and wellness.

Stages of Change

People do not change overnight—it takes time. Psychologists working to help people stop smoking found that most smokers do not quit all at once but go through five stages to eventually quit. Later, exercise psychologists and nutrition scientists found that these five stages of change also apply to other lifestyle choices, such as physical activity and nutrition. Understanding these stages can help you make positive changes in your lifestyle.

Healthy lifestyle behaviors—such as being active, eating well, and managing stress—are within your control. With effort, almost anyone can make healthy lifestyle changes. There are

My grandpa smoked for years and tried to quit many times. I told him that lots of people have tried to quit many times. He tried again and he did it. I am proud of him.

Jack LaPrada

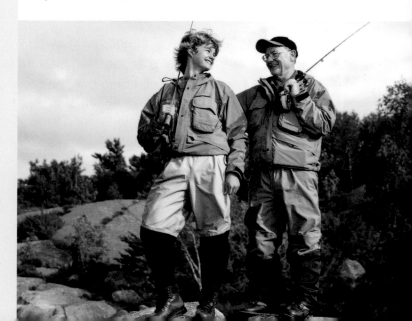

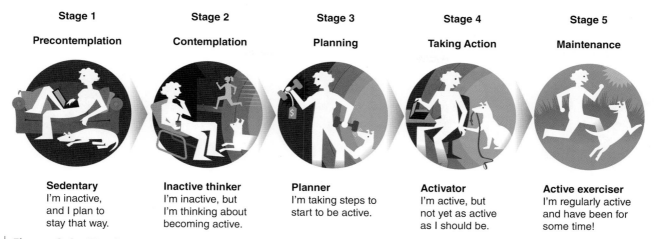

Stage 1
Precontemplation

Stage 2
Contemplation

Stage 3
Planning

Stage 4
Taking Action

Stage 5
Maintenance

Sedentary
I'm inactive,
and I plan to
stay that way.

Inactive thinker
I'm inactive, but
I'm thinking about
becoming active.

Planner
I'm taking steps to
start to be active.

Activator
I'm active, but
not yet as active
as I should be.

Active exerciser
I'm regularly active
and have been for
some time!

Figure 2.4   The five stages of change for physical activity.

five stages of change for modifying behaviors: precontemplation (not thinking of change), contemplation, planning for change, taking action to change, and maintaining change. Figure 2.4 shows the five stages of change for physical activity. The following describes the stages of change for a person becoming more active.

• *Stage 1: Precontemplation.* A person at stage 1 chooses to be inactive and has no intention of changing. An inactive person does not meet national goals for any type of physical activity. This means that they move very little and mostly sit during their waking hours. Nearly one-third of American adults are considered inactive. You might think there are no inactive teens, but nearly one in five teens can also be included in this group. In an ideal world, all people would be active exercisers, but sometimes people move slowly from one stage to the next.

• *Stage 2: Contemplation.* In stage 2, the person still does little physical activity but is thinking about becoming active. They might read about the importance of physical activity but do not take action yet. This person has moved from being sedentary to being an inactive thinker.

• *Stage 3: Planning.* At stage 3, a person starts planning to be active. For example, they might visit an exercise facility or buy a new tennis racket. The person has now become a planner, even though they are not yet active.

• *Stage 4: Action.* Stage 4 involves actually becoming active. The person, now an activator, goes to the exercise facility to work out or plays tennis with a friend.

• *Stage 5: Maintenance.* Stage 5 involves maintaining regular activity. This stage is reached when a person is regularly active for at least six months. The ultimate goal is to help all people progress to the stage of the active exerciser.

These stages of change can also apply to other healthy lifestyle choices. For example, figure 2.5 shows the stages for eating well. Only 9 percent of teens eat the recommended servings of fruits and 2 percent eat the recommended servings of vegetables each day, and about 1 in 10 have avoided eating meals for as long as 24 hours. Teens who do not eat well and do not want to change are at stage 1, whereas those who eat well on a regular basis are at stage 5.

You can be at one level of change in one area and at another level in a different area. For example, perhaps you're not active on a regular basis but are thinking about becoming more active; therefore, you're at stage 2 for physical activity. At the same time, you might regularly eat well and therefore be at stage 5 for healthy eating. For any healthy lifestyle choice, the goal is to move to stage 5.

FIT FACT
Physical activity refers to movement that uses your large muscles and includes a wide range of pursuits, such as sport, dance, recreational activities, and activities of daily living. **Exercise** is a form of physical activity specifically designed to improve your fitness.

Happiness lies, first of all, in health.

George William Curtis, author and social reformer

FIT FACT
Changes in behavior don't always occur from stage 1 to 5 without interruption. Sometimes people move forward a few stages, then fall back a stage, and then move forward again. With effort, progress is made gradually from one stage to another.

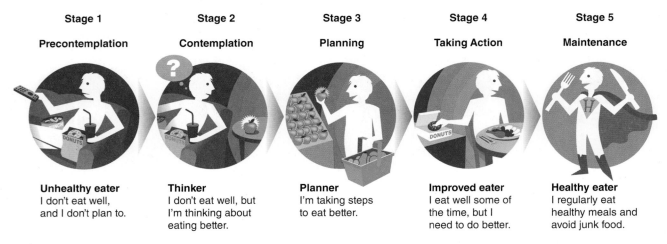

Stage 1	Stage 2	Stage 3	Stage 4	Stage 5
Precontemplation	**Contemplation**	**Planning**	**Taking Action**	**Maintenance**

Unhealthy eater I don't eat well, and I don't plan to.	**Thinker** I don't eat well, but I'm thinking about eating better.	**Planner** I'm taking steps to eat better.	**Improved eater** I eat well some of the time, but I need to do better.	**Healthy eater** I regularly eat healthy meals and avoid junk food.

Figure 2.5   The five stages of change for eating well.

Self-Management Skills

How do you change your lifestyle? How do you move from stage 1 to stage 5? The best way is to learn **self-management skills**. Self-management skills are abilities that help you change your lifestyles. Like any other skill, the more you practice it, the more you improve. There are three kinds of self-management skills: those that help you begin to change, those that help you make change, and those that help you maintain change (see figure 2.6).

Table 2.1 lists 21 self-management skills that can help you live an active, healthy life. These skills can help you begin to change, help you make changes, and help you maintain changes. One self-management skill is emphasized in the Taking Charge and Self-Management features in each chapter of this book.

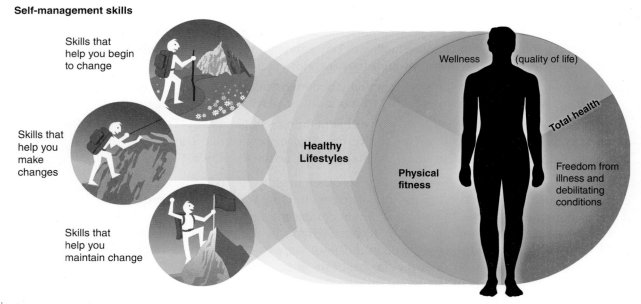

Self-management skills

Skills that help you begin to change

Skills that help you make changes

Skills that help you maintain change

Healthy Lifestyles

Wellness (quality of life)

Physical fitness

Total health

Freedom from illness and debilitating conditions

Figure 2.6   Self-management skills help you change your lifestyles to improve your fitness, health, and wellness.

TABLE 2.1   **Self-Management Skills for Fitness, Health, and Wellness**

Skills that help you begin to change	
Effective communication	This skill helps you effectively receive information and pass it on to others.
Self-assessment	This skill helps you see where you are and what to change in order to get where you want to be.
Building self-confidence	This skill helps you build the feeling that you're capable of making healthy lifestyle changes.
Building knowledge and understanding	This skill helps you solve problems—such as how to make healthy changes in your life—using a modified form of the scientific method.
Improving self-perception	This skill helps you think positively about yourself so that you're more likely to make healthy lifestyle choices and feel that they will make a difference in your life.
Building positive attitudes	This skill helps position you to succeed in adopting healthy lifestyles.
Skills that help you make change	
Setting goals	This skill creates a foundation for developing your personal plan by helping you set goals that are SMART (specific, measurable, attainable, realistic, and timely).
Overcoming barriers	This skill helps you find ways to overcome barriers to making healthy lifestyle choices, such as lack of time, temporary injury, lack of safe places to be active, inclement weather, and difficulty in selecting healthy foods.
Managing time	This skill helps you be efficient so that you have time for the important things in your life.
Improving performance	This skill helps you enjoy and stay interested in being physically active for a lifetime.
Finding social support	This skill enables you to get help and support from others (such as your friends and family) as you adopt healthy behaviors and try to stick with them.
Managing competitive stress	This skill involves preventing or coping with the stresses of competition.
Choosing good activities	This skill involves selecting the activities that are best for you so that you will enjoy and benefit from doing them.
Skills that help you maintain change	
Resolving conflicts	This skill helps you adapt when confronted with problems with other people.
Self-monitoring	This skill involves keeping records or logs to see whether you are in fact doing what you think you're doing.
Preventing relapse	This skill helps you stick with healthy behaviors even when you have problems getting motivated.
Developing tactics	This skill helps you focus on a specific plan of action and successfully execute the plan.
Saying no	This skill helps keep you from doing things you don't want to do, especially when you're under pressure from friends or other people.
Thinking success	This skill helps you adapt your way of thinking to help you believe that you can achieve success.
Thinking critically	This skill enables you to find and interpret information that helps you make good decisions and solve problems.
Positive self-talk	This skill helps you perform your best and make healthy lifestyle choices by thinking positive thoughts rather than negative ones that detract from success.

Skills That Help You Begin to Change

The first type of skills are especially helpful to people who need to make changes but have not begun a plan of action (people in stages 1 and 2). Self-assessment skills, for example, help you see that you need to make changes and determine what changes to make. Others are described in table 2.1.

Skills That Help You Make Change

The second type of self-management skills, which include setting goals and managing your time, help you prepare for and move toward action. Others are described in table 2.1.

Skills That Help You Maintain Change

Once you have taken action (stage 4), skills such as self-monitoring help you keep track of your behavior and keep you at the maintenance stage (stage 5). The descriptions in table 2.1 will help you understand how each self-management skill can benefit you.

Using Multiple Skills to Promote Change

Although different self-management skills work best at certain stages, many have benefits at all stages of change. For example, finding social support is listed as a skill for helping you make change, but it can also help you get started and maintain change. If friends and family encourage you, you may be more willing to try something new. Encouragement from others can also help you keep trying new things by making you feel like a part of the group. Using a variety of self-management skills can ultimately result in behavior changes that promote good fitness, health, and wellness.

Self-Management Skills and Social–Emotional Learning

Health and wellness have five different components: intellectual, social, physical, emotional–mental, and spiritual. Learning that focuses on the social and emotional components is referred to as **social–emotional learning**. SHAPE America, an organization of health and physical education teachers, endorses social–emotional learning as a way to make connections among all of the five components of health and wellness.

Effectively using the self-management skills described in table 2.1 promotes social–emotional learning. Three important components of social–emotional learning include making responsible decisions, building self-awareness, and establishing positive relationships. They are described in more detail in the following sections.

Making Responsible Decisions

Several self-management skills help you collect, process, and use information to make responsible decisions and solve problems according to the scientific method. Examples include learning to communicate effectively, building knowledge and understanding, learning to think critically, and learning to self-assess.

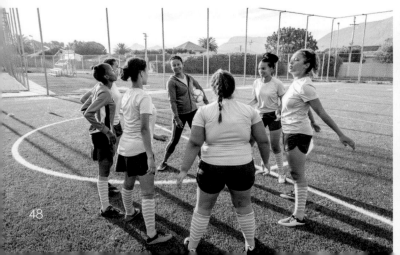

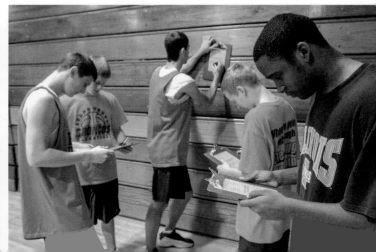

Building Self-Awareness

Awareness means being informed about things around you or having an accurate picture of the situations in which you find yourself. *Self-awareness*, therefore, refers to the ability to see yourself accurately and know your own strengths and weaknesses. It helps you to be aware when in social situations so that you can act appropriately. Many of the self-management skills promote self-awareness, including learning to self-assess, improving self-perception, building self-confidence, building positive attitudes, and thinking success.

Establishing Positive Relationships

Having good relationship skills is an important goal of social–emotional learning. The word *relationship* refers to the way people behave toward each other. It refers to the bonds and connections they have with others and the regard they have for each other. Several self-management skills can help you establish and maintain healthy social relationships. Examples of relationship skills include communicating effectively, finding social support, resolving conflict, and learning to say no.

Practicing these skills helps you move through the five stages of change to promote healthy lifestyles and social–emotional learning.

LESSON REVIEW

1. What are the five stages of change, and how do they help you adopt healthy lifestyles?
2. What are the three types of self-management skills, and what are some examples of each?
3. How can you benefit from using multiple self-management skills to promote change?
4. What are the three components of social–emotional learning, and how do self-management skills promote social–emotional learning?

TAKING CHARGE: **Self-Assessment**

Self-assessment is a self-management skill that enables you to test yourself to see where you are succeeding and what needs improvement. You can perform self-assessments in many areas, such as physical fitness, eating patterns, stress level, health risks, knowledge, and sport skills. This book includes many self-assessments focused on physical fitness, as well as some that address

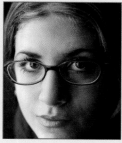

health, wellness, and healthy lifestyle choices. The following example focuses on health-related physical fitness.

Julia and Troy were friends who wanted to know more

about their health-related physical fitness. They had taken fitness tests in school but had learned little about why they were doing the tests or how to test themselves.

Julia remembered some of the tests she had taken in elementary school, such as running a 50-yard dash and performing a "shuttle run." Troy had not taken a fitness test

>continued

>continued

in physical education, but he had been tested for his baseball team to see how far he could throw a ball and how fast he could run to first base.

Julia and Troy thought about doing a self-assessment that included all of the tests they had previously taken, but they weren't sure how to do the tests correctly, and they weren't sure that these were the best tests. What they really wanted to learn was how to do a self-assessment for health-related physical fitness.

FOR DISCUSSION

Discuss a self-assessment plan that Julia and Troy could follow to determine their health-related physical fitness. Did the tests Julia performed in elementary school assess health-related physical fitness? Did the tests Troy performed for his baseball team measure health-related physical fitness? What do you think these tests really measured? Consider the guidelines in the following Self-Management feature as you answer these discussion questions and as you try the various self-assessments included in this book.

SELF-MANAGEMENT: Skills for Self-Assessment

Before you go on a trip, you use a map to plan where you want to go. Assessing your own fitness is much like using a map. You can assess your current fitness and physical activity in order to help you learn where you need to improve and make your plans for doing so. You can also use your assessment information to develop strategies to commit to your plan. Use the following guidelines as you learn to do personal fitness and activity self-assessments.

- *Try a wide variety of tests.* Fitness and physical activity include many components, and performing a variety of self-assessments enables you to get a total picture of your fitness and activity needs. You will learn various self-assessment techniques in this class.

- *Choose self-assessments that work best for you.* You'll try all the self-assessments you learn in this book, but ultimately you won't need to use them all. You should choose at least one assessment for each type of health-related physical fitness and one assessment to determine your current activity level. After you've tried them all, you'll be prepared to select the ones that work best for you.

- *Practice.* When you first drive a car, it's not easy, but your skill improves with practice. Similarly, the first time you do self-assessments, you'll make mistakes, but the more you practice, the better you'll get. Once you decide which assessments to use on a regular basis, practice using them!

- *Use self-assessments for personal improvement.* Once you've learned to use self-assessments, repeat them from time to time to monitor your progress. It takes several weeks to see improvement after starting a new activity program, so avoid daily or even weekly self-assessments in favor of self-assessing after several weeks, when improvement is more likely.

- *Use health standards rather than comparing yourself with others.* Sometimes people are discouraged when they get test results because they had unrealistic expectations. Rather than comparing yourself with others, evaluate yourself in relation to health standards and to your own previous performances. This type of comparison helps you stay realistic. The standards used in this book are based on the level of fitness needed for good health and wellness—not on comparisons of one person with another.

- *Information from self-assessments is personal.* Self-assessments are done to gain information that will help you build an accurate personal profile and plan for healthy active living. When paired up for assessments, partners must agree to keep test results private. Information may be submitted to an instructor, parent, or guardian—again, with the expectation that information is kept private. Information should not be shared with others without the permission of the person being tested.

Taking Action: **Fitness Trails**

Fresh air, nature, and fitness? Yes, please! Most communities have natural spaces where you can walk, jog, run, or bike. Some communities have also created fitness trails—pathways through parks or woodlands designed especially for walking, jogging, and running. Some fitness trails include human-made or natural structures intended for particular exercises. These structures allow walkers, joggers, and runners to mix their movement activity with muscle fitness and flexibility exercises. Fitness trails are sometimes considered outdoor gyms, and there's probably one near you!

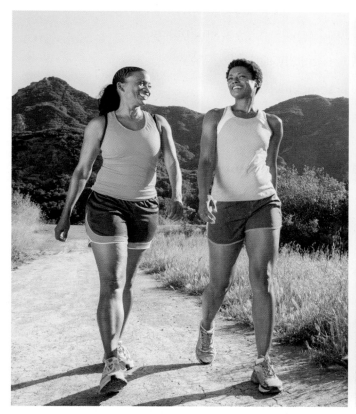 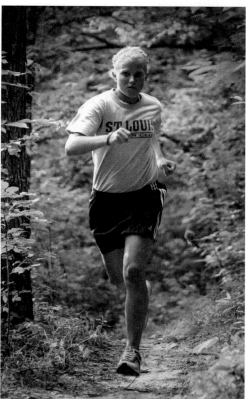

Being outdoors dramatically increases the amount of activity that people perform.

Take action by learning about, visiting, or even helping create a fitness trail near you. Many fitness trails are already well established by city or county parks and recreation departments or federal agencies such as the U.S. National Park Service. Although they may differ from remote trails, urban areas can also have fitness trails.

CHAPTER REVIEW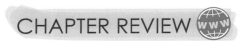

Reviewing Concepts and Vocabulary

Answer items 1 through 5 by correctly completing each sentence with a word or phrase.

1. Factors that affect your fitness, health, and wellness are called _____.

2. The factors influencing fitness, health, and wellness over which you have the least control are _____.

3. The factors influencing fitness, health, and wellness over which you have the most control are _____.

4. The steps that lead you from dependence to independence are referred to together as the _____.

5. The fitness test used to assess cardiorespiratory endurance by running when signaled by a beep is called the _____.

For items 6 through 10, match each term in column 1 with the appropriate phrase in column 2.

6. sedentary person   a. just bought exercise equipment

7. inactive thinker   b. is regularly active

8. planner   c. is sometimes active

9. activator   d. is considering becoming active

10. active exerciser   e. is inactive

For items 11 through 15, respond to each statement or question.

11. Explain what a self-management skill is and why it can be useful.

12. What are some of the fitness test items used in batteries such as FitnessGram, and what do they measure?

13. Describe the five stages of change.

14. What is social–emotional learning, and what are three of its components?

15. What are some guidelines for learning to do effective self-assessment?

Thinking Critically

Write a paragraph to answer the following question.

Of all the self-management skills described in lesson 2.2, which one would most help *you* be more active or eat better? Give the reasons for your answer.

Project

Assume that you are the head of a marketing company assigned to create an ad campaign promoting healthier eating and more active living. Prepare a script for a television commercial for the promotion. If resources are available, create a video of the commercial.

Goal Setting and Program Planning

3

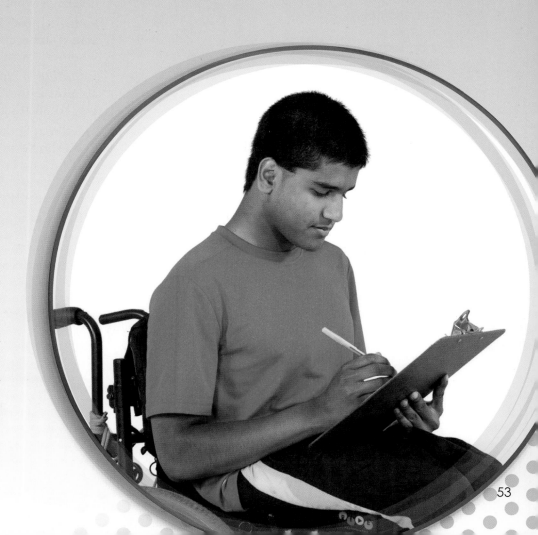

Goal Setting

Lesson Objectives

After reading this lesson, you should be able to

1. explain the SMART formula for setting goals;

2. describe short-term goals and explain when they are best used;

3. describe long-term goals and explain when they are best used; and

4. describe process and product goals and explain how they differ.

Lesson Vocabulary

acronym
goal setting
long-term goal
mnemonic
process goal
product goal
short-term goal
SMART goal

How do you turn your dreams into realities? Successful people use **goal setting** as part of their overall planning to achieve success. You can use goals to plan a personal fitness program, a healthy diet plan, or any other type of program. In this lesson, you'll learn to use long-term and short-term goals. You'll also learn about other goals that can help you make good lifestyle choices, such as being physically active and eating well.

SMART Goals

You may have learned about **SMART goals** in middle school. Here's a quick review to help you remember the five rules for setting goals as you work your way through this book.

S: Specific. Your goal should include specific details of what you want to accomplish.

M: Measurable. You should be able to measure your progress and accurately determine whether you've accomplished your goal.

A: Attainable. You should make them attainable by setting short-term goals first on the way to meeting long-term goals.

R: Realistic. Your goals should challenge you. They should not be too easy or too hard.

When I was a kid I read *The Little Engine That Could*. It was a corny story, but I thought about it when I was trying to reach my goals. If you think you can do something and keep trying, little by little you can do what you set out to do. I did.

Silvia Garcia

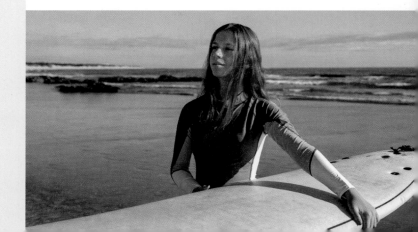

T: Timely. Your goal should have a specific time line in which to be accomplished and be useful to you at this time in your life.

SMART Short-Term Goals

Long-term goals take months or even years to accomplish, whereas **short-term goals** can be reached in a short time, such as a few days or weeks. It is best to begin with short-term goals that help you move toward meeting your long-term goals. Let's consider an example. Anna needs $2,400 for her first year of college. But this amount seems overwhelming because she will start college in two years. Anna can keep the $2,400 long-term goal in mind, but experts agree that it is best to start with SMART short-term goals. Rather than worry about how much money she could make, Anna set a short-term goal of working five hours a week for the next four weeks. Now let's see whether this would be a SMART short-term goal for Anna.

Specific. Five hours a week is a specific amount of work time and a good specific short-term goal.

Measurable. The goal of working five hours a week for four weeks is measurable. Anna can keep a log each week to see if she is reaching the goal.

Attainable. Working five hours per week is a short-term goal. Meeting the short-term goal will help her as she works toward her long-term savings goal.

Realistic. For someone else, the goal might not be realistic. But Anna has a job and knows that if she sticks with it she can save money for college. After four weeks, Anna can adjust the number of hours she works upward or downward as necessary.

Timely. The goal of working five hours a week for four weeks has a specific and workable time line. The hours of work fit her schedule and allow her to do other important things in her life.

SMART Long-Term Goals

Anna reached the short-term goal of working five hours a week for four weeks. She felt good because even after spending some of her earnings she was able to save $100. So she set a

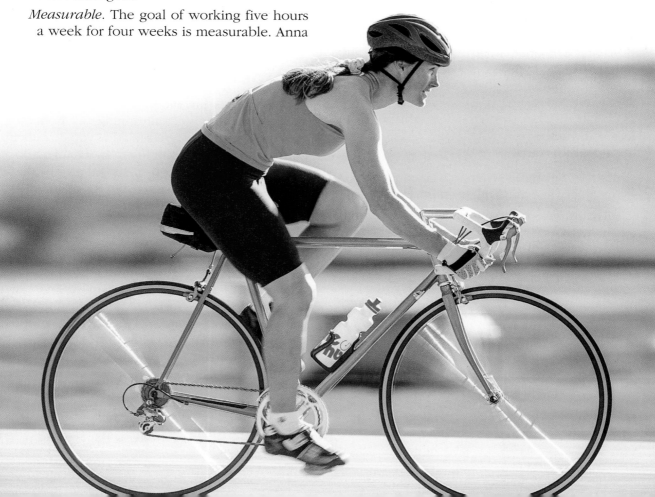

ACADEMIC CONNECTION: **Mnemonics and Acronyms**

A **mnemonic** (pronounced ni-mon'-ik) is a tool that helps you remember something. There are many types of mnemonics. Examples include rhymes, songs, and patterns of letters. For example, a rhyme is commonly used as a mnemonic to remember how many days there are in each month ("Thirty days hath September, April, June, and November") and the alphabet song is a mnemonic that helps children learn their ABCs. An **acronym** is a type of mnemonic that uses the first letter of several words to form a new word. Two examples used in this book are SMART and FIT. SMART helps you remember the characteristics of goal setting and FIT helps you remember the *frequency, intensity,* and *time* of physical activity (when the type of activity is already established).

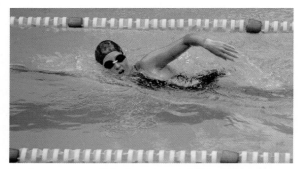

Swimmers on this team used the acronym TEAM (Together Everyone Achieves More) to help them achieve their goals.

STUDENT ACTIVITY

Create a mnemonic or an acronym related to your study in *Fitness for Life.* Briefly describe the mnemonic or acronym and explain how it might be useful.

---

new goal of continuing to work for five hours a week for the next eight weeks. Over the next eight weeks, Anna met her goal and was able to save $240. At this point she had saved $340 and felt confident about setting a long-term goal of saving $100 per month over the next nine months if she sticks to her schedule. If Anna meets her long-term goal, she will have saved at least $1,240 for the year ($340 + $900), more than half of what she needs for college. Now let's see whether this would be a SMART long-term goal for Anna.

Specific. Saving $100 a month for nine months is a very specific long-term goal.

Measurable. The goal of saving $100 a month is measurable. Anna can count her money every month to see how close she is to reaching the long-term goal.

Attainable. Anna set short-term goals and met them twice, so the long-term goal is likely to be attained.

Realistic. For someone else, the goal of $100 a month might not be realistic, but for Anna it is not unreasonable. She has saved at least $100 a month for three months, and if she continues to save at that rate she will meet the long-term goal as scheduled.

Timely. The goal of saving $100 a month for nine months ($900 total) has a specific and workable time line, fits her schedule, and over two years will provide the funds that she will need for college.

Product and Process Goals

Process goals involve performing a behavior, such as working a certain number of hours to earn money. *Process* refers to what you do rather than to the product resulting from what you do. Examples of process goals for fitness, health, and wellness include exercising for 60 minutes and eating five servings of fruits and vegetables every day (figure 3.1*a*). Process goals make good short-term goals because you can easily monitor your progress. In contrast, product goals do not make especially good short-term goals, because they typically take a while to achieve and can be discouraging, especially for a person who is just beginning to change. For example, if you chose a product goal of being able to perform 25 push-ups, it might (depending on your current fitness level) take you so long to meet the goal that you would give up. But a short-term process goal—such as performing 5 to 10 push-ups each day for two weeks—would be possible for you

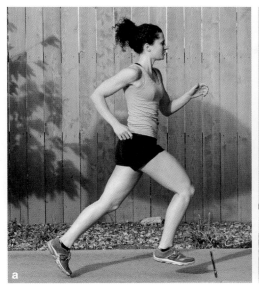 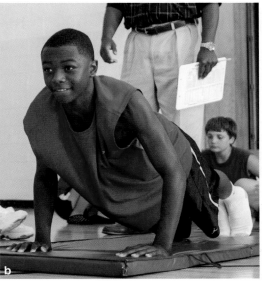

Figure 3.1 Process and product goals: *(a)* doing 60 minutes of physical activity a day is a process goal, and *(b)* being able to perform 25 push-ups is a product goal.

to achieve with effort. Thus, as you meet a series of short-term process goals, you work toward meeting long-term product goals.

The long-term goal of earning $900 is a **product goal**. A product is something tangible that results from work or effort. In other words, it's not what you do, but what you get as a result of what you do. Examples of product goals for fitness, health, and wellness include being able to perform 25 push-ups, being able to run a mile in six minutes, and losing five pounds (figure 3.1*b*). Product goals make

TECH TRENDS: **Software Applications (Apps)**

Smartphones and other smart devices such as computer tablets use software called *applications* (also known as *apps*). Software companies have developed many different apps that can help you plan and monitor your physical activity and nutrition. For example, you can create a physical activity schedule, track your exercise, and monitor your food intake.

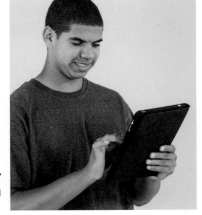

Smartphone and computer tablets have apps that help you meet healthy lifestyle goals.

USING TECHNOLOGY

Create an idea for a fitness or health app. Describe the app and how it would be used.

SCIENCE IN ACTION: **Optimal Challenge**

Scientists in many fields have collaborated to find ways to help people stay active, eat well, and stick with other healthy lifestyle behaviors. They have discovered that in order to be successful, you must set goals that provide optimal challenge. If a challenge is too easy, there's no need to try hard—it's not really a challenge. On the other hand, if a goal is too hard, we fail, which may lead us to give up because our effort seems hopeless (see figure 3.2).

An optimal challenge requires reasonable effort. Meeting an optimal challenge allows us to experience success and makes us want to try again. In fact, optimal challenge is one reason that video games are so popular. They challenge you by making the task more difficult as you improve, which makes you want to play again and again. You can use optimal challenge when setting your own goals to help you succeed.

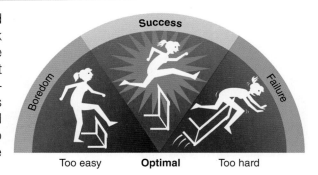

Figure 3.2   Some challenges can lead to boredom or failure, but optimal challenges can lead to success.

STUDENT ACTIVITY

Imagine that you want to help a friend learn a skill—for example, hitting a tennis ball. How could you use optimal challenge to help your friend learn the skill?

> If you want to live a happy life, tie it to a goal, not to people or things.
>
> *Albert Einstein,*
> *Nobel Prize–winning*
> *physicist*

appropriate long-term goals because it may take you a fair amount of work and time to reach them.

The Taking Charge and Self-Management features in this chapter focus on setting goals for nutrition and fitness. Elsewhere in the book, you'll get the chance to set long-term goals for making healthy lifestyle changes (product goals). You'll also get the chance to set short-term goals (process goals) that help you move toward achieving your long-term goals.

LESSON REVIEW

1. What is the SMART formula for setting goals?
2. What are short-term goals, and how are they best used?
3. What are long-term goals, and how are they best used?
4. What are process and product goals, and how do they differ?

SELF-ASSESSMENT: **Assessing Muscle Fitness**

Chapter 2 introduced you to national and international fitness test batteries and gave you a chance to practice test items to make sure that you know how to do them properly. In this self-assessment, you'll perform four tests that measure your muscle fitness: curl-up, push-up, handgrip strength, and long jump. For each item, you'll learn how to rate your performance. Later, when you've taken all of the tests included in FitnessGram, you can use your scores and ratings to prepare a FitnessGram report. For the tests included in this chapter, you'll record your scores and ratings as directed by your teacher so that you can use the information when you plan your personal fitness program. If you're working with a partner, remember that self-assessment information is confidential and shouldn't be shared without the permission of the person being tested.

CURL-UP (abdominal muscle strength and muscular endurance)

1. Lie on your back on a mat or carpet. Bend your knees approximately 140 degrees. Your feet should be slightly apart and as far as possible from your buttocks while still allowing your feet to be flat on the floor. Your arms should be straight and parallel to your trunk with your palms resting on the mat.

2. Place your head on a piece of paper. Place a strip of cardboard (may also substitute rubber, plastic, or tape) 4.5 inches (about 11.5 centimeters) wide and 3 feet (about 1 meter) long under your knees so that the fingers of both hands just touch the near edge of the strip.

3. Keeping your heels on the floor, curl your shoulders up slowly and slide your arms forward so that your fingers move across the cardboard strip. Curl up until your fingertips reach the far side of the strip.

4. Slowly lower your back until your head rests on the piece of paper.

5. Repeat the curl-up procedure so that you do one curl-up every three seconds. A partner could help you by saying "up, down" every three seconds. You are finished when you can't do another curl-up or when you fail to keep up with the three-second count.

6. Record the number of curl-ups you completed, then find your rating in table 3.1 and record it.

The curl-up assesses fitness of the abdominal muscles.

TABLE 3.1   Rating Chart: Curl-Ups (Number of Repetitions)

	13 years old		14 years old		15 years or older	
	Male	**Female**	**Male**	**Female**	**Male**	**Female**
High performance	≥41	≥33	≥46	≥33	≥48	≥36
Good fitness	21–40	18–32	24–45	18–32	24–47	18–35
Marginal fitness	18–20	15–17	20–23	15–17	20–23	15–17
Low fitness	≤17	≤14	≤19	≤14	≤19	≤14

Data based on *FitnessGram*.

PUSH-UP (upper body strength and muscular endurance)

1. Lie facedown on a mat or carpet with your hands (palm down) under your shoulders, your fingers spread, and your legs straight. Your legs should be slightly apart and your toes tucked under.

2. Push up until your arms are straight. Keep your legs and back straight. Your body should form a straight line from your head to your heels.

3. Lower your body by bending your elbows until your upper arms are parallel to the floor (elbows at a 90-degree angle), then push up until your arms are fully extended.

4. Do one push-up every three seconds. You may want to have a partner say "up, down" every three seconds to help you. You are finished when you are unable to complete a push-up with proper form for the second time or are unable to keep the pace for a second time.

5. Record the number of push-ups you performed, then find your rating in table 3.2 and record it.

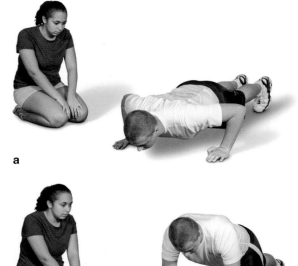

a

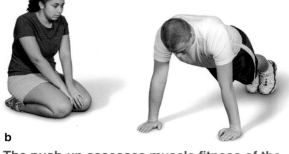

b

The push-up assesses muscle fitness of the upper body.

TABLE 3.2   Rating Chart: Push-Ups (Number of Repetitions)

	13 years old		14 years old		15 years old		16 years or older	
	Male	**Female**	**Male**	**Female**	**Male**	**Female**	**Male**	**Female**
High performance	≥26	≥16	≥31	≥16	≥36	≥16	≥36	≥16
Good fitness	12–25	7–15	14–30	7–15	16–35	7–15	18–35	7–15
Marginal fitness	10–11	6	12–13	6	14–15	6	16–17	6
Low fitness	≤9	≤5	≤11	≤5	≤13	≤5	≤15	≤5

Data based on *FitnessGram*.

HANDGRIP STRENGTH (isometric hand and arm strength)

1. Adjust the dynamometer to fit your hand size.

2. With your arm extended and your elbow nearly straight, squeeze as hard as possible for two to five seconds. Do not touch your body with your arm or hand.

3. Repeat with each hand. Alternate hands to allow a rest between each attempt.

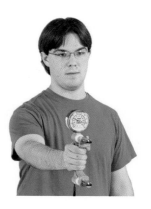

The handgrip strength test assesses isometric hand and arm strength.

4. Results are most often reported in kilograms (a kilogram equals about 2.2 pounds). To get your score in pounds, multiply your score in kilograms by 2.2. Add your best right-hand score to your best left-hand score, then divide the total by two to get your average score.

5. Record your average score, then find your rating in table 3.3 and record it.

TABLE 3.3   Rating Chart: Handgrip Strength (Pounds)

	13 years old		14 years old		15 years old		16 years old		17 years or older	
	Male	Female	Male	Female	Male	Female	Male	Female	Male	Female
High performance	≥65	≥57	≥80	≥60	≥91	≥61	≥107	≥62	≥112	≥71
Good fitness	58–64	54–56	71–79	58–59	82–90	59–60	100–106	60–61	104–111	65–70
Marginal fitness	52–57	50–53	63–70	55–57	74–81	56–58	93–99	57–59	97–103	59–64
Low fitness	≤51	≤49	≤62	≤54	≤73	≤55	≤92	≤56	≤96	≤58

Ratings are based on the average of the best right-hand and left-hand scores.

Based on ALPHA-FIT

STANDING LONG JUMP (leg power or explosive strength)

1. Mark a line on the floor with masking tape.

2. Stand with your feet shoulder-width apart behind the line. Bend your knees and hold your arms straight out in front of you.

3. Swing your arms backward, then jump forward as far as possible while vigorously swinging your arms forward and extending your legs.

4. Land on both feet and try to maintain your balance on landing. Do not run or hop before jumping.

5. Perform the test two times. Record the better of your two scores in inches (1 inch equals 2.54 centimeters), then find your rating in table 3.4 and record it.

The standing long jump assesses leg power.

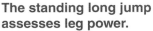

TABLE 3.4   Rating Chart: Standing Long Jump (Inches)

	13 years old		14 years old		15 years old		16 years old		17 years or older	
	Male	Female	Male	Female	Male	Female	Male	Female	Male	Female
High performance	≥73	≥59	≥80	≥60	≥85	≥61	≥88	≥62	≥91	≥68
Good fitness	67–72	57–58	73–79	58–59	78–84	59–60	82–87	60–61	86–90	63–67
Marginal fitness	61–66	54–56	67–72	55–57	73–77	56–58	77–81	57–59	80–85	58–62
Low fitness	≤60	≤53	≤66	≤54	≤72	≤55	≤76	≤56	≤79	≤57

Based on ALPHA-FIT

Program Planning

Lesson Objectives

After reading this lesson, you should be able to

1. describe how to prepare a personal needs profile and explain why it is important;

2. describe how to prepare a list of program options and explain why it is important;

3. describe how to prepare a list of SMART goals and explain why it is important; and

4. describe how to structure, write, and evaluate a program plan.

Lesson Vocabulary

personal needs profile
personal program

Have you ever prepared a written plan for adopting a healthy lifestyle? If not, would you know how to prepare a good plan? In this lesson, you'll learn the five steps that will help you prepare personal plans for adopting a healthy lifestyle. As you will see, the steps used in program planning are similar to the steps in the simplified scientific method. Program planning is a self-management skill like the others described in chapter 2. Because it is especially important, this entire lesson is devoted to helping you learn about program planning.

Step 1: Determine Your Personal Needs

The first step toward preparing a good **personal program** is to collect information about your personal needs. Throughout this book, you'll

> Last year when I was on the soccer team, I was very active. Now I am not on the team anymore and I am much less active. Planning got me going and kept me going after I quit playing soccer.
>
> *Mason Bettencourt*

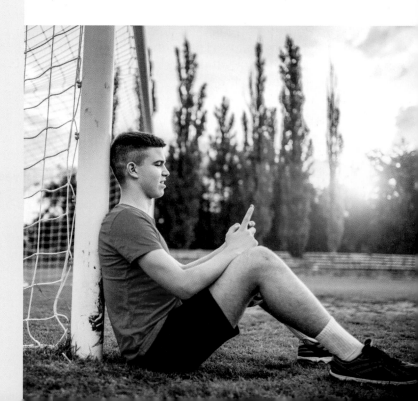

do many self-assessments of fitness, physical activity patterns, diet, and other health-related areas. You'll use this information to build a personal fitness, physical activity, or nutrition profile. This personal profile will help you focus on your needs as you plan your program. For example, before planning a fitness and activity program, you assess your current fitness level and physical activity patterns. Before planning a nutrition program, you assess your eating habits. In fact, before you plan to change *any* aspect of your lifestyle, you should perform a self-assessment in that particular area. If you don't know your needs, it will be difficult to perform the next steps in personal program planning, such as considering program options (step 2) or setting goals (step 3).

Once you complete your self-assessment in a specific lifestyle area, summarize your scores and ratings in a chart called a **personal needs profile**. You'll build a personal needs profile for each healthy lifestyle plan you develop as you work your way through this book. The following example will help you see what a personal needs profile looks like.

Jordan is a freshman in high school. She had always wanted to play on the lacrosse team and felt that improving her muscle fitness would help her be a better player. She also felt that building muscle fitness would help her look better. To evaluate her current muscle fitness, Jordan performed three self-assessments: the curl-up, the push-up, and the long jump. She also answered some questions about her current muscle fitness activities. She summarized her results in a personal needs profile (see table 3.5).

TABLE 3.5   **Jordan's Personal Needs Profile**

Activity self-assessment	Yes	No	Comment
Do you do muscle fitness exercises 2–3 days per week?		✓	Stretch every day for 10 min

Fitness self-assessments	Score	Rating	
Push-up	6	Marginal fitness	
Curl-up	19	Good fitness	
Standing long jump	57 in. (145 cm)	Marginal fitness	

Step 2: Consider Your Program Options

After determining your personal needs, the next step is to consider your program options. For physical activity, determine what types of activities are available to you. Because Jordan was interested in muscle fitness, she used a checklist of muscle fitness activities. As you can see from the chart (table 3.6), there are many types of muscle fitness exercises. Jordan checked elastic band exercises, calisthenics, and isometric exercises because she could do them at home and had the necessary equipment. She decided to hold off on considering other types of exercise until she learned more about them.

CONSUMER CORNER: **Too Good to Be True**

Ripped abs in 4 weeks!
Drop 30 pounds without getting off the couch!
Get a perfect body in just 4 minutes a day!

These are just a few examples of headlines you'll see in magazines, newspapers, and TV and web ads. The fitness and health industry is big business. Unfortunately, many companies try to make money by promising big results with little effort. They use marketing campaigns that prey on people who want quick results. As a student of *Fitness for Life*, you're in the process of becoming a critical consumer of fitness, health, and wellness information. Use the tips presented here to make good decisions and avoid falling victim to false claims.

Consumer guideline	Consumer action
Evaluate the source of the information.	Avoid testimonials by famous people (such as athletes and movie stars) who are not experts.
	Use information from experts in health, medicine, nutrition, and kinesiology.
	Use information from government sources (such as the U.S. Food and Drug Administration) and reliable professional organizations (such as the American Heart Association).
	Use the scientific method to evaluate information.
Be suspicious of claims that promise quick results and are inconsistent with information presented in this book.	Compare claims with facts you've learned from this book and other reliable sources.
	Beware: If a claim seems too good to be true, it probably isn't.
Be suspicious of "special offers" that say you must take advantage immediately or they will no longer be available.	Avoid quick action. Offers that quickly expire are designed to get you to act fast without taking the time to make a good decision.
Check the credentials of the person or company doing the promotion.	Check to see if people who claim to be experts really are. Do they have a college degree or advanced degree? Are they certified by a well-known, legitimate organization? People with university degrees in kinesiology, physical education, and physical therapy are generally well equipped to give you sound advice about exercise. The same is true for a certified strength and conditioning specialist (CSCS), American College of Sports Medicine certified personal trainer (CPT), certified health fitness specialist (CHFS), certified group exercise instructor (CGEI), or registered clinical exercise physiologist (RCEP). For nutrition needs, a registered dietitian (RD) is well qualified to give you information.

TABLE 3.6   Jordan's Exercise Options for Muscle Fitness

Elastic band exercises		Calisthenics		Free weights	Resistance machine exercises	Isometric exercises	
✓	Arm curl	✓	Prone arm lift	Bench press	Bench press	✓	Biceps curl
✓	Arm press	✓	Push-up	Biceps curl	Biceps curl	✓	Bow exercise
✓	Upright row	✓	Bridge	Dumbbell row	Lat pull-down	✓	Hand push
✓	Leg curl	✓	Curl-up	Seated French curl	Seated row	✓	Back flattener
✓	Two-leg press	✓	Trunk lift	Seated press	Triceps press	✓	Knee extender
✓	Toe push	✓	High-knee jog	Half squat	Hamstring curl	✓	Leg curl
		✓	Side leg raise	Hamstring curl	Heel raise	✓	Toe push
		✓	Stride jump	Heel raise	Knee extension	✓	Wall push
				Knee extension			

Step 3: Set Goals

The next step in your planning is to set SMART goals. Jordan reviewed the example of writing SMART goals to save money for college from lesson 3.1, then used the SMART formula to write down her own long-term and short-term goals (see table 3.7). She chose exercise (process) goals for her short-term goals and fitness (product) goals for her long-term goals.

You are never too old to set another goal or to dream a new dream.

C.S. Lewis, author

TABLE 3.7   Jordan's Short-Term and Long-Term Goals

Short-term goals	Long-term goals
1. Perform the push-up and elastic band arm curl exercises three days a week.	1. Perform 10 push-ups.
2. Perform the long jump, elastic band leg curl, and elastic band toe push exercises three days a week.	2. Perform a 59-in. long jump (about 1.5 m).
3. Perform the curl-up exercise for the abdominal muscles three days a week.	3. Perform 25 curl-ups.

Specific. Jordan set her goals for muscle fitness and physical activity by choosing specific exercises and a specific number of exercise days per week. She grounded these decisions in the information recorded in her personal needs profile.

Measurable. Jordan made her goals measurable by deciding the number of weeks and the number of exercise days per week for her short-term goals, and the number of repetitions or distance for each outcome for her long-term fitness goals.

Attainable. To keep her goals attainable, Jordan's short-term goals addressed only activity (not fitness). She took this approach because muscle fitness takes time to build, which means that short-term fitness goals are often not attainable. For her short-term activity goal, Jordan chose two weeks of exercise. In this way, she will first focus on her short-term goal as a step toward achieving her long-term goal. For her long-term fitness goals, she chose scores that are higher than she can currently perform—but not too high. That makes this goal an optimal challenge. Jordan also sought out help from her physical education teacher in selecting her exercises and setting attainable goals.

Realistic. Because Jordan has various types of commitments—such as homework, family activities, and school activities—she limited the number of her goals and chose exercises that were not too hard or too easy so that she has a realistic chance to meet them all. As she becomes more experienced she can consider more goals.

Timely. Jordan also set a specific amount of time for reaching both her long-term and her short-term goals. Because she needs more muscle fitness to make the lacrosse team her goals are timely for her.

Steps 4 and 5: Create a Written Program and Evaluate It

In the fourth step, you use information gained during steps 1, 2, and 3 to structure your program. Once you establish your goals, you prepare a detailed written plan. As you work through this book, you'll create written plans for several programs; they will all be similar to Jordan's planning.

Jordan used a chart to prepare her exercise plan for muscle fitness. Because muscle fitness exercises should not be done every day, Jordan's teacher helped her decide which days to do each exercise and how many to do. Her teacher also helped her select the right elastic band to use in her exercises. Jordan decided on the best time of day based on her free time and the times when she most enjoyed exercising. She also considered times when she was not likely to be interrupted. A sample of Jordan's written plan is shown in table 3.8. The last column allowed Jordan to check off each day she completed her exercises.

After you've tried your program for some time (the exact amount of time depends on your goals), evaluate it. Did you meet your goals? Was your program a good one? After your evaluation, make a new plan using the program planning steps.

Jordan tried her plan for two weeks. As you can see in table 3.8, she missed her planned exercises on only one day during the two-week period. Given this success, she decided to keep doing the same plan for another two weeks on her way to meeting her long-term goals. She hoped to reach her long-term goal in eight weeks.

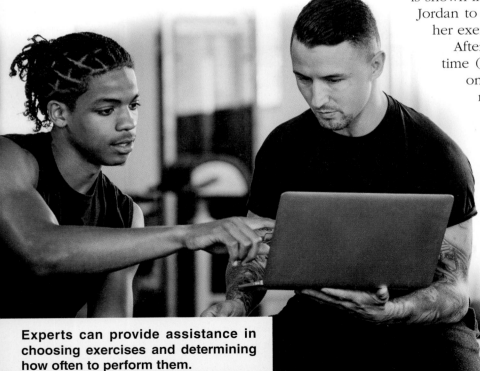

Experts can provide assistance in choosing exercises and determining how often to perform them.

TABLE 3.8   **Jordan's Two-Week Written Program Plan**

Day	Activity (exercise)	Time	Repetitions	Completed Week 1	Completed Week 2
Mon.	Warm-up (jog)	4 p.m.	5 min	✓	✓
	Biceps curl (exercise band)		3 sets of 10	✓	✓
	Toe push (exercise band)		3 sets of 10	✓	✓
	Curl-up		2 sets of 15	✓	✓
	Long jump		3 sets of 10	✓	✓
Tues.	Warm-up (walk)	4 p.m.	5 min	✓	✓
	Push-up		2 sets of 5	✓	✓
	Leg curl		3 sets of 10	✓	✓
Wed.	Warm-up (jog)	4 p.m.	5 min	✓	✓
	Biceps curl (exercise band)		3 sets of 10	✓	✓
	Toe push (exercise band)		3 sets of 10	✓	✓
	Curl-up		2 sets of 15	✓	✓
	Long jump		3 sets of 10	✓	✓
Thurs.	Warm-up (walk)	4 p.m.	5 min	✓	
	Push-up		2 sets of 5	✓	
	Leg curl		3 sets of 10	✓	
Fri.	Warm-up (jog)	4 p.m.	5 min	✓	✓
	Biceps curl (exercise band)		3 sets of 10	✓	✓
	Toe push (exercise band)		3 sets of 10	✓	✓
	Curl-up		2 sets of 15	✓	✓
	Long jump		3 sets of 10	✓	✓
Sat.	Warm-up (walk)	4 p.m.	5 min	✓	✓
	Push-up		2 sets of 5	✓	✓
	Leg curl		3 sets of 10	✓	✓
Sun.	No exercise				

You can use the five steps presented in this lesson to help you plan your own program. Once you've developed a personal program, you're on your way to becoming independent.

LESSON REVIEW

1. How do you prepare a personal needs profile?
2. How do you prepare a list of program options?
3. How do you prepare a list of SMART goals?
4. How do you structure, write, and evaluate a program plan?

TAKING CHARGE: **Setting Goals**

You probably know people who are sedentary or who eat a lot of unhealthy food. They may have tried to make lifestyle changes but been ineffective because they failed to set good goals. This feature highlights SMART goals for nutrition.

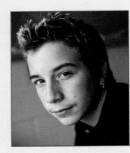

Ms. Booker, a physical education teacher, noticed that Kevin seemed a bit listless in class. She stopped by his desk and asked, "Are you all right, Kevin? You seem a bit tired."

Kevin said, "I'm okay. I was in a hurry this morning so I missed breakfast."

Later, as she passed through the cafeteria, Ms. Booker couldn't help noticing that Kevin was eating food from a vending machine for lunch. They were sitting by themself at an isolated table.

Ms. Booker walked over, sat down, and asked, "Are you feeling better now?"

Kevin replied, "Yes, but I know I need to eat better."

Ms. Booker said, "Maybe you need to make a plan to eat better. Do you remember the SMART formula we learned in class? Maybe you could use the formula to set some goals." Kevin agreed that this was a good idea.

FOR DISCUSSION

How could Kevin use the SMART formula to set good nutrition goals? What might be some good long-term goals for them? What might be some good short-term goals? What kinds of advice do you think Ms. Booker gave Kevin about goal setting? What advice would you have for Kevin? Consider the guidelines in the following Self-Management feature as you answer these discussion questions.

SELF-MANAGEMENT: **Skills for Setting Goals**

Now that you know more about different types of goal setting, you can begin developing some goals of your own. Use the following guidelines to help you as you identify and develop your personal goals.

- *Know your reasons for setting your goals.* People who set goals for reasons other than their own personal improvement often fail. Ask yourself, *Why is this goal important to me?* Make sure you're setting goals based on your own needs and interests.

- *Choose a few goals at a time.* As you work your way through this book, you'll establish goals for fitness, physical activity, food choices, weight management, stress management, and other healthy lifestyle behaviors. But rather than focusing on all of them at once, you'll choose a few goals at a time. Trying to do too much often leads to failure.

- *Use the SMART formula.* The SMART formula helps you to set goals that are specific, measurable, attainable, realistic, and timely.

- *Set long-term and short-term goals.* The SMART formula helps you establish both long-term and short-term goals. When setting short-term goals, focus on process goals—that is, focus on making good lifestyle changes, not on results.

- *Put your goals in writing.* Writing down a goal represents a personal commitment and increases your chances of success. You'll get the opportunity to write down your goals as you do the activities in this book.

- *Self-assess and keep logs.* Doing self-assessments helps you set your goals and determine whether you've met them. Focus on improvement by working toward goals that are slightly beyond your current results.

- *Reward yourself.* Achieving a personal goal is rewarding. Allow yourself to feel good. Congratulate yourself for your accomplishment.

- *Revise if necessary.* If you find that a goal is too difficult to accomplish, don't be afraid to revise it. It's better to revise your goal than to quit.

- *Consider maintenance goals.* Improvement is not always necessary. Once you reach the highest level of change, setting a goal of maintenance can be a good idea. For example, an active, fit person cannot continue to improve in fitness forever, and following a regular workout schedule to maintain good fitness is a reasonable goal. Likewise, once you achieve the goal of eating well, maintaining your healthy eating pattern is a worthwhile goal.

Taking Action: **Exercise Circuits**

An exercise circuit consists of several stations, each of which features a different exercise. Typically, you move from one station to the next without resting. They also have the advantage of not requiring a lot of equipment, though you might enjoy bringing some music to listen to while working out. Exercise circuits are popular because the variety of exercises helps make the workout interesting. Circuits can be designed to focus on either health-related or skill-related fitness components, and they can be performed in a variety of places—indoors or outdoors, at home or elsewhere. **Take action** to create an exercise circuit using the following tips:

- Before starting the circuit, perform a dynamic warm-up.
- Plan stations that address all parts of your body: lower, middle, and upper.
- Avoid having two stations in a row that challenge the same body part.
- Pace yourself so that you can move continuously through the stations without stopping.
- Use correct technique at each station; if your technique fails due to fatigue, take a break.
- After doing the circuit, perform a cool-down.

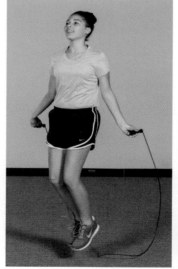
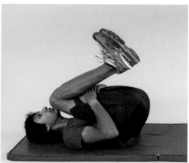

Exercise circuits use a variety of exercises at several stations.

CHAPTER REVIEW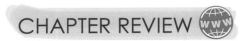

Reviewing Concepts and Vocabulary

Answer items 1 through 5 by correctly completing each sentence with a word or phrase.

1. The acronym used to remember the characteristics of effective goals is _____.

2. Deciding to exercise three days a week for two weeks is an example of a _____-term goal.

3. Deciding to walk 30 minutes a day for the next three months is an example of a _____-term goal.

4. Being able to run a mile in six minutes (a kilometer in four) is an example of a _____ goal.

5. Doing a behavior such as performing flexibility exercises three days a week is an example of a _____ goal.

For items 6 through 10, match each term in column 1 with the appropriate phrase in column 2.

6. step 1   a. set goals

7. step 2   b. consider program options

8. step 3   c. structure your program

9. step 4   d. determine your personal needs

10. step 5   e. evaluate your program

For items 11 through 15, respond to each statement or question.

11. What are some tests you can use to assess and rate your muscle fitness?

12. Describe the five rules for setting SMART goals.

13. Describe the five steps in program planning.

14. What are exercise circuits, and why are they useful for staying active?

15. What are some guidelines for using the self-management skill of goal setting?

Thinking Critically

Write a paragraph to answer the following question.

Why is it important to understand the concept of optimal challenge when setting goals? Provide an example.

Project

Imagine that you are hired as a health consultant to help clients make New Year's resolutions for eating better and being more active. Prepare a brief booklet that contains advice for making effective New Year's resolutions.

UNIT II

Safe and Smart Health-Enhancing Physical Activity

CHAPTER 4   Safe and Smart Physical Activity
CHAPTER 5   Social, Health, and Wellness Benefits of Physical Activity
CHAPTER 6   How Much Is Enough?

Healthy People 2030 Goals and Objectives

Overarching Goals
- Attain healthy, thriving lives and well-being, free of preventable disease, disability, injury, and premature death.
- Eliminate health disparities, achieve health equity, and attain health literacy to improve the health and well-being of all.

Objectives
- Promote healthy development, healthy behaviors, and well-being across all life stages.
- Reduce risk, incidence, and early death from chronic illness such as heart disease, stroke, cancer, diabetes, high blood pressure, osteoporosis, and back problems.
- Reduce unintentional injuries including brain injuries.
- Increase the proportion of schools that have policies and practices that promote health and safety.
- Increase the proportion of adolescents who have preventive health care visits.
- Reduce the proportion of people who do no physical activity in their free time.
- Increase the proportion of adolescents and adults who do enough aerobic and muscle building physical activity for health benefits.
- Increase the proportion of teens who play sports and walk or bike to get places.
- Increase the proportion of teens who limit screen time.
- Reduce the proportion of teens with obesity.

Self-Assessment Features in This Unit
- Body Composition and Flexibility
- Modifying Rules in Games
- PACER and Trunk Lift

Taking Charge and Self-Management Features in This Unit

- Overcoming Barriers
- Conflict Resolution
- Learning to Self-Monitor

Taking Action Features in This Unit

- Safe Exercise Circuit
- Team Building
- Physical Activity Pyramid Circuit

Safe and Smart Physical Activity

In This Chapter

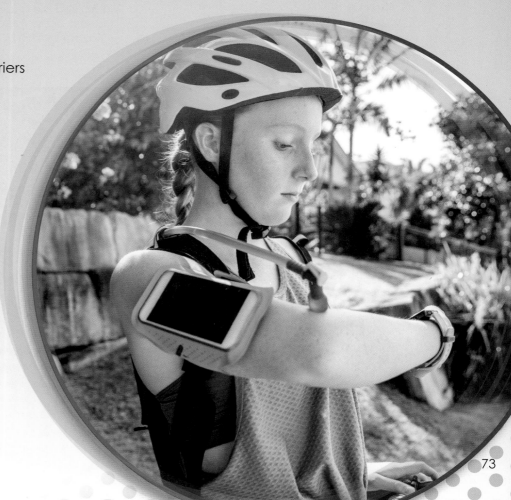

Readiness for Physical Activity

Lesson Objectives

After reading this lesson, you should be able to

1. describe medical readiness and explain how to assess it;

2. explain the dangers of performing physical activity in hot, humid conditions and describe some guidelines for avoiding these dangers;

3. explain the dangers of performing physical activity in cold, windy, wet conditions and describe some guidelines for avoiding these dangers;

4. explain the dangers of performing physical activity in polluted or high-altitude conditions and describe some guidelines for avoiding these dangers; and

5. describe some guidelines for dressing appropriately for physical activity.

Lesson Vocabulary

air quality index
electrolytes
graded exercise test
heat index
humidity
hyperthermia
hypothermia
Physical Activity Readiness
 Questionnaire for Everyone (PAR-Q+)
windchill factor

Are you prepared to be active? Whether you're a beginner or you've been physically active for some time, you need to know how to exercise safely in all conditions. If you're a beginner, the first step is to be physically and medically ready. As a young person, you probably won't have a problem with physical and medical readiness, but you should answer some simple questions just to be sure. You should also be ready for a variety of environmental conditions—such as heat, cold, pollution, and altitude—that could necessitate a change in your exercise habits. In this lesson, you'll learn how to prepare yourself for physical activity.

I didn't think much about the dangers of exercising in the heat until Sonja had to go to the emergency room for heatstroke after a long hike. It scared me and made me more aware of the need to take steps to stay safe when I exercise.

Zach Bender

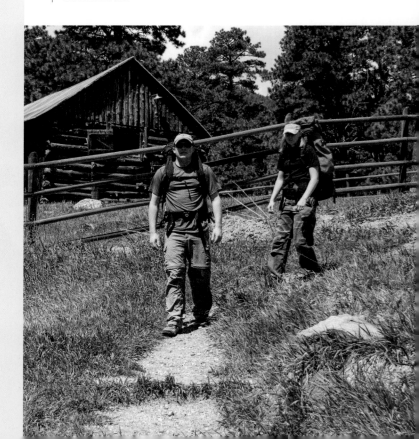

Medical Readiness

> An ounce of prevention is worth a pound of cure.
>
> *Benjamin Franklin, statesman and scientist*

Have you ever been injured during physical activity? Do you know how to prepare yourself for exercise in order to participate safely and avoid injury? Before you begin a regular physical activity program for health and wellness, you should assess your medical and physical readiness. For this purpose, experts have developed a seven-item questionnaire called the **Physical Activity Readiness Questionnaire for Everyone (PAR-Q+)**. If you answer yes to any of the questions, you are advised to seek medical consultation before beginning or continuing an exercise program. You should also consider any current health problems that might alter your plans for exercise, including short-term illnesses such as a cold or the flu. Those with chronic conditions such as asthma and diabetes should consult their doctor. You may want to encourage older adults who are important to you to answer the PAR-Q+ questions before they begin an exercise program, because older people are more likely to be at risk when doing exercise.

As for yourself, you may even be required to have a medical examination to participate in school sports or other community athletic programs. Medical exams help ensure that you are free from disease and can also help you prevent health problems in the future. You should also answer the questions included in the PAR-Q+.

Later in life, you may need to do a **graded exercise test** (sometimes called an *exercise stress test*), which is administered by a health professional (figure 4.1). The test is done on a treadmill and can help identify potential problems that may put a person at risk of a heart attack. It is an expensive test and is not necessary for everyone. Health professionals typically administer a physical exam and assess heart disease risk factors to determine when a graded exercise test is appropriate.

Readiness for Physical Activity in Different Environmental Conditions

Whether you are just beginning a physical activity program or have been exercising for a while, it is important to understand how environmental conditions can affect

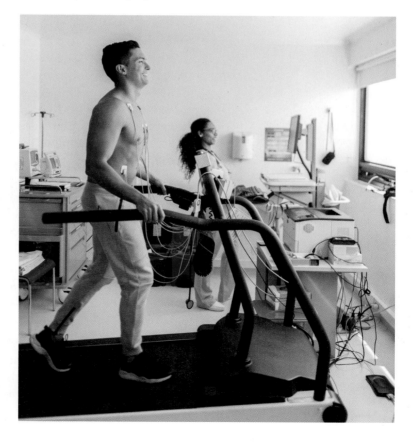

Figure 4.1 The treadmill graded exercise test can be used to screen adults with risk factors.

FIT FACT

Hyper means too much or excessive, and *thermia* refers to heat, so *hyperthermia* means too much heat. *Hypo* means too little or less than normal, so *hypothermia* means too little heat.

your body during exercise. With appropriate preparation you can be ready to safely navigate environmental factors such as heat, cold, wind, precipitation, air quality, and altitude that are discussed in the following sections.

Readiness for Hot and Humid Weather

Performing physical activity in high heat and **humidity** can cause your body temperature to rise too high—a situation referred to as **hyperthermia**, or overheating. When exercise causes your body temperature to rise, you start to perspire (sweat), which cools your body as it evaporates. But when the humidity is high, evaporation is less effective in cooling your body, and hyperthermia is more likely to occur. Hyperthermia causes three main conditions, which are described in table 4.1.

Use the following guidelines to prevent and cope with heat-related conditions.

TABLE 4.1   **Heat-Related Conditions**

Condition	Definition
Heat cramps	Muscle cramps caused by excessive heat exposure and low water consumption.
Heat exhaustion	Condition caused by excessive heat exposure and characterized by paleness, clammy skin, profuse sweating, weakness, tiredness, nausea, dizziness, muscle cramps, and possibly vomiting or fainting. Body temperature may be normal or slightly above normal.
Heatstroke	Condition caused by excessive heat exposure and characterized by high body temperature up to 106 °F (41 °C); hot, dry, flushed skin; rapid pulse; lack of sweating; dizziness; and possibly unconsciousness. This serious condition can result in death and requires prompt medical attention.

- *Begin gradually.* As your body becomes accustomed to physical activity in hot weather, it becomes more resistant to heat-related injury. Start with short periods of activity and gradually increase the duration.

- *Drink water.* In hot weather, your body perspires more than usual to cool itself. In order to replace the water your body loses through perspiration, you need to drink plenty of water before, during, and after activity. The recommended water consumption for teens is two or more quarts per day, or 8 to 10 eight-ounce glasses. Active teens should consume extra fluid to replace water lost in sweat.

- *Wear proper clothing.* Wear breathable and moisture-wicking fabric that allows air to pass through and keeps you cool. Choose light-colored clothing—lighter colors reflect the sun's heat, whereas darker colors absorb it.

- *Rest frequently.* Physical activity creates body heat. Periodically stop to rest in a shady area to help your body lower its temperature.

- *Avoid extreme heat and humidity.* The heat index chart (shown in figure 4.2) uses the temperature and the humidity to determine whether the environment is safe for activity. If the **heat index** is too high, you should postpone

Heat index
As humidity increases, air can feel hotter than it actually is.
This chart shows how hot it feels as humidity rises.

Relative humidity (%)	70	75	80	85	90	95	100	105	110	115	120
100	72	80	91	108	132						
90	71	79	88	102	122						
80	71	78	86	97	113	136					
70	70	77	85	93	106	124	144				
60	70	76	82	90	100	114	132	149			
50	69	75	81	88	96	107	120	135	150		
40	68	74	79	86	93	101	110	123	137	151	
30	67	73	78	84	90	96	104	113	123	135	148
20	66	72	77	82	87	93	99	105	112	120	130
10	65	70	75	80	85	90	95	100	105	111	116
0	64	69	73	78	83	87	91	95	99	103	107

Air temperature (°F)

☐ Caution zone
■ Danger zone

Figure 4.2 Heat index chart.

or cancel your activity. Perform physical activity in the caution zone only if you are well adapted to hot environments and follow all of the basic guidelines. The amount of time it takes to adapt to these conditions varies from person to person.

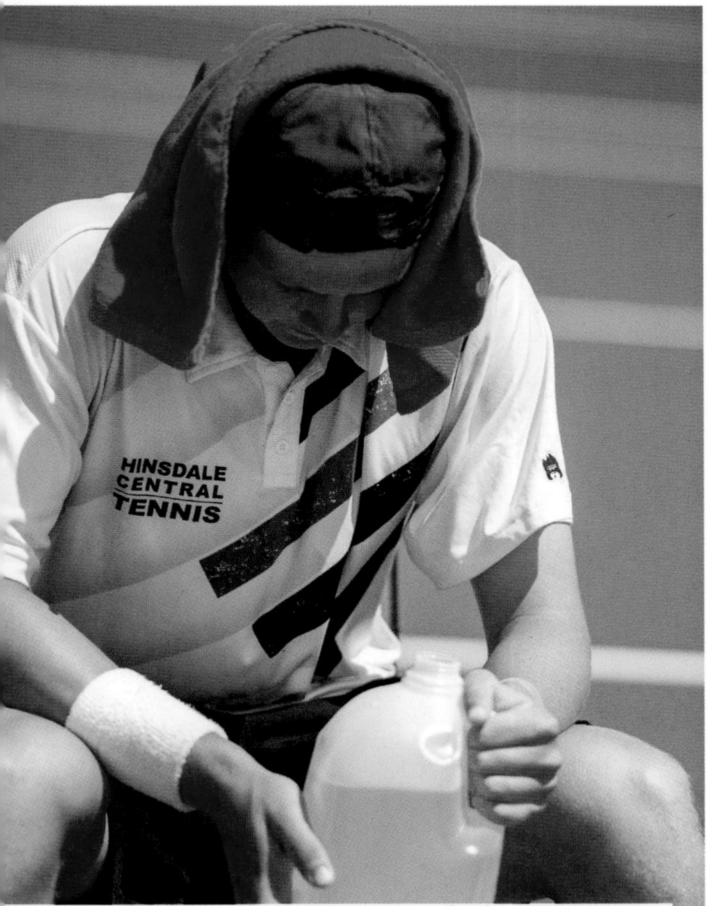

- *Monitor weather conditions.* Conditions can change rapidly, so it is important to keep track of heat and humidity during an exercise session.
- *If heat-related injury occurs, get out of the heat and cool your body.* Find shade; apply cool, wet towels to your body; spray your body with water; drink water; and seek medical help if heatstroke occurs.

Readiness for Cold, Windy, and Wet Weather

Heat and humidity are two conditions that can affect safety and performance in physical activity. It can also be dangerous to exercise in cold, windy, and wet weather. Extreme cold can result in **hypothermia**, or excessively low body temperature. Hypothermia is accompanied by shivering, numbness, drowsiness, muscular weakness, and confusion or disorientation. Extreme cold can also cause a condition called *frostbite*, in which a body part becomes frozen. A person with frostbite often feels no pain, thus making the condition even more dangerous. Use the following guidelines when exercising in cold, windy, and wet weather.

When you exercise in hot weather, wear light-colored clothing and drink plenty of water to help cool your body.

SCIENCE IN ACTION: **Sport and Energy Drinks**

Regardless of the weather, you need to keep your body hydrated during exercise to prevent conditions such as heat exhaustion and heatstroke. To replenish the body, researchers have developed flavored sport drinks that contain important minerals called **electrolytes**. When appropriate ingredients are used, these drinks can help adults keep their body hydrated during exercise. Energy drinks are also popular, but they are not intended primarily to replace fluids lost during exercise. They may contain ingredients similar to those in sport drinks, but they often also contain large amounts of sugar and relatively large amounts of caffeine.

The American Academy of Pediatrics (AAP) has expressed concern about sport and energy drinks because they are often marketed to children and teens via TV, magazines, and the Internet. The AAP discourages use of these drinks by children and teens and notes that high-caffeine energy drinks have "no place in the diet of children and adolescents." The group further states that sugars in these drinks may be linked to increases in weight and even obesity. The AAP indicate that sport drinks (not energy drinks with caffeine) can be helpful to young athletes who are engaged in "prolonged, vigorous physical activity, but in most cases they are unnecessary on the sport field or in the school lunch room." For most teens who perform the amount of activity recommended by national guidelines, plain water is best.

A separate group of medical doctors has asked the U.S. Food and Drug Administration (FDA) to restrict the amount of caffeine in energy drinks to protect youth from medical problems. Indeed, each year more than 20,000 ER visits involve health problems in which energy drink consumption was a contributing factor. Common problems caused by too much caffeine include fast heart rate, inability to sleep, stomach upset, anxiety, and headache. The FDA has issued warnings indicating that mixing alcohol and caffeine is especially dangerous.

STUDENT ACTIVITY

Research a sport or energy drink. Find out its key ingredients and prepare a report about the possible benefits and dangers associated with the drink.

- *Avoid extreme cold and wind.* Exercising when the temperature is cold and the wind is blowing is especially dangerous because the air feels colder. Before dressing for physical activity, use the chart in figure 4.3 to determine the **windchill factor**. This chart shows how long it takes to get frostbite when your skin is exposed to various windchill levels. Experts agree that if the time to frostbite is 30 minutes or less, you should postpone activity. If you're active when the windchill factor is excessive, be sure to dress properly and be aware of the symptoms of frostbite:

  - Skin becomes white or grayish yellow and looks glossy.

  - Pain may be felt early and then subside, though often feeling is lost and no pain is felt.

- Blisters may appear later.

- The affected area feels intensely cold and numb

- *Dress properly.* Wear a hat with ear flaps or a knit cap. If possible, wear mittens (which keep hands warmer than gloves do). Consider a ski mask to cover the face in extreme conditions. Wear several layers of lightweight clothing rather than a heavy jacket or coat. Wearing layers allows you to make adjustments—you can take off or add a layer as necessary. The clothing closest to your body (base layer) should be moisture wicking to keep you warm and dry. Silk and synthetic fibers such as Polartec are good for this layer; cotton is not recommended. The second layer (insulating layer) helps retain body heat but should also wick away moisture.

Temperature (°F)

Wind (mph)	30	25	20	15	10	5	0	−5	−10	−15	−20	−25
5	25	19	13	7	1	−5	−11	−16	−22	−28	−34	−40
10	21	15	9	3	−4	−10	−16	−22	−28	−35	−41	−47
15	19	13	6	0	−7	−13	−19	−26	−32	−39	−45	−51
20	17	11	4	−2	−9	−15	−22	−29	−35	−42	−48	−55
25	16	9	3	−4	−11	−17	−24	−31	−37	−44	−51	−58
30	15	8	1	−5	−12	−19	−26	−33	−39	−46	−53	−60
35	14	7	0	−7	−14	−21	−27	−34	−41	−48	−55	−62
40	13	6	−1	−8	−15	−22	−29	−36	−43	−50	−57	−64
45	12	5	−2	−9	−16	−23	−30	−37	−44	−51	−58	−65
50	12	4	−3	−10	−17	−24	−31	−38	−45	−52	−60	−67
55	11	4	−3	−11	−18	−25	−32	−39	−46	−54	−61	−68
60	10	3	−4	−11	−19	−26	−33	−40	−48	−55	−62	−69

Frostbite occurs in 30 minutes or less

Figure 4.3   Windchill chart.

Polyester fleece and wool are good for this layer. The outer layer should protect you against wind, rain, and snow but also allow heat and moisture to be released. For this reason, jackets made of breathable synthetic fibers (for example, Gore-Tex) are recommended; plastic, rubber, or other materials that do not "breathe" are not. Wearing a jacket with a zipper allows you to retain and release heat as needed. Wear a high collar on one of the inner layers.

• *Avoid exercising in weather that is icy or wet.* These conditions can cause special problems. Your shoes, socks, and pant legs can get wet, which increases your risk of foot injuries and falls.

Pollution and Altitude

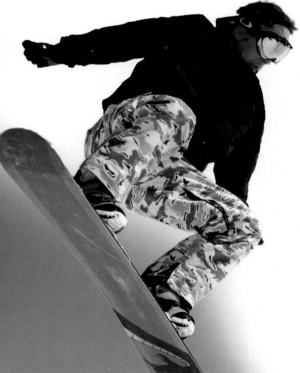

The effectiveness and safety of exercise can also be affected by environmental conditions other than weather, such as air pollution and altitude. Experts have identified levels of pollution (ozone and particulate matter) that are unhealthy and can affect your ability to breathe. Pollution levels are rated by means of an **air quality index** that ranges from good to hazardous. When the air pollution level is high, you can find warnings on radio, television, and reliable websites. During such times, avoid exercising outdoors.

People who live at high altitude are usually able to exercise there with little trouble, but people who live at lower altitude may have trouble adjusting to being active at higher altitude, even if they are very fit. If you exercise at a higher altitude than you are used to (for example, if you go skiing), adjust the intensity of your physical activity until your body adapts.

FIT FACT
A popular myth suggests that not covering your head in cold weather results in 40 to 80 percent of the heat loss from the body. In fact, heat lost from the head is similar to the heat loss from any other body part of similar surface area (about 10 percent). Still, the head is often the most exposed part of the body and it is important for it to be covered in cold, windy, and wet weather.

CONSUMER CORNER: Dressing for Physical Activity

As you've seen, special environmental circumstances—such as intense heat and cold—require special dress for physical activity. But even under normal circumstances, the way you dress has a lot to do with your comfort and enjoyment. Consider the following general guidelines when dressing for physical activity.

- *Wear comfortable and appropriate clothing for the environmental conditions.* Guidelines for dressing for cold and hot weather were presented earlier. In addition to following these guidelines, wearing comfortable clothing will make your workout more enjoyable.

- *Wash exercise clothing regularly.* Clean clothing is more comfortable than soiled clothing, and it reduces the chance of fungal growth and infection.

- *Dress in layers when exercising outdoors.* You can remove layers of clothing as you become warmer while exercising and put them back on when you cool down.

- *Wear proper socks.* Moisture-wicking fabrics are now frequently used in making socks and other apparel. Socks made with these fabrics reduce foot moisture and can help prevent blisters. Thick socks made of cotton or another traditional fabric can help cushion your feet but are not as effective at keeping them dry.

- *Wear proper shoes.* Most people can use a good pair of multipurpose exercise or sport shoes for physical activity. However, if you plan to do certain activities, you might prefer specialized shoes. Before buying shoes, try them on (while wearing the kind of socks you will wear for the activity) and walk around to see how the shoes feel. They should not feel too heavy, because extra weight makes exercise more tiring. Avoid vinyl or plastic shoes that do not let air pass through to help cool your feet. As an alternative to cloth and leather shoes (which do allow some air passage), shoes made from moisture-wicking fabric have proven effective in keeping feet dry. Before buying shoes, consider the features shown in figure 4.4.

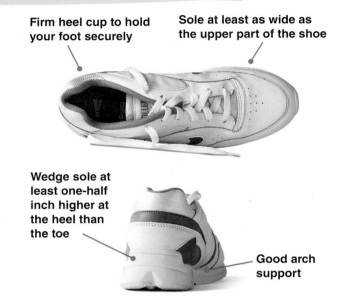

Firm heel cup to hold your foot securely

Sole at least as wide as the upper part of the shoe

Wedge sole at least one-half inch higher at the heel than the toe

Good arch support

Figure 4.4   Characteristics of proper shoes.

- *Consider protective equipment.* Various types of protective equipment can be used to prevent injury in physical activity. More information on injury prevention is presented in lesson 4.2.

- *Consider clothing made from high-tech fabrics.* Modern technology has produced clothing that is good for exercising in both hot and cold weather. As noted in the

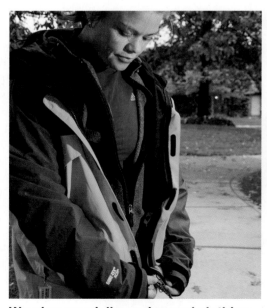

Wearing specially engineered clothing can help you when you exercise in the heat or cold.

guidelines for exercising in hot or cold environments, clothing made of special synthetic fibers can wick moisture away from the body to help it stay cool (e.g., Coolmax) or warm (e.g., Polartec). Breathable synthetic material such as Gore-Tex blocks the wind but allows body heat to be released, making it an ideal outer layer in cold weather. These synthetic fibers are engineered to function in different ways.

CONSUMER ACTIVITY

Research one type of synthetic fiber used in making exercise clothing in hot or cold environments. What are the special characteristics of the fiber you selected?

LESSON REVIEW

1. What are some steps you can take to make sure you're medically ready to participate in physical activity and sports?
2. What are some of the dangers of performing physical activity in hot, humid environments and in cold, windy, wet conditions, and what are some guidelines for avoiding these dangers?
3. What are some of the dangers of performing physical activity in cold, windy, wet conditions, and what are some guidelines for avoiding these dangers?
4. What are some of the dangers of performing physical activity in polluted or high-altitude conditions, and what are some guidelines for avoiding these dangers?
5. What are some ways that you can dress properly for physical activity?

SELF-ASSESSMENT: **Body Composition and Flexibility**

In this activity, you'll perform two self-assessments: the back-saver sit-and-reach and the body mass index (BMI). These are two self-assessments commonly included in FitnessGram.

BACK-SAVER SIT-AND-REACH (flexibility of the hip)

1. Place a yardstick or meter stick on top of a box that is 12 inches (30 centimeters) high, with the stick extending 9 inches (23 centimeters) over the box and the lower numbers toward you. You may also use a flexibility testing box if one is available.

2. To measure the flexibility of your right leg, fully extend it and place your right foot flat against the box. Bend your left leg, with the knee turned out and your left foot 2 to 3 inches (5 to 8 centimeters) to the side of your straight right leg.

3. Extend your arms forward over the measuring stick. Place your hands on the stick, one on top of the other, with your palms facing down. Your middle fingers should be together with the tip of one finger exactly on top of the other.

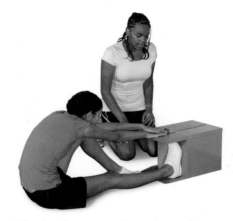

The back-saver sit-and-reach assesses flexibility.

4. Lean forward slowly; do not bounce. Reach forward, then slowly return to the starting position. Repeat four times. On the fourth reach, hold the position for three seconds and observe the measurement on the stick below your fingertips.

5. Repeat the test with your left leg.

6. Record your score to the nearest inch (1 inch equals 2.54 centimeters). Consult table 4.2 to determine your fitness rating for each side of your body.

TABLE 4.2   Rating Chart: Back-Saver Sit-and-Reach (Inches)

	13 or 14 years old		15 years or older	
	Male	**Female**	**Male**	**Female**
High performance	≥10	≥12	≥10	≥14
Good fitness	8–9	10–11	8–9	12–13
Marginal fitness	6–7	8–9	6–7	10–11
Low fitness	≤5	≤7	≤5	≤9

To convert centimeters to inches, divide by 2.54.

Data based on *FitnessGram*.

BODY MASS INDEX

The BMI uses height and weight as an indicator of body composition. However, BMI is not a definitive tool for assessing body composition; it is simply a method of screening to see if you need further testing. For example, the BMI does not take muscle mass into account, so muscular people may receive a score suggesting that they are not in the good fitness zone when they really are. The FitnessGram advisors suggest that students who have scores that are not in the good fitness zone consider follow-up testing (see chapter 14).

1. Measure your height in inches (or meters) without shoes.

2. Measure your weight in pounds (or kilograms) without shoes. If you're wearing street clothes (as opposed to lightweight gym clothing), subtract two pounds (0.9 kilogram) from your weight.

3. Calculate your BMI using figure 4.5 or either of the following formulas.

$$\frac{weight\ (lb)}{height\ (in.) \times height\ (in.)} \times 703 = BMI \qquad \frac{weight\ (kg)}{height\ (m) \times height\ (m)} = BMI$$

4. Use table 4.3 to find your BMI rating. Record your BMI score and rating.

TABLE 4.3   Rating Chart: Body Mass Index

	13 years old		14 years old		15 years old		16 years old		17 years old		18 years old	
	Male	**Female**	**Male**	**Female**	**Male**	**Female**	**Male**	**Female**	**Male**	**Female**	**Male**	**Female**
Very lean	≤15.4	≤15.3	≤16.0	≤15.8	≤16.5	≤16.3	≤17.1	≤16.8	≤17.7	≤17.2	≤18.2	≤17.5
Good fitness	15.5–21.3	15.4–22.0	16.1–22.1	15.9–22.8	16.6–22.9	16.4–23.5	17.2–23.7	16.9–24.1	17.8–24.4	17.3–24.6	18.3–25.1	17.6–25.1
Marginal fitness	21.4–23.5	22.1–23.7	22.2–24.4	22.9–24.5	23.0–25.2	23.6–25.3	23.8–25.9	24.2–26.0	24.5–26.6	24.7–27.6	25.2–27.4	25.2–27.1
Low fitness	≥23.6	≥23.8	≥24.5	≥24.6	≥25.3	≥25.4	≥26.0	≥26.1	≥26.7	≥27.7	≥27.5	≥27.2

Data based on *FitnessGram*.

Height

	90	95	100	105	110	115	120	125	130	135	140	145	150	155	160	165	170	175	180	185	190	195	200	205	210	215	220	225	230	235	240	245	250
4'6"	25	25	26	26	27	28	29	30	31	32	34	35	36	37	39	40	41	42	43	45	46	47	48	49	51	52	53	54	56	57	58	59	60
4'7"	24	24	25	25	26	27	28	29	30	31	32	34	35	36	37	38	39	40	41	43	45	46	47	48	49	50	51	52	54	55	56	57	58
4'8"	23	23	24	24	25	26	27	28	29	30	31	32	34	35	36	37	38	39	40	42	43	44	45	46	47	48	49	50	52	53	54	55	56
4'9"	22	22	23	23	24	25	26	27	28	29	30	31	32	34	35	36	37	38	39	40	42	42	43	44	45	47	48	49	50	51	52	53	54
4'10"	21	22	22	23	23	24	25	26	27	28	29	30	31	32	34	35	36	37	38	39	40	41	42	43	44	45	46	47	48	49	50	51	52
4'11"	20	21	21	22	22	23	24	25	26	27	28	29	30	31	32	33	34	35	36	37	38	39	40	41	42	43	45	46	46	47	48	49	50
5'0"	19	20	20	21	21	22	23	24	25	26	27	28	29	30	31	32	33	34	35	36	37	38	39	40	41	42	43	44	45	46	47	48	49
5'1"	18	19	19	20	21	22	23	24	25	26	26	27	28	29	30	31	32	33	34	35	36	37	38	39	40	41	42	43	43	44	45	46	47
5'2"	18	18	18	19	20	21	22	23	24	25	26	27	27	28	29	30	31	32	33	34	35	36	37	37	38	39	40	41	42	43	44	45	46
5'3"	17	18	18	19	19	20	21	22	23	24	25	26	27	27	28	29	30	31	32	33	34	35	35	36	37	38	39	40	41	42	43	43	44
5'4"	17	17	17	18	19	20	21	21	22	23	24	25	26	27	27	28	29	30	31	32	33	33	34	35	36	37	38	39	39	40	41	42	43
5'5"	16	17	17	17	18	19	20	21	22	22	23	24	25	26	27	27	28	29	30	31	32	32	33	34	35	36	37	37	38	39	40	41	42
5'6"	15	16	16	17	18	19	19	20	21	22	23	23	24	25	26	27	27	28	29	30	31	31	32	33	34	35	36	36	37	38	39	40	40
5'7"	15	15	16	16	17	18	19	20	20	21	22	23	23	24	25	26	27	27	28	29	30	31	31	32	33	34	34	35	36	37	38	38	39
5'8"	14	15	15	16	17	17	18	19	20	21	21	22	23	24	24	25	26	27	27	28	29	30	30	31	32	33	33	34	35	36	36	37	38
5'9"	14	15	15	15	16	17	18	18	19	20	21	21	22	23	24	24	25	26	27	27	28	29	30	30	31	32	32	33	34	35	35	36	37
5'10"	13	14	14	15	16	17	17	18	19	19	20	21	22	22	23	24	24	25	26	27	27	28	29	29	30	31	32	32	33	34	34	35	36
5'11"	13	14	14	15	15	16	17	17	18	19	20	20	21	22	22	23	24	24	25	26	26	27	28	29	29	30	31	31	32	33	33	34	35
6'0"	13	13	14	14	15	16	16	17	18	18	19	20	20	21	22	22	23	24	24	25	26	26	27	28	28	29	30	31	31	32	33	33	34
6'1"	12	13	13	14	15	15	16	16	17	18	18	19	20	20	21	22	22	23	24	24	25	26	26	27	28	28	29	30	30	31	32	32	33
6'2"	12	12	13	13	14	15	15	16	17	17	18	19	19	20	21	21	22	22	23	24	24	25	26	26	27	28	28	29	30	30	31	31	32
6'3"	11	12	12	13	14	14	15	15	16	17	17	18	19	19	20	21	21	22	22	23	24	24	25	26	26	27	27	28	29	29	30	31	31
6'4"	11	12	12	13	13	14	15	15	16	16	17	18	18	19	20	20	21	21	22	23	23	24	24	25	26	26	27	27	28	29	29	30	30

Weight

Figure 4.5   BMI calculation table. Locate your height in the left column and your weight in pounds in the bottom row. The box where the selected row and column intersect is your BMI score.

ACADEMIC CONNECTION: Metrics and the U.S. Measurement System

The metric system is a measurement system that uses units of measurement (e.g., meters, kilograms) that are related by factors of 10—for example, 1,000 milligrams equals one gram, 1,000 grams equals one kilogram, and so on. The United States is the only industrialized country in the world that does not use this system for making typical daily measurements. In the United States, the U.S. Customary System is used. It uses units such as yards, pounds, and miles. There is no consistent factor for converting one type of unit to another (for example, ounces to pounds). Although Americans do not use metrics for common measurements, metrics are used by scientists, for track and field and swimming events (e.g., 100-meter dash), and by devices such as dynamometers for measuring strength and calipers for measuring body composition. Some formulas are based on the metric system (e.g., body mass index). For these reasons, it is useful to know how to convert units of measure from one system to another.

STUDENT ACTIVITY

It is now easy to make conversions using calculators available on the web (search metric conversion calculator). It is interesting that an effort was made in the 1970s and 1980s to adopt the metric system in the United States, but it was abandoned when most Americans failed to endorse the change. Comment on why you think the effort to convert to metrics failed and if you think that the United States should try again.

Safe and Injury-Free Physical Activity

Lesson Objectives

After reading this lesson, you should be able to

1. list and describe some common activity-related physical injuries;

2. list some guidelines for preventing injury during physical activity;

3. explain how to apply the RICE formula for caring for physical injuries; and

4. identify risky exercises and explain why they are risky.

Lesson Vocabulary

biomechanical principles
extension
flexion
ligament
microtrauma
overuse injury
RICE
side stitch
sprain
strain
tendon

Would you know what to do if you sprained your ankle? If you were performing a risky yoga pose, would you know it? Physical activity provides many benefits for your health and wellness, but it also carries a risk of injury if performed improperly. Fortunately, most injuries are minor and can be prevented by being careful.

In the previous lesson, you learned preparations and guidelines for exercising safely. In this lesson, you'll learn about some common minor injuries, as well as some basic precautions you can take to avoid them. You'll also learn about some exercises that are considered too risky and about safer alternatives that you can use.

Common Activity-Related Injuries

If you've ever suffered a sport or exercise injury, you may already know that an injury can be quite painful even if it's not serious. Some of the more common minor injuries related to sport and exercise are sprains, strains, blisters,

When I woke up in the hospital, I had a concussion. I was riding my bike wearing a helmet. I was in the bike lane waiting for the light to change. The long arm mirror on the bus hit me in the back of the head. The doctors say it would have been much worse if I hadn't been wearing a helmet.

Jade Lee

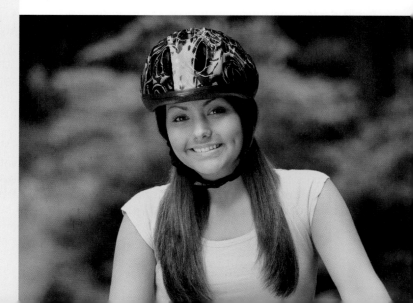

bruises, cuts, and scrapes. More serious and less common injuries include joint dislocation and bone fracture. The body parts injured most commonly in physical activity are the skin, feet, ankles, knees, and leg muscles (see figure 4.6). Parts less likely to be injured are the head, arms, trunk, and internal organs, such as the liver and kidneys.

Common Minor Injuries

One type of injury, called an **overuse injury**, occurs when you repeat a movement so much that your body suffers wear and tear. You're most likely familiar with one very common overuse injury—a blister. Another example is shin splints, which involves soreness in the front of the lower leg, likely caused by small muscle tears or spasms resulting from overuse. Runner's heel also involves soreness and is especially common among long-distance runners and other people whose activities involve the heel repeatedly hitting the ground.

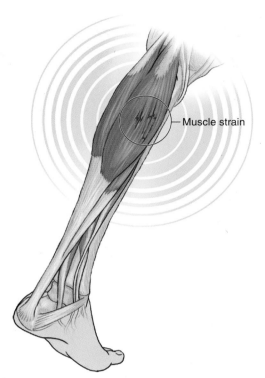

Figure 4.6   Muscle strains are a common injury in sport and physical activity.

A **side stitch** is a pain in the side of the lower abdomen that people often experience with exertion. Its cause is not known, but one theory is a spasm in the diaphragm (the muscle tissue involved in breathing). Side stitches are most common among people who are not accustomed to vigorous activity. To help relieve a side stitch, press firmly at the point of the pain with your hand while bending forward or backward. Luckily, a side stitch is not really an injury and will go away if you stop the activity or continue at a more moderate pace.

Another type of injury is called **microtrauma**. *Micro* means small—so small it may not show up on an X-ray or exam—and *trauma* is another word for injury. This injury often causes no immediate pain, but with repeated use, symptoms of the damage eventually appear. Many adults today experience back problems, neck aches, and stiff or painful joints caused by microtrauma suffered when they were younger. Some risky exercises that can cause microtrauma are discussed later in this chapter.

Concussions

Although head injuries are not as common as some of the minor injuries discussed previously, they can have serious short- and long-term effects. One serious head injury is concussion, which occurs when a blow to the head causes the brain to crash into the bones of the skull. Concussions can range from mild to severe. A mild concussion may result in dizziness and confusion. A more severe concussion can cause you to pass out; it can also result in temporary or long-term loss of functions such as speaking or moving your muscles. Although many concussions are not severe, experts caution that all head injuries should be treated as serious

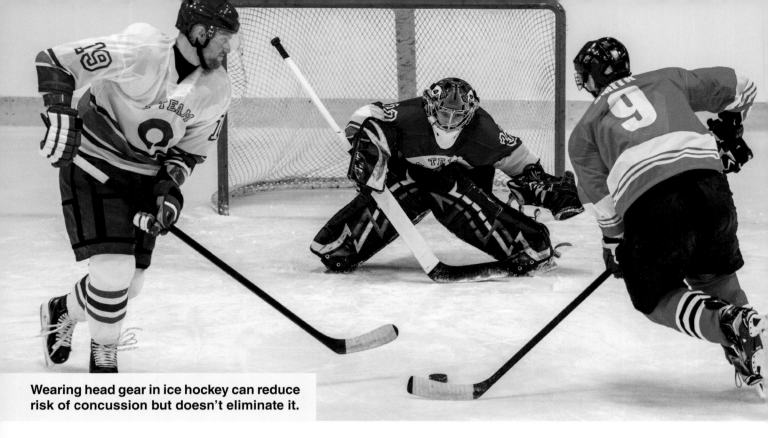

Wearing head gear in ice hockey can reduce risk of concussion but doesn't eliminate it.

until medical screening indicates otherwise. Experts also indicate that having one concussion increases the risk of having another.

Concussions are more prevalent in collision sports such as hockey and football, but they also occur in other sports. They can result from head-to-head contact in football and soccer, head-to-ball contact in soccer, and falls and blows to the head in basketball. Repeated concussions increase the risk of suffering permanent brain damage; repeated blows or jolts to the head can also cause cumulative damage even when a concussion is not present. Sports medicine experts have developed guidelines for preventing concussions and for allowing athletes to return to action after a concussion. For more information, search the websites of the American College of Sports Medicine (ACSM), the National Athletic Trainers Association, and the Centers for Disease Control and Prevention (CDC) HEADS UP Resource Center. See figure 4.7 for the signs and symptoms of concussion.

Preventing Injury

Your body is made up of more than 200 bones, which connect at joints. Different kinds of joints allow different types of movement. For example, synovial joints allow free movement; they include hinge joints (such as your knees and elbows) that allow only **flexion** and **extension**, as well as ball and socket joints (such as your hips and shoulders) that allow movements such as rotation. Cartilaginous joints (such as the vertebrae in your back) allow only limited movement. Fibrous joints are referred to as *immoveable* or *fixed*; examples are the joints where the bones of your skull connect.

When your muscles contract, they pull your tendons and make your bones move. Your bones act as levers to allow body movement. For example, contracting the muscles at the top of your upper arms (your biceps) provides force that pulls on the tendons connecting to the bones (levers) of your lower arms, thus causing your elbows (hinge joints) to bend, as shown in figure 4.8. When used

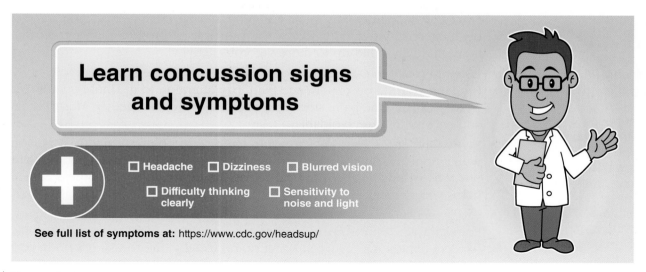

Figure 4.7 The signs and symptoms of concussion.

properly, the levers of your body help you move efficiently, but when used incorrectly, they can produce forces that cause injury to a joint or other body part.

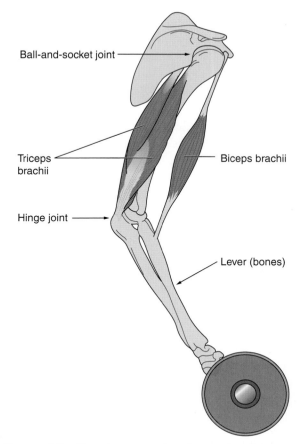

Figure 4.8 Your bones act as levers to allow body movement.

Different types of injury can affect different types of tissue. An injury to a **ligament** is called a **sprain**. As illustrated in figure 4.9, ligaments are tough tissues that hold your bones together. A sprain typically results in swelling and pain around a joint. The other types of tissue you see in the figure are muscles, bones, and **tendons** (which connect muscles to bones). A **strain**, sometimes called a *pulled muscle*, is an injury to tendon or muscle resulting from tears in the tissues. Like sprains, strains often result in pain and swelling.

Experts in sports medicine have developed the following guidelines to help prevent sports-related injury.

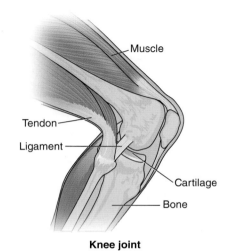

Knee joint

Figure 4.9 These tissues are commonly injured.

- *Start slowly.* Injuries are more common among beginners. If you haven't been exercising regularly, follow the principle of progression: start slowly, then gradually build up to more vigorous activity.

- *Listen to your body.* Injury can occur when you ignore signs that your body is giving you. If you experience pain, pay attention to it. Until you address what is causing the pain, slow your exercise or stop altogether. Most blisters and shin splints are avoidable.

- *Be fit!* One of the best ways to avoid injury is to be physically fit. A person with a fit heart and lungs and strong muscles is less likely to be injured than one who is unfit. Proper physical activity builds total physical fitness, which helps you prevent injury.

- *Use moderation.* Overuse causes many minor injuries in physical activity. For example, about 40 percent of regular runners and 50 percent of aerobic dancers experience injury at some point, usually due to using a body part too intensely or for too long a time.

- *Dress properly.* Some injuries are caused by improper dress—for example, wearing poor shoes and socks can cause blisters or runner's heel. Make sure you dress properly following the guidelines from the previous lesson.

- *Avoid risky exercises.* Injury can be caused by certain exercises that violate the rules of biomechanics (see the discussion of risky exercises later in this lesson).

- *Wear safety equipment when appropriate.* Proper head gear is important for collision sports such as hockey and football and for high-speed activities such as biking and skateboarding. Hand, elbow, and knee guards also help prevent injuries in skateboarding. Lace-up ankle braces can help prevent ankle injuries during activities that involve quick changes in direction such as basketball and racquetball, especially among those who have a history of these injuries (some also prefer high-top shoes).

- *Learn proper sports techniques.* Performing sports skills properly can help prevent injuries. For example, proper tackling techniques are useful in preventing concussions.

Simple Care for Minor Injuries

When injury occurs, it is often necessary to seek medical help. However, you can take immediate steps to reduce pain and prevent complications if you know basic first aid. For muscle strains, sprains, and bruises, which are common in sport and other activities, you can follow the **RICE** formula. Each letter in the formula represents a step taken to treat a minor injury:

- *R is for rest.* After first aid has been given, the injured body part should be immobilized for two or three days to prevent further injury. The length of rest depends on the severity of the injury and the response to treatment.

- *I is for ice.* A body part that has been sprained or strained should be immersed in cold water or covered with ice that is wrapped in a towel or placed in a plastic bag. Icing for 20 minutes immediately after injury helps reduce swelling and pain. Apply ice or cold several times a day for one to three days. To relieve the pain of shin splints, apply the ice bag and towel to the front of your leg until the pain subsides (no longer than 20 minutes at a time).

• *C is for compression.* Use an elastic bandage to wrap the injured area in order to help limit swelling. For a sprained ankle, keep the shoe laced and the sock on the foot until compression can be applied with a bandage (the shoe and sock compress the injury). To avoid restricting blood flow, remove the bandage for a few minutes or loosen it if you feel throbbing or it feels too tight.

• *E is for elevation.* Raise the injured body part above the level of your heart to help reduce swelling.

Risky Exercises

Some exercises are considered *risky* because they cause your body to move in ways that violate basic **biomechanical principles**. As you know, biomechanics is a branch of kinesiology that studies the human machine in motion. Biomechanical principles are rules that help you move efficiently and avoid injury.

Applying Biomechanical Principles

Understanding and applying biomechanical principles can also help you avoid risky exercises. Risky exercises can result in pain, joint problems, excessive wear of joint cartilage, and wear-and-tear injuries such as inflammation of tendons and bursas (cushioning tissues in your joints). They may not cause immediate injury and pain, but over time, microtrauma caused by risky exercise can result in arthritis or back and neck pain—a leading medical complaint in the United States.

Several biomechanical principles that help you avoid risky exercises are listed here. In the next section, examples of exercises that violate these principles and safer alternatives are provided.

• *Principle 1: Movements that overstretch ligaments can reduce joint stability.* Ligaments connect bones and keep your joints stable. If overstretched, ligaments become less effective in supporting and protecting joints.

• *Principle 2: Movements that force your joints to move in unnatural ways or that twist them can cause trauma or microtrauma to joints.* Twisting results in forces that can damage tissues of the joints (e.g., ligaments, cartilage).

• *Principle 3: Movements that use your body's levers improperly can result in trauma or microtrauma to joints and body tissues.* Your bones serve as levers that produce movement when your muscles contract. Some exercises use the levers in ways that put the joints and tissues at risk.

If any exercise causes you pain, even if not listed here, stop doing it. If pain persists, seek medical help.

Hyperflexion Exercises to Avoid

Hyper means too much, and *flexion* refers to bending at the joint. Hyperflexion exercises violate principle 1 because they bend your joints too far and may overstretch your ligaments. For example, the shoulder stand (figure 4.10) causes hyperflexion to the neck (safer substitute: plank). The similar yoga plow (safer substitute: back and hip stretch) and the bicycle exercise (safer substitute: leg change) also cause neck hyperflexion. Another example is the full squat, which studies show can be done without injury with proper technique and adequate supervision; however, most people can get the benefits they need by performing

FIT FACT
People who are just beginning a physical activity program sometimes get a type of soreness called *delayed onset muscle soreness* (DOMS), which is caused by microscopic muscle tears. This soreness occurs 24 to 48 hours after a vigorous workout. Unlike microtrauma, these tears do not cause permanent damage. To avoid DOMS, progress gradually when you begin an exercise program. It is okay to continue to exercise when you're sore, but if pain persists or is sharp rather than general in nature, stop exercising and seek medical advice.

The more injuries you get, the smarter you get.

Mikhail Baryshnikov, professional dancer

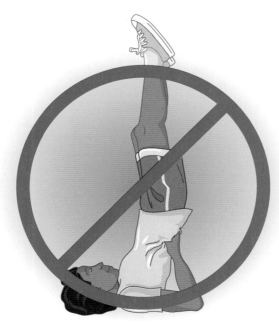

Figure 4.10 Avoid hyperflexion exercises, such as shoulder stand.

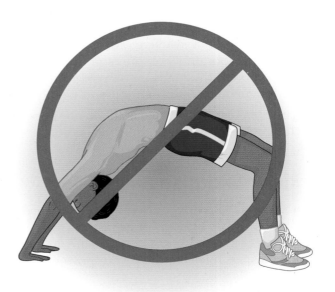

Figure 4.11 Avoid hyperextension exercises, such as back bends.

the half squat, which does not cause knee hyperflexion. Other hyperflexion exercises to avoid include duckwalks (safer substitute: half squat), sit-ups with the hands behind the neck (safer substitutes: curl-ups with hands across the chest, plank), and knee pull-downs with hands over the shins (safer substitute: same exercise with hands behind the thighs).

Hyperextension Exercises to Avoid

Hyperextension is the opposite of hyperflexion: increasing the angle of the joint too much. For example, having some curve in the back is normal, but arching the lower back more than normal involves hyperextension. Exercises that create hyperextension cause joints to move in ways for which they are not intended and the levers of the body to apply force inappropriately— violating principles 2 and 3, respectively.

Risky hyperextension exercises include back bends (figure 4.11), straight-leg sit-ups, rocking horses, cobras, prone swan positions, excessive upper-back lifts, and incorrect weightlifting positions in which the back is arched. Safe alternatives include the curl-up, plank, knee-to-nose touch, and the hip and thigh stretch. Some other exercises that hyperextend the spine

are neck circling to the rear (figure 4.12), neck hyperextensions, rear double-leg lifts, donkey kicks, landing from a jump with the back arched, wrestler's bridges, and backward trunk circling. Exercises that cause hyperextension are especially risky for people with swayback, weak abdominal muscles, a protruding abdomen, or back problems. You can learn more about swayback and other back problems in chapter 11, Muscle Fitness Applications.

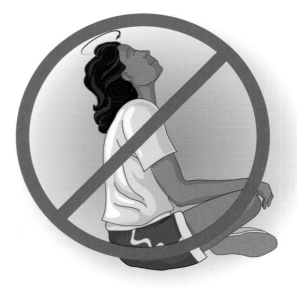

Figure 4.12 Avoid hyperextension exercises that cause friction, such as neck circling to the rear.

SCIENCE IN ACTION: **Protecting Your Skin**

Excessive exposure to the sun can put you at risk for skin-related injuries. Each year millions of people are treated for skin cancer and the principal cause is exposure to ultraviolet radiation in sunlight. Scientists have identified two types of sunlight radiation: ultraviolet A radiation (UVA), which is associated with premature skin aging, and ultraviolet B radiation (UVB), which is associated with sunburn and skin cancer. There is also a link between skin cancer and the use of indoor tanning beds, which cause similar UVA and UVB exposure. Scientists have developed the following guidelines to reduce the risk of skin cancer, premature skin aging, and sunburn resulting from UVA and UVB exposure:

- Limit exposure to the sun (especially at midday).
- Use a broad-spectrum, water-resistant sunscreen that screens both UVA and UVB rays. The American Academy of Dermatology (AAD) recommends a skin protection factor (SPF) of at least 30. Consult the required label on a sunscreen to determine its characteristics (see figure

4.13). The Food and Drug Administration (FDA) website includes current information about national sunscreen regulations and also revises guidelines for sunscreens periodically, so search online for the latest information.

- Apply sunscreen liberally at least 20 to 30 minutes before sun exposure. Reapply after sweating heavily, swimming, or after drying with a towel.
- Cover up to avoid excessive sun exposure. Wear a hat, sunglasses, long pants, and long sleeve shirts with a high collar. The American Cancer Society recommends that you "Slip, Slop, Slap, and Wrap": Slip on a shirt, slop on sunscreen, slap on a hat, and wrap on sunglasses.
- Take precautions when exposed to sunlight, even in cold weather and on cloudy days.
- Avoid the use of tanning salons and tanning lights. The Skin Cancer Foundation indicates that people who use tanning beds or lights before the age of 35 increase risk of melanoma by 75 percent.

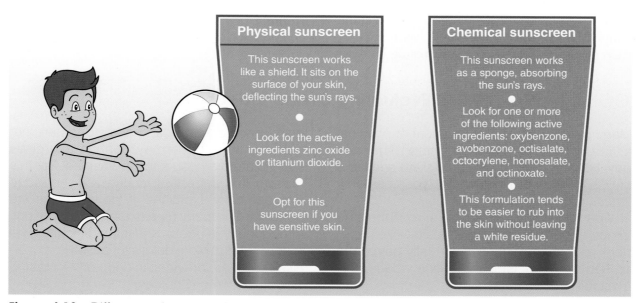

Figure 4.13   Differences between physical and chemical sunscreens.

STUDENT ACTIVITY

Every year 5 million Americans are treated for skin cancer, yet researchers have found that men, people of lower income, and non-Hispanic black people are less likely than others to use sunscreen. Comment on why you think this is true and what might be done to get more people to use sunscreen.

Joint-Twisting, Compression, and Friction Exercises to Avoid

Some exercises violate principle 2 because they cause the joints to twist excessively. Examples include hero stretches, as shown in figure 4.14 (no substitute: no exercise should twist the knee) and standing windmill toe touches (safer alternative: back-saver sit-and-reach).

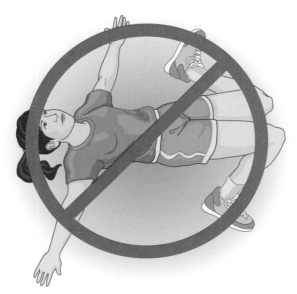

Figure 4.14 Avoid exercises that twist your joints.

Other exercises can cause compression at the joints or cause certain structures to rub against each other, creating friction that results in wear and tear. Examples of exercises in this category are hurdle sits, double-leg lifts, sit-ups with the hands behind the head, standing straight-leg toe touches, and arm circling with the palms down. Safe alternatives include the back-saver hamstring stretch, the reverse curl, the curl-up, the plank, knee-to-nose touch, and the hip and thigh stretch.

The double-leg lift (see figure 4.15) is an example of an exercise that can cause compression, especially for people with weak abdominal muscles. If the abdominals are weak, lifting the

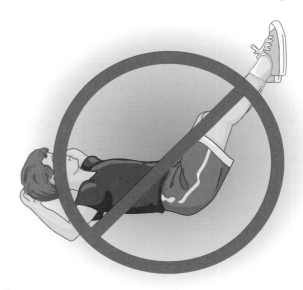

Figure 4.15 Avoid exercises that cause compression of the joints.

CONSUMER CORNER: **Evaluating Online Videos**

Many people get limited amounts of physical activity and a large amount of screen time each day. However, many great tools are available online to help you implement your personal fitness program.

Video-sharing websites like YouTube and Vimeo and other social media sites like Facebook and Instagram allow virtually anyone to upload video, including exercise videos. The availability of so many videos can be a good thing if the quality is good. However, because many people who post these videos are not experts, the videos may contain exercises that violate biomechanical principles. For this reason, it is important to check if the video includes risky exercises, if the exercises are performed properly (see exercise descriptions throughout this book), and if the difficulty level is appropriate. More details for assessing exercise videos are provided in chapter 19, Making Good Consumer Choices.

STUDENT ACTIVITY

Search the web for a video that contains fitness or yoga exercises. Check it for any risky exercises that violate the biomechanical principles discussed in this lesson.

legs (long levers) causes the back to arch, resulting in disc compression in the lower back. Most people perform the exercise with the intent of building the abdominal muscle, but it primarily builds the hip flexor muscles. Safer substitutes for building the abdominals include the plank and the curl-up with the arms across the chest.

Using Proper Technique

Generally speaking, you should avoid risky exercises and replace them with safe substitutes. Of course, some athletes may find it impossible to avoid all potentially harmful exercises—for example, gymnasts must perform stunts that require arching the back, and softball and baseball catchers must do full squats. Athletes who expect to perform potentially risky movements should participate in supervised exercises that build adequate flexibility and muscle fitness to prepare their bodies for these activities. Correct technique when performing these exercises is essential to maintain control of movement and to reduce the stress associated with risky movements.

LESSON REVIEW

1. What are some activity-related physical injuries, and what are their characteristics?
2. What steps can you take to prevent injury during physical activity?
3. How can the RICE formula be used to care for activity-related injuries?
4. What are some types of risky exercise, and why are they considered risky?

TAKING CHARGE: Overcoming Barriers

When some people face a problem beyond their control, they use it as an excuse for not being physically active. Someone might say, "I'm too short to be a basketball player, so I'm not going to try out for any sports." To be physically active, focus not on what you can't change but on what you *can* do.

Connie stood at the window. "It's pouring out there! How can we go hiking?"

Bridgette sighed. "I guess we're stuck spending the afternoon here."

Yesterday it was too hot to go hiking; now it was too rainy. It seemed as if they were never going to have good weather. But the weather was not the only

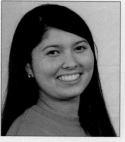

problem. The last time they tried hiking at the state park, it was sunny, but the paths were too crowded.

"I bet Alanzo is at the fitness center right now," Bridgette said. "He can exercise no matter what the weather is. I wish we could afford to go there!"

Connie glanced down at her sweats. "I'd need to buy more than a membership to go there. They wear expensive exercise clothes at that club. I'd get laughed out of the place in these clothes."

Bridgette smiled. "You don't look so bad—and the rain's starting to let up now. What if we put on older clothes, take rain gear, and hike around the park for a while?"

"You're right!" Connie said. "So what if we get a little damp?"

FOR DISCUSSION

What reasons do Connie and Bridgette give for not being active? Which of these problems can they control? They eventually decide not to let the weather stop them; what other strategies could they use to cope with the problems they've identified? Consider the guidelines in the following Self-Management feature as you answer these discussion questions.

SELF-MANAGEMENT: **Skills for Overcoming Barriers**

People face many barriers to becoming and staying active. Some barriers involve the environment (such as areas unsafe for exercise, lack of nearby exercise facilities, bad weather, expense), some involve personal physical characteristics (lack of physical size or skill), and some are psychological (low self-confidence, perceived lack of time). People who are active throughout life overcome such barriers, often with the help of government or community programs. Use the following strategies to overcome the barriers you face.

- *Find a way to exercise at home or at school.* If parks, fitness clubs, and other places for exercise are too expensive, too far away, or unsafe, find another way to exercise. Buy some equipment that you can use at home. If possible, use school facilities to exercise before or after school. Start a fitness club at school and ask school officials to help you find facilities and equipment.
- *Develop alternate plans.* Make multiple plans for activity. That way, for example, if it rains, you can switch to your alternate plan indoors. If something interferes with your planned exercise time, find another time.
- *Get active in community or school affairs.* Many communities have developed community centers; trails for biking, walking, and jogging; and other recreational facilities, such as tennis courts, basketball courts, and sport fields. If these options are not available in your community, write to your city or county officials or contact school officials and see what you can help create.
- *Use self-management skills to develop realistic plans that you will stick with.* Practice skills such as goal setting, program planning, self-monitoring, and time management.
- *Develop a new way of thinking.* Accept yourself as you are. If negative self-talk is an issue, use the strategies presented in this book to adjust your self-perceptions and boost your self-confidence.

Taking Action: **Safe Exercise Circuit**

In this lesson, you learned how to replace risky exercises with safe substitutes. You can **take action** by trying some of these exercises using a safe exercise circuit. The exercises in the circuit give you the benefits of risky exercises without the risk. Additional safe exercises are described throughout this book.

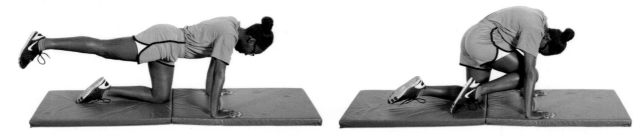

Take action by doing a safe exercise circuit that includes only safe alternatives to risky exercises.

CHAPTER REVIEW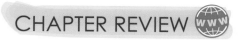

Reviewing Concepts and Vocabulary

Answer items 1 through 5 by correctly completing each sentence with a word or phrase.

1. The seven-item questionnaire used to determine readiness for physical activity is called the _____.

2. The two factors used to determine the heat index are _____ and _____.

3. The measure used to determine whether it is too cold to exercise is called the _____.

4. Invisible body damage caused by heavy repetition of a movement is called _____.

5. Hot, dry, flushed skin; rapid pulse; and lack of sweating are symptoms of _____.

For items 6 through 10, match each term in column 1 with the appropriate phrase in column 2.

6. electrolytes   a. holds bones together at the joint

7. ligament   b. body composition measure

8. hyperextension   c. minerals that help keep the body hydrated

9. hypothermia   d. extremely low body temperature

10. BMI   e. increasing the angle of the joint too much

For items 11 through 15, respond to each statement or question.

11. What is the PAR-Q+ and how is it useful?

12. Describe the three types of heat-related conditions.

13. What are the symptoms of frostbite?

14. Explain how to follow the RICE formula when caring for an activity-related injury.

15. Describe two risky exercises and explain why they are risky.

Thinking Critically

Write a paragraph to answer the following question.

How would you convince a friend that they need to take steps to avoid skin damage and potential skin cancer associated with sun or tanning light exposure?

Project

You have been asked to give a speech to a local civic club on preparing for physical activity. Prepare a presentation using 10 or more slides.

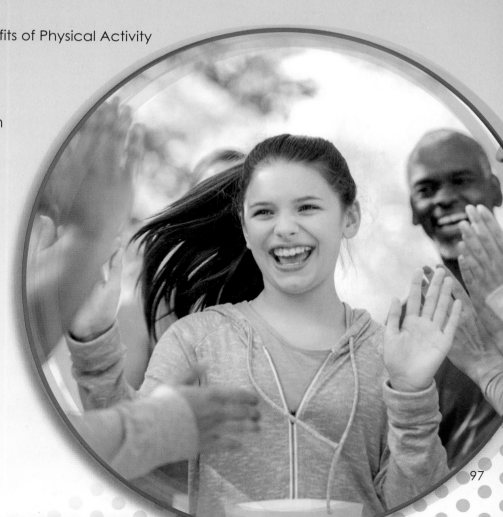

5

Social, Health, and Wellness Benefits of Physical Activity

Benefits of Social Interactions in Physical Activity

Lesson Objectives

After reading this lesson, you should be able to

1. define *leadership* and describe important leadership skills,
2. define *teamwork* and *group cohesiveness* and describe the guidelines for building teamwork;
3. define *rule*, *etiquette*, and *sportspersonship* and explain how they are important in sport and physical activity; and
4. define *diversity*, *sensitivity*, *trust*, *empathy*, and *bullying* and explain how these factors are important in sport and physical activity.

Lesson Vocabulary

bullying
diversity
empathy
equity
etiquette
group cohesiveness
inclusion
leadership
rule
sensitivity
social justice
sportspersonship
teamwork
trust

One goal of this book is to help you move from dependence to independence, whether you're making a personal plan to get fit or making decisions about what to eat. This chapter provides guidelines to help you to build skills and make responsible choices that lead to achieving the many social, emotional, and physical benefits of physical activity.

Leaders and Leadership Skills

Leadership involves actively assuming the role of a leader. You can't be a leader just because you want to be; becoming a leader requires leadership skills. Some of the most important leadership skills are presented in table 5.1. Like all skills, these must be practiced in order to be mastered.

One way to get leadership experience is to play sports and games. Another way is to participate in physical education class; for example, in sport education, students are grouped into teams whose members serve as leaders, team members, and referees. In the workplace, companies often use cooperative games to train managers and executives.

> When I first joined my volleyball club, I was the rookie. I depended on others to lead and to help the team succeed. Now I am one of the older team members and I realize that I have to step up and help the younger members to be respectful and to work together to achieve the goals of the team.
>
> *Elana Kieffer*

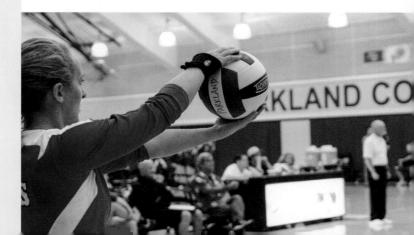

TABLE 5.1 **Leadership Skills**

Skill	Description	Tips for building
Integrity	Integrity means being fair; for a leader, it means directing while adhering to rules and standards of the group. Not all leaders have integrity, but good leaders do.	Integrity is built over time. You establish a reputation based on your actions.
Communication	Good leaders are good listeners. They listen in order to understand the group's needs, then speak clearly to be understood. Good leaders also inspire and persuade.	Practice listening even when you have much to say. Keep track of what others say. Ask for clarification to be sure you understand. Ask for confirmation that others understand you. Get the facts to help you make good arguments.
Strategy and planning	Creating a strategy requires creating a clear vision of your goals. It also involves developing tactics for carrying out the plan.	Practice using the steps for developing a strategy and carrying out a plan. Get the facts before planning.
Management	Leaders help group members work together to meet goals. Keys include building teamwork (group unity) and building trust based on integrity. Relevant skills include directing and supervising others, resolving conflicts, and negotiating.	Study the information presented in this chapter about teamwork and conflict resolution.
Other	Other characteristics of a good leader include self-confidence, optimism, enthusiasm, decisiveness, and being proactive. Good leaders can also accept criticism and are willing to learn better ways to reach group goals.	Most of these characteristics are built through experience. It also helps to practice the self-management skills presented in this book.

Teams and Teamwork

The Greek philosopher Aristotle stated, "the whole is greater than the sum of its parts"— meaning that when people work together, they can accomplish things that they otherwise could not accomplish working independently. **Teamwork** is effective, cooperative work by all team members to achieve a common goal. In order to experience teamwork, group members often have to sacrifice personal recognition in favor of team goals. For this reason, sport teams often use the slogan "there is no I in team" to emphasize that individual goals are secondary to team goals (figure 5.1).

Consider the following guidelines for effective teamwork:

• *Learn your role.* What tasks are you best able to perform that will help the team? A team

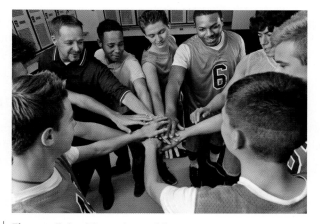

Figure 5.1 There is no I in team.

has a few common goals but many different roles. Though some roles are more prominent (for example, pitcher on a softball team), all must be performed well for the team to succeed.

If your actions create a legacy that inspires others to dream more, learn more, do more, and become more, then you are an excellent leader.

*Dolly Parton,
singer and actor*

• *Accept your role.* The role you want may not be the role you get. Teams can function effectively even if a member does not like their role—and even when team members don't get along well—as long as members *accept* their roles. In addition, carrying out a role that you don't prefer can lead to more desirable roles in the future.

• *Practice your role.* As with being a leader, being an effective team member requires practice. Every role requires specific skills. For example, the pitcher on a softball team may not be an especially good hitter. For this reason, the pitcher may be called on to perform a sacrifice bunt to move a runner into scoring position, so pitchers often practice bunting more than other players. Of course, roles are often assigned by leaders on the basis of team members' special skills.

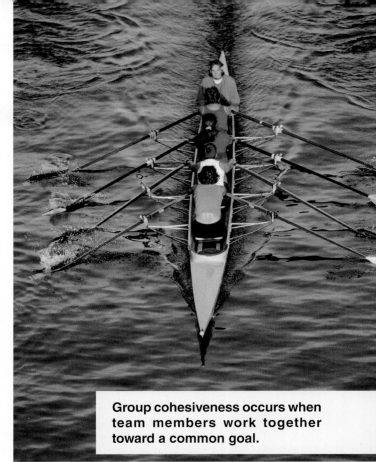

Group cohesiveness occurs when team members work together toward a common goal.

• *Carry out your role.* It's one thing to practice your role but another to carry it out effectively. Even when everyone does their job as practiced, success may not follow. It's important not to get discouraged if you and your team are not successful every time. However, if you accept your role and practice it, the chances of success are improved.

• *Adapt as necessary.* If a team's strategy and tactics are not working, adjustments need to be made, and those adjustments could mean a change in some team members' roles. To be successful, your role may change as well.

Rules, Etiquette, and Sportspersonship

In an orderly society, consideration for all group members is important. The same is true in physical activity settings such as sports and recreation. Information about rules, etiquette, and sportspersonship are discussed in the paragraphs that follow.

Making and Enforcing Rules

A **rule** is a guideline or regulation for conduct or action. Rules help bring order and fairness to sports and games. They can be very formal, as with the official rules of baseball, or they can be informal, as is the case for conduct within a group of friends.

There are many kinds of rules, ranging from societal laws (for example, the rules of the road) to the laws of physics. Classrooms have rules, as do business

SCIENCE IN ACTION: **Group Cohesiveness**

Cohesion means sticking together tightly. In chemistry, it means uniting particles to form a single mass. **Group cohesiveness** occurs among people when members of a group work together to achieve a common goal. Group cohesiveness contributes to good teamwork, as described earlier. Scientists have studied group cohesiveness in a variety of sports and found that several factors help groups stick together, including small group size, friendship among members, commitment to the group's goals, group success or failure, and competitiveness of group members.

It's easier to achieve group cohesiveness in small groups because fewer people have to coordinate their efforts. For example, it's easier for 5 people on a basketball team to work together than for 11 people on a football team to do so. It's also easier for small groups to agree on common goals.

In addition, if team members know and like each other, it's easier to work together. How-ever, studies also show that some teams win championships despite dissension among their members because team members are strongly committed to the group's goals. Several studies of rowers, for example, show that personal feelings can be overcome if team members want strongly enough to win. Thus, competitiveness is also a factor that creates desire among team members to work togeth-er. However, this can cut both ways: Winning a competition can help members get along, but losing sometimes leads to disagreements between team members (see this chapter's Taking Charge feature).

Research also shows that it's important for group members to recognize that everyone makes mistakes sometimes. This acknowl-edgment reduces blaming when the team does poorly and increases the chances for achieving group cohesiveness in the future. It's crucial to support fellow team members when they're down.

STUDENT ACTIVITY

Search websites, magazines, or newspapers to find a true story about group cohesiveness. Describe how the group members worked together to achieve a common goal.

meetings. Sport teams have rules for remaining in good standing with the team, and religions have rules of moral conduct. Violating a rule typically results in some sort of punishment, whereas regular adherence to rules is usually rewarded. Rules are enforced in a variety of ways—for example, police officers enforce laws, referees enforce sport rules, and coaches and team leaders enforce team rules.

Experts agree that for rules to be effective, they must be consistently enforced. They should also be appropriate for the situation, and punishment should be con-sistent with the violation. Rules must be fair to all members of the group.

In some cases, not much can be done to change rules—at least not quickly. In sport, for example, teams are bound by existing rules as they are enforced by officials. Team and school rules, however, can be changed more quickly if they are not serving their intended purpose. Team members can modify bad rules by using a version of the scientific method. After identifying the rules that seem to need changing, the group can collect information, then use it to articulate clear reasons (evidence) for changing the rules. Group members should consult with each other and debate the evidence, after which either the group as a whole or its leaders can make a decision. Once the decision is made, the group's effectiveness depends on whether group members comply with the new rules. A group member who finds the rules unacceptable doesn't have to continue to be a member.

FIT FACT
A national survey of Americans found that nearly 85 percent of adults agree that bending or breaking the rules in sport is cheating and should not be tolerated. A similar percentage agree that bending or breaking the rules is cheating even if no one notices. In spite of this finding, however, one in five admits to breaking rules in sports, and nearly half say they know someone who has bent or broken rules.

Etiquette in Physical Activity

Etiquette involves acting in a way that is consistent with the typical or expected behavior of a social group. In Western society, for example, etiquette for eating indicates when to use a knife, a fork, or a spoon. In some Asian cultures, however, dining etiquette involves chopsticks. Sport also involves social situations subject to a code of etiquette.

Some rules of sport etiquette are informal and unwritten. In golf, for example, it is considered poor etiquette to talk while another player is swinging. Other rules of etiquette are more formal. For example, it is considered unacceptable to make negative comments to a referee or umpire. Players sometimes test the rules of etiquette, however. Coaches may remove a player from the game for violations and, if extreme, comments to officials can result in penalties or expulsion from the game.

Most people agree that following rules of etiquette, whether formal or informal, generally helps make social situations more enjoyable. Knowing the etiquette of a particular sport or social group can also help you feel more comfortable in the group, whereas not knowing it can make you quite uncomfortable.

Sportspersonship

Sportspersonship is a term used to describe respect for opponents and grace in winning or losing. A good sport exhibits good ethical conduct and plays by the rules. An overemphasis on winning can sometimes result in acts of poor sportspersonship such as attempting to hurt an opponent or intentionally violating the rules. You'll find that if you participate in games and sports for fun, health benefits, stress reduction, and social interaction, you'll enjoy yourself much more than if you focus only on winning.

▌ Respect for Others

The American College of Sports Medicine (ACSM) released a statement on diversity, equity, and inclusion. The ACSM notes that *all* people deserve the right to be able

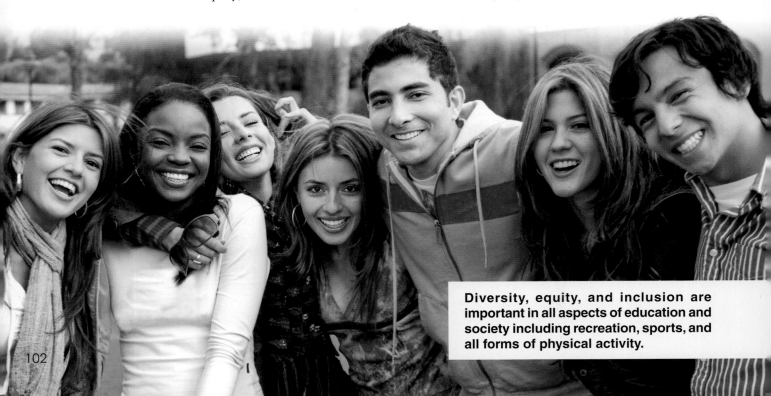

Diversity, equity, and inclusion are important in all aspects of education and society including recreation, sports, and all forms of physical activity.

to safely participate in physical activities, receive proper nutrition, have appropriate health care, and have access to other basic human needs. The statement asks that all people "go about their daily lives, making decisions with social justice in their hearts and minds." The ACSM statement is about respect for others--all others. Respect for others is important for enjoyment in sports, as well as meaningful interactions in life. Several factors that promote respect for others are described in the following paragraphs.

Social Justice

The National Education Association (NEA) defines **social justice** as a "concept in which equity or justice is achieved in every aspect of society rather than in only some aspects or for some people." Both the ACSM and NEA point out the importance of social justice and emphasize diversity, equity, and inclusion in all aspects of education and society.

Diversity, Equity, and Inclusion

The word *society* refers to a large group of people who have a history of working and living together. It can refer to a neighborhood, a school, a community, a nation, or an even larger group (for example, Western society). Characteristics of a society include traditions, organized laws and rules, and standards for living and conduct (social etiquette).

Societies provide for the common interests of all members and protect them from outside threats. **Diversity** refers to the **inclusion** of different types of people in society regardless of race, ethnicity, age, disability, culture, socioeconomic status, sex, or gender identity. **Equity** refers to the personal quality of being fair and impartial (free of bias or favoritism). To achieve diversity and social justice it is important for each individual to show equity by treating all members of society equally and fairly and including everyone in all aspects of life. The vocabulary terms relating to social justice have similar but distinct meanings as described in the following section.

Sensitivity and Trust

Sensitivity refers to paying attention to the feelings and concerns of others. Ways to build sensitivity include listening (for example, hearing what others have to say rather than only telling others what to do) and communicating in nonthreatening language (for example, giving positive feedback rather than harsh criticism). **Trust** refers to the belief that others are honest and reliable. Demonstrating honesty and reliability in your actions helps others learn to trust you. People who are trustworthy and sensitive to others' needs typically earn the respect of others.

Empathy

Empathy refers to the ability to understand and be sensitive to the feelings of others. An empathetic person can imagine what it is like to be in another person's shoes and acts with compassion. True empathy is the result of an internal desire to help people rather than acting because of external pressures. Empathic people listen, challenge prejudice, and take action to aid others.

FIT FACT

Jackie Robinson and Patsy Mink are examples of pioneers who fought for social justice in sports. Jackie Robinson was the first Black man to play major league baseball in the modern era of the sport. He joined the Brooklyn Dodgers in the summer of 1947 and was elected to the Hall of Fame. Patsy Mink was the first Asian-American woman to serve in Congress (Hawaii). She was a principal author of Title IX Legislation that stated "no person in the U. S. shall, on the basis of sex, be excluded from participation in, be denied the benefits of, or be subjected to discrimination under any education program or activity receiving Federal financial assistance." The law opened the door for sports opportunities for females who had previously been denied equity in sports and education.

Bullying

Bullying is a serious problem among teens. Experts in sport sociology indicate that half of all teens say they have been bullied, and nearly as many say they have bullied someone else. A U.S. government website (StopBullying.gov) describes several types of bullying, including verbal (name calling, teasing), social (spreading rumors, exclusion, breaking friendships), physical (hitting, punching, shoving), and cyber (using the web and tech devices to do harm). Bullying shows disrespect for individuals and for the rules of the social group. You will learn more about bullying in chapter 17, Stress Management.

LESSON REVIEW

1. What is leadership, and what are some important leadership skills?
2. What are teamwork and group cohesiveness, and what are some guidelines for building teamwork and being a good team member?
3. What are rules, etiquette, and sportspersonship, and how are they important in sport and physical activity?
4. How are diversity, sensitivity, trust, empathy, and bullying defined, and how are they important in sport and physical activity?

SELF-ASSESSMENT: Modifying Rules in Games

This activity will help you assess the importance of fair rules when playing games. Perform the activity as described, then, as directed by your instructor, record information about the activity.

1. Each person in the class writes their name on a small piece of paper. Place the names in a box or bag. One member of the class draws the names of six people.
2. The people whose names are drawn come to the front of the class. The first three drawn form one team, and the second three form the other. Members of each team spread out in a defined game area in front of the class. They may stand wherever they want within the game area, but once their location is determined they cannot move their right foot from that spot.
3. The name of an additional person is drawn to be the referee. The referee tosses a small ball into the air within the playing area. When a player on either team touches the ball, the referee awards a point to one team. The referee decides which team gets the point and does not have to explain why the point was given. Points do not have to be awarded for the same reason for each throw. The referee retrieves the ball and continues to throw it and award points until the ball is thrown 10 times. The team with the most points is the winner. If the score is tied, the team that scores the next point wins.
4. Ask team members to explain how they felt about the game and its rules.
5. After the discussion, draw names for additional teams and referees, so that several games are played at the same time, involving all members of the class. Before each group plays the game, both teams must agree on two or three rules for awarding points. The referee writes down the rules and uses them when throwing the ball and awarding points.
6. After all teams have finished playing their game, each group comes up with ideas for improving the game.
7. Each group then presents and justifies its list of rules to the rest of the class.
8. If time allows, play the game using rules created by one of the groups.

Adapted from an activity developed by the College of Education at the University of North Carolina.

Health and Wellness Benefits of Physical Activity

Lesson Objectives

After reading this lesson, you should be able to

1. describe some types of cardiovascular disease and explain, using examples, how physical activity can reduce the risk of these conditions;

2. describe several other hypokinetic conditions and explain, using examples, how physical activity can reduce the risk of these conditions;

3. describe some wellness benefits of physical activity; and

4. explain, using examples, how physical activity is related to hyperkinetic conditions.

Lesson Vocabulary

atherosclerosis
blood pressure
cardiovascular disease (CVD)
diabetes
diastolic blood pressure
eating disorder
exercise addiction
heart attack
hyperkinetic condition
hypertension
metabolic syndrome
osteoporosis
peak bone mass
risk factor
stroke
systolic blood pressure

Have you ever wondered why people today often live twice as long as people did a few hundred years ago? Do you know the leading causes of death today? Do you understand the roles played by physical activity and nutrition in living a long, high-quality life?

Prior to 1900, the leading cause of death in the United States and other developed countries was pneumonia; other common causes of death included infection from other bacteria and viruses. With cures or vaccinations now existing for many of these conditions, the leading health threats today are hypokinetic conditions (i.e., caused in part by sedentary living), such as cardiovascular disease, cancer, stroke, and diabetes. In this lesson, you'll learn more about how physical activity reduces your risk of hypokinetic conditions and increases your personal wellness.

The COVID-19 pandemic showed that even in our time of advanced medical science, infectious diseases can be the source of extensive

At my great grandma's 99th birthday party I asked how she stays so healthy. She said, "I worked hard on the farm and learned to stay active, eat well, and surround myself with the people I care most about. Good health for me and my family is the most important thing in the world."

Noah Felder

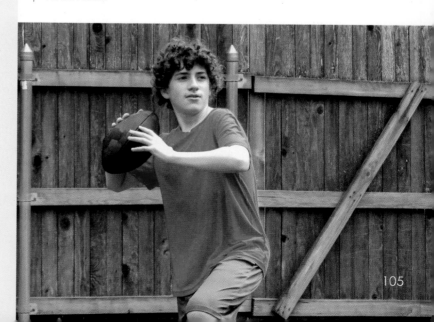

illness and death. The pandemic also revealed that hypokinetic conditions such as obesity and diabetes increased risk for getting the virus.

Cardiovascular Disease, Stroke, and Related Risk Factors

Sedentary living costs the United States billions of dollars each year in health care expenses and loss of productivity. Even more alarming, thousands of people die prematurely every year from conditions caused in part by inactivity. Reports issued by major health organizations, including the U.S. Office of the Surgeon General, the Centers for Disease Control and Prevention (CDC), and the American Heart Association (AHA), indicate that regular physical activity is one of the best ways to reduce illness and increase wellness in American society. The American College of Sports Medicine (ACSM) lists dozens of different health benefits of regular exercise. Sometimes teenagers feel that these statistics are not relevant to them; they think illness happens only to old people. As you'll see next, however, many hypokinetic diseases are now prevalent among teens.

Cardiovascular Diseases

Cardiovascular diseases have been the leading cause of death in the United States each year since 1920, and in fact have been a primary or contributing cause of more than one-third of all deaths in the United States. Currently, nearly one-half of American adults have at least one form of heart disease.

Heart disease is a commonly used term. However, the term **cardiovascular disease (CVD)** is more descriptive and inclusive because it includes diseases of the heart (cardio) as well as diseases of the blood vessels (vascular). As shown in figure 5.2, your heart is a muscle that acts as a pump. When you have problems with the heart muscle's ability to pump blood, you have heart disease. When you have problems with your blood vessels (arteries and veins), you have vascular disease. Together heart disease and vascular disease are considered to be cardiovascular diseases.

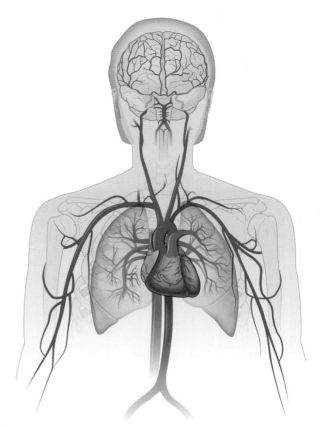

Figure 5.2   The heart pumps blood to all areas of the body.

Heart Attack

A **heart attack** is one type of CVD. A heart attack occurs when the blood supply within the heart is severely reduced or cut off; as a result, an area of the heart muscle can die. The main reason for heart attacks is a blockage of the arteries within the heart. This happens when a blood clot blocks an artery or when spasms in the muscle of the artery occur, or a combination of these causes. During a heart attack, the heart may beat abnormally or even stop beating (cardiac arrest). Treatments often include medicines that stabilize the heartbeat and cardiopulmonary resuscitation (CPR) to restore circulation of oxygen. Regular physical activity has been shown to reduce the risk of heart attack, and it is also used to help people recover after a heart attack.

Atherosclerosis

Another type of CVD is **atherosclerosis**. It occurs when substances such as cholesterol

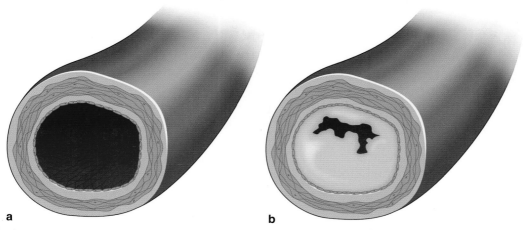

Figure 5.3 *(a)* A healthy heart has open arteries. *(b)* An unhealthy heart has clogged arteries that can cause a heart attack.

build up on the inside walls of the arteries inside of the heart, narrowing the openings through the arteries. As a result, the heart must work harder to pump blood. Figure 5.3 illustrates the difference between a clear artery and one that is partially blocked with atherosclerosis. Atherosclerosis typically develops with age, but it can begin early in life. Regular physical activity can reduce the risk of atherosclerosis.

High Blood Pressure (Hypertension)

A primary risk factor for heart attack is **hypertension**, commonly known as high blood pressure. Each time your heart beats, it forces blood through your arteries. The force of the blood pushing against the artery walls is called **blood pressure**. When the doctor checks your blood pressure, they look for two readings. The higher number is the pressure in your arteries immediately after your heart beats, called **systolic blood pressure**. The lower of the two numbers, your **diastolic blood pressure**, is the pressure in your arteries just before the next beat of your heart.

The American Heart Association and the American Stroke Association have developed blood pressure standards (see table 5.2), which include normal (healthy), elevated, stage 1 hypertension, stage 2 hypertension, and hypertensive crisis (requires immediate care).

It is important to have your blood pressure checked regularly, especially as you grow older. When you have your blood pressure checked, you should be rested and relaxed. Blood pressure will be higher if you exercise immediately before taking a reading and is often elevated when you're excited or anxious.

Medications are now available to help people with elevated or high blood pressure. The incidence of high blood pressure has decreased in recent years because of improved medicines and early screening. Because high blood pressure is a hypokinetic condition, regular physical activity can help decrease it, as can a healthy low-sodium diet.

> **FIT FACT**
> An automated external defibrillator (AED) is an electronic device used to restore a normal heartbeat in a person who has suffered cardiac arrest. AEDs are available in airports and other public places, and the fact that they are automated makes them usable even by someone who is untrained.

TABLE 5.2 **Blood Pressure Readings**

	Normal	Elevated	Stage 1	Stage 2	Crisis
Systolic	≤119	120–129	130–159	160–179	≥180s
Diastolic	≤79	80–89	90–99	100–109	≥110

ACADEMIC CONNECTION: Statistics

Statistics is a branch of mathematics dealing with the collection, analysis, and interpretation of data (numerical information). Mathematic literacy is important for meeting college and career readiness standards. Understanding and using some basic statistical concepts will not only help you prepare for a career or further studies but also allow you to understand health risks.

The typical person is said to be average. In math, *average* refers to measures of central tendency such as

- the mean, or the sum of all scores divided by the number of scores (11 scores in the following example);
- the median, or the middle score in a number of scores (in the following example, the sixth score from the lowest or sixth score from the highest); and
- the mode, or the most common score in a number of scores (in the following example, the only score that was common to two people).

STUDENT ACTIVITY

Calculate the mean, median, and mode for a group of 11 people with the following systolic blood pressure readings in mmHg: 120, 125, 130, 130, 135, 140, 145, 150, 155, 160, 165. Remember that systolic blood pressure is the higher of the two blood pressure numbers and reflects the pressure in your arteries just after the heart beats.

A systolic blood pressure of 120 mmHg is considered to be healthy. Knowing this, would you want to have your blood pressure equal to the average for this group (using any of the three measures of central tendency)?

CHECK YOUR ANSWERS

Mean = 141.36; median = 140; mode = 130

Stroke

Stroke is a condition that results from lack of blood supply to the brain (see figure 5.4). It occurs when a vessel that supplies blood to the brain bursts or is blocked by a blood clot or atherosclerosis. Because a stroke damages the brain, it can affect a person's ability to move, think, or speak and can be fatal. Stroke is the fifth leading cause of early death in the United States. Because regular physical activity reduces risk of atherosclerosis, it also reduces risk of stroke.

Risk Factors for Cardiovascular Disease and Stroke

People get cardiovascular disease and stroke for many reasons, each of which is called a **risk factor**. The more risk factors you have, the more chance you have of getting a disease. Two kinds of risk factors exist: modifiable and non-modifiable (personal). The AHA has identified

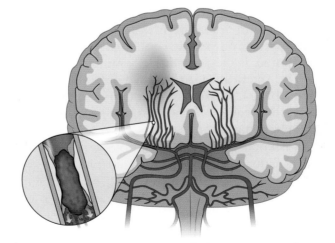

Figure 5.4   A clot in the brain is one cause of stroke.

"Life's Simple 7," a list of lifestyle-related risk factors that are under your control (see figure 5.5). Being active and eating well have double benefits because they help you maintain a healthy body weight and also improve other

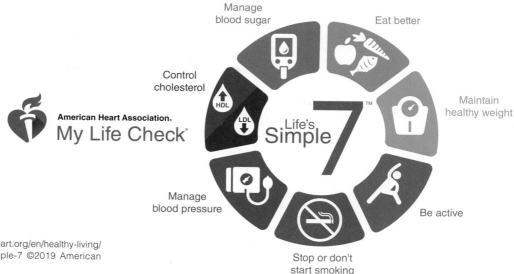

Figure 5.5   Life's Simple 7.

Reprinted with permission https://www.heart.org/en/healthy-living/healthy-lifestyle/my-life-check--lifes-simple-7 ©2019 American Heart Association, Inc.

risk factors such as high blood pressure, high cholesterol, and high blood sugar. Quitting (or not starting) smoking is another major modifiable risk factor that can prevent cardiovascular disease. In addition to the Simple 7, other modifiable risk factors include getting adequate sleep, avoiding excessive use of alcohol, and managing stress.

Personal (nonmodifiable) risk factors include heredity, age, sex, and race. People with a family history of cardiovascular disease, older people, males, and people with other conditions such as kidney disease are at higher than normal risk of cardiovascular disease. African Americans have a higher risk of high blood pressure than people of other racial backgrounds. People with risk factors that are nonmodifiable can especially benefit from modifying lifestyles.

Teens typically have fewer risk factors than adults, but in recent years the prevalence of elevated blood pressure, blood sugar, and cholesterol has increased among teens. There has also been an increase in the number of teens that are overweight. Because of this increase, doctors now check risk factors as part of a regular medical exam beginning in the teens.

Physical Activity, Cardiovascular Disease, and Stroke

An active and fit person has a strong heart muscle capable of pumping adequate blood through healthy unobstructed arteries, including those in the heart, brain, muscles, and other organs. The active and fit person also has blood that is low in fat, such as cholesterol, and has blood pressure in the healthy range. Regular physical activity not only reduces your risk of heart attack and stroke but is often prescribed by doctors to help people recovering from these conditions. Figure 5.6 illustrates some ways in which regular physical activity reduces the risk of hypokinetic conditions, including CVD.

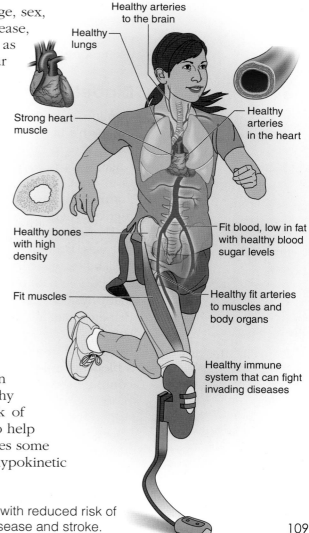

Figure 5.6   Physical activity benefits associated with reduced risk of hypokinetic conditions such as cardiovascular disease and stroke.

In the United States, physical inactivity is the biggest health problem of the 21st century.

Dr. Steven Blair, past president of the American College of Sports Medicine

Cancer, Diabetes, and Other Hypokinetic Conditions

It has long been known that cardiovascular diseases are hypokinetic conditions. More recently, evidence indicates that other conditions can be caused in part by inactivity. Some of these hypokinetic diseases and conditions are described in the following sections.

Cancer

According to the American Cancer Society, there are more than 100 types of cancer, all characterized by the uncontrollable growth of abnormal cells. Cancer's uncontrolled cells invade normal cells, steal their nutrition, and interfere with the cells' normal functioning.

Cancer is the second leading cause of death in the United States. Many of the risk factors for cancer are the same as those for cardiovascular disease. Certain forms of cancer (breast, colon, prostate, and rectal) are considered hypokinetic conditions because people who are physically active are less likely to get them than people who are inactive. The death rate from all forms of cancer is also lower in active people than in inactive people. It is not clear why physical activity helps reduce the risk of cancer, but, as shown in figure 5.6, one of the health benefits of physical activity is an immune system that is more capable of fighting diseases that invade the body. Another good way to help prevent or minimize cancer is to get regular physical exams, including a full-body skin exam (skin cancer is on the rise among teens).

Diabetes

Insulin is a hormone made in the pancreas that helps control blood sugar. When a person's body cannot produce enough insulin or use it effectively, the person has a disease called **diabetes**. A person with diabetes has excessively high blood sugar, which can lead to coma or death unless the person gets medical assistance. Over time, diabetes can also damage the blood vessels, heart, kidneys, and eyes. Fortunately, several effective medical treatments can help people with diabetes regulate their blood sugar and lead a normal life.

There are two types of diabetes. Type 1, which accounts for about 10 percent of cases, is not a hypokinetic condition and is often hereditary. People with type 1 diabetes typically do not produce enough insulin. At one time, it was thought that people with type 1 diabetes should avoid physical activity, but we now know that physical activity can help people manage diabetes. Most people with type 1 diabetes take a blood sample one or more times a day in order to test their blood sugar. If the level is high, they must take insulin injections or oral medications to lower their blood sugar. In the past, it was necessary to puncture the skin to take a blood sample, but new technology allows some people with diabetes to wear a computerized watch that automatically tests blood sugar without having to draw blood.

The most common kind of diabetes, type 2, occurs when the body resists the effects of insulin. In some cases, type 2 diabetics take medicines or insulin to regulate blood sugar levels. However, many can regulate the disease by being active and eating well. Exercise helps reduce your risk of type 2 diabetes by lowering your blood sugar level, helping your body tissues use insulin more efficiently and helping control body fat. Having too much body fat, especially abdominal fat around

FIT FACT

Type 2 diabetes used to be called *adult-onset diabetes* because adults got it, not teens and children. This name is no longer used because the disease has become more common among youth in recent years.

the organs, is a risk factor for type 2 diabetes. In fact, so many obese people have diabetes that one expert coined the term *diabesity*—a combination of the words *diabetes* and *obesity*.

Obesity

Obesity, in which a person has a high percentage of body fat, often results from inactivity, though many other factors can contribute. The American Medical Association now classifies obesity as a disease. Having too much body fat, especially internal abdominal fat, contributes to conditions such as cardiovascular disease and diabetes. Since 1980, the incidence of obesity among teens ages 12 to 19 in the United States has quadrupled, rising from 5 percent to nearly 21 percent, and a similar upward trend is found in other developed nations. Regular physical activity expends calories, and when combined with healthy eating, results in body fat loss. Regular physical activity also increases muscle mass, which burns more calories at rest.

Osteoporosis

Osteoporosis exists when the structure of bones deteriorates (see figure 5.7) and bones become weak. It is most common among older people but has its beginnings in youth. It is in youth that you develop your greatest bone mass, also called **peak bone mass**. People who do the right kind of exercise on a regular basis develop a greater peak bone mass than those who are sedentary. Choose activities that cause you to bear weight and thus stress your bones in a healthy way, such as walking, running, jumping, and resistance training. As a result, even if you lose bone mass as you get older, you'll have stronger bones than if you hadn't exercised while young.

One contributor to osteoporosis is a lack of sufficient calcium in the diet, especially during youth. Women are more likely to have osteoporosis than men because the hormonal changes they experience later in life cause their body to absorb calcium less efficiently. No matter what you sex or gender identity, you can maximize your bone health throughout life by getting good nutrition, regular activity, and proper medical attention.

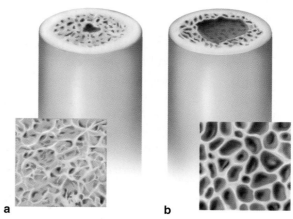

Figure 5.7 Osteoporosis involves a decrease in bone density: *(a)* healthy bone in an active person; *(b)* unhealthy bone (osteoporosis), more common among sedentary people.

Additional Hypokinetic Conditions

Evidence suggests that regular physical activity can also reduce the risk or relieve the symptoms of the following diseases and conditions.

• *Mental health conditions.* One-third of all adults report that they often feel depressed or anxious. Many teens (nearly 1 in 3) feel sad for more than a few days in a row. People who do regular physical activity are less likely to be depressed, anxious, and sad. More information is provided in chapter 17, Stress Management.

• *Back problems.* Back pain is one of the most common hypokinetic conditions. According to the ACSM, as many as 84 percent of adults experience low back pain at some point in their lives. Recent studies indicate that as many as 58 percent of teens experience back pain at some point in their teen years. Regular physical activity can help prevent back pain by improving core muscle fitness, maintaining good flexibility, and helping in healthy body fat management. Emphasizing good lifting mechanics can also be important in preventing low back pain.

• *Metabolic health conditions. Metabolism* is a word that refers to the many chemical reactions that allow the body and cells to live and function effectively. You are metabolically healthy when the chemical reactions work normally, allowing the cells to function well. A condition called **metabolic syndrome** can occur when the systems are not working well. People who have at least three of five specific hypo-kinetic conditions are considered to have metabolic syndrome. These conditions include high blood sugar levels, high blood pressure, high blood cholesterol, high blood triglycerides, and a large waist size. Metabolic syndrome is associated with cardiovascular disease, diabetes, and other hypokinetic diseases. Regular exercise can improve metabolic health and reduce the symptoms of metabolic syndrome.

• *Immune system conditions.* Regular physical activity, in appropriate amounts, has been shown to enhance the function of the immune system. This enhanced function allows the body to resist infections such as the common cold and the flu.

• *Arthritis.* Moderate activity has been shown to help reduce symptoms of some forms of arthritis.

• *Alzheimer's disease and dementia.* Research shows that regular physical activity and challenging mental tasks can improve brain health and reduce the risk of memory loss disorders.

Physical Activity and Wellness

As you can see, physical activity plays an important role in preventing hypokinetic diseases and conditions and thus is a key to good health. But remember—health is more than freedom from disease; it also includes wellness, the positive component of health. As a result, the U.S. Healthy People 2030 report incorporates wellness as one of its major goals.

As you learned in an earlier chapter, there are social, emotional–mental, intellectual, physical, and spiritual components of wellness. Being regularly active can help you achieve all of these benefits. In the first lesson of this chapter you learned about some of the social–emotional benefits of interactions in physical activity. These and other wellness benefits of physical activity are illustrated in figure 5.8.

Being active helps you to become physically fit, which in turn leads to other physical benefits such as effective and efficient daily functioning. During the teen years, when you are in school, regular physical activity provides intellectual benefits as well. For example, regular physical activity stimulates the brain, which enables better performance on tests and better attention span in the classroom.

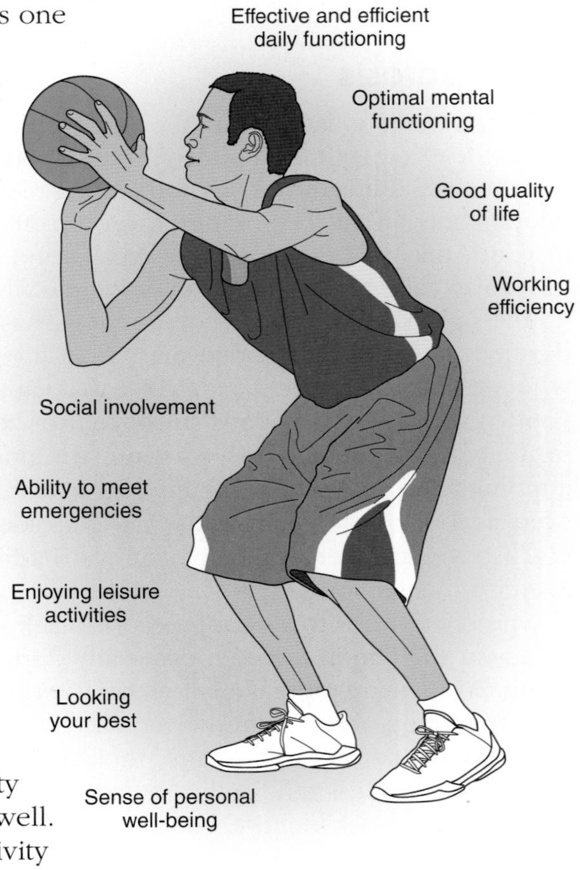

FIT FACT
Studies conducted by experts in exercise physiology, exercise psychology, and physical activity show that teens who are fit and active are less likely to be absent or cause discipline problems than unfit, inactive teens.

Effective and efficient daily functioning
Optimal mental functioning
Good quality of life
Working efficiency
Social involvement
Ability to meet emergencies
Enjoying leisure activities
Looking your best
Sense of personal well-being

Figure 5.8 The wellness benefits of regular physical activity.

Hyperkinetic Conditions

You've probably heard the saying "too much of a good thing can be bad." This can even be true of physical activity. The fact that some physical activity is good does not mean that more activity is always better. In some cases, people experience **hyperkinetic conditions**—health problems caused by doing too *much* physical activity.

Overuse Injuries

As discussed in the previous chapter, overuse injuries occur when you do so much physical activity that you suffer damage to a bone, muscle, or other tissue. Examples include stress fractures, shin splints, and blisters.

Exercise Addiction

Exercise addiction is a term that refers to uncontrollable excessive exercise that leads to harmful conditions such as injury and damaged social relationships. Exercise addiction is also known as compulsive exercise because people who have it are overly concerned about getting enough exercise. They feel upset if they miss a regular workout and often continue physical activity when they are sick or injured. Exercise addiction is more common among aerobic dance instructors, bodybuilders, and runners than other active groups. Aerobic dance instructors often teach many classes and also take classes to improve their dance skills, which can lead to a compulsive need to exercise. Some bodybuilders seek perfection and continue to do more exercise in pursuit of this ideal. Runners may overexercise because of a desire to improve running times or distance.

Body Image Disorders

People with body image disorders try to achieve their idea of an ideal body by controlling their diet and often excessive exercise. Anorexia nervosa and bulimia are body image disorders that are more commonly called **eating disorders**. Both are associated with an extreme desire to be thin, disturbed eating patterns, and excessive exercise. Anorexia athletica is a body image disorder that affects athletes. It is characterized by compulsive exercise and disordered eating. These and other body image disorders are discussed in detail in chapter 14.

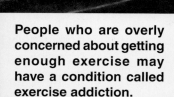

People who are overly concerned about getting enough exercise may have a condition called exercise addiction.

113

LESSON REVIEW

1. What are some types of cardiovascular disease, and how can physical activity reduce the risk of these conditions?
2. What are some other types of hypokinetic conditions, and how can physical activity reduce the risk of these conditions?
3. What are some of the wellness benefits of physical activity?
4. What are some hyperkinetic conditions, and how are they related to physical activity?

TAKING CHARGE: **Conflict Resolution**

Monica and Juana made a plan to walk to school five days a week for one month. However, their friend Miguel kept offering them a ride to school. The third time Miguel offered, Monica accepted and left Juana to walk alone. Juana did not accept because she wanted to walk as planned. Juana then was mad at both Monica and Miguel and didn't speak to them at school. The next

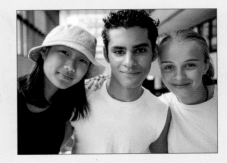

day, Monica didn't stop by to walk with Juana—she just rode with Miguel. The friends did not speak at school. In

fact, Monica said something to other friends about Juana that upset her.

FOR DISCUSSION

What could the friends have done to avoid the conflict? What steps should they take to resolve it? Consider the guidelines in the following Self-Management feature as you answer these discussion questions.

SELF-MANAGEMENT: **Skills for Conflict Resolution**

All of us have disagreements with our friends at times. The disagreements are usually over small things and can be easily resolved. A conflict is typically bigger than a disagreement. When a conflict occurs, one or more of the people involved come to feel threatened, whether physically or emotionally. In sport, for example, one player may get angry with another, and strong emotions may lead to angry words. In extreme cases, the anger can result in fighting. Whether the conflict occurs in sport or daily life, the following steps can help you resolve it.

- *Keep emotions under control.* When working with others to resolve conflict, remember to be calm, patient, and respectful.
- *Communicate.* To resolve a conflict, you need good communication. Watch what you say and be willing to listen. Words

can hurt, and it's crucial not to make the conflict worse.

- *Recognize that there is a conflict.* Don't ignore it. Avoiding a conflict can cause it to get worse.
- *Consider a meeting.* Although a conflict can sometimes be resolved on the phone, by e-mail, through social media, or in other ways, it's often best to meet in person. The meeting should be held in a neutral and safe setting for all involved.
- *Set the scene.* Define the problem and restate it if necessary. Each person should describe the problem without interruption, then the parties can try to find a statement of the problem that all can agree to.
- *List possible solutions.* Make a list of possible solutions based on ideas from people on all sides of the conflict.

- *Consider the options.* Once options have been proposed, communicate respectfully to find the options that best meet the needs of all parties concerned.

- *Compromise.* If the people involved have very different ideas about the conflict, it may be necessary for each person to give up something in order to find a resolution.

- *Seek help.* If the parties involved cannot resolve the conflict on their own, they may need to use an independent arbitrator. In sport, a coach or referee can resolve some conflicts, and others may be resolved with the help of a common friend, but difficult conflicts may call for a professional arbitrator.

Taking Action: **Team Building**

The TEAM concept (Together Everyone Achieves More) can help you succeed in all aspects of your life. It's an exciting challenge to build a team of individuals who work well together in pursuit of a common goal. **Take action** by performing a team-building activity in your physical education class.

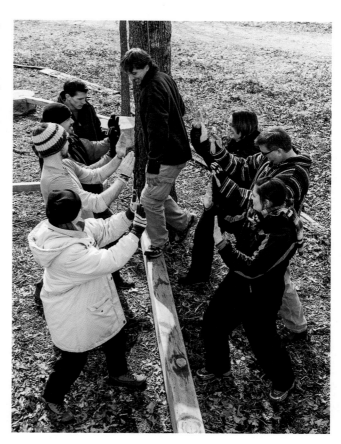

Take action by trying team-building activities.

115

CHAPTER REVIEW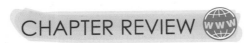

Reviewing Concepts and Vocabulary

Answer items 1 through 5 by correctly completing each sentence with a word or phrase.

1. The word used to describe being fair and following the rules is _____.

2. A guideline or regulation for conduct or action is called a _____.

3. _____ involves acting in a way that is consistent with expected behavior in a group.

4. The disease caused by clogged arteries is called _____.

5. Deterioration or weakness of the bones is called _____.

For items 6 through 10, match each term in column 1 with the appropriate phrase in column 2.

6. exercise addiction   a. inability to regulate blood sugar

7. diabetes   b. paying attention to the feelings of others

8. sportspersonship   c. high blood pressure

9. sensitivity   d. respect for opponents

10. hypertension   e. overconcern with exercise

For items 11 through 15, respond to each statement or question.

11. What are some guidelines for building teamwork?

12. What are some steps you can take to resolve conflicts?

13. What are the benefits of physical activity in preventing cardiovascular disease?

14. Describe two hyperkinetic conditions.

15. Describe two wellness benefits of physical activity.

Thinking Critically

Write a paragraph to answer the following question.

What are some of the risk factors for cardiovascular disease and stroke that are most in your control?

Project

Investigate the programs in your school designed to promote social–emotional learning. Work with others to create a plan to expand these programs. Prepare a report of your findings and the plan for expansion.

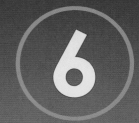

How Much Is Enough?

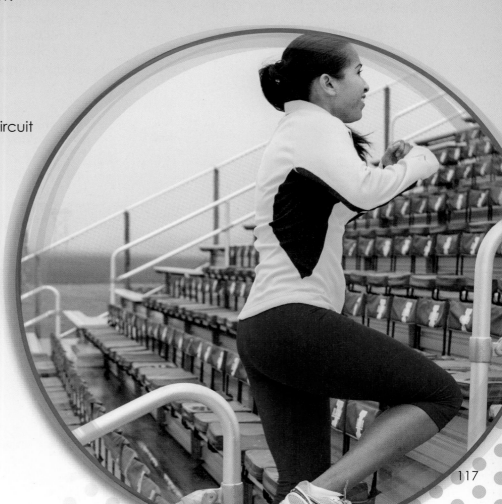

117

How Much Physical Activity Is Enough?

Lesson Objectives

After reading this lesson, you should be able to

1. name and describe the guidelines for physical activity for people of different ages;

2. name and describe the three principles of exercise, threshold of training, target zone, and target ceiling;

3. describe the four parts of the FITT formula and describe the importance of volume and patterns of physical activity; and

4. describe the five types of physical activity included in the Physical Activity Pyramid.

Lesson Vocabulary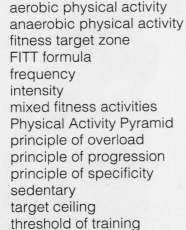

aerobic physical activity
anaerobic physical activity
fitness target zone
FITT formula
frequency
intensity
mixed fitness activities
Physical Activity Pyramid
principle of overload
principle of progression
principle of specificity
sedentary
target ceiling
threshold of training
time
type

How much physical activity is enough? This question might seem very simple, but the answer can be complicated, especially if you're just beginning an activity program. In this lesson, you'll learn how much physical activity is right for you.

Physical Activity Guidelines for Americans

Every 10 years the U.S. Department of Health and Human Services releases its Physical Activity Guidelines for Americans. The first guidelines were published in 2008 and the most recent guidelines were published in 2018. Some guidelines for people of different ages are described in table 6.1.

The original guidelines indicated that only activity in bouts of 10 minutes or more counted toward your daily 60-minute goal. The new guidelines removed this requirement, allowing shorter bouts to count and encouraging people to do physical activity whenever they can. All activity counts.

> I think the best way to be active for 60 minutes a day is to find activities that you really enjoy. If it is fun, you will do it.
>
> *Zara Arain*

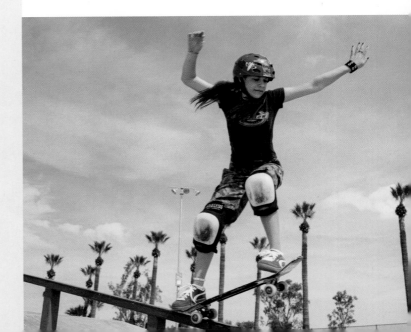

TABLE 6.1   **Physical Activity Guidelines for Americans**

Age group	Guidelines
Preschool (ages 3–5)	Participate in a variety of physical activities throughout the day to enhance growth and development.
Children and teens (ages 6–17)	Participate in a variety of enjoyable, age-appropriate, moderate to vigorous physical activities for 60 minutes or more each day. • *Aerobic activity.* Most of the 60 minutes should be in moderate or vigorous aerobic activity. Vigorous physical activity should be performed at least 3 days per week. • *Muscle fitness activity.* Exercise that enhances all aspects of muscle fitness (strength, muscular endurance, power) should be part of the daily 60 minutes of activity at least 3 days per week. • *Bone-strengthening activity.* Exercise that strengthens the bones should be part of the daily 60 minutes of activity at least 3 days per week.
Adults (ages 18 and up)	Adults should move more and sit less throughout the day. Some activity is better than none. • *Aerobic activity.* Adults should participate in at least 150 to 300 minutes of moderate or 75 to 150 minutes of vigorous aerobic activity each week. Moderate and vigorous activity can be combined to meet the guideline. Preferably, the activity should be spread out through the week. • *Muscle fitness activity.* Adults should participate in muscle fitness exercise (for all major muscle groups) on two or more days per week.
Older adults	The key guidelines for younger adults also apply to older adults. Additional guidelines also apply. • *Functional fitness.* Older adults should include activities that promote fitness for daily living, including balance exercise. • *Age-appropriate activity.* Older adults should adapt activity based on health status and fitness level.

Adapted from the Physical Activity Guidelines for Americans (USDHHS).

Other new information in the report includes the following:

- An emphasis on sitting less, including less screen time
- Activity guidelines for very young Americans (see table 6.1)
- Activity information for people with chronic health conditions and disabilities
- Activity information for those who are pregnant or have just given birth
- New evidence about the health benefits of physical activity, such as reduced cancer risk, reduced fall risk among older people, improved sleep, improved functional fitness, enhanced wellness, and the sense of "feeling good"

Principles of Physical Activity

Consider this example. Mia has been exercising for several months. Every day, she does the same physical activities for about 15 minutes. Initially, Mia saw some positive results from her program: She was no longer tired at the end of her exercise, and a self-assessment showed that her cardiorespiratory endurance had improved. Lately, however, Mia has felt disappointed because her strength and flexibility haven't been improving as much as they did at first. Mia wants to know what she's doing wrong. For some clues to the answer, let's look at the three principles of exercise: overload, progression, and specificity.

FIT FACT
In 2020, the World Health Organization (WHO) released its physical activity guidelines, which are very similar to the Physical Activity Guidelines for Americans. The guidelines recommend that teens get vigorous physical activity at least three days a week. The WHO indicates that four to five million lives could be saved worldwide if people were active enough to meet the guidelines.

Principle of Overload

The most basic law of physical activity is the **principle of overload**, which states that the only way to produce fitness and health benefits through physical activity is to require your body to do more than it normally does. Increased demand on your body—overload—forces it to adapt. Your body was designed to be active, so if you do nothing (underload), your fitness will decrease, and you will increase your risk of hypokinetic disease.

Because Mia is no longer overloading when she exercises, she is maintaining but no longer gaining fitness and health benefits. If she wants to continue improving her strength and flexibility, she'll have to increase the amount of her physical activity.

Principle of Progression

The **principle of progression** states that the amount and intensity of your exercise should be increased gradually. After a while, your body adapts to an increase in physical activity (load), and the activity gets easier for you to perform. When this happens, you can gradually increase your activity.

Figure 6.1 shows the minimum overload you need in order to build physical fitness, called your **threshold of training**. Performing activity above your threshold builds your fitness, whereas exercise below the threshold is not enough to produce benefits. Because Mia has exercised for several months at the same level, she may now be exercising below her threshold of training for at least some parts of fitness.

This correct range of physical activity is called your **fitness target zone**, typically shortened to just *target zone*. It begins with the threshold of training and has an upper limit called the **target ceiling**. Activities above the target ceiling (excessive exercise) can increase risk of injury and soreness and may produce less than optimal benefits. Some people think you have to experience pain in order to gain fitness, but the principle of progression makes clear that "no pain, no gain" is a myth. If you experience pain when you exercise, you're probably overloading too much or too quickly for your body to adjust.

Principle of Specificity

The **principle of specificity** states that the particular type of exercise you perform determines the particular benefit you receive. Different kinds and amounts of activity produce different benefits and may not be equally good at promoting all types of fitness. For example, Mia jogs on a track several days a week, but she does not do stretching exercises as often as she should. She may also need to use more resistance in her muscle fitness exercises.

In addition, exercises performed for specific body parts, such as the calf muscles, may provide benefits only for those parts. For example, if Mia does exercises only for her calf muscles, she will not build the muscles in her back, shoulders, arms, or other parts of her legs.

Applying the FITT Formula

You now know that you must do more physical activity than normal to build fitness and that

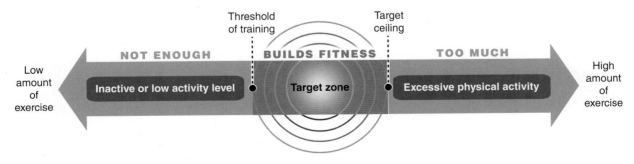

Figure 6.1   The fitness target zone.

120

you should gradually increase your physical activity in order to stay within your fitness target zone. But how much physical activity do you need?

To help you apply the principles of exercise, you can use the **FITT formula** to determine the right amount of physical activity.

The FITT Formula

Each letter in the acronym FITT represents a key factor in determining how much physical activity is enough: frequency, intensity, time, and type. The four factors in the FITT formula are described here.

• *Frequency refers to how often you do physical activity.* For physical activity to be beneficial, you must do it several days a week. Optimal **frequency** depends on the type of activity you're doing and the part of fitness you want to develop. To develop strength, for example, you might need to exercise two days a week. To lose fat, you should exercise daily.

• *Intensity refers to how hard you perform physical activity.* If the activity is too easy, you will not build fitness or gain other benefits. But remember— extremely vigorous activity can be harmful if you don't work up to it gradually. **Intensity** is determined differently depending on the activity and the type of fitness you want to build. For example, you can use your heart rate to determine your intensity of activity for building cardiorespiratory endurance, whereas you would use the amount of weight lifted to determine the intensity for building strength.

• *Time refers to how long you do physical activity.* As with frequency and intensity, the length of **time** for which you should do physical activity depends on the activity. For example, to build flexibility you should exercise muscles in each muscle group for 15 seconds or more, but to build cardiorespiratory endurance you need to be vigorously active for a minimum of 20 minutes.

• *Type refers to the kind of activity you do to build a specific part of fitness or gain a specific benefit.* One **type** of activity may be good for building one part of fitness but not another. For example, doing vigorous aerobics builds your cardio-respiratory endurance but does little to develop your flexibility. Throughout this book, you'll learn how to apply the FITT formula to different activities that build specific parts of physical fitness. Once you determine the type of activity, you can drop the second *T* in FITT and determine the frequency, intensity, and time (or FIT) for each specific activity. FIT information is given for each type of activity included in the Physical Activity Pyramid (see figure 6.2).

Volume and Progression

The American College of Sports Medicine (ACSM) uses the FITT formula for prescribing how much physical activity is enough but also includes the letters VP

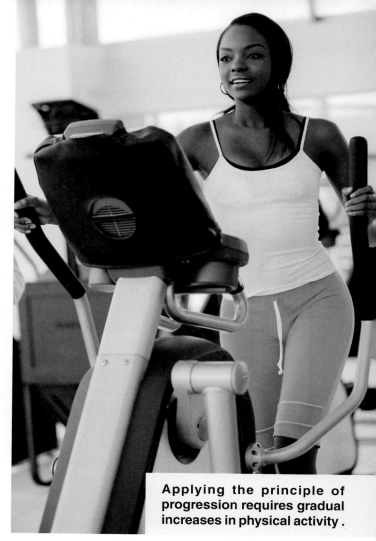

Applying the principle of progression requires gradual increases in physical activity.

FIT FACT
FITT is a mnemonic used to remember the four key factors in applying the principles of physical activity: frequency, intensity, time, and type.

after FITT (FITT-VP). In this version, V stands for the volume (total amount) of exercise, determined both by how long you are active and the intensity of your activity. For example, you can do the same total volume of activity by either performing a moderate activity for a longer time or a vigorous activity for a shorter time. As you learn more about the FITT formula, you will learn how volume of exercise can be adjusted by altering the intensity and time of the workout. Over a longer time, the frequency of exercise also contributes to volume (e.g., doing a workout four days a week will have twice the volume as doing the same workout two days a week).

The P in FITT-VP is to remind people of the importance of progression—that is, applying the FITT formula gradually. As you work through this book, you'll see only the acronyms FIT and FITT, but you should also keep volume and progression (VP) in mind as you develop your personal activity plan.

Patterns of Physical Activity

A pattern is a schedule you use to accumulate minutes of physical activity. One pattern is continuous activity, in which you do all of your physical activity for the day in one continuous session (for example, taking a 30-minute walk).

The second pattern is accumulated activity, in which you do a few minutes of activity many different times during the day rather than doing all activity at once. This pattern is acceptable if daily and weekly activity guidelines are met.

The third pattern is that of the "weekend warrior." This pattern is marked by a long bout of physical activity (often several hours at a time) performed one day a week. The person is then inactive on the remaining days of the week. Adults often do extended activity on weekends because of their work commitments during the week—thus the name "weekend warrior." The newest physical activity guidelines suggest that it is best to have physical activity spread throughout the week. However, recent research indicates that activity done in long sessions one or two days a week can be beneficial if the person is otherwise fit and healthy.

The Physical Activity Pyramid

The second T in FITT is for the type of activity that you perform. For each type of activity, there is a FIT formula. To make it easy for you to remember the different types of activity, the **Physical Activity Pyramid** was developed (see figure 6.2). Each step of the Physical Activity Pyramid includes descriptions and examples of

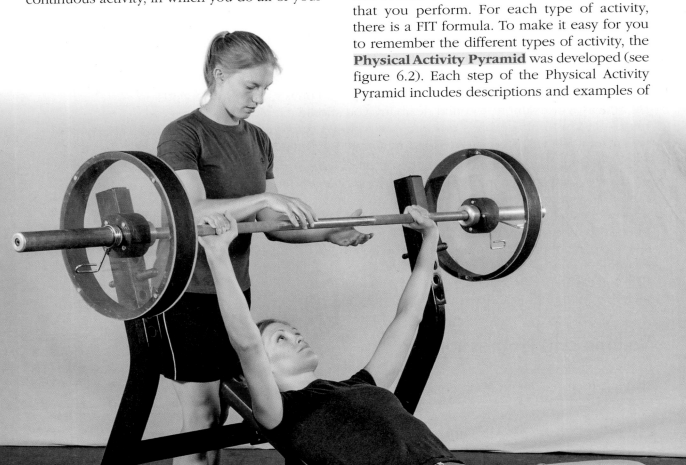

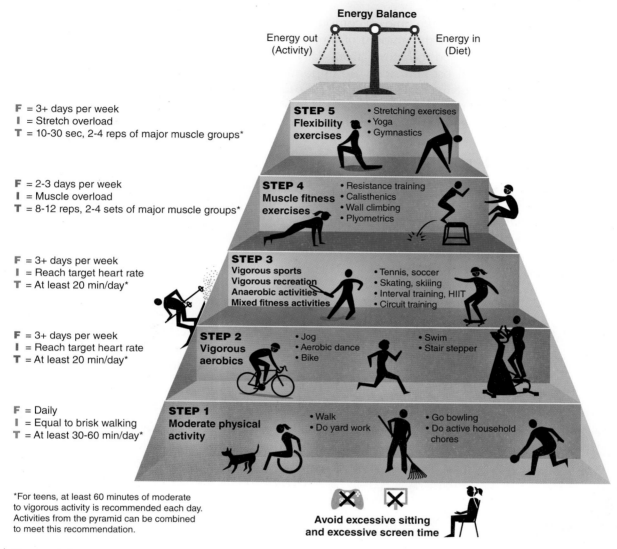

Figure 6.2 The new Physical Activity Pyramid for Teens.

© C.B. Corbin, from *Fitness for Life*, 7th ed. (Champaign, IL: Human Kinetics, 2021).

the five types of physical activity. A summary of the FIT formula is provided for each type of activity to help you decide how much activity to perform. To meet the recommended 60 minutes of daily activity, you can choose from the different types of activity. For optimal benefits, you should perform activities from all steps of the pyramid each week, following the FIT formula for each step.

Avoiding Sedentary Living and Inactivity

Just below the Physical Activity Pyramid (see figure 6.2) you'll notice three pictures intended to emphasize the importance of avoiding sedentary and inactive behavior. A person is **sedentary** when doing low-energy activities such as lying down and sitting. The pictures below the pyramid are meant to discourage too much sitting and excessive screen time during the day. A recent survey of children and teens in the United States found that they watch TV for an average of nearly four hours a day. Sixty-eight percent of teens have a TV in their room, and of course many also spend screen time on computers, video games, movies, and cell phones, more than doubling the amount of time they spend watching a screen.

We all need to recover from daily stresses and prepare for new challenges, so periods of rest and sleep are important for good health. Some activities of daily living involving inactivity—such as studying, reading, and even a moderate amount of screen time—are appropriate. However, excessive sedentary behavior is harmful to your health.

Moderate Physical Activity

Moderate physical activity, the first step in the Physical Activity Pyramid, should be performed daily or nearly every day. It involves physical activities equal in intensity to brisk walking. It includes some activities of normal daily living (also called *lifestyle activities*), such as yardwork and housework (e.g., raking leaves, mopping). It also includes sports that are not vigorous, such as bowling and golf. Some sports can be either moderate or vigorous—for example, shooting basketballs is typically a moderate activity, whereas playing a full-court game is vigorous. National guidelines recommend 60 minutes of moderate to vigorous activity each day for teens. Moderate activity is the most common type of physical activity for most people and accounts for the biggest share of daily activity. It is well suited for people of varying abilities and is associated with many of the health benefits of activity described in this book, such as controlling body fat levels.

Vigorous Aerobics

Step 2 of the Physical Activity Pyramid represents vigorous aerobics, such as jogging, swimming, biking, and aerobic dance. Activities at this step are intense enough to increase your breathing and heart rate and make you sweat, but not so vigorous that your body cannot supply enough oxygen to perform the activities for long periods of time without stopping. Like moderate activity, they provide many health and wellness benefits, and they're especially helpful for building a high level of cardiorespiratory endurance. You should perform vigorous activities at least three days a week in order to meet national activity guidelines.

Vigorous Sports, Recreation, Anaerobics, and Mixed Fitness Activities

Like vigorous aerobics, vigorous recreation and sport activities (represented in step 3 of the Physical Activity Pyramid) require your heart to beat faster than normal and cause you to breathe faster

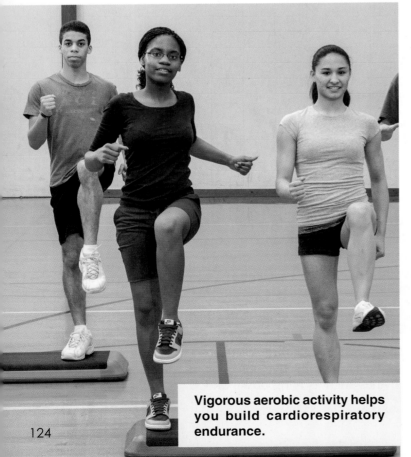

Vigorous aerobic activity helps you build cardiorespiratory endurance.

and sweat more. Unlike vigorous aerobics, vigorous sport and recreation often involve short bursts of activity (anaerobic activity) followed by short periods of rest (as in basketball, football, soccer, and tennis). These activities provide similar fitness, health, and wellness benefits to those of vigorous aerobics. They also help you build motor skills and contribute to healthy weight management. As with vigorous aerobics, you can use vigorous sport and recreation to meet the national activity recommendation when performed at least three days a week.

Other anaerobic activities can also be performed to meet national physical activity guidelines, such as interval training, which involves repeated bouts of vigorous activity alternated with rest periods. **Mixed fitness activities** consist of several types of activities, such as vigorous aerobics, anaerobics, and muscle fitness exercises (step 4). You will learn more about anaerobic and mixed fitness activities in chapter 9.

Muscle Fitness Exercises

Step 4 in the Physical Activity Pyramid represents muscle fitness exercises, which build strength, muscular endurance, and power. Muscle fitness exercises include both resistance training (with weights or machines) and moving your own body weight (as in rock climbing, calisthenics, and jumping). This type of exercise produces general health and wellness benefits, as well as better performance, improved body appearance, a healthier back, better posture, and stronger bones. These exercises can be used to meet national activity guidelines and should be performed at least three days a week.

Flexibility Exercises

Step 5 of the Physical Activity Pyramid represents flexibility exercises. The ACSM indicates that poor flexibility is related to low back pain. Evidence also indicates that flexibility exercises and other activities that improve flexibility, such as yoga (see figure 6.3) and tai chi, can benefit functional fitness, improve postural stability

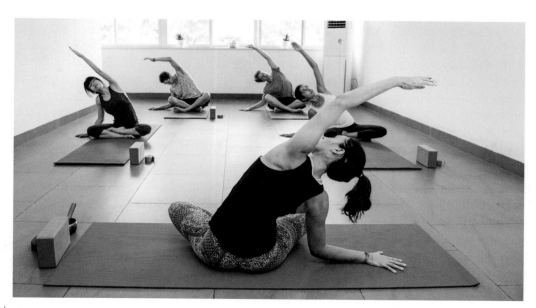

Figure 6.3 Yoga is one type of physical activity for improving flexibility.

and balance, and reduce risk of falling among older people. There is also some evidence that flexibility exercises may reduce soreness and prevent injuries. In addition, flexibility exercises improve your performance in activities such as gymnastics and dance and are used in therapy to help people who have been injured. You will learn more about stretching exercises to improve flexibility in chapter 12. To build and maintain flexibility, you should perform flexibility exercises at least three days a week.

Balancing Energy

The top of the pyramid presents a balance scale, illustrating the need for energy balance—meaning that the calories in the food you eat each day are equal to the calories you expend in exercise each day. Energy balance is essential to maintaining a healthy body composition.

LESSON REVIEW

1. What are the guidelines for physical activity for people of different ages?
2. What are the three principles of exercise, and how are they related to the threshold of training, the target zone, and the target ceiling?
3. What are the four parts of the FITT formula, and how are they related to volume and patterns of physical activity?
4. What are the five types of activity included in the Physical Activity Pyramid, and what are some examples of each?

SELF-ASSESSMENT: **PACER and Trunk Lift**

In this assessment, you'll perform two tests: one to assess your cardiorespiratory endurance and another to measure the flexibility and fitness of your back and trunk muscles. If you have not done so already, practice each test before performing them for a score. Record your scores and fitness ratings for the two tests as directed by your teacher. Performing these tests will provide information that you can use in preparing a personal fitness profile and a personal physical activity plan. If you're working with a partner, remember that self-assessment information is confidential and shouldn't be shared without the permission of the person being tested.

PACER (Progressive Aerobic Cardiovascular Endurance Run, or 20-meter shuttle run)

Originally called the 20-meter shuttle run (still used in many countries), Dr. Jack Rutherford submitted the name PACER in a contest designed to create a new name for the test that would be easy to remember.

The test can be scored in two different ways. In this book, you'll use the number of laps performed to determine your fitness rating score. Using laps makes it easy for you to see if you improve after performing your personal activity plan.

The objective of the test is to run back and forth across a distance of 20 meters (almost 22 yards) as many times as you can at a predetermined pace (pacing is based on signals from a special audio recording provided by your instructor). This measures cardiorespiratory endurance, and higher scores are related to reduced risk of conditions such as heart disease.

1. Start at a line located 20 meters from a second line. When you hear the beep from the audio track, run across the 20-meter area and touch the second line with your foot just before the audio track beeps again. Turn around and get ready to run back.

2. At the sound of the next beep, run back to the line where you began. Touch the line with your foot. Again, make sure to wait for the beep before running back.

3. Continue to run back and forth from one line to the other, touching the line each time. The beeps will come faster and faster, causing you to run faster and faster. The test is finished when you twice fail to reach the opposite side before the beep.

4. Your score is the number of times you ran the 20-meter distance from one line to the other before your test was finished. Using laps as your score allows you to easily test yourself to see how you improve over time. This method of scoring provides you with a good indicator of your cardiorespiratory endurance, which is a measure of functional fitness—your ability to function effectively in daily living.

5. Use table 6.2 to determine your rating. Record your score and rating.

6. If you want to do a FitnessGram report, you'll need to convert your laps score to an aerobic capacity score. A chart for the conversion is available on the FitnessGram website and may be available from your teacher. Aerobic capacity is discussed further in chapter 8, Cardiorespiratory Endurance.

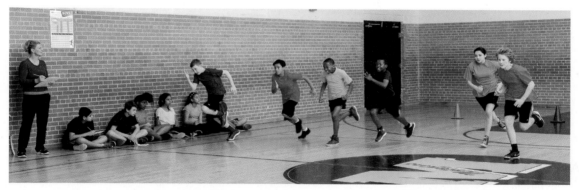

The PACER test assesses cardiorespiratory endurance and can be used to estimate aerobic capacity.

TABLE 6.2   Rating Chart for PACER (Laps)

	13 years old		14 years old		15 years old		16 years old		17 years or older	
	Male	Female	Male	Female	Male	Female	Male	Female	Male	Female
High performance	≥36	≥31	≥45	≥34	≥54	≥38	≥60	≥40	≥67	≥50
Good fitness	29–35	25–30	36–44	27–33	42–53	30–37	47–59	32–39	54–66	38–49
Marginal fitness	23–28	19–24	28–35	21–26	32–41	23–29	36–46	25–31	42–53	30–37
Low fitness	≤22	≤18	≤27	≤20	≤31	≤22	≤35	≤24	≤41	≤29

Based on data provided by G. Welk.

TRUNK LIFT (back muscle fitness and back and trunk muscle flexibility)

1. Lie facedown with your arms at your sides and your hands under or just beside your thighs.

2. Lift the upper part of your body very slowly so that your chin, chest, and shoulders come off the floor. Lift your trunk as high as possible, to a maximum of 12 inches (30 centimeters). Hold this position for three seconds while a partner measures how far your chin is from the floor. Your partner should hold the ruler at least 1 inch (2.5 centimeters) in front of your chin. Look straight ahead so that your chin is not tipped abnormally upward.

3. Perform the trunk lift twice for the required three seconds. Do not record scores above 12 inches (30 centimeters).

   Caution: The ruler should not be placed directly under your chin, in case you have to lower your trunk unexpectedly.

4. Use table 6.3 to determine your fitness rating. Record your score and rating.

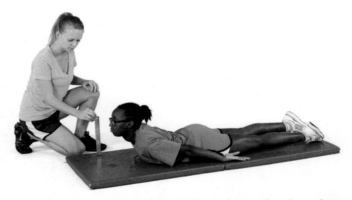

The trunk lift measures the fitness and flexibility of your back and trunk muscles.

TABLE 6.3   Rating Chart for Trunk Lift

Rating	Inches
High performance	11–12
Good fitness	9–10
Marginal fitness	7–8
Low fitness	≤6

To convert centimeters to inches, divide by 2.54.

Data based on *FitnessGram*.

How Much Fitness Is Enough?

Lesson Objectives

After reading this lesson, you should be able to

1. define *test battery* and describe several different types of fitness test batteries;

2. describe the four fitness rating categories and how they apply to your physical activity program;

3. describe four factors that influence physical fitness; and

4. explain how a person can attain good health and fitness even if some factors make it difficult to succeed.

Lesson Vocabulary

criterion-referenced health standard
maturation
test battery

You now know that physical activity is necessary to build each part of physical fitness. But exactly how much fitness do you need? In this lesson, you'll learn some ways to decide how much fitness is enough for you.

The Types of Health-Related Fitness Assessments

This book includes many different types of health-related fitness self-assessments, most of which are part of formal fitness test batteries such as FitnessGram, ALPHA-FIT, and Eurofit. In the following paragraphs, several fitness test batteries are described. From the different tests, you will choose self-assessments that work best for you as you prepare your own personal fitness **test battery**.

National and International Fitness Test Batteries

Experts in physical education and exercise physiology have worked together to develop various physical fitness test batteries. A test battery is a group of tests designed to assess all parts of physical fitness. As you've learned, FitnessGram

Being fit makes me healthier, but I want to be fit enough to do the things I enjoy doing like rock climbing, mountain biking, and skiing.

David Riordan

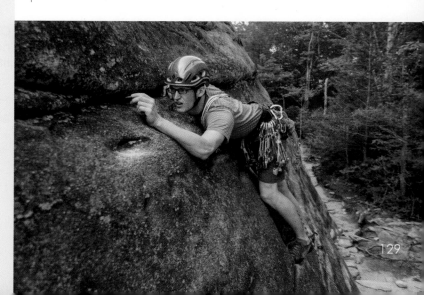

129

is a widely used fitness test battery that has been adopted as the national assessment program for both the President's Council on Sports, Fitness, and Nutrition (PCSFN) and the Society of Health and Physical Educators (SHAPE America). FitnessGram includes the PACER, 90-degree push-up, curl-up, back-saver sit-and-reach, trunk lift, and BMI. ALPHA-FIT and Eurofit are similar fitness test batteries widely used in Europe. Both include the PACER and the BMI as well as grip strength, standing long jump, and skinfold measurements.

Your Personal Fitness Test Battery

In this book, you'll try many assessments that are included in popular fitness test batteries. You will perform the test items in the FitnessGram, ALPHA-FIT, and Eurofit batteries, as well as several other tests. For all tests in this book, you'll use the *Fitness for Life* rating system, but you can also learn how to use standards and ratings from other test batteries. What's most important is that you learn to test your own fitness and use the results to plan for your own fitness and physical activity.

Fitness Standards and Rating Categories

Sometimes people judge their fitness by comparing themselves with others. If they score higher on a fitness test than other people, they consider themselves fit. This type of comparison creates several problems. First, it suggests that only a few people can be fit. Second, it suggests that only high test scores are adequate for being fit. In this lesson, you'll learn why neither of these suggestions is true.

Experts agree that you should judge fitness using **criterion-referenced health standards**. The word *standard* refers to an established amount or quantity, and the word *criterion* is a marker used to establish the standard. A criterion-referenced standard for health-related fitness therefore refers to the amount of fitness you need in order to achieve good health. This type of standard does not require you to compare yourself with others. It does require you to have enough fitness to

- enjoy your free time,
- achieve wellness benefits,
- function effectively in your daily life,
- meet emergencies, and
- reduce your risk of health problems.

As described in the first section of this lesson, you'll learn to do many self-assessments for each of the health-related parts of physical fitness. In this book, we use a rating system based on criterion-referenced health standards. It is similar to the rating systems used in test batteries such as FitnessGram, and we use it here so that you can rate your fitness in all of the tests included in this book by means of the same system.

To rate yourself in each of the six parts of health-related physical fitness, you'll use one of the four categories shown in figure 6.4. If you attain a rating of "good fitness" for all six fitness areas, you'll achieve the basic health and wellness standards of physical fitness.

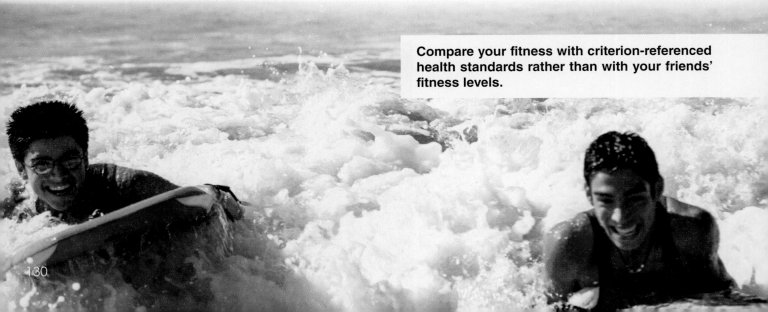

Compare your fitness with criterion-referenced health standards rather than with your friends' fitness levels.

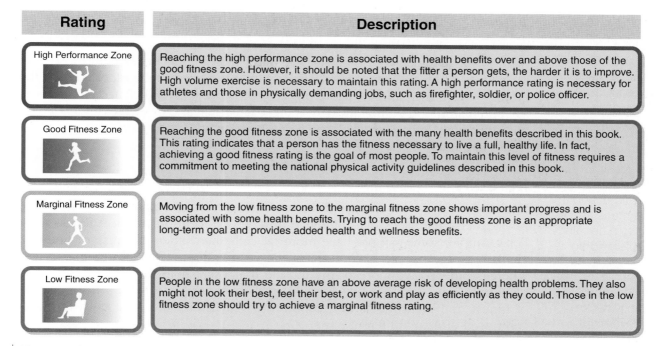

Rating	Description
High Performance Zone	Reaching the high performance zone is associated with health benefits over and above those of the good fitness zone. However, it should be noted that the fitter a person gets, the harder it is to improve. High volume exercise is necessary to maintain this rating. A high performance rating is necessary for athletes and those in physically demanding jobs, such as firefighter, soldier, or police officer.
Good Fitness Zone	Reaching the good fitness zone is associated with the many health benefits described in this book. This rating indicates that a person has the fitness necessary to live a full, healthy life. In fact, achieving a good fitness rating is the goal of most people. To maintain this level of fitness requires a commitment to meeting the national physical activity guidelines described in this book.
Marginal Fitness Zone	Moving from the low fitness zone to the marginal fitness zone shows important progress and is associated with some health benefits. Trying to reach the good fitness zone is an appropriate long-term goal and provides added health and wellness benefits.
Low Fitness Zone	People in the low fitness zone have an above average risk of developing health problems. They also might not look their best, feel their best, or work and play as efficiently as they could. Those in the low fitness zone should try to achieve a marginal fitness rating.

Figure 6.4   Rating zones for health-related fitness.

Factors Influencing Physical Fitness

Physical activity is the most important thing you can do to improve or maintain your health-related physical fitness. Fortunately, it is also something that you can control. You can choose the kinds of activity you want to do and schedule a regular time to do them. But as figure 6.5 shows, physical activity is not the only factor that contributes to your physical fitness. Other important factors are maturation, age, heredity, environment, and lifestyle choices such as nutrition and stress management.

Maturation

Physical **maturation** means becoming physically full grown and developed. It begins in earnest in your early teen years because of hormones that promote growth and development. Some people mature earlier than others, and early developers often do better on physical fitness tests than those who mature later. But ultimately, time is the great equalizer. We all develop fully over time, and it is not unusual for late developers to achieve fitness levels that equal or exceed those who develop early.

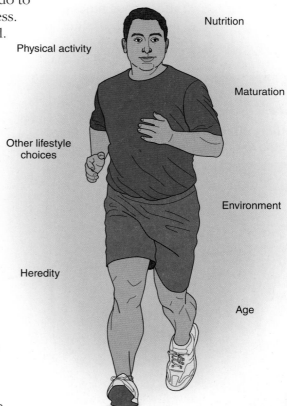

Figure 6.5   Various factors influence your physical fitness.

Age

Studies show that older teens perform better on fitness tests than younger teens. Even in the same class, those who are older typically do better than those who are younger. This difference results mostly from the fact that the older you are, the more you've grown and the more physically mature you're likely to be. However, age and maturation do not always parallel each other, and in such cases a younger but more physically mature person could have an advantage in performing physical fitness tests.

Heredity

Heredity involves the characteristics we inherit from our parents, including the physical characteristics that influence how we perform on physical fitness tests. For example, some people have more fat cells than others because of heredity. Similarly, some people have more of the muscle fibers that help them run fast, whereas others have more of the muscle fibers that help them run a long time without fatigue. Each person's heredity enables better performance in some areas of fitness and makes it harder to perform well in others. Fortunately, fitness is composed of many different parts.

Environment

Your fitness is also affected by environmental factors, such as where you live (city, suburbs, country), your school environment, and the availability (or lack) of places to play and do other types of physical activity. Even your social environment can affect your fitness, including the friends you choose. For example, people who live near parks and those who have active friends are typically more active than those who don't.

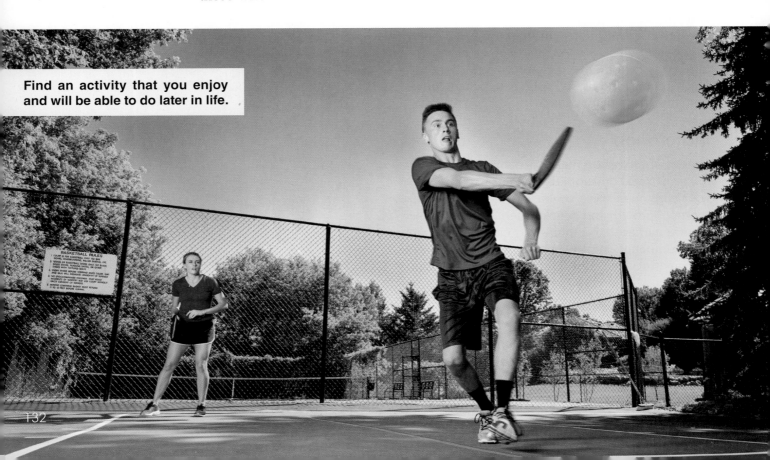

Find an activity that you enjoy and will be able to do later in life.

Anyone Can Succeed

Because many factors contribute to physical fitness, it is possible for some people who do relatively little physical activity to achieve relatively good fitness scores while in their teens. These people probably matured early and inherited physical characteristics that help them do well on physical fitness tests. However, they may also be in danger of concluding that they don't need to do physical activity. This may be true if they care only about doing well on fitness tests while they're young, but it will not be true for a lifetime. As people get older, they can no longer gain a fitness advantage from early physical maturation or the energy of youth. Physical inactivity will affect everyone sooner or later. Therefore, if you want lifetime fitness, health, and wellness, you need to perform regular physical activity and make healthy lifestyle choices.

Just as some people enjoy fitness advantages because of age, maturation, and heredity, others face disadvantages. Some find it hard to get high fitness scores even if they do physical activity, and they may become discouraged. If you're one of these people, avoid comparing yourself with others. Try to achieve a good fitness rating rather than worrying about getting a high performance rating. In fact, studies show that people who are good at sports in school but do not remain active later in life are less healthy and die earlier than those who do regular activity throughout their lives, even if they were not especially good performers when they were young.

Anyone can do physical activity. And no matter who you are, physical activity is crucial to your fitness, health, and wellness. With regular physical activity, you can achieve a good fitness rating in all parts of fitness.

> Do not let what you cannot do interfere with what you can do.
>
> *John Wooden,*
> *basketball coach*

FIT FACT

Teens who walk or ride a bicycle to school are more active overall than those who do not. Specifically, they get an average of 16 minutes more activity each day, and that difference in itself is more than 25 percent of the recommended amount of daily activity.

LESSON REVIEW

1. What is a fitness test battery, and what are two popular batteries?
2. What are the four fitness rating categories, and how do they apply to your physical activity program?
3. What are the four factors that influence physical fitness?
4. How can a person attain good health and fitness even if they have factors that make it difficult to build a high level of fitness?

TAKING CHARGE: **Learning to Self-Monitor**

An activity log is a written account of your physical activities during a specified time. It's a way to keep track of what you do so that you can tell whether you're meeting your activity goals. *Self-monitoring* refers to any of a variety of techniques for keeping track of your behavior (for example, a log, diary, or step counter).

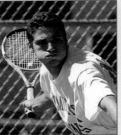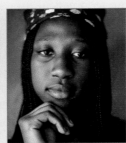

Mark enjoyed playing tennis on the weekends. He would start out full of energy, but he lacked the endurance to play well for a complete match. His instructor suggested that he do some daily activities to improve his endurance. For several weeks, Mark reported that he faithfully engaged in the activities. But Mark's instructor was a little skeptical based on his lack of improvement. Finally, she suggested that Mark keep a log of all the times that he did the activities, and the results were eye opening: "Boy, was I surprised," said Mark. "I usually didn't spend as much time as I thought on each activity. I really thought I was doing well until I saw the results written down."

Erica's situation was different. She had knee surgery and was ordered to limit both the kinds and the amount of her activity and to follow a schedule of rehabilitation exercises. She was also told to elevate her leg whenever possible. Her leg was often sore and swollen at the end of the day, so her physical therapist suggested that she keep a daily log. Erica discovered that she was spending much more time on her feet than she had intended. As a result, she realized that she had to curtail her activities so that her knee could heal.

FOR DISCUSSION

How did keeping a log help Mark and Erica? What are some other ways in which a log might help someone? What other ways might Mark and Erica self-monitor their physical activity levels? Consider the guidelines in the following Self-Management feature as you answer these discussion questions.

SELF-MANAGEMENT: **Skills for Self-Monitoring**

Most adults tend to underestimate how much they eat and overestimate how much physical activity they get. People also make other errors in estimating what they do. For example, we often underestimate how much television we watch and how much money we spend on nonessential items. One name for keeping track of what we do is *self-monitoring*. We all self-monitor our behavior in informal ways, but sometimes it's necessary to make formal assessments if we want accuracy. You can self-monitor your behaviors to help you set goals and then evaluate to see if you're meeting your goals. Self-monitoring of physical activity is sometimes referred to as *record keeping*. Use the following guidelines to effectively monitor your physical activity.

- *Keep a written log.* Make a formal record of your physical activities by using an activity log.

- *Consider using an activity monitor.* Many different watchlike devices that include internal computer chips (e.g., Apple watch, Fitbit) can be used to count daily steps, time in physical activity, and sometimes heart rate. Pedometers are similar devices that are typically less expensive and are worn on your belt, your arm, or carried in your pocket. They count the number of steps you take and sometimes time spent in activity. Either of these devices gives you objective information that you can record in your activity log.

- *Record information as frequently as you can.* The longer you wait before you write down what you do, the more likely you are to make an error. Write things down as soon as possible after you do them.
- *Start by monitoring your current activity pattern.* To get an accurate picture of your activity level, monitor yourself for at least three days. At least one of the days should be a weekend day; most people's activity pattern is different on weekends than on weekdays.
- *Use your current activity pattern to help you determine your goals and plans.* People who are already active can set higher goals than those who are less active (or just beginning).
- *Determine how much activity you do in each area of the Physical Activity Pyramid.* For each type of activity included in the pyramid, determine your frequency, intensity, and time (FIT).
- *Write down your goals and plans and keep records to see whether you fulfill them.* Putting your goals and plans in writing can help you self-monitor. Keep records to see whether you did what you planned to do. Keep a diary or an activity chart.

You can also use these guidelines to monitor other behaviors, such as your eating patterns.

ACADEMIC CONNECTION: **Percentages**

The term *percentage* is used to express a portion or part of a whole. The whole is 100 percent. In a group of 100 people, one person represents 1 percent of the whole group. As an example, we often describe the activity levels of teens and adults in terms of percentages.

Among adults in the United States, 20 percent meet national activity guidelines (150 minutes a week) and 80 percent do not. Among teens, 29 percent meet national activity guidelines (60 minutes a day); 71 percent do not.

STUDENT ACTIVITY

You can calculate the percentage of a group that meets a health standard by dividing the number of people in the group who meet the standard by the total number of people in the group. Scores for the trunk lift test for one group of teens are presented in table 6.4. A score of 9 or higher (shown in bold) is required to meet the good fitness standard for this test. To determine the percentage of teens meeting the good fitness standard for the trunk lift, count the number who met the standard and divide it by the total number of teens in the group. What percentage of teens in the group meet the good fitness standard?

TABLE 6.4 **Distribution of Trunk Lift Test Scores for One Group**

					8				
				7	8				
				7	8	**9**	**10**		
			6	7	8	**9**	**10**	**11**	
		5	6	7	8	**9**	**10**	**11**	
3	4	5	6	7	8	**9**	**10**	**11**	**12**
3	4	5	6	7	8	**9**	**10**	**11**	**12**

CHECK YOUR ANSWERS

40 percent (16 students met the standard, and there are 40 total students; 16 ÷ 40 = 0.40)

Taking Action: **Physical Activity Pyramid Circuit**

The Physical Activity Pyramid illustrates how much of each type of physical activity you need in order to build fitness, health, and wellness. For example, you need to perform moderate physical activity (the first step of the pyramid) almost every day to get health benefits, whereas you need to perform muscle fitness activities only three times per week. The area *below* the pyramid represents inactivity or sedentary living. Aside from sleeping, you should minimize your daily sedentary time. **Take action** by performing the Physical Activity Pyramid circuit, an exercise circuit that includes activities from each step of the Physical Activity Pyramid.

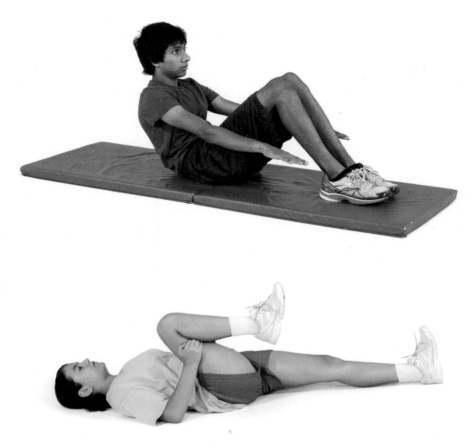

The Physical Activity Pyramid circuit includes activities from each step of the pyramid, including step 4 (muscle fitness) and step 5 (flexibility).

CHAPTER REVIEW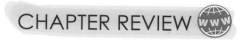

Reviewing Concepts and Vocabulary

Answer items 1 through 5 by correctly completing each sentence with a word or phrase.

1. The diagram with five steps that helps you understand the types of physical activity is called the _____.

2. The minimum amount of overload needed to achieve physical fitness is called the _____.

3. In addition to healthy lifestyle choices such as being active and eating well, age, maturation, _____, and the environment are factors that affect your physical fitness.

4. If you achieve a _____ fitness rating, you're probably at the level of fitness you need in order to live a full, healthy life.

5. The preferred standard used to rate fitness based on health is called a _____.

For items 6 through 10, match each term in column 1 with the appropriate phrase in column 2.

6. target ceiling
7. intensity
8. progression
9. specificity
10. overload

a. how hard you perform physical activity
b. gradual increase of exercise
c. upper limit of beneficial physical activity
d. performing more exercise than you normally do
e. exercising for one fitness part

For items 11 through 15, respond to each statement or question.

11. What is the FITT formula, and what does each of the four letters mean?

12. Describe the four health-related fitness ratings (zones).

13. Explain why your physical activity program should include activities from all steps of the Physical Activity Pyramid.

14. What are some guidelines for self-monitoring physical activity?

15. Explain why you shouldn't compare yourself with others when assessing fitness.

Thinking Critically

Write a paragraph to answer the following question.

A friend tells you that it's important for everyone to attain a high performance fitness rating. Your friend says that if a good rating is the goal, then a high performance rating must be even better. How would you respond? Write a paragraph to explain your answer.

Project

Investigate places in your school and community that offer facilities and equipment you can use to perform activities in the Physical Activity Pyramid. Compile a directory of places, their addresses and phone numbers, their websites, and their facilities and equipment. Distribute the directory to class members or post it on a website that other students can access.

UNIT III

Moderate and Vigorous Physical Activity

CHAPTER 7 **Moderate Physical Activity and Avoiding Sedentary Living**
CHAPTER 8 **Cardiorespiratory Endurance**
CHAPTER 9 **Vigorous Physical Activity**

Healthy People 2030 Goals and Objectives

Overarching Goals

- Attain healthy, thriving lives and well-being, free of preventable disease, disability, injury, and premature death.
- Eliminate health disparities, achieve health equity, and attain health literacy to improve the health and well-being of all.

Objectives

- Reduce the proportion of people who do no physical activity in their free time.
- Increase the proportion of adolescents and adults who do enough aerobic physical activity for health benefits.
- Increase the proportion of teens who participate in daily school physical education.
- Increase the proportion of teens who play sports.
- Increase the proportion of teens who walk or bike to get places.
- Increase the proportion of teens who limit screen time.
- Improve cardiovascular health and reduce the risk of heart related conditions (e.g., high blood pressure, high blood lipids, heart attack).
- Reduce unintentional injuries including brain injuries.

Self-Assessment Features in This Unit

- Walking Test
- Step Test and One-Mile Run Test
- Assessing Jogging Techniques

Taking Charge and Self-Management Features in This Unit

- Learning to Manage Time
- Self-Confidence
- Improving Performance Skills

Taking Action Features in This Unit

- Performing Your Moderate Physical Activity Plan
- Target Heart Rate Workouts
- Performing Your Vigorous Physical Activity Plan

7

Moderate Physical Activity and Avoiding Sedentary Living

In This Chapter

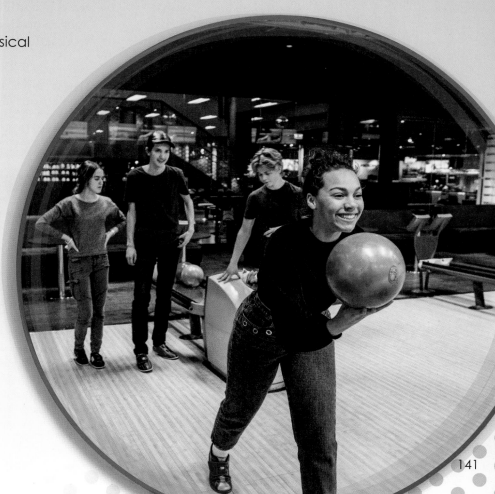

Moderate Physical Activity Facts

Lesson Objectives

After reading this lesson, you should be able to

1. define *moderate physical activity* and the term *MET* and describe several types of moderate physical activity;

2. describe several reasons why you should perform regular moderate physical activity;

3. describe the FIT formula and how to apply it to moderate physical activity; and

4. describe several methods for self-monitoring moderate physical activity.

Lesson Vocabulary

accelerometer
lifestyle physical activity
metabolic equivalent (MET)
MET minute
moderate physical activity
pedometer
physical activity compendium

Have you ever wondered if you can be active without feeling uncomfortable and sweaty? You can, and moderate physical activity is a good way to do it. These activities are easy to do and can be performed by people of all ages and ability levels. They are sometimes considered the foundation of health-enhancing physical activity and thus are appropriately placed at the base of the Physical Activity Pyramid (see figure 7.1).

What Are Moderate Physical Activities?

The term **metabolic equivalent (MET)** comes from the word *metabolism*, which refers to the amount of energy (oxygen) necessary to sustain life, and is used to measure the intensity of exercise. One MET represents the energy expended sitting quietly. Physical activities are rated according to their MET value, from very light to maximal exertion. The harder the body works, the higher the MET value.

I know I need 60 minutes of aerobic physical activity each day. I enjoy walking to school and it helps me to reach my daily activity goal.

De'Wayne Jackson

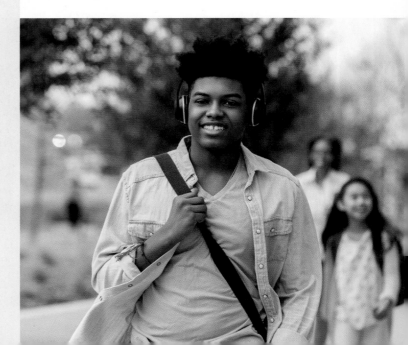

The Physical Activity Guidelines for Americans indicate that **moderate physical activity** requires you to use three to six times as much energy (3 to 6 METs) as sitting quietly (1 MET). A commonly used example of moderate physical activity is brisk walking. The American College of Sports Medicine suggests 100 steps per minute as a good pace for brisk walking.

Moderate physical activities are often divided into the following categories: **lifestyle physical activities**, or tasks done as part of daily life (such as walking to school and doing housework), moderate sports (such as bowling and golf), moderate recreational activities (such as social dancing and biking at a leisurely pace), moderate fitness activities (such as calisthenics), and occupational activities (such as carpentry or landscaping). Table 7.1 presents examples in each of these categories, along with the MET values for each activity. Some of the activities can require more than 6 METs, at which point they are considered vigorous activities.

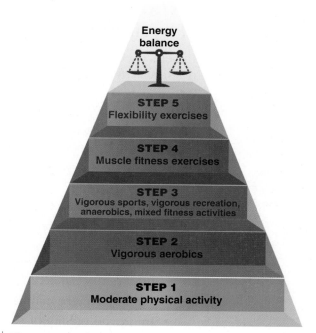

Figure 7.1 Moderate activity provides a foundation for all other activities.

TABLE 7.1 **Moderate Physical Activities for Teens**

Activity type	Description	METs
Lifestyle activities	Walking (brisk)	3.0–5.5
	Yardwork	
	Push mower (no power)	5.0–6.0
	Push mower (power)	4.0–5.0
	Leaf raking	3.0–4.0
	Shoveling	4.0–6.0
	Housework	
	Dusting and sweeping	3.0–4.0
	Laundry	3.0–4.0
	Mopping	3.0–4.0
Moderate sports and recreation	Bowling	3.0–5.0
	Golf (walking)	3.5–4.5
	Basketball (shooting only)	4.0–5.0
	Baseball (playing catch)	3.5–4.5
	Bicycling (slow)	3.0–5.0
	Bicycling (brisk)	5.0–6.0
	Fishing while standing	3.0–4.0
Moderate fitness activities	Jumping jacks	4.0–5.0
	Aerobic dance (low intensity)	4.5–6.0
Occupational activities	Bricklaying	3.5–5.5
	Carpentry	3.0–6.0

MET values may vary for people of different fitness levels.

Walking is [our] best medicine.

Hippocrates, Greek physician and originator of modern medicine

FIT FACT

The amount of energy (the number of METs) used in an activity depends in part on your fitness level. Fit people use fewer METs than unfit people for the same activity.

What Are Some of the Benefits of Moderate Physical Activities?

Experts used to think that in order to gain health benefits you had to do vigorous physical activity (using more than 6 METs). We now know that many health benefits can be achieved by doing moderate physical activity (3 to 6 METs). The benefits of moderate physical activity include the following:

- Improved wellness and functional fitness, including feeling good, enjoying free time, and doing the things you want to do without undue fatigue
- Improved mental and academic performance
- Reduced risk of hypokinetic disease, such as heart disease, cancer, and diabetes
- Improved bone health
- Improved fitness for people in the low and moderate fitness zones (vigorous activity is required for fitness improvement for those in the good fitness and high performance zones)
- Healthy weight maintenance
- Improved quality of sleep

What Is the FIT Formula for Moderate Physical Activity?

Some of the recommended 60 minutes of daily activity for teens should be vigorous activity performed at least three times a week, and some should be activity that promotes muscle fitness and bone building performed at least three times a week. But for most people, moderate activity is the most common type of daily activity, and for most teens it will be the easiest way to meet the 60-minute daily recommendation. For adults, the recommendation is 150 minutes of moderate activity per week, which translates to 30 minutes per day, five days a week.

Table 7.2 provides details for the FIT formulas for moderate physical activity for both teens and adults. The teen guidelines apply, of course, while you're in school. The adult guidelines will apply for the rest of your life after school.

What Are Some Ways to Self-Monitor Moderate Physical Activity?

People who self-monitor their physical activity are more likely to meet national guidelines than those who don't. Self-monitoring refers to keeping track of your behavior—in this case, how much physical activity you perform. Consider the following ways to self-monitor your moderate physical activity.

Counting Minutes of Physical Activity

As indicated in table 7.2, activity guidelines are based on minutes of physical activity per day or per week. For many longer activities you can use a watch or a smartphone to keep track—for example, walking 15 minutes to school, doing 20 minutes of yardwork, or riding a bike for 30 minutes. For shorter bouts of activity,

TABLE 7.2 **FIT Formulas for Health and Wellness Benefits of Moderate Physical Activity**

FIT formula	Threshold of training	Target zone
Teens		
Frequency	Most days of the week	Daily
Intensity	3 METs Moderate activity equal to walking briskly or raking the yard	3–6 METs At least as intense as brisk walking but less intense than normal jogging
Time	60 min of total activity accumulated throughout the day (some or all moderate)	60 min to several hours of total activity (some or all moderate)
Adults		
Frequency	Most days of the week	Daily or most days of the week
Intensity	3 METs* Moderate activity equal to walking briskly or raking the yard	3–6 METs At least as intense as brisk walking but less intense than normal jogging
Time	At least 30 min accumulated throughout the day**	30–60 min accumulated throughout the day**

*Less fit adults may use activities of less than 3 METs.

**At least 150 minutes per week, spread over multiple days.

such as walking from one classroom to another or doing intermittent activity at home, tracking using a phone or watch is more difficult. Most fitness trackers automatically record minutes of activity for you; however, these can be expensive. A less expensive option is keeping a written activity log during the day.

Counting Steps and Movement

Another way you can determine how much moderate physical activity you perform is to count the steps you take each day. You can do so by using a pedometer (see the Tech Trends feature), which automatically tracks your step count; the disadvantage is that a pedometer counts *all* steps that you take, regardless of intensity. Still, wearing a pedometer can help you see how active you really are, especially if you do a lot of moderate activity during the day.

If you're just beginning or don't regularly meet activity guidelines, apply the principle of

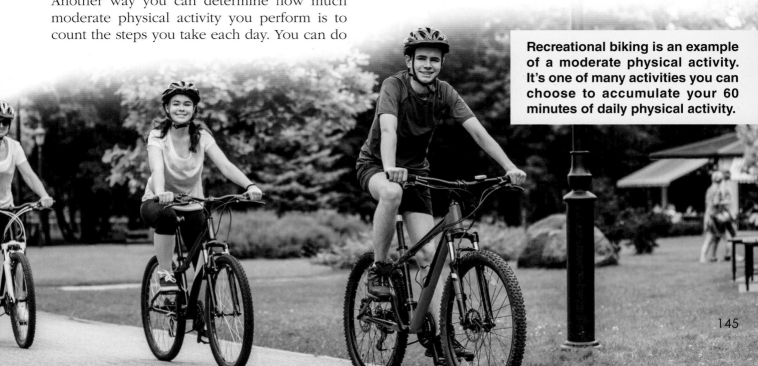

Recreational biking is an example of a moderate physical activity. It's one of many activities you can choose to accumulate your 60 minutes of daily physical activity.

progression. Instead of starting with a high goal such as 10,000 steps per day, which some experts recommend for adults, increase your step count gradually. Monitor your activity for a full week and then determine your average daily step count. Each week add 500 to 1,000 steps to your daily step count. The average teen takes about 10,000 steps a day (11,000 for boys and 9,000 for girls), and those involved in sports activities often accumulate 12,000 to 15,000 steps per day. Experts indicate that 12,000 steps per day is a reasonable long-term step goal for teens.

Tracking Energy Expended

Another way to determine whether you perform enough moderate activity is to track the energy you expend in activity. Some activity trackers estimate the calories you expend during physical activity. To allow the counters to estimate calories, you enter personal data such as your age and weight. The counter then uses this information as well as the time and intensity of your activity to estimate the calories expended during the day. During 60 minutes of moderate activity, such as brisk

TECH TRENDS: Pedometers and Activity Trackers (Accelerometers)

As described in chapter 6, a **pedometer** is a small, battery-powered device that counts each step you take and displays the running count on a meter. You simply open the face of the pedometer or push a button to see how many steps you've taken. If you choose a pedometer to monitor physical activity, additional information can be useful. Some pedometers allow you to enter the length of your step (your stride length) and your body weight so that the computer can estimate the distance you walk and the number of calories you expend. More expensive pedometers can also track the total time you spend in activity during the day. Less expensive pedometers must be reset at the end of the day, but some more expensive ones can store steps for several days. Pedometers are good for counting steps when walking but are not as good for tracking other forms of activity.

Activity trackers such as the Fitbit and the Apple Watch contain an **accelerometer**, which tracks body movements (forward and backward, up and down, and side to side). The accelerometer uses a formula determine how

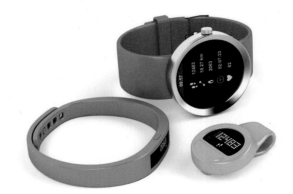

A pedometer counts steps and is a good way to self-monitor moderate activity.

much you move each day. Activity trackers are similar to pedometers but measure physical activity in more detail, including the intensity of your movements (METs) and the amount of time you spend at different intensities. With these measurements, most activity trackers can estimate the energy you expend in many types of activity. Accelerometers are now available in watches, phones, and devices worn on your belt or carried in your pocket.

USING TECHNOLOGY

Check your pedometer for accuracy (you may also use a smartphone app or fitness monitor). Set the counter to zero, count as you take 100 steps, and check the pedometer to see how many steps it counted. If it is within 3 steps (97-103) it is counting well. Next, estimate the number of steps you take on a typical weekday and a typical weekend day. Then wear a pedometer to see how many steps you actually take on these days. See if you're as active as you think you are!

walking, a teen who weighs 150 pounds (68 kilograms) would expend 300 to 400 calories. A heavier person would expend more calories and a lighter person would expend fewer.

You can also determine energy expenditure by using a physical activity compendium. A compendium is a document that includes a comprehensive list of information about a topic. A **physical activity compendium** lists many different activities and the energy expended in METs for each. Table 7.1 is an example of a small compendium. Search "physical activity compendium" online to access a more complete list of activities. Once you have determined the number of METs expended during an activity, you can determine your expenditure for a specific bout of that activity using MET minutes (see Academic Connection).

ACADEMIC CONNECTION: **MET Minutes**

MET minutes can be calculated to determine energy expended when you know the MET value of the activity and the amount of time spent doing it. As you have learned, 1 MET is equal to energy expended while sitting quietly. To get MET minutes for an activity, multiply the minutes in the activity by the MET value. The following is an example for a teen who walked for 60 minutes:

60 minutes × 3.0 METs (brisk walk) = 180 MET minutes

During the brisk walk the teen met the minimum number of minutes (60) and the minimum activity intensity (3.0 METs) for meeting the daily activity requirement and accumulated a score of 180 MET minutes. Therefore, 180 MET minutes is the standard for meeting teen activity guidelines each day. If the teen did 60 minutes of activity at a 6 MET intensity, such as mowing the lawn with a nonpowered push mower, the MET minutes would double (see the following worked example).

60 minutes × 6.0 METs = 360 MET minutes

To meet national physical activity goals, a teen would need to do 60 minutes of activity 7 days a week (420 minutes) at an intensity of at least 3 METs. This amounts to at least 1,260 MET minutes of activity per week.

STUDENT ACTIVITY

Refer to table 7.1. Find the MET value for baseball (playing catch). Using the lower MET value in the table, calculate the MET minutes for 30 minutes of playing catch. Next, find the MET value for dusting and sweeping. Using the upper MET value in the table, calculate the MET minutes for 15 minutes of dusting and sweeping.

CHECK YOUR ANSWERS

Playing catch: 105 MET minutes; dusting and sweeping: 60 MET minutes

LESSON REVIEW

1. What is a MET, what is moderate physical activity, and what are some examples of moderate physical activity?
2. What are some of the benefits of moderate physical activity?
3. What is a FIT formula, and how do you apply it to moderate physical activity?
4. What are some methods of self-monitoring moderate activity?

SELF-ASSESSMENT: **Walking Test**

Many of the self-assessments you perform in this course require very intense physical activity. If you're active and fit, the mile run or PACER may be the best way to estimate your cardiorespiratory endurance, but the walking test is especially good for beginners, those who haven't done a lot of recent activity, or those who are regular walkers but do not regularly get more vigorous activity. The walking test is also good for older people and for those who cannot do running tests due to joint or muscle problems. As directed by your teacher, record your scores and fitness ratings for the walking test. You can then use the information in preparing your personal physical activity plan. If you're working with a partner, remember that self-assessment information is confidential and shouldn't be shared without the permission of the person being tested.

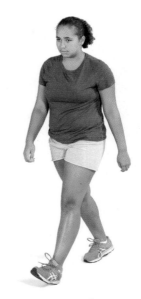

The walking test is a good assessment for beginners or people who don't do a lot of vigorous activity.

1. Walk a mile at a fast pace (as fast as you can go while keeping approximately the same pace for the entire walk).

2. Immediately after the walk, count your heartbeats for 15 seconds. (For information about counting heart rate, see chapter 8.) Multiply the result by four to calculate your one-minute heart rate.

3. Use the appropriate chart to determine your walking rating.

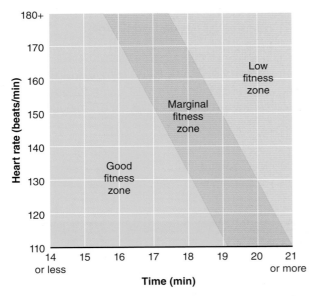

Rating chart for the walking test (for females).

Adapted from the *One Mile Walk Test* with permission of author James M. Rippe, M.D.

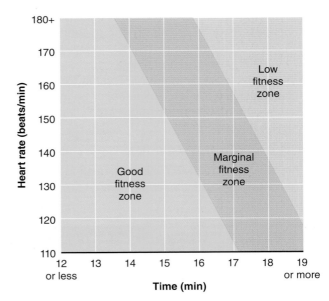

Rating chart for the walking test (for males).

Adapted from the *One Mile Walk Test* with permission of author James M. Rippe, M.D.

Preparing a Moderate Physical Activity Plan

Lesson Objectives

After reading this lesson, you should be able to

1. define sedentary, very light, and light activities;
2. describe the moderate physical activity patterns of inactive, active, and highly active teens;
3. describe the dangers of sedentary living; and
4. describe the steps for planning a moderate physical activity program.

Lesson Vocabulary

inactive

In the first lesson of this chapter you learned about how much moderate physical activity is enough to get health and wellness benefits. In this lesson, you will learn about healthy 24-hour activity patterns of teens, including the need for sleep, useful low-intensity activity, and participation in activities of many types and intensities. In addition, you'll have the opportunity to develop a moderate physical activity plan that will help you to meet national physical activity guidelines and avoid the dangers of being sedentary.

Meeting Daily Activity Guidelines

During each 24-hour day the typical teenager performs activities that range from being sedentary to being very active. *Sedentary* refers to behaviors that involve very little movement or energy expenditure (1 to 1.5 METs). Activities requiring 1 to 1.9 METs include sedentary behaviors and are considered to be very light—for example, eating, reading, using a computer, or sitting while playing a video game. Activities requiring 2 to 2.9 METs are considered to be light—for example, slow walking, grocery shopping,

> I read that too much sitting is not good for you. So now when I'm on the phone, I walk while I talk.
>
> *Quinn Metal*

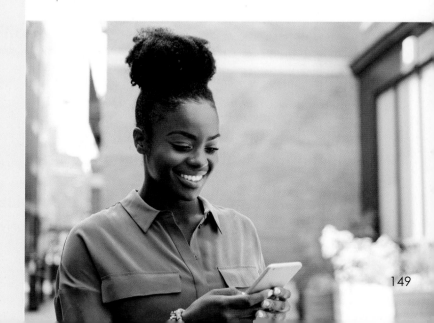

or active arcade games such as air hockey. These activities are not intense enough to contribute to the 60 minutes of daily physical activity necessary to meet teen guidelines. However, as you've learned, research has shown that some activity is better than none, and performing light or very light activity does expend some energy.

Healthy 24-Hour Activity Patterns

An **inactive** person is one who fails to meet national physical activity guidelines. An inactive teen (see red bars in figure 7.2) is one who fails to accumulate 60 minutes of moderate to vigorous daily activity (less than 180 MET minutes per day). The bars in the graph that are relatively small indicate that some activity was performed, but it was light or very light. As pointed out earlier, sedentary refers to sitting or standing or performing very light activity. Both active and inactive people spend time being sedentary. The shortest bars in figure 7.2 represent periods of sedentary behavior. A good portion of the inactive teen's day is spent sitting. However, not all of the short bars represent unproductive behavior—teens need time to study, attend school, and engage in hobbies. Some of the short bars therefore represent productive activities, but in many cases they also represent unhealthy sedentary behavior.

The blue bars represent sleep. Healthful sleep (0.9 MET) is important for teens; in fact, the American Academy of Pediatrics recommends that teens regularly get 8 to 10 hours of sleep each night. One important finding of the National Physical Activity Guidelines report is that regular physical activity helps people get sound and healthful sleep.

The activity patterns of an active teenager are illustrated by the gold bars in figure 7.2. Like the inactive teen, there are some periods of low-intensity activity during the day, including time spent in healthful sleep. However, this teen accumulated 60 minutes of moderate to vigorous physical activity, the standard for being active (180 or more MET minutes per day). The moderate to vigorous activity is indicated by the taller bars. Several tall bars in a row indicate relatively long bouts of moderate to vigorous activity. The activities can be counted toward the daily 60-minute goal. Very tall bars indicate vigorous activity, which is recommended at least three days per week for teens (360 or more MET minutes per day).

The activity patterns of a highly active person are illustrated by the series of green bars. This person does several bouts of physical activity that is intense enough to be considered moderate to vigorous. In this case, the vigorous activity totals more than 120 minutes during the day. There are fewer short green bars because

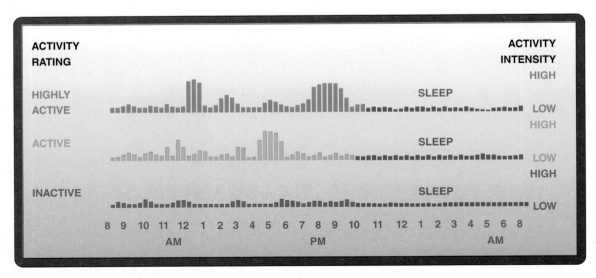

Figure 7.2 Activity patterns of inactive, active, and highly active teens.

the highly active person spends more time in moderate to vigorous activity than active and inactive teens. Still, the active teen makes time for healthful sleep and other restful activities.

FIT FACT
Teens who watch three or more hours of TV a day have a 65 percent higher chance of becoming obese.

The Dangers of Sedentary Behaviors

For the first time, the recent *Physical Activity Guidelines for Americans* report includes information on the dangers of being sedentary. The report indicates that Americans spend 55 percent of their waking hours being sedentary. Other reports indicate that teens spend an average of six hours and 40 minutes per day using a device with a screen. The average teen spends more than two hours a day watching TV, and 70 percent of teens own a smartphone and use it several hours per day.

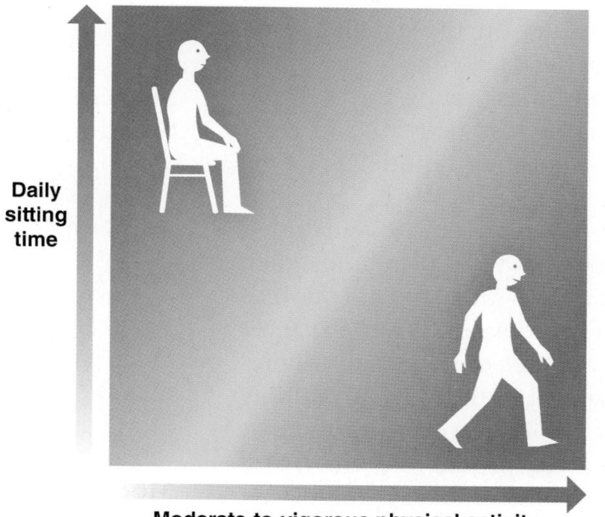

Figure 7.3 Risks of too much sitting and too little physical activity.

From U.S. Department of Health and Human Services, *Physical Activity Guidelines for Americans*, 2nd ed. (Washington, DC: U.S. Department of Health and Human Services, 2018).

You already know that performing too little moderate to vigorous physical activity increases risk of disease and early death. You may not know that long periods of sedentary activity add to that risk. Figure 7.3 shows that both doing regular moderate to vigorous activity and reducing daily sitting time have effects on longevity, health, and wellness.

In figure 7.3, the person in the upper left does little activity and a lot of sitting—this person is at the greatest health risk. The person at the bottom right does considerable activity and little sitting—this person has the lowest risk of early death as well as reduced risk of chronic disease and improved wellness. Because it is important to avoid excessive sitting, you may want to do a self-assessment of your daily sitting time in addition to preparing your moderate physical activity plan.

Preparing a Moderate Physical Activity Plan

In chapter 3 you learned about the five steps in program planning. In this chapter you have learned about moderate physical activities and their benefits. You can now prepare your own personal moderate physical activity plan using the five planning steps. Your instructor will provide you with worksheets that you can use to plan a two-week program.

Like you, Javier was assigned to prepare a two-week moderate physical activity program. Notice that Javier did his planning using steps similar to those of the scientific method. Follow these five planning steps to prepare your two-week plan.

Walking is the best possible exercise. Habituate yourself to walk very fast.

Thomas Jefferson, U.S. president

Step 1: Determine Your Personal Needs

To get started, Javier collected some basic information about his moderate physical activity levels in the past week and his fitness test results that related to moderate physical activity. He recorded his results on the activity sheet provided by his teacher (see table 7.3).

Javier had a good fitness rating for both the PACER and the walking test (see table 7.3). He also met the national activity guideline of 60 minutes a day on three days of the previous week. His moderate activity mostly included walking to and from school (20 minutes each weekday) and riding his bike for 10 minutes two days a week (Tuesday and Thursday). He also performed 10 minutes of home calisthenics (Tuesday, Thursday, and Saturday). On Saturday he played tennis in addition to his calisthenics. Still, his physical activity profile told him that if he wanted to meet national activity guidelines, he needed to increase his physical activity.

Step 2: Consider Your Program Options

Javier looked at the list of moderate physical activities presented in table 7.1 and created a list including other moderate activities that were easily available to him.

Lifestyle activities (e.g., walking to school)

- Walking to and from school
- Additional walking
- Yardwork at home

Moderate sports and recreation (e.g., bowling)

- Bowling
- Shooting baskets
- Fishing
- Bike riding

Occupational or school activities (e.g., PE class)

- Physical education class

Moderate fitness activities

- Calisthenics

Step 3: Set Goals

Because two weeks is too short to accommodate long-term goals, Javier developed only short-term goals for his moderate physical activity

TABLE 7.3   **Javier's Moderate Physical Activity and Fitness Profiles**

Physical fitness profile			
Fitness self-assessment	**Score**	**Rating**	
Walking test	Time: 15:00 Heart rate: 140	Good fitness	
PACER	41 laps	Good fitness	
Physical activity profile			
Day	**Moderate activity (min)**	**All activity (min)**	**Met guideline**
Mon.	30	30	
Tues.	30	60	✓
Wed.	30	30	
Thurs.	30	60	✓
Fri.	30	60	✓
Sat.	30	30	
Sun.	0	0	

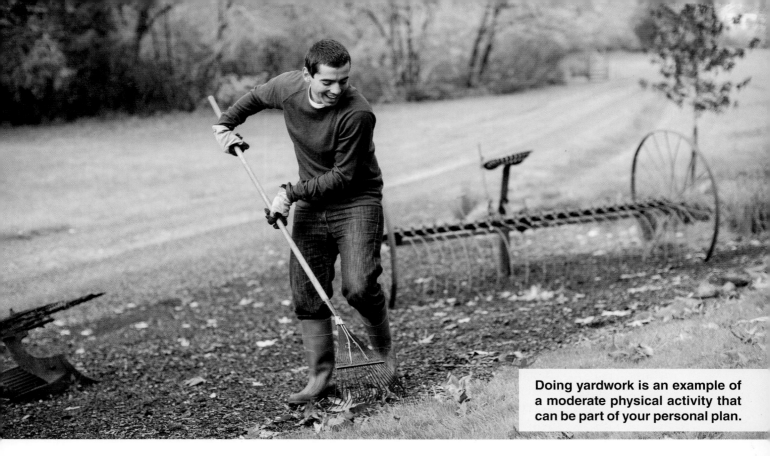

plan. As a result, all of his goals were activity goals (process goals), which work best as short-term goals. Later, when he prepares a longer plan, Javier will develop long-term goals, including fitness (product) goals. He also knew that if he met his short-term activity goals, he would be making progress toward his long-term fitness goals. For these first two weeks, Javier decided to focus on moderate activity through the following goals.

Short-term activity goals

- Continue to perform regular activities, including physical education (30 min three days per week), biking with friends (30 min two days per week), and walking to and from school (30 min per day).
- Rake the yard (30 min) and mow the neighbor's yard (60 min) once every two weeks.
- Shoot baskets (30 min) two days a week.
- Go fishing one day a week (includes walking for 60 min).
- Do moderate calisthenics (15 min) two days a week.

Javier remembered to use SMART goals. His goals listed *specific* activities and amounts of time because he wanted to be able to *measure* his progress. He also tried to make his goals challenging but *attainable* and *realistic*. Finally, he wanted to be able to reach his goals in the time available.

Step 4: Create a Written Program

Javier's plan included a minimum of 60 minutes of moderate physical activity on each day during the two-week period. On several days, he planned to do more than 60 minutes. As shown in table 7.4, he wrote down the activities and the times when he planned to perform them.

FIT FACT
Walking, a moderate physical activity, is the most popular type of activity in the United States. More than 145 million adults report walking regularly, most commonly for transportation, for fun, for exercise, or for walking the dog. People who have a dog walk more frequently than people who don't.

FIT FACT
Canadian laws provide tax incentives for increasing regular physical activity. Families that enroll children and teens in youth activity programs get an income tax break, and people who buy bicycles get a reduction in sales tax.

TABLE 7.4   **Javier's Two-Week Moderate Physical Activity Plan**

Day	Week 1 Activity	Time	✓	Week 2 Activity	Time	✓
Mon.	Walk to school* Walk home* Shoot baskets	7:45–7:55 a.m. 3:30–3:40 p.m. 3:45–4:15 p.m.		Walk to school* Walk home* Shoot baskets	7:45–7:55 a.m. 3:30–3:40 p.m. 3:45–4:15 p.m.	
Tues.	Walk to school* Physical education class* Walk home*	7:45–7:55 a.m. 10:00–10:30 a.m. 3:30–3:40 p.m.		Walk to school* Physical education class* Walk home*	7:45–7:55 a.m. 10:00–10:30 a.m. 3:30–3:40 p.m.	
Wed.	Walk to school* Walk home* Ride bike	7:45–7:55 a.m. 3:30–3:45 p.m. 3:45–4:00 p.m.		Walk to school* Walk home* Ride bike	7:45–7:55 a.m. 3:30–3:45 p.m. 3:45–4:00 p.m.	
Thurs.	Walk to school* Physical education class* Walk home* Calisthenics	7:45–7:55 a.m. 10:00–10:30 a.m. 3:30–3:40 p.m. 6:30–6:45 p.m.		Walk to school Physical education class* Walk home* Calisthenics	7:45–7:55 a.m. 10:00–10:30 a.m. 3:30–3:40 p.m. 6:30–6:45 p.m.	
Fri.	Walk to school* Physical education class* Walk home*	7:45–7:55 a.m. 10:00–10:30 a.m. 3:30–3:45 p.m.		Walk to school Physical education class* Walk home*	7:45–7:55 a.m. 10:00–10:30 a.m. 3:30–3:40 p.m.	
Sat.	Mow the grass* Ride bike	9:00–9:30 a.m. 1:00–1:30 p.m.		Rake the yard* Ride bike	9:30–10:30 a.m. 1:00–1:30 p.m.	
Sun.	Bowling Calisthenics	2:30–3:30 p.m. 6:30–6:45 p.m.		Bowling Calisthenics	2:30–3:30 p.m. 6:30–6:45 p.m.	

*Activities that Javier was already doing.

Step 5: Keep a Log and Evaluate Your Program

Over the next two weeks, Javier will monitor his activities and place a checkmark beside each activity he performs. At the end of the two-week period, he'll evaluate his performance to see whether he met his goals, then use that evaluation to help him make another activity plan.

LESSON REVIEW

1. How many METs are used in activities considered to be sedentary, very light, or light?
2. What do the moderate physical activity patterns of active and highly active teens look like, and how do they differ from patterns of inactive or sedentary teens?
3. What are the dangers of sedentary living?
4. What steps did Javier take to plan his moderate physical activity program?

TAKING CHARGE: Learning to Manage Time

Why can some people always find time for another activity, but others barely have time to do everything in their regular schedule? For a lot of people, the answer is time management. Good time managers know how to make the best use of their time and efficiently control their schedule in order to complete activities without wasting a minute. These people are more likely to find time for regular physical activity.

Here's an example of poor time management: Jennifer lives near some good cross-country ski trails. In the winter, her friends spend a few hours skiing every Monday and Wednesday after school; they also go skiing on weekends.

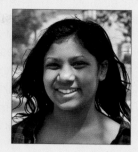

Although they always ask her to join their fun, Jennifer usually refuses. Her common excuse is, "I just don't have the time. I really love skiing, but with three honors classes, homework, and my job at the mall, I barely have time to eat, let alone ski. I wish I could go with you, but I can't. It's impossible! I'll ski next year when my schedule is easier. Then I'll have more spare time."

Jennifer's friends are used to her excuses. In fact, she used many of the same ones last year. Her friends have the same classes and work hours that Jennifer has, but they complete their homework assignments and handle their jobs with time to spare. They do not understand why Jennifer can't manage to find the time to go skiing with them.

FOR DISCUSSION

What can Jennifer do to manage her time better so that she can do things with her friends? What can her friends do to help? What suggestions can you make to help anyone who would like to manage time better? Consider the guidelines in the following Self-Management feature as you answer these discussion questions.

SELF-MANAGEMENT: Skills for Managing Time

How many times do you hear yourself and others say, "I don't have the time"? If you're one of the many people who seem to have too little time, how can you remedy the problem? Many experts believe that time management is a good solution. In this lesson, you'll learn how to manage your time so that you can be more active.

In 1900, the average person worked more than 60 hours a week. Now the average workweek is less than 40 hours. Similarly, in 1900, many young people were not enrolled in school and were already working long hours in factories and on farms. Now most teens are in school, and those who work limit their work hours.

Fewer working hours has made free time much more abundant now than it was years ago. But work and school aren't the only things that take time; most of us make other time commitments as well. For example, you might have to care for a sibling, or you might have committed to a school or community activity such as a club, band, chorus, or sport team. And of course you also spend time on necessary activities such as eating, sleeping, dressing, and getting to and from school or work. The time you spend in all of these activities is called *committed time*.

Free time, on the other hand, is the time left over after accounting for school, work, and other committed time. Some people make so many commitments that they have very little free time. Often, people who say they don't have time for physical activity have not planned their time carefully. Active people manage their time effectively so that they can commit to

>continued

>continued

regular activity. If you're in the group of people who often say, "I don't have time," the following guidelines can help you.

- *Keep track of your time.* The best way to start managing your time more efficiently is to see what you're doing with it now. You can do this by self-monitoring: Write down what you do during the course of each day. Record when you sleep, when you eat, when you're in school, when you're at work, and when you do all of the other things you do. You might use three categories: school and work, other committed time, and free time. Most people who keep records of their time use are surprised by the results. For example, some people who say they don't have time to exercise spend several hours a day watching television or are otherwise unoccupied.

- *Analyze your use of time.* Once you've tracked your time for several days, review your records to see how many hours you spend in each of the three categories. You can also identify exactly how you spend your committed time and your free time. Doing so will help you decide whether you're using your time in the way you really want to use it.

- *Decide purposefully what to do with your time.* After you determine how much time you spend doing various activities, decide whether you're managing your time efficiently. Efficient time management enables you to do the things you think are most important. To decide what's most important to you, answer the following questions.

- What activities did you spend more time on than you wanted to?
- How much less time could you spend on these activities?
- What activities do you want to spend more time on?
- How much more time would you like to spend on these activities?
- Are the activities you would like to change under your control?

- *Schedule your time.* After you decide how you would like to spend your time, create a schedule to ensure that you make time for the things you identified as most important. If you feel that regular physical activity is important, you will commit time to doing it. Plan a schedule for one day, making sure you have time to do the most important things.

Sometimes good scheduling allows you to do two things at once. For example, you have to get to school somehow—what if you did so by walking or riding a bicycle? Thus, you would be effectively committing that time to two different purposes. Similarly, if you join a sport team or activity club, the time you commit to that group is also committed to doing physical activity.

Taking Action: **Performing Your Moderate Physical Activity Plan**

Use the worksheet provided by your teacher to prepare a two-week moderate physical activity plan using the five steps described in this chapter. Like Javier, consider moderate activities from each activity category: lifestyle activity, moderate sports and recreation, moderate fitness activities, and occupational or school activity. The goal is to accumulate at least 60 minutes of activity each day, including a considerable portion that involves moderate activity. Prepare a written plan and carry out it over a two-week period. Your teacher may give you time in class to do some of the activities in your plan. Consider the following suggestions for **taking action** to build moderate activity into your plan.

- *Lifestyle activity.* Walk or bike to school. If driving, park away from your destination and walk the rest of the way. When you have a choice, take the stairs. Walk while talking on the phone. Work in the yard.

- *Moderate sports and recreation.* Consider playing catch, shooting baskets, or bowling with friends.
- *Moderate fitness activities.* Consider moderate fitness activities such as low-intensity aerobic dance or moderate-intensity calisthenics.
- *Occupational or school activity.* Do yardwork for pay, take an optional physical education class, participate in intramural activities, or start a walking club.

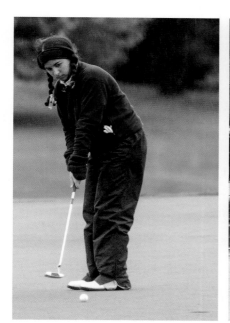
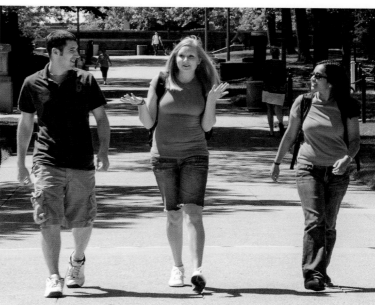
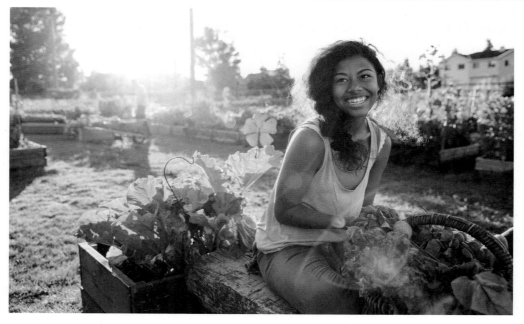

Lifestyle activities can be part of your plan for taking action.

CHAPTER REVIEW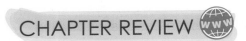

Reviewing Concepts and Vocabulary

Answer items 1 through 5 by correctly completing each sentence with a word or phrase.

1. Activity that is equivalent to brisk walking in intensity is considered to be _____ physical activity.

2. An activity done as part of daily life is called a/an _____ activity.

3. A device worn on your belt that counts steps is called a/an _____.

4. Intensity of activity can be expressed in units called _____.

5. The recommended amount of nightly sleep for teens is _____ hours.

For items 6 through 10, match each term in column 1 with the appropriate word or phrase in column 2.

6. inactive   a. low energy expenditure

7. sedentary   b. body weight activities

8. MET minute   c. fails to meet activity guidelines

9. calisthenics   d. counts active movements

10. accelerometer   e. energy expended × time

For items 11 through 15, respond to each statement or question.

11. What does *sedentary* mean, and what can be done to reduce sedentary living among teens?

12. Describe several devices that can be used to self-monitor physical activity.

13. How much moderate physical activity is enough?

14. List and describe the five steps for planning a moderate physical activity program.

15. Describe several guidelines for managing time effectively.

Thinking Critically

Write a paragraph to answer the following question.

Teens are often more vigorously active than adults. For this reason, some people say that teens should begin to do more moderate activity to increase their chance of staying active later in life. Do you think you will become more or less active as you grow older? What types of activity do you think you'll do as you grow older?

Project

National polling groups regularly conduct surveys to learn people's opinions about various issues, including health and fitness. Assume that you work for a polling company. Develop a list of questions about moderate activity and ask at least six people to answer them. Try to interview people from different age groups. Analyze your results and prepare a brief news article reporting the results.

Cardiorespiratory Endurance

In This Chapter

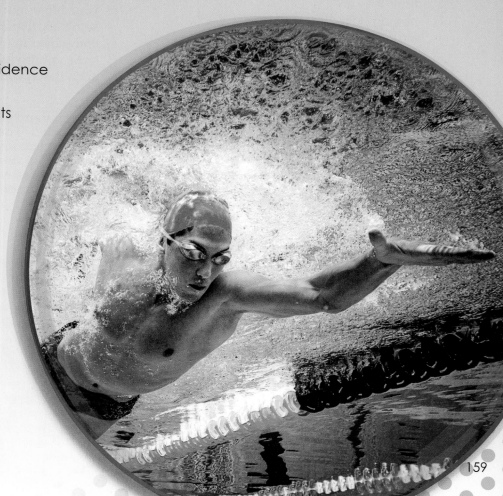

Cardiorespiratory Endurance Facts

Lesson Objectives

After reading this lesson, you should be able to

1. define cardiorespiratory endurance and identify other terms often used to describe this part of fitness;

2. describe the benefits of physical activity and cardiorespiratory endurance;

3. describe several methods for assessing your cardiorespiratory endurance; and

4. explain how much cardiorespiratory endurance the typical person needs.

Lesson Vocabulary

aerobic capacity
cholesterol
fibrin
hemoglobin
high-density lipoprotein (HDL)
low-density lipoprotein (LDL)
maximal oxygen uptake test

Do you have good cardiorespiratory endurance? Do you do enough regular vigorous physical activity to build good cardiorespiratory endurance? Of the 11 parts of fitness, cardiorespiratory endurance is considered to be the most important by many experts. As shown in figure 8.1, cardiorespiratory endurance requires fitness of your heart, lungs, blood vessels, and muscles. In this lesson, you'll learn how proper physical activity improves your cardiorespiratory endurance. You'll also learn how to assess your cardiorespiratory endurance.

What Is Cardiorespiratory Endurance?

Cardiorespiratory endurance is the ability to exercise your entire body for a long time without stopping. It requires a strong heart, healthy lungs, and clear blood vessels to supply your large muscles with oxygen. Examples of activities that require good cardiorespiratory endurance are distance running, swimming, and cross-country skiing. Cardiorespiratory endurance is sometimes referred to by other names,

> My best friend's mother had breast cancer. We wanted to participate in a 5K run to raise money for cancer research. Because this was important to us, we trained to improve our cardiorespiratory endurance. We did the run, and it was great. Now we want to try a 10K.
>
> *Morgan Whittaker*

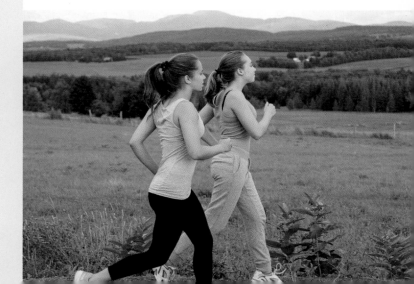

including *cardiovascular fitness, cardiovascular endurance*, and *cardiorespiratory fitness*. The term **aerobic capacity** is also used to describe good cardiorespiratory function, but it is not exactly the same as cardiorespiratory endurance (see this chapter's Science in Action feature).

Cardiorespiratory endurance involves two vital systems: your cardiovascular system, made up of your heart, blood vessels, and blood, and your respiratory system, made up of your lungs and the passages that bring air to your lungs from outside of your body. These systems work together to bring your cells the materials they need and rid the cells of waste. *Endurance* refers to the ability to sustain effort, which depends on fitness of the cardiovascular (cardio) and respiratory systems. Together, the two systems help you function both effectively (with the most benefits possible) and efficiently (with the least effort).

The importance of good cardiorespiratory endurance can be illustrated by the case of professional hockey player Richard Zednik. His high level of fitness helped him perform well in hockey, but it became crucial to his survival when his carotid artery was cut by an opponent's skate during a game. For most people, this would be a deadly injury. However, the doctor who performed the rescue surgery reported that because of Zednik's fitness level, he had very healthy and elastic arteries that were large and easy to repair. Because of his good cardiorespiratory endurance, Zednik made a full recovery.

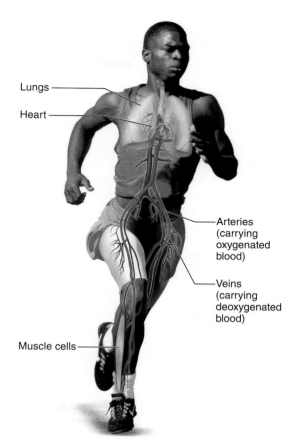

Lungs

Heart

Arteries (carrying oxygenated blood)

Veins (carrying deoxygenated blood)

Muscle cells

Figure 8.1 Cardiorespiratory endurance requires fitness of many parts of the body, including the heart, lungs, muscles, and blood vessels.

What Are the Benefits of Having Good Cardiorespiratory Endurance?

Doing regular physical activity can help you look better by controlling your weight, building your muscles, and helping you develop good posture. Regular physical activity also produces changes in your body's organs, such as making your heart muscle stronger and your blood vessels healthier, and enhancing your brain and other bodily functions. These changes improve your cardiorespiratory endurance and reduce your risk of hypokinetic diseases, especially heart disease and diabetes.

Physical activity provides benefits for both your cardiovascular and respiratory systems. In this lesson, you'll learn how each part of these systems benefits and how all the parts work together to promote optimal functioning and good health.

Physical Activity Strengthens the Heart Muscle

Because your heart is a muscle that acts as a pump to deliver blood to cells throughout your body, it benefits from exercise such as jogging, swimming, and long-distance hiking. When you do vigorous physical activity, your muscle cells need

FIT FACT
In the early 1900s, medical doctors referred to an enlarged heart as the "athlete's heart" because athletes' hearts tended to be large and, at that time, a large heart was associated with disease. By midcentury, research showed that the large heart muscle of a trained athlete was a sign of health, not disease.

more oxygen and produce more waste products. Therefore, your heart must pump more blood to supply the additional oxygen and remove the additional waste. If your heart is unable to pump enough blood, your muscles will be less able to contract and will fatigue more quickly.

Your heart has two ways to get more blood to your muscles: by beating faster and by sending more blood with each beat (this is called *stroke volume*). Because a fit heart has a greater stroke volume, it pumps more blood with each beat than a less fit heart (figure 8.2).

Physical Activity Helps the Lungs Function Efficiently

When you inhale, air enters the lungs, causing them to expand. In the lungs, oxygen is transferred from the air to the blood for transport to the tissues of the body. When you exhale, air leaves the lungs. The diaphragm (a band of muscular tissue located at the base of your lungs) and abdominal muscles (which help move the diaphragm) work to allow you to breathe in and out (figure 8.3a). Because they have more

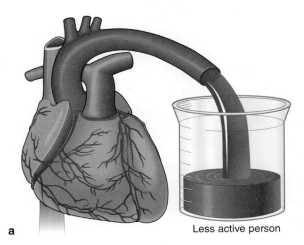

Figure 8.2   The heart of a less active person *(a)* pumps less blood per beat than the heart of a more active person *(b)*.

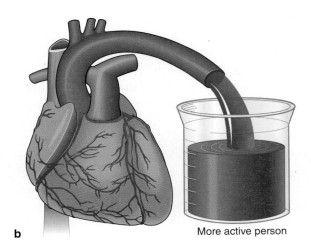

Air enters the lungs when your diaphragm and other respiratory muscles contract and create an area of low pressure.

Inhale

Exhale

The average lung holds 3 to 5 liters of air.

Trained individuals take bigger breaths, thus requiring fewer breaths to get the same amount of oxygen.

Untrained individuals take shallow breaths and thus need more breaths to get sufficient oxygen.

Figure 8.3   *(a)* The lungs and diaphragm during inhalation and exhalation; *(b)* fit people can breathe more efficiently than unfit people.

efficient respiratory muscles, fit people can take in more air with each breath than unfit people and therefore can transport the same amount of air to the lungs in fewer breaths (figure 8.3b). Healthy lungs also have the capacity to easily transfer oxygen to the blood. Together, healthy lungs and fit respiratory muscles contribute to good cardiorespiratory endurance.

Arteries

The arteries carry blood away from your heart to other parts of your body (e.g., lungs, vital organs, muscles). The beating of your heart forces blood through your arteries. Healthy arteries are open and free from blockage (see figure 8.4). Arteries become unhealthy when fatty deposits on the inner walls of an artery lead to atherosclerosis. Atherosclerosis in an artery in the heart muscle can lead to a heart attack. Regular physical activity can help keep your arteries healthy and free from atherosclerosis and reduce risk of heart attack.

Regular physical activity also provides other cardiovascular benefits. Figure 8.5 shows that the heart muscle has its own arteries (coronary arteries), which supply it with blood and oxygen. Scientists have found that people who exercise regularly develop more branching of the arteries in the heart. This richer network of

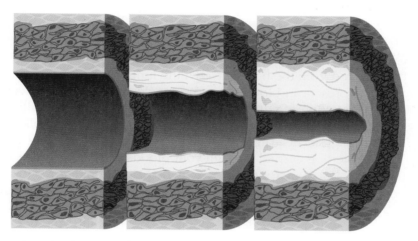

Figure 8.4   Atherosclerosis clogs arteries and can lead to a heart attack.

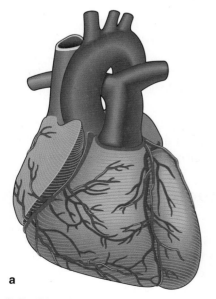
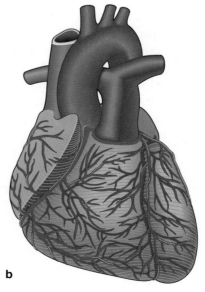

a   b

Figure 8.5   Blood vessels of (a) the heart of a typical person and (b) the heart of a person who exercises regularly.

blood vessels is important because when an artery is blocked, as in a heart attack, the extra artery branches continue to supply blood and oxygen to the part of the heart that is affected. For example, doctors found that one of the major arteries in an astronaut's heart was completely blocked due to atherosclerosis. However, because of all the physical training that astronauts perform, extra branching of arteries occurred in the heart muscle, limiting the damage to the heart muscle.

Veins

The veins carry blood from the tissues back to the heart using one-way valves to keep the blood from flowing backward. Your muscles squeeze the veins to help pump the blood back to your heart. Regular exercise helps your muscles squeeze your veins efficiently. Lack of physical activity can cause the valves, especially those in your legs, to stop working efficiently, thereby reducing circulation.

Physical Activity Promotes Healthy Blood

Your blood carries nutrients to the cells and waste away from the cells. It has red blood cells that contain **hemoglobin**, a protein that picks up oxygen for delivery to the cells via the arteries. It also carries carbon dioxide away from the cells to be removed from the body through the lungs. It is normal for a certain amount of fat to be present in blood. However, as described earlier, excessive amounts can trigger formation of fatty deposits along your artery walls. **Cholesterol**—a waxy, fatlike substance found in meat, dairy products, and egg yolk—can be dangerous because high levels can build up in your body without your noticing it.

Cholesterol is carried through your bloodstream by particles called *lipoproteins*. One kind, **low-density lipoprotein (LDL)**, is often referred to as "bad cholesterol" because it carries cholesterol that is more likely to stay in your body and contribute to atherosclerosis. According to the American College of Sports Medicine, an LDL count below 100 is considered optimal for good health. Another kind, **high-density lipoprotein (HDL)**, is often referred to as "good cholesterol" because it carries excess cholesterol out of your bloodstream and into your liver for elimination from your body. Therefore, HDLs appear to help prevent atherosclerosis. An HDL count above 60 is considered optimal for good health. Regular physical activity helps you improve your health and resist disease by reducing your LDL (bad cholesterol) and increasing your HDL (good cholesterol).

In addition to being free of fatty deposits, healthy arteries are free from inflammation, which contributes to arterial clogging. Blood tests can pick up markers of inflammation. Regular physical activity helps reduce inflammation in your arteries and can help prevent the formation of blood clots by reducing the amount of fibrin in your blood. **Fibrin** is a substance involved in making your blood clot, and high amounts of fibrin can contribute to the development of atherosclerosis.

Physical Activity Positively Affects Nerves That Control Heart Rate

Your heart muscle is not like your arm and leg muscles. When your arm and leg muscles contract, nerves respond to a message sent by the conscious part of your brain. In contrast, your heart is not controlled voluntarily; it beats regularly without your consciously telling it to do so. Your heart rate is controlled by two types of nerves. One type (parasympathetic) slows the heart rate and the other (sympathetic) speeds it. Factors such as stress, fear, consuming caffeinated drinks,

If you don't do what's best for your body, you're the one who comes up on the short end.

Julius "Dr. J" Erving, Hall of Fame basketball player

and participating in physical activity cause the release of hormones that increase heart rate. Factors such as slow breathing, yoga, and relaxation exercises release hormones that slow the heart rate. Regular long-term physical activity also has a slowing effect on heart rate and helps you function more effectively during emergencies and during vigorous physical activity.

Physical Activity Promotes Healthy Muscle Cells

In order to do physical activity for a long time without getting tired, your muscle cells must function efficiently. Regular physical activity helps your cells use oxygen and get rid of waste materials effectively. Physical activity also helps your muscle cells use blood sugar, with the aid of insulin, to produce energy. This function is important for good health.

Summary of Benefits

Figure 8.6 illustrates how the cardiovascular and respiratory systems work together to help you function effectively in daily living and in physical activity. You breathe in air that is high in oxygen content, which is delivered to your lungs. In the lungs, oxygen is transferred to the blood and then pumped by the lower left side

- Lungs work more efficiently
- Deliver more oxygen to blood
- Healthy lungs allow deeper and less frequent breathing

- Healthy elastic arteries allow more blood flow
- Less risk of atherosclerosis
- Lower blood pressure
- Less risk of a blood clot leading to heart attack
- Development of extra blood vessels
- Healthy veins with healthy valves

- Use oxygen efficiently
- Get rid of more wastes
- Use blood sugars and insulin more effectively to produce energy

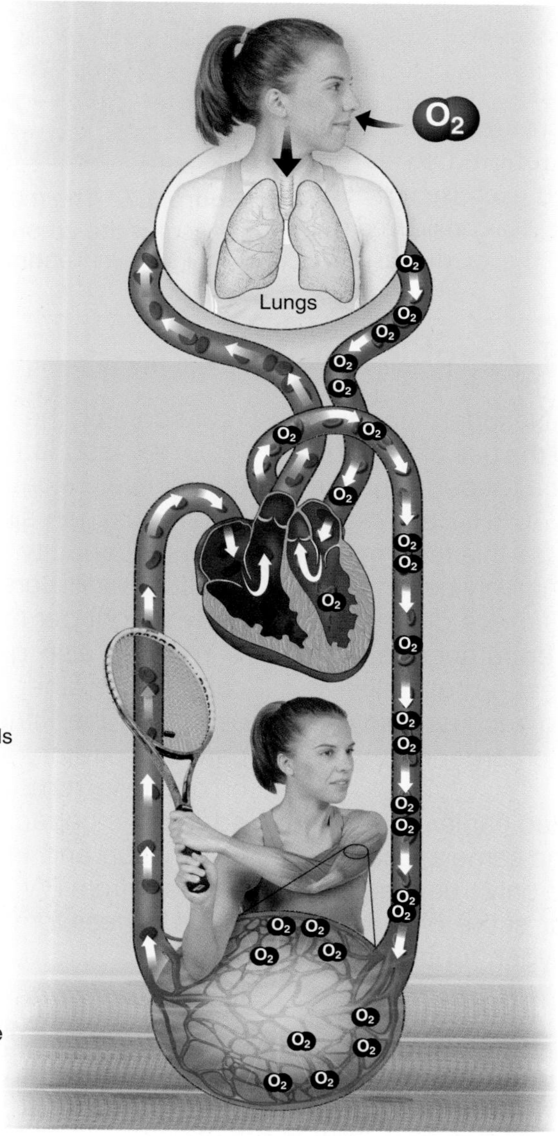

- Heart muscle gets stronger
- Pumps more blood with each beat (stroke volume)
- Beats slower
- Gets more rest
- Works more efficiently
- Helps the nerves slow your heart rate at rest
- Builds muscles and helps them work more efficiently

- Less bad cholesterol (LDL) and other fats in the blood
- More good cholesterol (HDL) in the blood
- Reduces inflammatory markers in the blood
- Fewer substances in the blood that cause clots (fibrin)

Figure 8.6 Benefits of physical activity for the cardiovascular and respiratory systems.

of the heart to be used by the rest of the body (e.g., organs, muscles). Carbon dioxide, a waste product of bodily functions, is picked up in the blood and returned to the lungs through the pulmonary vein to be expelled from the body when you exhale.

Cardiorespiratory Assessments

You might be curious about your own cardiorespiratory endurance. How good is it? You can assess the fitness of your cardiorespiratory systems in two settings: in the laboratory or in the field (such as in a gym and or on an athletic field).

Laboratory Tests

Two types of laboratory tests are the maximal oxygen uptake test (also referred to as the $\dot{V}O_2$max test) and the graded exercise test. The **maximal oxygen uptake test** is considered the best for assessing fitness of the cardiovascular

and respiratory systems. It measures how much oxygen you can use when you're exercising very vigorously. To take the test, you run on a treadmill while connected to a special gas meter (figure 8.7). The difficulty increases as the

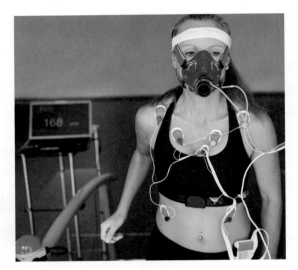

Figure 8.7 The maximal oxygen uptake test measures the amount of oxygen you use while running on a treadmill.

SCIENCE IN ACTION: Aerobic Capacity

As you learned earlier, the National Academy of Medicine recommended the use of the term *cardiorespiratory endurance* for performance on field tests such as the PACER. Because of this recommendation, we use this term rather than some of the other commonly used terms (such as *cardiovascular fitness* or *aerobic fitness*). Cardiorespiratory endurance reflects a person's functional fitness—the ability to perform tasks of daily living such as enjoying leisure activities and meet emergencies without undue fatigue.

Aerobic capacity, as noted earlier, is a term similar to, but not exactly the same as, cardiorespiratory endurance. The only true measure of aerobic capacity is your score on a laboratory-based maximal oxygen uptake test.

Your score on the maximal oxygen uptake test ($\dot{V}O_2$max test) is recorded in liters of oxygen per minute. Because larger people use more liters of oxygen simply because of their size, aerobic capacity scores are commonly reported as milliliters of oxygen per kilogram of body weight per minute (mL/kg/min).

You can also get an idea of your aerobic capacity in other ways. For example, when used with the FitnessGram report card, your cardiorespiratory endurance score (PACER or one-mile run) is converted to an estimated aerobic capacity score. You can find more information and tables for estimating aerobic capacity from PACER and one-mile run scores at the *Fitness for Life* web resource.

STUDENT ACTIVITY

Estimate your aerobic capacity score in milliliters of oxygen per kilogram of body weight per minute (mL/kg/min) using your PACER or one-mile run score. Tables for converting PACER and one-mile run scores to aerobic capacity scores are available at the *Fitness for Life* web resource.

treadmill goes faster and you begin to run uphill. As you exercise, the gas meter measures the amount of oxygen you use each minute; fit individuals are able to use more oxygen than less fit people. The amount (volume) of oxygen you can use during the hardest minute of exercise is considered your $\dot{V}O_2$max score (see the Science in Action feature).

As you learned earlier, medical doctors and exercise physiologists sometimes use another laboratory test called a *graded exercise test* (or *exercise stress test*) to detect potential heart problems. During the test, your heart is monitored by an electrocardiogram while you run on a treadmill.

Field Tests

Both the graded exercise test and the maximal oxygen uptake test are done in a laboratory and require special equipment and people who are trained to administer them. Most people, however, assess their cardiorespiratory endurance using practical tests called *field tests*. These tests require little equipment and can be done at home or at school. Scores are determined based on your ability to function (your functional fitness) rather than on the amount of oxygen you can use. Examples such as the PACER, the walking test, the step test, and the one-mile run test are included as self-assessments in this book.

Self-assessments are not as accurate as laboratory tests of fitness; therefore, you should perform more than one self-assessment for cardiorespiratory endurance. However, self-assessments do give a good estimate of your fitness level, and each assessment has its own strengths and weaknesses. For example, the results of the PACER and the one-mile run (included in this chapter) are influenced by your motivation; if you don't try very hard, you won't get an accurate score. Because these tests require a high level of exertion, they may not be the best tests for people who have not been exercising regularly or who have low fitness.

The walking test, on the other hand, is a good indicator of fitness for most people but is not best for assessing very fit people. It would be a good test for a beginner or for a person with a low level of fitness. The step test (included in this chapter) assesses heart rate and therefore motivation does not influence its results as much as other tests; however, results can be distorted if you've done other exercise that might elevate your heart rate before doing the assessment. Your heart rate can also be influenced by emotional factors (stress) and nutritional factors (caffeine) that cause it to be higher than normal, and fatigue associated with daily activities may result in poorer scores late in the day.

Regardless of which tests you do, practice them before using them to assess your fitness. Practice allows you to pace yourself and perform the tests properly so that you get accurate assessments. Because you may get different ratings on different tests of cardiorespiratory endurance, consider the strengths and weaknesses of each test when making decisions about which score best represents your fitness. After you've done regular exercise over time, test yourself again to see how much you've improved.

How Much Cardiorespiratory Endurance Is Enough?

The risk of hypokinetic diseases is greatest for people in the low fitness zone. Moving out of the low fitness zone and into the marginal fitness zone provides

FIT FACT

Studies show that endurance athletes—such as cross-country skiers, cyclists, and distance runners—typically have very high aerobic capacity and score well on field tests of cardiorespiratory endurance.

some health benefits, but to get optimal health and wellness benefits associated with cardiorespiratory endurance, you should achieve the good fitness zone. You can use the rating charts that accompany each self-assessment in this book to determine your ratings.

Some people aim for especially high cardiorespiratory endurance because they want to perform at a high level in a sport or a physically demanding job, such as being a Marine or a police officer. To be properly fit for such challenges, you must train harder than most people. Achieving the high performance zone will be difficult for some people, and doing so is not necessary in order to get many of the health benefits of fitness. Nevertheless, the higher your cardiorespiratory endurance score, the lower your risk of hypokinetic disease.

LESSON REVIEW

1. What is cardiorespiratory endurance, and what are other terms often used to describe this part of fitness?
2. What are some of the benefits of physical activity and cardiorespiratory endurance?
3. What are some of the different methods of assessing cardiorespiratory endurance?
4. How much cardiorespiratory endurance does a typical person need?

SELF-ASSESSMENT: **Step Test and One-Mile Run Test**

As you've learned, the maximal oxygen uptake test is the best test of fitness of the cardiovascular and respiratory systems. But if you want a quicker, easier, and less expensive test, try the step test or the one-mile run test. Then, after you've done regular exercise over time, test yourself again to see how much you've improved. As directed by your teacher, record your scores and fitness ratings for either test (or both). You can then use the information to prepare your personal physical activity plan. If you're working with a partner, remember that self-assessment information is confidential and shouldn't be shared without the permission of the person being tested.

STEP TEST

1. Using a bench that is 12 inches (30 centimeters) high, step up with your right foot. Step up with your left foot. Step down with your right foot. Step down with your left foot.

2. Repeat this four-count pattern (up, up, down, down). Step 24 times each minute for three minutes.

3. As soon as you are finished, sit and count your pulse. Begin counting within five seconds. Count for one minute.

4. Determine your cardiorespiratory endurance rating with table 8.1. Record your heart rate and rating.

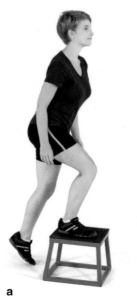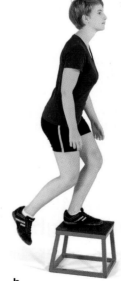

The step test assesses cardiorespiratory endurance.   **a**   **b**

Note: The height of the bench and the rate of stepping are crucial to getting an accurate test result. Sit calmly for several minutes before the test to assure that your resting heart rate is normal.

TABLE 8.1   Rating Chart for Step Test (Heartbeats per Minute)

	13 years old		14–16 years old		17 years or older	
	Male	**Female**	**Male**	**Female**	**Male**	**Female**
High performance	≤90	≤100	≤85	≤95	≤80	≤90
Good fitness	91–98	101–110	86–95	96–105	81–90	91–100
Marginal fitness	99–120	111–130	96–115	106–125	91–110	101–120
Low fitness	≥121	≥131	≥116	≥126	≥111	≥121

Those who cannot step for three minutes receive a low fitness rating.

ONE-MILE RUN

An alternative test of cardiorespiratory endurance is the one-mile (1.6-kilometer) run. Remember that this test is for your own information; it's not a race. Your goal is a good fitness rating, which indicates reduced risk of hypokinetic disease and enough fitness to function effectively. Some people may strive to achieve a high performance rating, which provides additional health benefits and allows you to perform sports and jobs requiring strong cardiorespiratory endurance.

1. Run or jog for one mile (1.6 kilometers) in the shortest possible time. A steady pace is best. Try to set a pace that you can keep up for the full run. If you start too fast and then have to slow down at the end, you will probably not be able to run for the entire distance. You can use target heart rate or ratings of perceived exertion (RPE) to help you set a good pace. Another indicator is the talk test. If you are unable to talk comfortably with a friend while running, then you are probably running too fast.

2. Your score is the amount of time it takes you to run the full distance. Record your time in minutes and seconds.

3. Find your rating in table 8.2 and record it.

TABLE 8.2   Rating Chart for One-Mile (1.6-Kilometer) Run (Minutes:Seconds)

	13 years old		14 years old		15 years old		16 years old		17 years or older	
	Male	**Female**	**Male**	**Female**	**Male**	**Female**	**Male**	**Female**	**Male**	**Female**
High performance	≤7:45	≤8:40	≤7:30	≤8:25	≤7:15	≤8:10	≤7:00	≤7:45	≤6:50	≤7:35
Good fitness	7:46–10:09	8:41–10:27	7:31–9:27	8:26–10:15	7:16–9:00	8:11–9:58	7:01–8:39	7:46–9:46	6:51–8:26	7:36–9:31
Marginal fitness	10:10–12:29	10:28–13:03	9:28–11:51	10:16–12:48	9:01–11:14	9:59–12:27	8:40–10:46	9:47–12:11	8:27–10:37	9:32–11:54
Low fitness	≥12:30	≥13:04	≥11:52	≥12:49	≥11:15	≥12:28	≥10:47	≥12:12	≥10:38	≥11:55

Based on data provided by G. Welk.

Building Cardiorespiratory Endurance

Lesson Objectives

After reading this lesson, you should be able to

1. define *vigorous aerobic activity* and explain its relationship with cardiorespiratory endurance;

2. describe the frequency, intensity, and time (FIT) of physical activity for building cardiorespiratory endurance;

3. describe the methods for counting resting heart rate and for estimating maximal heart rate; and

4. explain how to use two methods of measuring heart rate and the RPE method for determining if your activity is intense enough to build cardiorespiratory endurance.

Lesson Vocabulary

heart rate reserve (HRR)
maximal heart rate
ratings of perceived exertion (RPE)
vigorous aerobic activity

You now know that physical activity is important to your cardiorespiratory endurance. But how much physical activity do you have to do to improve your cardiorespiratory endurance? In this lesson, you'll learn about the best types of activity for building cardiorespiratory endurance. You'll also learn to determine how much physical activity you need in order to build your own cardiorespiratory endurance.

Physical Activity and Cardiorespiratory Endurance

As you know, activity that is aerobic is steady enough to allow your heart to supply all the oxygen your muscles need. Moderate physical activities are considered to be aerobic because you can do them for a long time without stopping. These activities provide many health benefits and can build cardiorespiratory endurance in people with low fitness, but they are not intense enough to build cardiorespiratory endurance for most people.

I knew that my cardiorespiratory endurance wasn't as good as it should be. But I wasn't sure about the best way to improve it. Learning about the FIT formula helped me to get going.

Ben Metzger

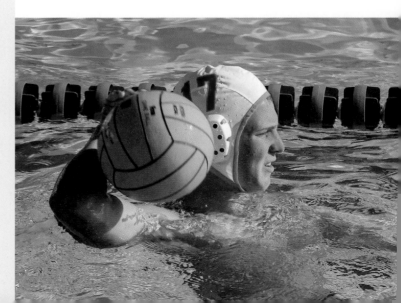

Vigorous aerobics, represented on the second step of the Physical Activity Pyramid, is the most effective way to build cardiorespiratory endurance. **Vigorous aerobic activities** are intense enough to elevate your heart rate above your threshold of training and into your target zone for cardiorespiratory endurance. National physical activity guidelines for teens recommend doing vigorous activity at least three days a week because they promote benefits beyond those provided by moderate activity.

Vigorous sport and recreation activities, represented on the third step of the Physical Activity Pyramid (figure 8.8), also build cardiorespiratory endurance. Vigorous sports often involve quick bursts of vigorous activity followed by rest, and for this reason they are not totally aerobic. However, they offer the same benefits as vigorous aerobic activity. To be considered vigorous, sports and recreation activities must be intense enough to elevate your heart rate above your threshold of training and into your target zone for cardiorespiratory endurance.

Energy balance

STEP 5
Flexibility exercises

STEP 4
Muscle fitness exercises

STEP 3
Vigorous sports, vigorous recreation, anaerobics, mixed fitness activities

STEP 2
Vigorous aerobics

STEP 1
Moderate physical activity

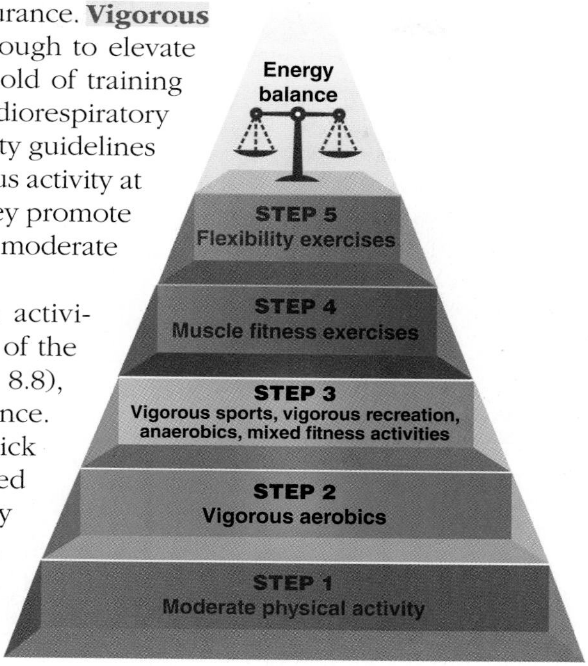

Figure 8.8 Vigorous activities (steps 2 and 3) are best for building cardiorespiratory endurance.

> To keep the body in good health is a duty; otherwise, we shall not be able to keep our mind strong and clear.
>
> *The Buddha*

How Much Vigorous Activity Is Enough?

National physical activity guidelines indicate that some of your recommended 60 minutes of daily activity should be of a vigorous nature. The FIT formula for vigorous physical activity is described in table 8.3. The threshold of training is listed first and represents the minimum values, followed by target zone values. Frequency (F) is determined in days per week and time (T) is determined by minutes per day. Intensity (I) is more complicated because it can be determined in several ways. The threshold and target zone heart rate values for intensity in table 8.3 are explained in the sections that follow.

FIT FACT

Activity guidelines for teens emphasize the importance of enjoyment and variety. You are more likely to meet activity guidelines if you choose activities that you enjoy. Selecting from a variety of activities helps promote enjoyment.

TABLE 8.3   **Threshold of Training and Target Heart Rate Zones (FIT Formula) for People Who Are Physically Active**

	Threshold of training	Target heart rate zone
Frequency	3 days a week	3–6 days a week
Intensity*		
Personal (HRR)	60%	60%–80%
General (% max HR)	80%	80%–90%
Time	20 min	20–90 min

*For inactive people, reduce the percentages by 10 (e.g., 60 becomes 50).

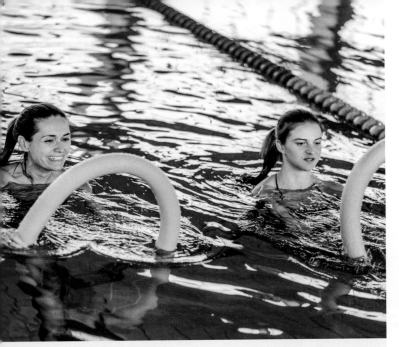

Water aerobics can be a good form of vigorous activity.

The ACSM recommends two methods of using heart rate to determine target zone intensity. The first, often called the *personal method* because you use personal resting heart rate values to calculate it, is officially known as the heart rate reserve (HRR) method. **Heart rate reserve (HRR)** refers to extra heartbeats available to you above your resting heart rate. Your heart rate reserve is calculated by subtracting your resting heart rate from your **maximal heart rate**, or the highest heart rate you can reach during the most vigorous exercise. You use a percentage of your heart rate reserve (%HRR) to determine threshold and target heart rate zone values (see table 8.3). For the second method, often called the *general method*, you use a percentage of your maximal heart rate (% of max HR) to determine adequate intensity (see table 8.3). As you can see, the percentages are different because the methods are different. You will learn more about these methods later in this lesson.

The values for intensity in table 8.3 are for healthy teens who participate somewhat regularly in vigorous physical activity. For those who do no regular vigorous activity, the intensity values should be reduced by 10. For teens who are highly active, the values can be increased by 10. The frequency and time values are the same as shown in table 8.3 for all teens, regardless of the regularity of their vigorous activity.

Determining Resting and Maximal Heart Rate

To determine your threshold of training and target heart rate zone using the personal method (HRR), you need to know your resting heart rate and your maximal heart rate. For the general method (% max HR) you only need your maximal heart rate. There are several methods of counting heart rate, including heart rate monitors or watches, using a stethoscope, or counting your pulse. Counting the pulse is easy to do and requires no special equipment other than a watch with a second hand.

Counting Your Resting Heart Rate (Pulse Counting Method)

Your resting heart rate is the number of times your heart beats when you are sitting at rest. For best results, you should sit quietly for several minutes before counting. Use the following instructions.

1. Sit and take your heart rate by using the first and second fingers of your hand to find a pulse at your opposite wrist (your radial pulse) (figure 8.9*a*). Do not use your thumb. Practice so that you can locate your pulse quickly.

2. Count the number of pulses for one minute. Record your one-minute heart rate. You can also count your pulse for 30 seconds and multiply by 2, or count for 15 seconds and multiply by 4, to get a one-minute resting heart rate.

3. Take your resting (seated) heart rate again, this time counting the pulse at your neck (your carotid pulse) (figure 8.9*b*). Place the index and middle fingers on the side of your neck. Move until you locate the pulse. Press only as hard as necessary to feel the pulse; be careful not to press too hard.

4. Have a partner take your pulse while sitting. Compare your self-counted heart rate with your heart rate as determined by your partner for both the radial (wrist) and carotid (neck) pulses.

5. As directed by your teacher, record your resting heart rate using each of the methods just described. Use your lowest resting heart rate value as your resting heart rate.

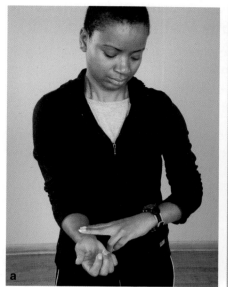 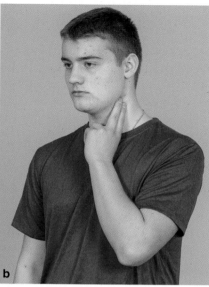

Figure 8.9 Use your index and middle finger to find a pulse *(a)* at your wrist and *(b)* at your neck.

Determining Maximal Heart Rate (max HR)

Maximal heart rate (max HR) is the highest possible heart rate that a person can reach during the most vigorous exercise. Because determining a true max HR requires very vigorous activity, it isn't appropriate for some people. For this reason, exercise physiologists have developed several formulas for estimating max HR without doing exercise. Several different formulas are listed by the ACSM. Each has advantages and disadvantages.

The Fox formula (220 – age) for calculating estimated max HR is the simplest and the most widely used method for adults. However, it overestimates maximal heart rate for children and teens. Recent research indicates that the Tanaka formula (208 – [0.7 × age in years]) is more accurate for youth. For this reason, we use the Tanaka formula. You can use table 8.4 to get your estimated max HR or calculate it using the Tanaka formula.

Determining Physical Activity Intensity

The ACSM provides guidelines for determining how much physical activity is enough for building cardiorespiratory endurance and aerobic capacity, shown in table 8.3. As noted earlier, the frequency of activity is easy to determine (days per week), as

TABLE 8.4 **Estimated Maximal Heart Rates**

Your age (years)	12	13	14	15	16	17	18	19
max HR	200	199	198	198	197	196	195	195

is the time of activity (minutes per day). Determining intensity is a bit more complicated. The most accurate method is using a percentage of a person's $\dot{V}O_2$max (aerobic capacity). However, the special equipment required makes this impractical for most people.

As you learned, there are two recommended methods of determining heart rate intensity. The ACSM also indicates that you can determine intensity using a rating of perceived exertion (RPE). All of these methods for determining intensity of physical activity are described in the sections that follow.

The Heart Rate Reserve Method (HRR)

The heart rate reserve (HRR) method is the most accurate method because it uses your personal resting heart rate to make calculations, though it is a bit more difficult to calculate. To use this method, you must know your resting and maximal heart rates and your heart rate reserve (HRR).

Table 8.5 provides you with the steps for determining your threshold and target heart rate zone values using the percent of heart rate reserve (% HRR). The example values used are for a 16-year-old who is generally physically active. People who are generally inactive or

very active can use the values described in the footnote to table 8.3.

The Percent of Maximal Heart Rate Method (% max HR)

The percent of maximal heart rate (% max HR) method is not quite as accurate as the HRR method for determining target heart rate, but it is easier to calculate. In this method, you do not use your resting heart rate. Table 8.6 provides you with the steps for determining your threshold and target heart rate zone values using the percent of maximal heart rate (% max HR) method. The example values used are again for a 16-year-old who is generally physically active and has a resting heart rate of 67 beats per minute. People who are generally inactive or very active can use the values described in the footnote to table 8.3.

Ratings of Perceived Exertion (RPE)

An exercise physiologist named Gunnar Borg developed the first scale for estimating exercise intensity using **ratings of perceived exertion (RPE)**. His original RPE scale used numbers from 6 (no exertion) to 20 (maximal exertion). Since then, several other scales have been used.

TABLE 8.5 **Determining Target Heart Rate With the Heart Rate Reserve Method**

Steps	Calculations	Example
Resting heart rate	Count your pulse to determine a one-minute resting heart rate.	67 beats per minute
Maximal heart rate	208 − (.07 × age in years) = max HR	208 − (.07 × 16) 208 − (11.2) = 197 (rounded from 196.8)
Heart rate reserve	Maximal HR − resting HR = HRR	197 (max HR) − 67 (resting HR) = 130 (HRR)
Threshold heart rate	HRR × .60 (60%) + resting HR = threshold HR	130 (HRR) × .60 (threshold %) = 78 + 67 (resting heart rate) = 145 (threshold heart rate)
Target ceiling heart rate	HRR × .80 (80%) + resting HR = ceiling HR	130 (HRR) × .80 (ceiling %) = 104 + 67 (resting HR) = 171 (ceiling HR)
Target HR zone	Threshold to ceiling HR	145–171 beats per minute

TABLE 8.6 **Determining Target Heart Rate With the Percent of Maximal Heart Rate Method**

Steps	Calculations	Example
Maximal heart rate	208 – (.07 × age in years) = max HR	208 – (.07 × 16) = 208 – (11.2) = 197 (rounded from 196.8)
Threshold heart rate	Maximal HR × .80 (80%) = threshold HR	197 (max HR) × .80 (threshold %) = 158 (threshold HR)
Target range ceiling heart rate	Maximal HR × .91 (91%) = ceiling HR	197 (max HR) × .91 (ceiling %) = 179 (ceiling HR)
Target heart rate zone	Threshold to ceiling HR	158–179 beats per minute

A 10-point scale called the OMNI RPE scale has been shown to be effective for use with people of all ages, including teens. The OMNI scale (see figure 8.10) allows you to rate perceived exertion from 1 (no exertion) to 10 (maximal exertion). The RPE target zone range for building cardiorespiratory endurance in active teens is 6 to 8 (vigorous physical activity). For less active teens, the range is 5 to 7. Ranges of 3 to 6 for active teens and 3 to 5 for less active teens represent moderate physical activity.

Monitoring Vigorous Physical Activity Intensity

Now that you have learned about the different methods of determining physical activity intensity, you can use one or more of them to monitor your activity.

Heart Rate Monitoring

To use either the HRR or % HR method you must know if your heart rate during

physical activity gets you into the target zone. It can be difficult to count your pulse *during* vigorous activities, but you can get a good estimate of your heart rate during a physical activity by determining your heart rate immediately after exercising. To estimate, use the following instructions.

1. Immediately after exercise, locate your pulse (within 5 seconds).

2. Use either your wrist or neck pulse as described earlier to count your heart rate for 15 seconds. Multiply your count by 4 to get your one-minute heart rate. This method is useful because it is efficient and because your heart rate slows down quickly when you stop exercising, which

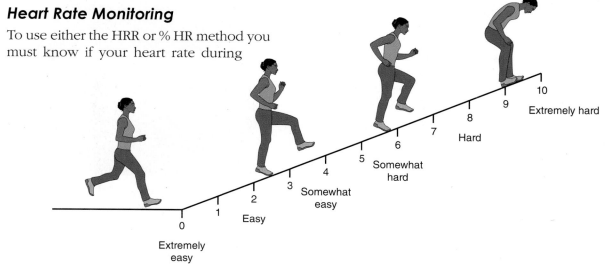

Figure 8.10 OMNI score for ratings of perceived exertion in physical activity.

Adapted from R. Robertson, *Perceived Exertion for Practitioners: Rating Effort With the OMNI Picture System* (Champaign, IL: Human Kinetics, 2004), 11. By permission of R. Robertson.

means longer counts may underestimate your heart rate during exercise. On the other hand, counting for a shorter time can result in error because a single counting mistake is multiplied. You can use table 8.7 to help you determine your one-minute heart rate from your 15-second count. While you count your heart rate, you may want to continue to walk slowly to help you recover faster.

TABLE 8.7   **Heart Rate in 15-Second and 1-Minute Intervals**

15-sec rate	1-min rate	15-sec rate	1-min rate	15-sec rate	1-min rate
15	60	27	108	39	156
16	64	28	112	40	160
17	68	29	116	41	164
18	72	30	120	42	168
19	76	31	124	43	172
20	80	32	128	44	176
21	84	33	132	45	180
22	88	34	136	46	184
23	92	35	140	47	188
24	96	36	144	48	192
25	100	37	148	49	196
26	104	38	152	50	200

Find your 15-second heart rate in a blue column; your 1-minute heart rate is in the yellow column to the immediate right of it.

TECH TRENDS: Smart Watches and Heart Rate Monitors

Smart watches have many functions in addition to telling time. Some versions of the Apple Watch have a sensor to detect electrical stimulation from your heart's nervous system (electrocardiogram or EKG) to count your heart rate during activity. You can use the watch to determine when you are in the target heart rate zone and to keep track of how many minutes you stay in your target zone. The Apple Watch can also detect abnormal heart rhythms and allows you to send a recording to your doctor.

However, the Apple Watch and many other smart watches are quite expensive. Less expensive heart rate monitors are available. If your school has heart rate monitors, you might have the opportunity to try one out.

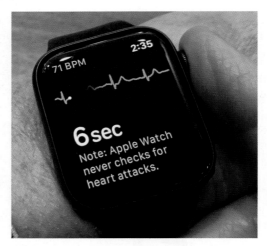

A heart rate watch is helpful for counting your pulse during activity.

USING TECHNOLOGY

Use a variety of sources to evaluate smart watches and heart rate monitors (e.g., physical education teacher, magazines such as *Consumer Reports*). Consider cost, reliability, and ease of use, then decide which monitor would be the best buy.

If you have trouble counting your heart rate while walking, stand still when you count, then begin moving.

3. Once you have established your heart rate after the activity, see if it is elevated into your target heart rate zone. You can use either your % HRR or your % max HR to determine your target heart rate zone.

Monitoring heart rate using this method is simple and inexpensive; it does not require any special equipment other than a watch or the timer on your smartphone. If available, you can also use a heart rate watch or a heart rate monitor to determine your actual heart rate during activity rather than using an estimate (see Tech Trends feature).

RPE Monitoring

As described earlier, you can also use the OMNI RPE scale as an alternative to heart rate for monitoring physical activity intensity.

LESSON REVIEW

1. What are vigorous aerobic activities, and how are they important for building cardiorespiratory endurance?
2. What is the frequency, intensity, and time (FIT) of physical activity necessary to build cardiorespiratory endurance?
3. How do you count your resting heart rate and estimate your maximal heart rate?
4. How can you use the two heart rate methods and rating of perceived exertion (RPE) to determine if your physical activity is intense enough to build cardiorespiratory endurance?

TAKING CHARGE: **Self-Confidence**

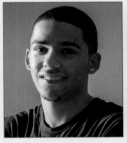

Self-confidence involves believing that you can be successful in an activity. If you think you'll succeed, you have more confidence than if you're unsure about how well you'll do. You're more likely to participate in an activity if your confidence is high.

Tony rarely takes part in any physical activity. He went through an awkward stage in his preteen years and thinks that people laugh at the way he runs: "My arms and legs don't seem to work together when I run. I think I look foolish."

Mei, on the other hand, loves any kind of physical activity. Every day, she shoots baskets or rides her bike, and she is a member of multiple teams. Even though she excels in sport, however, she feels shy around strangers and would like to socialize more: "I can't think of anything witty or even halfway intelligent to say. When I try to talk, I get tongue tied. It's easier for me to just avoid talking."

Tony and Mei lack self-confidence but in two different situations. Tony wants to participate in physical activity, and Mei wants to socialize, but they both avoid situations where they might get involved because they feel uncomfortable. Both need to find a way to build their self-confidence so they can succeed.

FOR DISCUSSION

People like Tony may avoid trying new activities or quit an activity prematurely. People like Mei who lack confidence in social situations may avoid them.

>continued

>*continued*

What are some reasons that people lack self-confidence? How can they increase their self-confidence? What advice can you give Tony to get him to try new activities and stick with them? What advice can you give Mei to help her be more comfortable in social situations?

Consider the guidelines presented in the following Self-Management feature as you answer these discussion questions.

SELF-MANAGEMENT: Skills for Building Self-Confidence

A recent study of teenagers found that one of the best indicators of who will be physically active is self-confidence. Some people are not very confident when it comes to physical activity because they think they are not very good at it or that others are better than they are. Does it surprise you to learn that self-confident people are not always the best performers and that some good performers lack confidence? In fact, research done with teenagers in schools shows that all students can find some type of activity in which they can be successful, regardless of physical ability. In addition, people who think they can succeed in activity are nearly twice as likely to be active as people who don't think they can succeed.

Building self-confidence is a self-management skill that you can learn. You may want to assess your self-confidence using the worksheet supplied by your teacher. Then, if necessary, you can use the following guidelines to improve your self-confidence.

- *Learn a new way of thinking.* One major reason some people lack self-confidence is that they think their own success depends on how they compare with others. Practicing a new way of thinking means setting your own standards of success rather than comparing yourself with others.

- *Set your own standards for success.* Assess yourself and set standards for success related to your own improvement. Comparing yourself with others is not necessary for success, and it can contribute to low self-confidence.

- *Avoid competition if it causes you a problem.* Some people like to compete, but others don't. If competition makes you feel less confident, try to find noncompetitive activities (such as walking, jogging, and swimming) that allow you to feel good about yourself.

- *Set small goals that you're sure to reach.* Setting goals that are a bit higher than your current level is a good idea, but don't set them too high. As you reach one small goal, you can set another. Reaching several small goals builds your self-confidence, whereas not reaching one unrealistic goal can make you less confident.

- *Think and act on positive—not negative—ideas.* When you're involved in a physical activity, think of how you can improve. Talk to yourself about what you did well and what you can practice to improve in the future. Avoid negative self-talk, such as berating yourself for what you didn't do well or referring to yourself in negative terms.

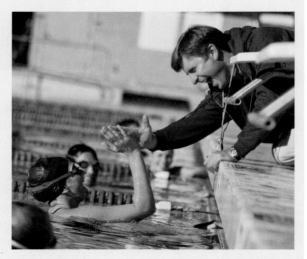

Setting a personal standard of success and getting reinforcement from others can help you build self-confidence.

Taking Action: **Target Heart Rate Workouts**

Cardiorespiratory endurance is important for living a long and healthy life. It's also essential for participating in your favorite physical activities and maintaining a healthy body weight. As you've learned in this chapter, you must do vigorous physical activity above your threshold of training and in your target zone to build cardiorespiratory endurance. **Take action** by doing vigorous activity that fulfills the FIT formula: at least three days each week (frequency), in your target heart rate zone (intensity), and for at least 20 minutes each session (time). Consider the following tips as you perform a target heart rate workout.

- Determine your target heart rate by using either the percent of heart rate reserve method or the percent of maximal heart rate method.
- Before choosing vigorous activities, consider your level of fitness.
- Before doing vigorous activity, perform a five-minute general warm-up.
- Check your pulse rate or rating of perceived exertion periodically to make sure you're maintaining the intensity of your workout in your target heart rate zone.
- After your vigorous workout, perform a cool-down.

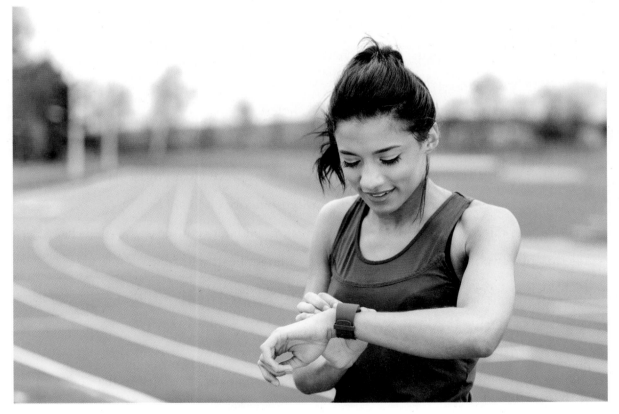

Take action by doing a workout that elevates your heart rate into the target zone.

CHAPTER REVIEW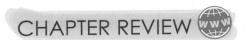

Reviewing Concepts and Vocabulary

Answer items 1 through 5 by correctly completing each sentence with a word or phrase.

1. Blood vessels that carry blood back to the heart are called _____.

2. The body system that includes your heart, blood vessels, and blood is the _____ system.

3. The substance in your blood that makes it clot is called _____.

4. The method for estimating exercise intensity without measuring it is called rating of _____.

5. The highest your heart rate ever gets is called your _____.

For items 6 through 10, match each term in column 1 with the appropriate phrase in column 2.

6. carotid   a. waxy, fatlike substance in blood

7. cholesterol   b. neck pulse

8. high-density lipoprotein   c. "bad" cholesterol

9. low-density lipoprotein   d. aerobic capacity

10. maximal oxygen uptake   e. "good" cholesterol

For items 11 through 15, respond to each statement or question.

11. Explain how cardiorespiratory endurance helps your cardiovascular and respiratory systems work more efficiently and therefore helps prevent cardiovascular disease.

12. How does aerobic capacity relate to cardiorespiratory endurance?

13. Describe the two field tests of cardiorespiratory endurance discussed in this chapter.

14. Describe two methods for determining your target heart rate zone.

15. Describe several guidelines for building self-confidence.

Thinking Critically

Write a paragraph to answer the following question.

Shante has a resting heart rate of 76 beats per minute. Bill has a resting heart rate of 54. Assuming that neither has a disease or illness, what are some possible reasons that their resting heart rates differ so much?

Project

In this chapter you learned two heart rate methods and the RPE method for monitoring the intensity of physical activity. Conduct a research study to determine if you get the same results with each method. On different days, perform the same vigorous workout. Determine if your workout was intense enough to build cardiorespiratory endurance with each method. Did you get similar results for each method? Which method do you think is best? Write a report and share it with others.

Vigorous Physical Activity

In This Chapter

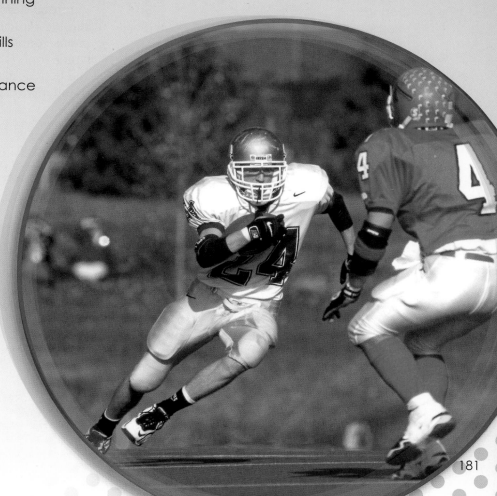

Vigorous Aerobics, Sports, and Recreation

Lesson Objectives

After reading this lesson, you should be able to

1. define *vigorous aerobics* and describe several examples of this type of activity;
2. define *vigorous sports* and describe several examples of this type of activity;
3. define *vigorous recreation* and describe several examples of this type of activity; and
4. describe several tips for safe participation in vigorous activities.

Lesson Vocabulary

aerobic
e-sports
exergaming
leisure time
lifetime sport
overexercising
recreation
sport
vigorous recreation
vigorous sports

How often do you engage in activities that make you breathe hard and sweat? As you know, activities such as vigorous aerobics, sports, and recreation are especially good for building cardiorespiratory endurance. They provide the same health benefits as moderate activity and help you perform well in athletic events and in certain careers (e.g., police, firefighters, military). Activities included in steps 2 and 3 of the Physical Activity Pyramid (see figure 9.1) are more vigorous (requiring 6 METs or more) than the moderate activities included in step 1 (3 to 6 METs).

Vigorous Aerobic Activity

Aerobic, meaning "with oxygen," refers to an activity for which the body can supply adequate oxygen to continue for long periods of time. Vigorous aerobic activities—such as jogging, aerobic dancing, cycling, and swimming—are intense enough to raise your heart rate into the target zone. They are among the most popular and beneficial of all the vigorous activities. Their popularity results from the following reasons.

> Dancing is in my blood. It relaxes me and makes me feel good about myself. Sometimes I lose myself in dance—it just makes me feel good.
>
> *Louie Aceves*

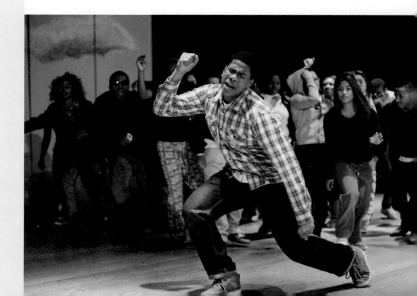

- They often do not require high levels of skill.
- They frequently are not competitive.
- They often can be done at or near home.
- They often do not require a partner or group.

There are many types of vigorous aerobic activity. Some of the most popular are briefly described in the following sections. Note that some activities could be classified in more than one section of the Physical Activity Pyramid. For example, swimming is a sport, a type of vigorous aerobic activity, and a type of vigorous recreation; in this book, it is classified as a vigorous aerobic activity. Each activity is described only once in this chapter, even if it could fit into multiple categories.

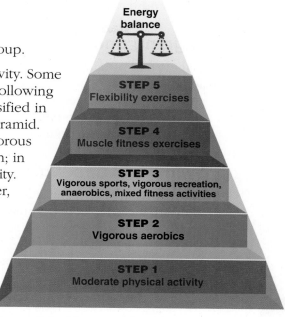

Figure 9.1 Vigorous physical activities (steps 2 and 3) build cardiorespiratory endurance and anaerobic capacity and enhance health and physical performance.

Aerobic Dance

Aerobic dance involves continuously performing various dance steps to music. Unlike social dancers, aerobic dancers typically dance by themselves, often following a leader or a video. Forms of aerobic dance include low-impact (one foot on the ground at all times), high-impact, and step aerobics.

Aerobic Exercise Machines

Types of aerobic exercise machines include treadmills, rowing machines, exercise bicycles, stair steppers, and ski machines. They can be used in your own home or in health clubs and schools. They can be effective if used properly, but some people do not find exercise on machines to be as enjoyable as activities that allow them to move more freely. For example, skiing may be more enjoyable than using a ski machine. Also machines for your home are expensive and those who can afford them may not have space for them. Joining a health club gives you access but not all people can afford a membership or have the time to travel to and from a club.

Bicycling

Bicycling can be classified as a competitive sport and as a recreational activity. If done at a steady pace for a sustained period, it can also be considered a form of moderate physical activity. It is included here because it is often done continuously at a consistent speed that elevates the heart rate. Some forms of cycling, such as BMX and downhill mountain biking, are considered extreme sports.

Dance

Dance is one of the oldest art forms and a means of expression in many cultures. Some dance forms are not only enjoyable but also excellent forms of vigorous aerobic exercise. More traditional dance activities include modern, ballet, folk, and square dance. Another category of dance is social dance, which includes both more traditional types (such as the waltz, country dancing, and Latin dancing) and newer forms (such as hip-hop and line dancing). Some dance activities use traditional steps in ways that are similar to aerobic dance; for example, Zumba uses Latin music and dance steps in ways that resemble aerobic dance.

Jogging and Running

Jogging and running consistently rank among the most popular forms of vigorous aerobic activity. Jogging is generally noncompetitive, whereas running is often done more seriously. Runners often participate in competitive events such as 5K and 10K races. Jogging and running are combined into one category here because they are very similar. You'll learn more about them in this chapter's Self-Assessment feature.

Swimming and Water Activities

Swimming and other water activities can be both a sport and a form of recreation. They are included here because they are among the most popular fitness activities among adults and can serve as a good way to improve cardiorespiratory endurance for almost all people when performed vigorously. Common activities include lap swimming and water aerobics. Water activities are a good choice for people who are overweight, elderly, or suffering from joint problems because they are not weight bearing.

Vigorous Sport

Sport involves physical activities that follow well-established rules. Typically, sports involve the large muscles of the body and moderate to vigorous physical activity. They are competitive and usually only one participant or team can win. Some sports, such as golf and bowling, are classified as moderate physical activity (step 1 of the Physical Activity Pyramid). **Vigorous sports** (Physical Activity Pyramid step 3) elevate the heart rate above the threshold level and into the target zone for cardiorespiratory endurance.

There are so many vigorous sports that it is impossible to mention them all here. However, general categories include team sports, partner sports, individual sports, and outdoor, challenge, or extreme sports. (Others exist but are not considered here because they have little relevance to a personal physical activity program, such auto racing and horse racing.)

Team Sports

Team sports such as basketball, football, hockey, volleyball, and soccer are among the most popular for high school students and for adult spectators. Cheerleading and competitive cheer are vigorous activities that are included in the team sport category. These activities can be very good for helping participants build fitness (though of course they do little for the fitness of spectators!). Team sports can be harder to participate in after your school years because they require teammates, as well as special equipment and facilities. Even though baseball and softball involve some vigorous activity and training for these sports is often vigorous, they are often considered to be moderate activities that include intermittent vigorous components.

Although team sports are very popular among youth, surveys indicate that they are often not among the most popular activities regularly performed by adults. The most popular adult activities are moderate physical activities (e.g., walking, gardening), vigorous aerobics (e.g., jogging, aerobic dance, swimming, spinning), or muscle fitness activities (e.g., resistance training, body weight exercise). Sports such as tennis, slowpitch softball, basketball, and soccer are among the most performed team sports among adults. Still, by comparison, relatively few people who played team sports when they were young continue to pursue them for a lifetime. For this reason, it will be important for you to actively seek opportunities if you want to continue team sports as you grow older. Another way to stay active is to begin learning an individual sport, a partner sport, an aerobic activity, or another activity that you can enjoy later in life.

Partner Sports

Partner sports are those you can do with just one other person (the person you are playing against) or with a partner against another set of partners (for example, tennis doubles). Tennis is often included in the top 10 participation activities in the United States, because it can be done with just one other person and because tennis courts are now widely available. Other examples of partner sports include badminton, pickleball, fencing, and judo. Because they require fewer people than team sports and therefore are easier to continue as you grow older, partner sports are often referred to as **lifetime sports**. However, some partner sports, such as wrestling, are not lifetime activities that many people continue as adults.

Individual Sports

Individual sports are those that you can do by yourself. Golf, gymnastics, bowling, and track and field are truly individual sports because you do not have to have a partner or a team to perform them. Many of these sports are also lifetime sports, although some, such as gymnastics, are not done by many people later in life (and gymnastics often requires a spotter). Skiing and skating are two forms of vigorous recreation that are also sometimes classified as individual sports.

Exergaming

Exergaming refers to digital games that involve using the large muscles of the body to perform physical activity that improves health-related physical fitness. Examples include video games that require you to perform movements shown on a screen or exercise that uses devices attached to a computer or game console (e.g., virtual tennis). Some allow you to track your heart rate and amount of exercise performed. Exergaming can be performed at home with special equipment or at video arcades or recreation facilities, though the expense is limiting to some. Research has shown that some forms of exergaming can be beneficial in developing physical fitness. Studies have also shown that exergaming increases motivation to be active. Exergames can be performed as an e-sport (see Tech Trends), although most current e-sport events do not include exergames.

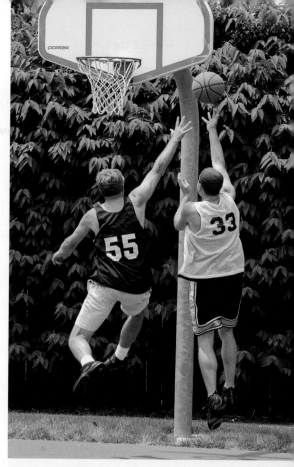

Basketball is one of the few team sports listed among the top 20 physical activities performed by adults in the United States.

FIT FACT

In *continuous* activities a person is active without stopping for relatively long periods of time (e.g., taking a 30-minute walk or jog). *Intermittent* activities involve bouts of activity followed by rest periods. Many sports include intermittent activity because of their stop-and-start nature (e.g., basketball rests during free shots). Activities such as interval training include short bouts of activity followed by rest periods, so they are considered to be intermittent activities.

TECH TRENDS: Electronic Sports (E-Sports)

The term **e-sports** (electronic sports) refers to organized competitive video gaming. In e-sports, individuals and teams compete against each other in leagues or at tournaments. Participants can compete at home using their own equipment or at events where equipment is provided. A variety of games on different platforms are used in e-sports competitions.

E-sports meet many of the criteria for being a sport. They follow set rules, are competitive, and require considerable skill. Some people contend that e-sports are really games similar to chess, not true sports. All are competitive and require skill, but none involve the vigorous activity similar to other sports described in this chapter and high levels of fitness are typically not required.

The National Federation of State High School Associations (NFHS) oversees and develops the rules for most high school competitions, including activities such as debate, speech, music, and theater—none of which meet all of the criteria for being a sport. Rules for e-sport competitions have been developed by the NFHS and now occur across the country.

Some critics express concern that video gaming is time consuming and contributes to sedentary lifestyles among teens. E-sports advocates note that nearly 75 percent of teens regularly play video games. They point out that e-sports has become a multimillion dollar industry, with televised national and world championships that draw millions of viewers and ever-expanding leagues and tournaments outside of schools. Advocates also argue that participation in e-sports prepares competitors for careers later in life. Given the large number of people who play e-sports, advocates argue that schools should have e-sports clubs as well as school teams to accommodate all who are interested.

STUDENT ACTIVITY

Prepare a statement that answers these questions: Do you think that e-sports are true sports? Do you think that participation in e-sports and video gaming affects your involvement in physical activities that improve your health-related fitness? Do you think that your school should have e-sports teams or clubs?

Outdoor, Challenge, or Extreme Sports

Many types of vigorous recreation can also be classified as sports. Some vigorous recreation activities are sometimes referred to as *outdoor* or *challenge sports*, such as mountain biking, rock climbing, sailing, and water skiing. Others are sometimes referred to as *extreme sports*, such as snowboarding, skateboarding, surfing, and BMX cycling.

Vigorous Recreation Activities

Vigorous recreation includes activities that are fun and typically noncompetitive. **Recreation** is something you do during your free time; therefore, recreational activities are sometimes called *leisure activities*. Recreation includes both physical activity and other pursuits, such as art and music. Here, of course, we focus on recreational activity that requires you to use your large muscles and involves considerable movement.

Many types of vigorous recreation are done outdoors because participants feel that the beauty of the setting and the fresh air helps rejuvenate them. Examples of vigorous recreation include the following.

Backpacking and Hiking

Hiking is particularly enjoyable because it takes place outdoors and can be done either independently or in a group. Most county, state, and national parks offer scenic trails for hikers of all levels of experience. Hiking usually involves a one-day trip, whereas backpacking often involves a multiday venture that requires you to carry food, shelter, and other supplies on your back.

Boating, Canoeing, Kayaking, and Rowing

Boating can be done in various forms that offer the enjoyment of water and the outdoors. When done vigorously, these activities also help you build fitness and promote good health. Kayaking and rowing can be especially vigorous, and they require considerable skill to perform well and safely. When not done vigorously, boating activities can be relaxing and refreshing.

Orienteering

Orienteering combines walking, jogging, and skilled map reading. It is usually done in a rural area and might include hiking through rugged terrain. Participants depart from a starting point in staggered fashion every few minutes (so that no participant can simply follow another). Each participant uses a compass and a map that describes a course up to 10 miles (16 kilometers) long. The compass is used to help locate several checkpoints marked by flags or other identifiers. At each checkpoint, the participant marks a card to indicate that they have located it. The activity can also be done competitively for time. Urban orienteering uses the same concept but in inner-city areas rather than rural settings.

Rock Climbing and Bouldering

Many schools now teach rock climbing using climbing walls. Learning on a climbing wall allows you to get proper instruction with good spotting (protection against falling). More advanced climbers are skilled in using special safety ropes and equipment. Beginners and intermediate climbers should always climb with the help of an expert. When rock climbing is done with proper equipment, it is a relatively safe activity. It's also a good activity for building muscle fitness.

Bouldering is a type of rock climbing in which the climber tries to reach the top of a boulder using only special shoes (no ropes or other equipment). Bouldering is most often done outside, but many clubs also have indoor bouldering walls. The height of climbs is typically limited to 15 feet (about 4.5 meters). As with rock climbing, bouldering requires special skills, so instruction is recommended for beginners.

> [Leave] all the afternoon for exercise and recreation, which are as necessary as reading; I will rather say more necessary, because health is worth more than learning.
>
> *Thomas Jefferson, U.S. president*

Canoeing can be a vigorous recreational activity that builds cardiorespiratory endurance and provides other health benefits.

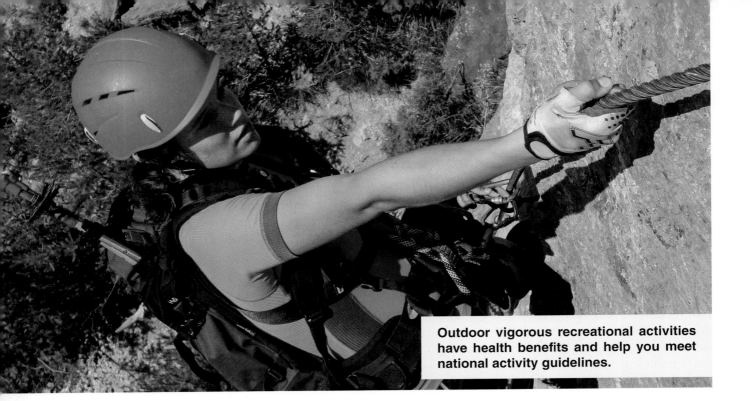

Outdoor vigorous recreational activities have health benefits and help you meet national activity guidelines.

Skateboarding

As you probably know, skateboarding is a popular recreational activity among teens. Competitive skateboarding is also considered an extreme sport. Like inline skating, skateboarding is a risky activity, so you should use proper safety equipment and seek proper instruction. You also need to find a proper place to perform skateboarding. Many skate hangouts are unsafe or located in places where skateboarding is prohibited, but many cities offer planned skate parks.

Skating

Types of skating include inline, ice skating, and roller skating. Inline skating was originally developed as a method of training for cross-country skiers in the summer, but its popularity has grown, and inline sports (for example, hockey) have been developed. One study by a sports medicine group found that inline skating was the most risky of the many participation activities studied, possibly because people fail to use proper safety equipment or because they try advanced skills too soon. Ice skating has some of the same risks as inline skating and is very popular in northern states. Roller skating is less popular and typically less risky than other forms of skating. The risk involved in skating activities makes it especially important for you to follow the safety guidelines described later in this chapter.

Skiing and Snowboarding

Kinds of skiing include cross-country skiing (a type of Nordic skiing), downhill skiing, snowboarding, and ski jumping. Cross-country skiing is typically done at a steady pace over a relatively long distance. For this reason, it could be considered a vigorous aerobic activity. Downhill skiing typically involves faster skiing, sometimes over moguls (bumps) and jumps. Snowboarding is similar to skateboarding on snow and has become extremely popular. It has joined the other forms of skiing as an Olympic sport, and some forms of snowboarding (halfpipe, superpipe, and slopestyle) can also be considered extreme sports. Ski jumping, also an Olympic sport, involves skiing down a ramp and jumping, trying to land as far down the hill as possible. All types of skiing could be considered sports, but they are included here because many of them are also popular activities for fun and recreation.

Guidelines for Safe Vigorous Activity

Participation in vigorous physical activities is not without risk. The following guidelines can help you perform these activities more safely.

- *Warm up before your workout.* Follow the warm-up guidelines described earlier in this book. Choose the appropriate warm-up for the type of activity you will perform.

- *Cool down after the workout.* A cool-down helps you recover more quickly.

- *Wear proper safety equipment.* For example, bikers and skaters should wear helmets, wrist guards, and elbow and knee pads. Dress appropriately for the weather.

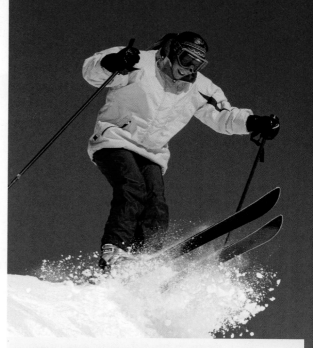

Skiing can be considered both a vigorous sport and a form of vigorous recreation.

- *Use safe equipment.* Bikes should have lights and reflectors. Backpacking equipment should fit your body size and loads should not be too heavy. Skis and other equipment should be in good repair, properly sized, and equipped with proper releases or other safety features. Boaters should wear life preservers. Rock climbers should use appropriate safety equipment. When doing any vigorous activity, especially in the heat, drink water regularly.

- *Get proper instruction.* Whether you're skiing, inline skating, boating, rock climbing, or doing any other activity, you should get proper instruction before participating. Performing an activity improperly has caused many people to get injured or have an accident.

- *Perform within the limits of your current skills.* Many injuries occur because people try to perform beyond their skill limits; for example, beginning skiers should not attempt to ski advanced slopes. For all activities, start with simple skills and then gradually attempt to perform more difficult skills as your abilities improve.

- *Don't overdo it.* Taking at least one day a week to rest can help you avoid injury, especially if you're participating in a vigorous aerobic activity such as aerobic dance or running. Most injuries can be prevented simply by not **overexercising** (doing so much exercise that you increase your risk of injury or soreness).

- *Plan ahead.* If you're going on a hike, make sure that you have a map and know where you're going. Carry an emergency phone. If you're going skiing, make sure that the trail is open, and don't ski in restricted areas. When backpacking, carry enough food and water to supply you if you get lost. When traveling in an unfamiliar area, stay with your group.

- *Get fit.* For most vigorous sport and recreation activities, you must have good fitness in order to perform well. For example, a baseball player must sprint between bases, slide into bases, and jump to catch the ball. Each of these actions could result in an injury if the player is not physically fit. Good or high-performance fitness is especially necessary for activities that involve physical contact (rugby, wrestling, ice hockey), sprinting (softball, soccer), sudden starts and stops (volleyball, racquetball), vigorous jumping (basketball, high jumping), danger of falling (skiing, skating, judo), and danger of overstretching muscles (tennis, football).

FIT FACT
Each year, participation in common recreational activities leads to two million medically treated injuries among youth in the United States. You can dramatically decrease your risk of injury by following simple safety tips when participating in physical activity.

LESSON REVIEW

1. What are vigorous aerobics, and what are some examples of this type of activity?
2. What are vigorous sports, and what are some examples of this type of activity?
3. What are vigorous recreation activities, and what are some examples of this type of activity?
4. What are some tips for safe participation in vigorous activities?

SELF-ASSESSMENT: **Assessing Jogging Techniques**

If you're looking for an excellent vigorous activity that requires little skill and no equipment—except for a good pair of running shoes and proper clothing—then jogging might be for you. Learning to jog properly will make the activity safe and fun. The following guidelines for jogging have been developed on the basis of the principles and concepts of biomechanics (e.g., leverage, stability) and exercise physiology (e.g., overload).

- Proper posture increases efficiency.
- Using the arms and legs (body levers) properly increases efficiency.
- Applying force in the direction of movement is more efficient than moving to the side.
- Friction is necessary in order to apply force and to prevent slipping.
- Action (foot striking) results in a reaction (impact to the sole of the foot or heel).
- Stability requires a wide base of support.
- Increasing speed (acceleration) is less efficient than maintaining a constant speed (velocity).
- Muscle contractions not used to produce movement are inefficient.
- You must do more than normal to improve.

Applying the Guidelines With a Partner

- Jog about 100 yards (90 meters) while your partner stands behind you to check your technique or takes a video of your performance.
- Have your partner answer the questions in table 9.1 after watching you jog, or answer them yourself after viewing the video. Your instructor may provide a worksheet that contains the questions.
- Have your partner jog while you evaluate their technique.
- Repeat a second time. Try to correct your technique.

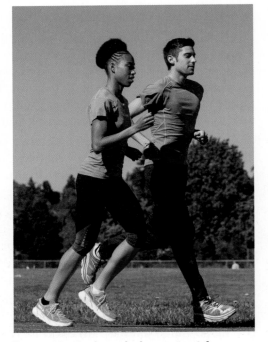

Proper technique is important for everyone, from beginning joggers to elite runners.

This self-assessment not only will help you jog more efficiently but also can reduce your risk of injury. Having your feet and legs out of alignment can cause unnecessary strain on your joints and muscles, causing injuries such as sore shins, sore calves, and even a sore back.

TABLE 9.1   Jogging Self-Assessment Guidelines and Checklist

Guideline	Principle/Concept	Checklist	✓
Use proper foot action. Land on your heel or your entire foot. Then rock forward and push off with the ball of your foot and your toes.	Leverage	Do you land on your heel or whole foot? Do you push off with the ball of your foot and toes?	
Swing your legs and feet forward. Do not let your feet turn out to the sides.	Force application	Do your legs and feet swing and land straight ahead?	
Swing your arms forward and backward. Do not swing them across your body or to the sides.	Force application	Do your arms swing straight forward and backward?	
Keep your trunk fairly erect. When jogging, do not lean forward as you would when starting to run fast. Keep your head and chest up.	Proper posture	Is your body erect or leaning forward only slightly? Are your head and chest up?	
Use a longer step than your normal walking step.	Leverage	Is your jogging stride longer than your walking stride?	
Keep your arms bent at the elbow and your hands relaxed. Try to keep your shoulders relaxed. Avoid jogging with a clenched jaw.	Efficient muscle use	Are your elbows bent properly (90 degrees) with your hands relaxed? Is your jaw relaxed?	
Jog at a steady pace. Avoid speeding up and slowing down. Correct jogging pace can vary from person to person. Find your own pace that elevates your heart rate into your target zone. If you are panting or gasping for breath, you are jogging too fast.	Velocity	Is your pace steady? Is your heart rate in your target zone after several minutes of jogging? Is your pace slow enough to prevent gasping for breath?	
Wear shoes with a wide sole and heel, good heel cushions, and tread designed for running.	Stability, friction	Do your shoes have a wide heel and sole and good tread?	

BEGINNER'S JOGGING WORKOUT

This workout helps you learn about how fast to jog to reach your target heart rate and get a fitness benefit. Try this workout after you've practiced your jogging technique.

1. Determine your target heart rate.
2. Jog for five minutes, trying to get your heart to the target level. Time your run—how long you run is more important than how far. Set your own course. Try to jog half the time moving away from your starting point and the other half returning to your starting point. If you are not near your starting point at the end of five minutes, walk the rest of the way back.
3. Focus on using the jogging techniques that you learned in this self-assessment.
4. At the end of five minutes, determine your one-minute exercise heart rate. Determine whether your rate was in your target heart rate zone.
5. Jog for five minutes again. If your exercise heart rate was lower than your target heart rate on the first jog, jog faster this time. If higher, jog slower. After your second run, count your exercise heart rate again.
6. Record your results.

Anaerobic Activities, Mixed Fitness Activities, and Vigorous Activity Planning

Lesson Objectives

After reading this lesson, you should be able to

1. define *anaerobic* and describe several types of anaerobic activities;

2. define *mixed fitness activities* and describe several types of these activities;

3. describe the health-related fitness benefits of vigorous activities and explain how to find an activity that you might enjoy; and

4. describe the steps you would take to prepare a personal vigorous activity program.

Lesson Vocabulary

anaerobic capacity
anaerobic physical activity
ATP-PC system
glycolytic system
mixed fitness activities
oxidative system

In this lesson, you'll learn about anaerobic and mixed fitness activities. You'll also learn to use the five steps of program planning to prepare your personal plan for vigorous physical activity. Creating your plan will help you meet national physical activity guidelines both now and later in life.

Anaerobic Physical Activity

Anaerobic physical activity is so intense that your body cannot supply adequate oxygen to sustain performance for more than a minute or so. Very vigorous anaerobic activity, such as an all-out sprint, can be sustained for only about 10 seconds. Other vigorous anaerobic activities are not "all-out" but are still very intense; these can be sustained for 11 to 90 seconds. Anaerobic activities are typically intermittent in nature

> When I was in elementary school I loved soccer. I still do! It is fun, keeps me fit, and active. I hope to play until I'm 100.
>
> *Taylor Malone*

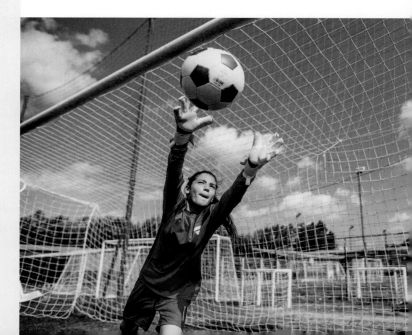

because time is necessary for recovery. Depending on the activity, recovery occurs during time-outs, rest periods, or breaks in the action.

Many vigorous sports (e.g., basketball, soccer) and vigorous recreational activities (e.g., skating, skiing) involve sprints or bursts of near maximal exertion. For this reason, these types of activities are both aerobic and anaerobic. The very vigorous bursts requiring maximal effort are anaerobic, whereas the less-intense continuous activity is aerobic.

Anaerobic Capacity and Interval Training

Aerobic activities are the preferred method of building cardiorespiratory endurance. Anaerobic activities also contribute to cardiorespiratory endurance but are mostly used to build **anaerobic capacity**, the ability to perform all-out exercise such as very vigorous sprinting or biking. Anaerobic capacity allows you to recover more quickly

The Wingate test measures anaerobic capacity.

from short, very intense bursts of exercise and therefore can help you to improve your performance in many different activities.

One of the most common tests of anaerobic capacity is the Wingate test, which is done on a bicycle ergometer (stationary bicycle) and requires an all-out effort to pedal as fast as possible. This test is typically reserved for very fit people interested in high-level anaerobic performance.

The FIT Formula for Anaerobic Activities and Building Anaerobic Capacity

The FIT formula for the most common types of anaerobic activity (e.g., high-intensity interval training) is shown in table 9.2.

People who train for vigorous sport and recreation activities often do anaerobic activity training, as do people in careers such as professional sports, police work, firefighting, and military service.

TABLE 9.2 **The FIT Formula for Anaerobic Physical Activity**

Frequency (F)	Three to six days a week
Intensity (I)	Upper level of the target heart rate zone (because exercise bouts are short)
Time (T)	Multiple exercise bouts of 10–60 sec alternated with 1- to 2-min rest periods

Interval Training

Interval training is a form of intermittent activity that typically involves repeated bouts of anaerobic exercise alternated with rest periods or bouts of lower-intensity exercise. The FIT formula for anaerobic interval training is provided in table 9.2. As intensity increases, duration of bouts decreases within the ranges shown in table 9.2. One of the most common forms of interval training, high-intensity interval training (HIIT), is a type of anaerobic training that uses very short and intense

FIT FACT
During anaerobic activities, your body builds up an "oxygen debt" because it can't take in enough oxygen to replenish the fuel needed to continue performance. After the activity is completed, adequate oxygen becomes available to replenish the fuel stores and repays the oxygen debt.

SCIENCE IN ACTION: **Energy Sources for Physical Activity**

The human body uses three systems to provide energy for physical activity (figure 9.2). However, different systems are used as the primary source of energy for different activities, depending on their intensity. For short bursts of very vigorous activity, such as sprinting (for 10 seconds or less), the body primarily uses a high-energy fuel called adenosine triphosphate (ATP) and phosphocreatine (PC), supplied by the **ATP-PC system**. When the high-energy fuel is used up, a second system called the **glycolytic system** takes over. This system uses glucose stored in the muscles and liver as glycogen to provide energy for vigorous activities that last between 11 seconds and about 90 seconds, such as running up and down a soccer field several times or lifting a heavy weight many times.

For sustained activity of moderate intensity, such as brisk walking, the body uses the **oxidative system** (also called the *aerobic system*) to provide energy. This system allows you to perform activity for many minutes or even hours. The oxidative system is able to use both glucose and glycogen stored in the body to produce energy.

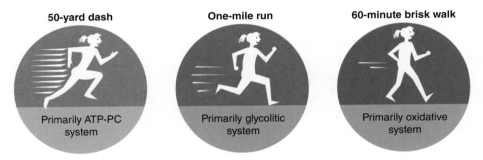

Figure 9.2   Energy systems used in activities of different intensities.

STUDENT ACTIVITY

Choose a vigorous physical activity that you especially enjoy. Do an analysis describing how the different energy systems are involved during a 10-minute bout of the activity.

bouts of activity followed by rest periods of low-intensity exercise. An example is swimming 10 25-yard sprints at 75 percent of maximum speed followed by one minute of rest. HIIT can be done using bouts of fast running, fitness stations, rope jumping, or exercise on machines such as treadmills, bikes, or stair steppers.

One of the benefits of anaerobic physical activity such as interval training is that workouts can be completed in a relatively short period of time, especially compared to continuous aerobic exercise such as jogging. It is most appropriate for people who have already achieved the good fitness zone for cardiorespiratory endurance and who regularly do vigorous activity. Before beginning this type of training, consult your teacher, coach, or other qualified expert in kinesiology.

Mixed Fitness Activities

Mixed fitness activities are activities that build many parts of fitness by combining several different types of activity into a single exercise bout. Some examples of mixed fitness activities are described here.

Circuit Training

Circuit training involves performing several different exercises one after another, with only a brief transition between exercises. The goal is to keep the heart rate in the target zone. Circuit training can use exercise machines, small equipment such as jump ropes or rubber bands, free weights, or no equipment at all (for example, calisthenics). Activities in the circuit can be both aerobic and anaerobic. Doing a variety of activities helps build muscle fitness as well as cardiorespiratory endurance and can keep you engaged. You can use music to determine how much time is spent on each exercise—a break in the music signals that it's time to move to the next exercise.

Martial Arts Exercise

Judo and karate (which can be classified as sports or recreational activities) are just two of the several hundred martial arts practiced around the world. Martial arts can build various parts of fitness, but they are not always good at building cardiorespiratory endurance because they may not involve enough continuous activity to keep the heart rate elevated. Some forms of martial arts, however, have been combined with aerobic dance to create martial arts exercises, such as Tae Bo and cardio kickboxing. While they are not true martial arts, they are included here because they have a martial arts component and they include a mix of different types of activities. They can build cardiorespiratory endurance, although they may not be as effective for self-defense as more traditional techniques.

Cross-Training

Cross-training was originally a type of training program that "crossed" or combined several different types of fitness activities in one workout—for example, jogging, jump rope, plyometrics, and calisthenics. More recently, combined fitness activities (e.g., CrossFit) and obstacle course racing (e.g., Tough Mudder) have emerged as competitive activities. In these competitions, various combinations of high-intensity anaerobic events, strength events, calisthenics such as burpees, and other types of activities are performed. Obstacle course races can cover distances ranging

> At the end of the day, if I can say I had fun, it was a good day.
>
> *Simone Biles, Olympic gymnast*

ACADEMIC CONNECTION: **Figurative Language**

Part of meeting standards for English language arts is being able to describe the meaning of words and phrases, including figurative and literal meanings. Figurative language describes a person or thing by comparing it to another thing. Literal language describes people and things as they actually are (in real terms).

When studying fitness, health, and wellness, you might have come across figurative language. Following are some examples of the use of figurative language from various categories.

- She is strong as an ox (simile: compares two things using the words *like* or *as*).

- He is a couch potato (metaphor: compares two things without using the words *like* or *as* to make a connection).

- He ran when he heard the crack of the bat (onomatopoeia: words that mimic sounds or sound like their meaning).

- I was so tired you could have knocked me down with a feather (hyperbole: exaggerating to emphasize a point).

- The team's bright uniforms screamed for attention (personification: things or ideas are described as if they had human characteristics).

STUDENT ACTIVITY

Prepare a list of five additional examples of figurative language associated with fitness, health, or wellness.

from 3 to over 15 miles and include a variety of obstacles and functional fitness challenges. Like circuit training, cross-training can provide variety. Like HIIT, these types of activities are often very vigorous and are most appropriate for people who perform with awareness of their current fitness and skill levels and who adhere to the guidelines for safe and effective participation.

Finding the Best Vigorous Activities for You

In this class, you'll get the opportunity to try many types of vigorous activity to help you discover which ones you like best. Try an activity more than once before you decide whether to do it in the future. It takes time to decide what you like and don't like. If you're going to stick with an activity over the long term, it must be enjoyable.

Table 9.3 provides information about the health benefits of different vigorous physical activities. You can use the table when planning your personal physical activity program to help you choose activities that benefit you the most.

Preparing a Vigorous Physical Activity Program Plan

Lin Su had been doing regular moderate activity but wanted to do more vigorous activity. She used the five steps of program planning to prepare a vigorous physical activity program. Her program is described in the following sections of this chapter.

In the Taking Action activity later in this lesson, you will use the same planning steps that Lin Su used to create a two-week personal plan for vigorous physical activity. Use table 9.4 to help you in your planning, then try out your program and see if you can meet your goals. The same steps can be used in the future to plan health goals or prepare for a special event, such as running a 10K race or participating on the cross-country team.

Step 1: Determine Your Personal Needs

To get started, Lin Su wrote down her fitness test results that related to vigorous physical activity and listed the vigorous physical activities that she had performed over the past week. Her results are shown in table 9.4.

Lin Su's cardiorespiratory endurance ratings showed that she was in the marginal category for each of the self-assessments that she performed and met the national activity guideline of 60 minutes per day on two days of the previous week. She did vigorous activity for 20 minutes on Tuesday and Thursday in her physical education class. On Friday she jogged for 20 minutes with her friend Eric, but she didn't do that regularly. She had also walked to and from school (20 minutes each way), and this moderate activity, combined with her physical education activities and jogging, totaled 60 minutes. On the other days, she did only moderate activity totaling less than 60 minutes. Lin Su knew that she needed to be more active and especially wanted to do more vigorous activity.

Step 2: Consider Your Program Options

Lin Su wanted to include activities that would help her build her cardiorespiratory endurance and offered other health-related benefits. She also wanted to focus

TABLE 9.3   **Health-Related Fitness Benefits of Selected Vigorous Physical Activities**

Activity	Develops cardiorespiratory endurance	Develops strength	Develops muscular endurance	Develops flexibility	Helps control body fat
Aerobic dance	Excellent	Fair	Good	Fair	Excellent
Aerobics machine	Excellent	Fair	Good	Poor	Excellent
Backpacking	Fair	Fair	Excellent	Poor	Good/Excellent
Badminton	Fair	Poor	Fair	Fair	Fair/Good
Baseball/Softball	Poor	Poor	Poor	Poor	Poor/Fair
Basketball, half-court	Fair	Poor	Fair	Poor	Poor/Fair
Basketball, full-court	Excellent	Fair	Good	Poor	Excellent
Biking	Good	Fair	Good	Poor	Good/Excellent
BMX cycling	Good	Good	Excellent	Fair	Good
Canoeing	Fair	Fair	Fair	Poor	Fair/Good
Cheerleading/ Competitive cheer	Good	Good	Good	Good/Excellent	Good
Circuit training/ Cross training	Good	Good/Excellent	Good/Excellent	Fair	Good/Excellent
Football	Fair	Good	Fair	Poor	Fair
Gymnastics	Fair	Excellent	Excellent	Excellent	Fair
Handball/Racquetball	Good/Excellent	Fair	Good	Poor	Good/Excellent
Hiking	Fair	Fair	Fair/Good	Poor	Good
Hip-hop dance	Good/Excellent	Fair	Good	Fair	Good/Excellent
Interval training	Excellent	Good	Good	Poor	Excellent
Kayaking	Good	Good	Good	Fair	Good
Martial arts	Good	Fair	Fair	Fair	Fair
Mixed fitness activities	Good/Excellent	Good	Good	Fair/Good	Good/Excellent
Mountain or rock climbing	Good	Good	Good	Poor	Good
Racquetball	Good/Excellent	Fair	Good	Poor	Good/Excellent
Rowing (crew)	Excellent	Fair	Excellent	Poor	Excellent
Skating (roller or ice)	Good	Fair	Good	Fair	Good
Skiing (cross-country)	Excellent	Fair	Good	Poor	Excellent
Skiing/Snowboarding (downhill)	Fair/Good	Fair	Good	Poor	Fair/Good
Soccer	Excellent	Fair	Good	Fair	Excellent
Social dance	Fair	Poor	Fair	Fair	Fair
Surfing	Fair	Poor	Good	Fair	Fair/Good
Swimming	Good	Fair	Good	Fair	Good/Excellent
Tennis	Good/Excellent	Fair	Good	Poor	Good/Excellent
Volleyball	Fair	Fair	Good	Poor	Fair/Good
Waterskiing	Fair	Fair	Good	Poor	Fair/Good

Benefits vary based on the specific activity performed.

TABLE 9.4   **Lin Su's Vigorous Physical Activity and Fitness Profiles**

Physical fitness profile			
Fitness self-assessment	**Score**	**Rating**	
Walking test	Time: 18:30 Heart rate: 150	Marginal fitness	
PACER	37 mL/kg/min	Marginal fitness	
Step test	Heart rate: 104	Marginal fitness	
One-mile (1.6 km) run	No score	No rating	
Physical activity profile			
Day	**Vigorous activity (min)**	**All activity (min)**	**Met guideline**
Mon.	0	40	
Tues.	20	60	✓
Wed.	0	40	
Thurs.	20	60	✓
Fri.	20	40	
Sat.	0	20	
Sun.	0	20	

on activities that she thought she would enjoy. To select vigorous activities, she used table 9.3, which illustrates the health-related fitness benefits of a wide variety of vigorous activities. However, this table includes only a sample of the most popular vigorous aerobics, sport, and recreation activities. A link to the full compendium of activities can be found at the Fitness for Life web resource.

After reviewing the list of activities, Lin Su wrote down her preferred activity options, which included her current activities and those she planned to include in her plan.

Vigorous aerobics

- Jogging
- Aerobic dance

Vigorous sports and recreation

- Hiking
- Inline skating
- Tennis
- Badminton

Anaerobics (e.g., interval training)
- Jumping rope

Mixed fitness activities

- Kickboxing in physical education class

Step 3: Set Goals

For this vigorous activity plan, Lin Su chose a time period of two weeks. Because two weeks is too short to accommodate long-term goals, she developed only short-term physical activity goals for the plan. Later, she will develop long-term goals, including some fitness goals, when she prepares a longer plan. For now, she referred to her activity preferences and chose several to develop her short-term goals. She also reviewed her work to be sure that she was setting SMART goals.

Short-term activity goals

- Continue current vigorous activity in physical education (20 min two days per week) and jogging (20 min one day per week).
- Play tennis (60 min) every other week.
- Hiking (60 min) every other week.
- Jump rope (10 min) one day a week.
- Aerobic dance (30 min) one day a week.

Step 4: Create a Written Program

Lin Su's written two-week plan for vigorous physical activity is shown in table 9.5. Lin Su included most of the preferred activities from her list in step 2. Her plan met the national activity guideline of at least 20 minutes of vigorous activity three days a week—in fact, it called for more than 20 minutes of vigorous activity on six days of the week. Lin Su decided to take a break from vigorous activity on Sunday. She also kept walking to and from school daily. Although this was moderate activity, she planned to keep doing it to help her meet the national activity goal.

TABLE 9.5 **Lin Su's Two-Week Vigorous Physical Activity Plan**

	Week 1			Week 2		
Day	**Activity**	**Time**	✓	**Activity**	**Time**	✓
Mon.	Jump rope	7:30–7:40 a.m.		Jump rope	7:30–7:40 a.m.	
Tues.	Physical education class	10:30–11:15 a.m.*		Physical education class*	10:30–11:15 a.m.*	
Wed.	Aerobic dance	4:00–4:30 p.m.		Aerobic dance	4:00–4:30 p.m.	
Thurs.	Physical education class	10:30–11:15 a.m.*		Physical education class	10:30–11:15 a.m.*	
Fri.	Jog	4:00–4:20 p.m.		Jog	4:00–4:20 p.m.	
Sat.	Tennis	9:00–10:00 a.m.		Hiking	9:00–10:00 a.m.	
Sun.	No planned activity			No planned activity		

*Only 20 minutes of the 45-minute class included vigorous kickboxing activity.

Step 5: Keep a Log and Evaluate Your Program

Over the next two weeks, Lin Su will monitor her activities and place a checkmark beside each activity she performs. At the end of the two-week period, she will evaluate her activity to see whether she met her goals, then use the evaluation to help her create another activity plan.

LESSON REVIEW

1. How do you define anaerobics, and what are some types of anaerobic activities?
2. How do you define mixed fitness activities, and what are some types of mixed fitness activities?
3. What are the health-related fitness benefits of vigorous activities, and how can you find an activity that you might enjoy?
4. What are the steps for preparing a personal vigorous physical activity program, and how would you implement them?

TAKING CHARGE: **Improving Performance Skills**

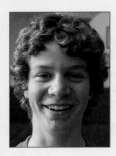

Performance skills such as kicking, throwing, hitting, and swimming can usually be learned with practice. It does, however, take some people longer than others to learn skills. Here's an example.

Zack felt that he was never really good at sports. He tried several activities and found that he was not as good at them as other people he knew. He even tried out for the soccer and swim teams at school but didn't make either one. His biggest problem was that he had not learned to play sports when he was young, and now he was behind others who had.

Zack wanted to learn a sport but was afraid that he'd be unsuccessful again and that his friends would

laugh at him. He performed a self-assessment of his skill-related abilities and was surprised to find that he did pretty well on most of the assessments. He did especially well in coordination and agility, though his speed was not very high.

Before trying out for another team, Zack thought it would be best to try to learn the skills needed for a sport that matched his abilities. His size seemed to be an advantage—he was over 6 feet (1.8 meters) tall and

weighed 180 pounds (82 kilograms)—but he wanted to get stronger, and he was not sure which sport would be best for him. He wanted to be on a team but also wanted to learn something that would be fun and interesting.

FOR DISCUSSION

What advice would you give Zack for choosing a sport? Once he makes his choice, what steps could he take to improve his performance skills? Who could he talk to for help? Zack knew that he needed to practice but wasn't sure exactly *what* to practice. What practice advice would you give him? Consider the guidelines in the Self-Management feature as you answer these discussion questions.

SELF-MANAGEMENT: **Skills for Improving Performance**

Experts in sport pedagogy and motor learning have studied the best ways to learn sport skills and developed guidelines that can help you as you work to improve your skills.

- *Get good instruction.* If you learn a skill incorrectly, it will be hard to improve, even with practice. Good instructors provide feedback that you can use to correct errors and improve your performance.

- *Practice.* Good practice is the key to improving your skills. It involves repeated performance focused on correct technique. Many people do not like to practice skills—they just want to play the game. But just playing the game doesn't provide practice in a particular skill, and if you play a game without the proper skills you

often develop bad habits that hinder your success.

- *Practice all skills, not just those that you already do well.* Sport requires more than a few skills to become proficient. For example, basketball requires shooting, dribbling, passing, catching, and defensive skills. In order to succeed, you must practice all necessary skills.

- *Don't try to fix everything at once.* When you first learn a skill, concentrate on the skill as a whole, then as you improve, concentrate on one detail at a time. If you try to concentrate on too many details at once, you may develop what is called "analysis paralysis," a condition in which you analyze an activity and try to correct several problems all at once. For example, if you're learning the tennis serve, don't try to work on your ball toss, grip, backswing, and follow-through at the same time. Instead, practice the parts of the skill one at a time, then put them all together.

- *Avoid competing while learning a skill.* Although competition can be fun, competing while you're learning a skill is stressful and does not promote optimal learning. When you compete, you are likely to only showcase skills that you are already good at, so you often don't make improvements in areas of need.

- *Think positively.* Experts have shown that if you think negatively, you're likely to

perform poorly. But if you think positively while you practice, you'll learn faster and become more confident in your abilities.

- *Choose an activity that matches your skill-related fitness.* Use the information from skill-related fitness assessments to help you determine which activities you might be best at performing.

- *Consider mental practice.* Research shows that practicing a skill mentally (i.e., imagining that you're performing the skill) can improve your performance. You can do mental practice even when you can't do regular practice due to factors such as bad weather or lack of a suitable facility.

Taking Action: **Performing Your Vigorous Physical Activity Plan**

Take action by preparing a vigorous physical activity plan using the five steps described in lesson 9.2. Like Lin Su, consider activities from all categories: vigorous aerobics, vigorous sport, vigorous recreation, anaerobic activities, and mixed fitness activities. Your goal should be to accumulate at least 20 minutes of vigorous physical activity on at least three days each week. Prepare a written plan and carry out it over a two-week period. Your teacher may give you time in class to do some of the activities included in your plan.

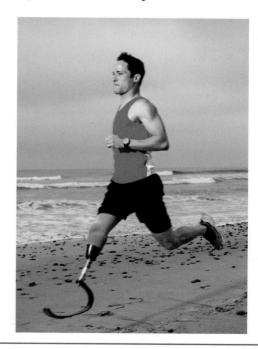

Take action by performing your vigorous physical activity plan.

CHAPTER REVIEW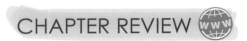

Reviewing Concepts and Vocabulary

Answer items 1 through 5 by correctly completing each sentence with a word or phrase.

1. Vigorous activity is exercise that raises your heart rate above the threshold level and into the _____.

2. Activities that are competitive and have rules are called _____.

3. Activities so intense that you can perform them for only a few seconds are called _____ activities.

4. Free time, or time free from work, is called _____.

5. Cardio kickboxing is a form of _____ exercise.

For items 6 through 10, match each term in column 1 with the appropriate phrase in column 2.

6. interval training
7. orienteering
8. inline skating
9. recreational activity
10. circuit training

a. a type of intermittent anaerobic activity

b. a common mixed fitness activity

c. done for fun during free time

d. uses map-reading skills

e. has relatively high injury risk

For items 11 through 15, respond to each statement or question.

11. What is the difference between individual and partner sports?

12. What are some examples of outdoor, challenge, and extreme sports? Why are these sports popular?

13. Describe the three systems that provide energy for sports and physical activities.

14. Describe the five steps in preparing a vigorous physical activity program and give examples of each step.

15. What are some guidelines for developing skills for improving performance?

Thinking Critically

Write a paragraph to answer the following question.

You have a friend who wants to avoid vigorous physical activity because of frequent injuries in the past. What advice would you give your friend to avoid such problems in the future?

Project

Create a vigorous aerobic exercise routine. Choose music paced at about 100 to 120 beats per minute and plan for the routine to last two to three minutes. You can do an aerobic dance routine, a hip-hop routine, or some other form of continuous exercise. Make a video of the activity and share it with others.

UNIT IV

Muscle Fitness and Flexibility

CHAPTER 10 **Muscle Fitness Basics**
CHAPTER 11 **Muscle Fitness Applications**
CHAPTER 12 **Flexibility**

Healthy People 2030 Goals and Objectives

Overarching Goals
- Attain healthy, thriving lives and well-being, free of preventable disease, disability, injury, and premature death.
- Eliminate health disparities, achieve health equity, and attain health literacy to improve the health and well-being of all.

Objectives
- Increase the proportion of adolescents and adults who do enough muscle fitness physical activity for health benefits.
- Reduce the proportion of people who do no physical activity in their free time.
- Increase the proportion of teens who participate in daily school physical education.
- Reduce the incidence of osteoporosis and increase osteoporosis screening.
- Reduce proportion of people with chronic pain that limits life or work activities.
- Reduce risk, incidence, and early death from chronic illness such as heart disease, stroke, cancer, and diabetes.
- Reduce unintentional injuries.
- Increase health literacy of the population.

Self-Assessment Features in This Unit
- Muscle Fitness Testing
- Healthy Back Test
- Arm, Leg, and Trunk Flexibility

Taking Charge and Self-Management Features in This Unit
- Preventing Relapse
- Finding Social Support
- Building Knowledge and Understanding

Taking Action Features in This Unit
- Resistance Machine Exercises
- Performing Your Muscle Fitness Exercise Plan
- Performing Your Flexibility Exercise Plan

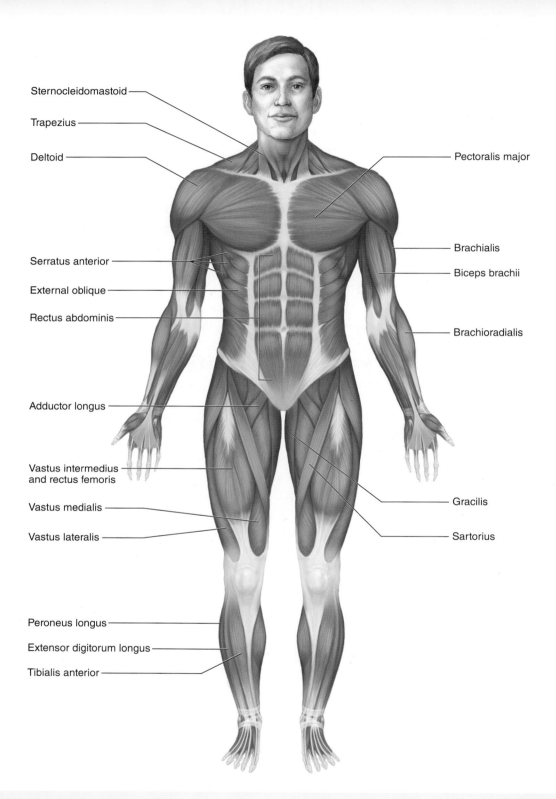

The major muscles of the body. The specific muscles addressed in the chapters that follow are described with each exercise. Refer to these two illustrations for exact muscle locations.

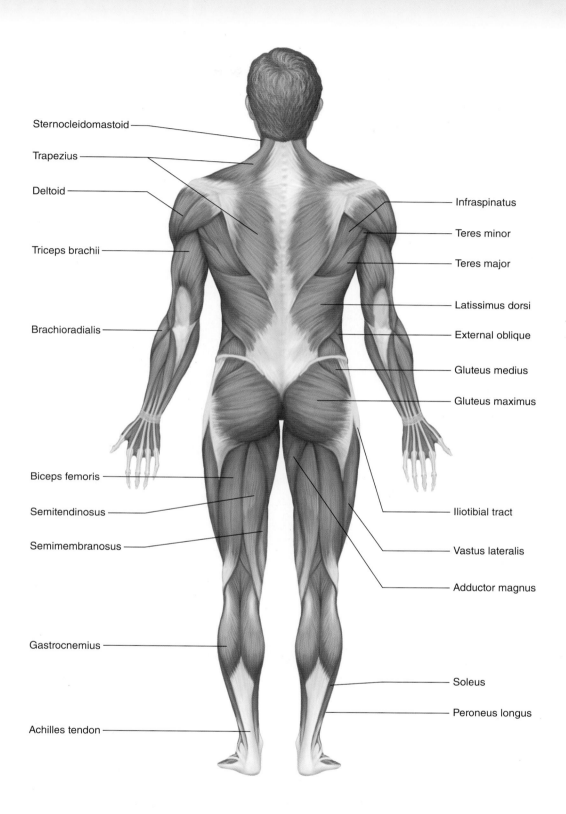

Sternocleidomastoid

Trapezius

Deltoid

Triceps brachii

Brachioradialis

Biceps femoris

Semitendinosus

Semimembranosus

Gastrocnemius

Achilles tendon

Infraspinatus

Teres minor

Teres major

Latissimus dorsi

External oblique

Gluteus medius

Gluteus maximus

Iliotibial tract

Vastus lateralis

Adductor magnus

Soleus

Peroneus longus

Muscle Fitness Basics

In This Chapter

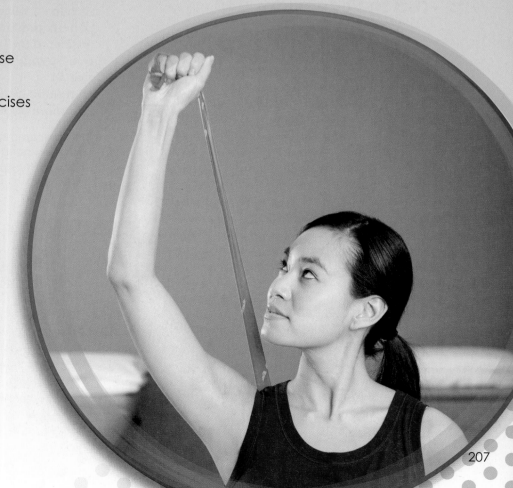

Muscle Fitness Facts

Lesson Objectives

After reading this lesson, you should be able to

1. explain the differences among strength, muscular endurance, and power;

2. explain how the basic principles of exercise apply to muscle fitness and describe some of the health benefits of muscle fitness exercise;

3. describe some different characteristics of muscles and identify and describe the major skeletal muscles; and

4. describe the different types of progressive resistance exercises and several methods for assessing each part of muscle fitness.

Lesson Vocabulary

absolute strength
bodybuilding
cardiac muscle
concentric
dynamometer
eccentric
fast-twitch muscle fiber
hypertrophy
intermediate muscle fiber
isokinetic exercise
isometric exercise
isotonic exercise
muscle contraction
Olympic weightlifting
one-repetition maximum (1RM)
plyometrics
powerlifting
principle of rest and recovery
progressive resistance exercise (PRE)
relative strength
rep
set
skeletal muscle
slow-twitch muscle fiber
smooth muscle

Earlier you learned about the various principles of physical activity. But do you know how the principles apply to building muscle fitness? Do you know about the different methods of building muscle fitness? In this lesson you will learn about muscle fitness definitions and principles, the characteristics of muscles, and the many methods of building muscle fitness.

Muscle Fitness Definitions

Together, strength, muscular endurance, power, and flexibility are referred to as *musculoskeletal fitness* because all are associated with the muscular and skeletal systems. In this book, *muscle fitness* is used to describe the three parts of musculoskeletal fitness that require the muscles to produce force—strength, muscular endurance, and power. Flexibility is discussed in chapter 12.

Strength is the amount of force that a muscle can exert. The highest amount of weight that a group of muscles can lift one time is called a **one-repetition maximum (1RM)**. This is considered the best measure of strength. Having good strength enables you to apply effective force in sports (such as football) and in tasks that require heavy lifting (figure 10.1a). You will learn more about 1RM later in this lesson.

> I thought muscle fitness exercises were just for athletes, but my mom tried them and now I know that they can be fun and help you look your best.
>
> *Tana Wenk*

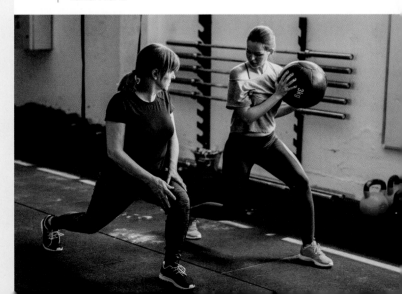

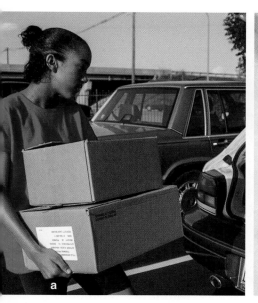
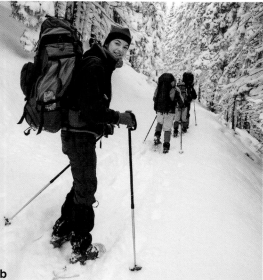
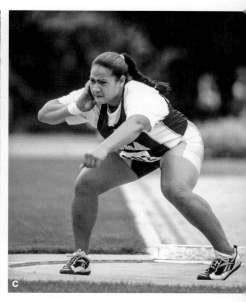

Figure 10.1 The parts of muscle fitness: *(a)* Lifting a heavy object requires strength; *(b)* using your muscles for a long time requires muscular endurance; and *(c)* doing activities that involve fast application of force requires power.

Muscular endurance is the ability to contract muscles many times or hold a muscle contraction for a long time without tiring. Muscular endurance allows you to resist muscle fatigue in recreational activities such as backpacking and to persist in work activities such as a nurse assisting people for hours at a time (figure 10.1*b*).

The third part of muscle fitness is power. Power is the ability to produce force quickly; thus it involves both strength and speed. It is often referred to as *explosive strength*. Examples of power include jumping high or far and throwing objects a great distance. Research has shown that power is especially important for bone health and that bone health built in the teen years provides lifelong benefits (figure 10.1*c*).

All three components of muscle fitness—strength, muscular endurance, and power—are important to both health and good performance. This chapter includes exercises to develop muscle fitness, step 4 of the Physical Activity Pyramid (figure 10.2).

Repetitions (Reps) and Sets

When performing muscle fitness exercise, it is important to know the meaning of two terms: reps and sets. The term **reps** (short for *repetitions*) refers to the number of consecutive times you do an exercise. A **set** is one group of reps. For example, suppose you do an exercise 8 times, then rest; repeat it 8 times, then rest again; and

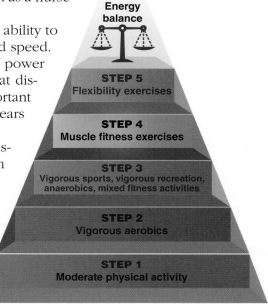

Figure 10.2 Muscle fitness activities fulfill step 4 of the Physical Activity Pyramid.

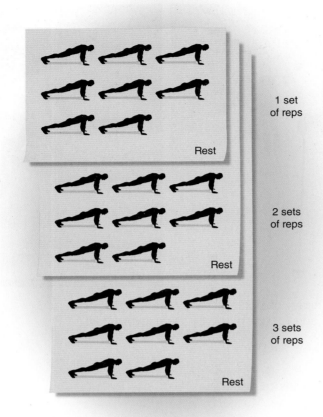

Figure 10.3 Muscle fitness exercises are typically done in reps and sets.

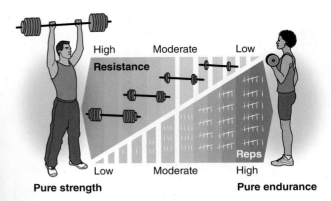

Figure 10.4 Muscular endurance–strength continuum.

repeat it another 8 times. You have just done 3 sets of 8 reps each. Figure 10.3 provides an illustration to help you understand these terms.

Muscle Fitness Interactions

Muscle fitness is a broad term that includes muscular endurance, power, and strength. These parts of health-related fitness are independent but related. Some of the interrelationships are described in the following paragraphs.

The Muscular Endurance– Strength Continuum

The exercises used to develop muscular endurance and strength differ only in the number of repetitions and the amount of resistance. The relationship between endurance and strength can be represented on a continuum such as the one shown in figure 10.4, which presents pounds of resistance on one side and number

of repetitions on the other. To develop strength, you use high resistance with fewer repetitions; to develop endurance, you use low resistance with more repetitions; and to develop both strength and endurance, you use the resistance and repetitions shown in the middle of the continuum. This continuum also shows that when you train for strength you will also develop some endurance, and when you train for endurance you will also develop some strength.

Cardiorespiratory Endurance and Muscular Endurance

Muscular endurance depends on the ability of your muscle fibers to keep working without getting tired. You can have good muscular endurance in one part of your body (such as your legs) without having it in another part of your body (such as your arms). Muscular endurance differs from cardiorespiratory endurance, which depends on your cardiovascular and respiratory systems to supply oxygen. Cardiorespiratory endurance is general (not specific to one area of the body) and allows your entire body to function for long periods of time without fatigue.

Strength and Power

As you learned earlier, power is sometimes referred to as *explosive strength* (strength × speed). For years, power was considered to be a skill-related part of fitness because it is important to sports activities such as jumping, kicking, and throwing. Today we understand that power, like strength, is also important for your health. Research indicates that adults who lack power have an increased risk of chronic disease, reduced life span, and poor functional health as they grow older. Exercise physiologists have also demonstrated that activities that produce power are very important for building healthy bones in youth. Because of these links to health, power is now classified as a health-related part of fitness.

Muscle Fitness: Principles

The basic principles of exercise you learned earlier can also be applied to muscle fitness exercise. They are reviewed here to show how they relate specifically to muscle fitness.

Principle of Overload

To improve muscle fitness, a muscle or muscle group must be challenged to perform more than in normal physical activities. High overload (resistance) builds strength, whereas more moderate overload repeated many times builds muscular endurance. Exercises for power require overload for speed and strength.

Principle of Reversibility

Overload is necessary to build muscle fitness. The reverse of the principle of overload also applies—if you don't use your muscles, you'll lose muscle fitness. "Use it or lose it!"

Principle of Progression

The principle of progression holds that you should gradually increase resistance or load over time in order to best improve your muscle fitness. If you try to use too much resistance too soon, you can injure yourself. Exercise that increases resistance until you reach the desired level of muscle fitness is referred to as **progressive resistance exercise (PRE)** or progressive resistance training (PRT). Many kinds of progressive resistance exercise—for example, weight training, resistance machine exercises, and plyometrics—are described later.

Principle of Specificity

Strength, muscular endurance, and power each have their own FIT formula. The specific type of training that you perform determines which part of muscle fitness you build. In addition, you build specific muscles by doing exercises specifically for those muscles (e.g., to build your arm muscles, you must overload your arm muscles). Examples of types of PRE for each part of muscle fitness and the basic exercises for specific muscle groups are discussed later in this chapter.

Principle of Rest and Recovery

The **principle of rest and recovery** holds that you need to give your muscles time to rest and recover after a workout. This is why muscle fitness exercises are typically performed on only two or three days per week. Because you need to perform exercises to build all of the important muscles of your body, some people

Where there is no struggle, there is no strength.

Oprah Winfrey, media personality

choose to work out every day but use different muscle groups on different days (upper body, lower body, etc.). For optimal results, you should also rest between sets (more information about rest is given throughout this chapter).

Health Benefits of PRE and Muscle Fitness

Many of the health benefits described throughout this book are a result of applying basic principles when using PRE to build good muscle fitness. Good muscle fitness helps reduce back problems, improves posture, reduces risk of muscle injury, and increases working capacity. In addition, muscle fitness exercises are very important for bone health (preventing osteoporosis), prevention of heart disease and diabetes, and rehabilitation from chronic diseases such as cancer. Muscle fitness exercises can also reduce your risk of becoming overweight or obese and provide mental health benefits such as looking and feeling your best and experiencing a high quality of life. Among older people, muscle fitness also helps reduce the risk of falling and improves a person's ability to do tasks of daily life.

Muscles and Muscle Fitness

The human body has three different types of muscles: smooth, cardiac, and skeletal. Smooth and cardiac muscles are involuntary muscles because you do not have to think to make them work—they function automatically. **Smooth muscles** are found in various body organs such as the walls of blood vessels and the lungs, eyes, and intestines. **Cardiac muscle** is located in the walls of the heart. The **skeletal muscles** are voluntary muscles—you consciously control them—and it is their contraction that produces movement involved in physical activity.

Skeletal Muscles and Movement

Your skeletal muscles are attached to your bones and make physical movement possible. Your muscles work together to allow your body parts to function efficiently and effectively. For example, when you contract your biceps muscle

(see figure 10.5*a*), your arm bends at the elbow, bringing your hand closer to your shoulder. At the same time, your triceps muscle relaxes to allow your biceps to do its work. The tendons of each muscle connect with bone in two places, the origin and the insertion. The origin is typically connected to the bone that is stationary during a movement, and the insertion is typically connected to the bone that moves. In figure 10.5, the origin of the biceps is at the shoulder, and the insertion is on the bone of the lower arm that moves during flexion and extension.

Skeletal Muscle Fibers

Skeletal muscles (e.g., arm and leg muscles) are made of many long, thin, cylindrical cells

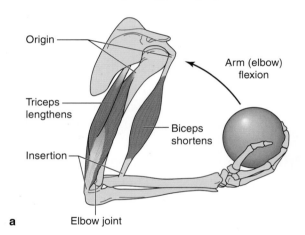

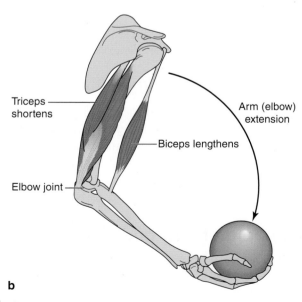

Figure 10.5   The origin, insertion, and action of the arm muscles: *(a)* flexion and *(b)* extension.

called *muscle fibers* (figure 10.6). The strength and endurance of skeletal muscles depend on whether the muscles are made of slow, fast, or intermediate fibers, as well as how much exercise they get.

Slow-twitch muscle fibers contract slowly and are usually red because they have a lot of blood vessels delivering oxygen to the muscle. These fibers generate less force than fast-twitch muscle fibers but are able to resist fatigue. **Fast-twitch muscle fibers** contract quickly and are white because they have less blood flow delivering oxygen. Fast-twitch fibers generate more force than slow-twitch fibers and, with training, account for growth in muscle size. Many factors influence performance, but muscles with many fast-twitch fibers favor enhanced strength and

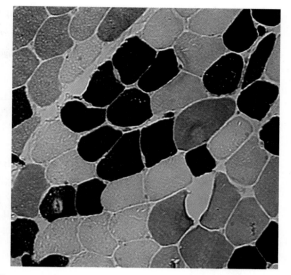

Figure 10.6 This photomicrograph shows slow-twitch (black) and fast-twitch (gray and white) muscle fibers.

Reprinted from W.L. Kenney, J.H. Wilmore and D.L. Costill, *Physiology of Sport and Exercise*, 7th ed. (Champaign, IL: Human Kinetics, 2019), 41. By permission of D.L. Costill, 1974.

power performance and muscles with many slow-twitch fibers favor muscular endurance performance.

Intermediate muscle fibers have characteristics of both slow- and fast-twitch fibers. You use them for activities involving both types of muscle fitness and cardiorespiratory endurance.

Your muscle capabilities are determined in part by heredity. People who inherit a large number of fast-twitch muscle fibers are especially likely to be good at activities requiring sprinting and jumping, whereas people who inherit a large number of slow-twitch muscle fibers are likely to be good at activities requiring sustained performance such as distance running and swimming. However, we now know that, regardless of your genes, you can increase your muscle strength, endurance, and power with proper training.

Muscle Hypertrophy

Muscle **hypertrophy** refers to growth in the size of muscles and muscle fibers. Hypertrophy is affected not only by overloading but also by heredity (because your inherited pattern of muscle fiber types affects how your body responds to training), as well as age, maturation, and sex.

As we age, our muscles grow, as do other tissues in the body. For preteens and young teens, who are not yet fully mature, the hormones responsible for hypertrophy (growth in muscle size) are not fully present until maturity. This occurs at different ages for different people, though typically earlier for females than for males. Prior to maturity, performing PRE does increase muscle size. However, gains in strength are also due to increased skill in performing the exercises or an increase in the number of muscle fibers called upon for a movement during exercise. In most exercises, only some of the available muscle fibers contract to cause a movement, but with regular PRE more fibers are called upon, increasing the number of exercises you can perform.

FIT FACT
New research indicates that a person's ability to perform push-ups is a good indicator of functional capacity and cardiovascular disease risk.

FIT FACT
Birds, like humans, have both fast-twitch and slow-twitch muscle fibers. The flying muscles (breast muscles) of ducks and geese are dark colored because they contain many slow-twitch fibers (which are typically red) that are needed for long-distance flights. In contrast, the breast of a chicken is made up of mostly fast-twitch fibers (typically white) because chickens typically don't fly long distances.

Preteens and teens who are late developers will see increases in muscle size with PRE but may not see the same gains as early developers. They should not get discouraged. When the body begins to produce more of the hormones that stimulate muscle growth, PRE will produce even more benefits, including greater muscle size.

Some people think that only males can build muscle fitness and increase muscle hypertrophy. This notion is false. Both males and females need strength in order to be healthy, avoid injury, look good, and be able to save themselves or others in an emergency. However, the hormones that promote muscle hypertrophy are not as prevalent in females as males, and adult females have a lower ratio of muscle to body fat than males. For this reason, the average female has less absolute strength than the average male. Even so, females who perform strength exercises do develop strong muscles, and building strength provides benefits, including self-confidence, for both females and males.

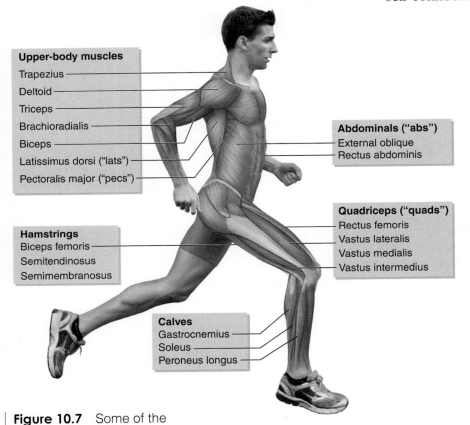

Upper-body muscles
Trapezius
Deltoid
Triceps
Brachioradialis
Biceps
Latissimus dorsi ("lats")
Pectoralis major ("pecs")

Hamstrings
Biceps femoris
Semitendinosus
Semimembranosus

Calves
Gastrocnemius
Soleus
Peroneus longus

Abdominals ("abs")
External oblique
Rectus abdominis

Quadriceps ("quads")
Rectus femoris
Vastus lateralis
Vastus medialis
Vastus intermedius

Figure 10.7 Some of the major muscles used in physical activity.

Major Skeletal Muscle Groups

There are hundreds of muscles in the human body. Some of the most frequently used muscles in physical activity are illustrated in figure 10.7. The muscle anatomy charts in the unit opener pages also illustrate the major skeletal muscles.

Types of Progressive Resistance Exercise (PRE)

The term **muscle contraction** (also called a *muscle action*) refers to activation of the muscle fibers. When the nerves stimulate the fibers, a chemical process begins and the fibers are activated. The different types of muscle contractions and actions are described in the paragraphs that follow.

Isotonic Exercise

As figure 10.8 indicates, your skeletal muscles are attached to bone on each side of a joint. The bones act as levers. When stimulated by a nerve, muscle fibers are activated to apply force. **Isotonic exercises** are those that use muscle actions to apply force to move bones (levers) and cause motion. The two types of isotonic muscle contractions are **concentric** (shortening action) and **eccentric** (lengthening action). Figure 10.8*a* shows the biceps muscle doing a concentric contraction, causing the elbow to flex. In figure 10.8*b*, as the arm is slowly straightened, the biceps is doing an eccentric action that causes the elbow to extend. An eccentric

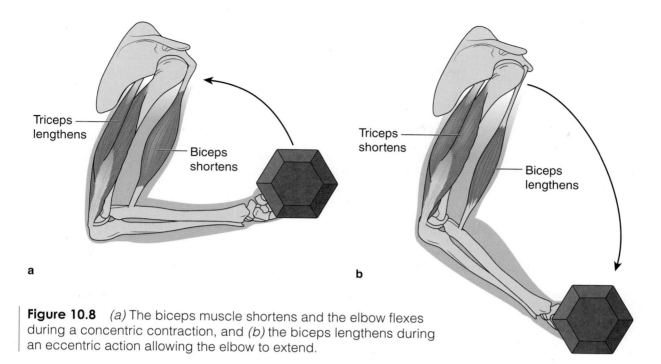

Triceps lengthens

Biceps shortens

a

Triceps shortens

Biceps lengthens

b

Figure 10.8 *(a)* The biceps muscle shortens and the elbow flexes during a concentric contraction, and *(b)* the biceps lengthens during an eccentric action allowing the elbow to extend.

contraction is sometimes called a *braking contraction* because the lengthening of a muscle works against gravity to slow the lowering of a weight (or "puts on the brakes") so that the weight does not drop too quickly.

Plyometric Exercise

Plyometrics is a type of muscle fitness exercise that is especially useful in building power but also contributes to strength development. This type of activity involves doing isotonic muscle actions explosively (as in jumping). You'll learn more about all forms of muscle fitness exercise later in this chapter.

Isokinetic Exercise

Isokinetic exercise is a type of isotonic PRE that uses special machines to produce a constant speed through the full range of movement (see Tech Trends feature). Because it requires special equipment, isokinetic exercise is less frequently used than other types of PRE.

Isometric Exercise

When performing **isometric exercises**, the muscles act with equal force in opposite directions so that no movement occurs. One example of an isometric contraction (sometimes called a

static contraction) involves pushing your hands together in front of your body. You push hard with each hand, applying force against the other, but no movement occurs. You can also do isometric calisthenics such as the wall sit, in which you hold your back against a wall in a seated position to strengthen the quadriceps. Several exercises that build the core muscles, such as the plank, are also isometric exercises. Isometric contractions are also common in yoga poses.

Other Definitions Related to Muscle Fitness

As you now know, PRE is a method of building muscle fitness. Although the following sports are not methods of building muscle fitness, all of them use PRE to improve performance.

Olympic weightlifting (also known as *Olympic-style weightlifting*) is a sport in which athletes use free weights to try lifting a maximum load. The sport includes only two lifts: the snatch and the clean and jerk. For those who train with weights but do not participate in Olympic weightlifting, the preferred terms are *weight training* or *progressive resistance training* (PRT) rather than *weightlifting*.

Powerlifting is another competitive sport that uses free weights. It includes only three lifts: the bench press, the squat, and the deadlift. Athletes in this sport try to make one maximal performance for each type of lift.

Bodybuilding is a competitive sport in which participants are concerned primarily with the appearance of their bodies. Judges rate competitors based on how large and well defined their muscles are, rather than how much they can lift.

Muscle Fitness Assessment

As you know, there are three different parts of muscle fitness—strength, muscular endurance, and power. In the following section, you will learn how to self-assess all three parts.

Strength Assessments

It is generally agreed that determining your one-repetition maximum (1RM) is a good way to assess isotonic strength. The 1RM test determines the amount of weight you can lift or resistance you can overcome in one repetition of an exercise. For example, if a person can lift 100 pounds once but can't lift more than 100 pounds one time, 100 pounds is the 1RM for that exercise.

The true 1RM test is commonly used by athletes and adults. Done properly, it can also be safe for teens, but a modified 1RM self-assessment is most often used in schools because it can be done quickly and does not require lifting maximal weight or using maximal resistance. In this chapter's Self-Assessment feature, you'll use the modified 1RM self-assessment using two isotonic exercises, one for the upper body (arm press) and one for the lower body (leg press).

Your 1RM score is an example of **absolute strength**, which is measured by how much total weight or resistance you can overcome regardless of body size. Big people typically have more absolute strength than smaller people. **Relative strength**, on the other hand, is strength per pound of body weight (absolute strength divided by weight). Relative strength scores are considered to be fairer

TECH TRENDS: Muscle Fitness Exercise Machines

In recent years, tremendous technological advances have been made in resistance exercise machines. Innovations include adjustable benches and chairs that fit people of all sizes and computer-based systems that make it simple to program resistance settings. Another innovation, variable resistance machines, use special hydraulics or electronics to regulate movement velocity (isokinetic exercise) and allow full exertion at all angles of joint movement during an exercise. With traditional free weights or resistance machines, resistance is often greater during the first part of a movement than at the end of the movement, and speed may vary as well.

Variable resistance machines can be used to develop power by using high-speed movements. They are considered quite safe and are often used by researchers and people who are rehabilitating injuries. Their disadvantages include being expensive and often not allowing eccentric contractions, which are used frequently in sport performance.

USING TECHNOLOGY

If your school has muscle fitness exercise machines with high-tech features, ask for a demonstration and try it out. If not, see if you can find a machine to try locally or to view on the Internet.

assessments of strength for those who are not large. For this reason, relative strength is used for the ratings in this chapter's Self-Assessment feature.

In chapter 2 you had the opportunity to try the grip dynamometer test (figure 10.9). It assesses isometric rather than isotonic strength. This test is easy to do but does require a grip **dynamometer**. (Dynamometers are also available for testing other muscle groups, such as leg muscles, but they are more expensive and harder to use than grip dynamometers and thus are used less frequently.) This test is used in national fitness assessments in Canada and Japan and in the ALPHA-FIT and Eurofit batteries often used in Europe.

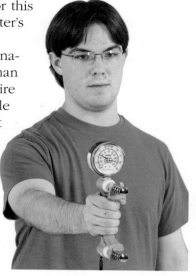

Figure 10.9 The grip dynamometer is used to measure isometric strength.

Muscular Endurance and Power Assessments

You've already tried several self-assessments for muscular endurance and power that are used in common fitness test batteries. Muscular endurance tests typically include calisthenics, such as the push-up, curl-up, and trunk lift exercises that you learned about in previous chapters, as well as the side stand, trunk extension, sitting tuck, leg change, and flexed-arm hang (see the Self-Assessment feature at the end of this lesson). Common tests of power include the standing long jump for leg power (see chapter 2 for details) and the medicine ball throw for upper-body power (see Self-Assessment).

LESSON REVIEW

1. What are strength, muscular endurance, and power, and how do they differ?
2. How do the basic principles of exercise apply to muscle fitness, and what are some of the health benefits of muscle fitness exercise?
3. What are some characteristics of muscles, and what are the names and locations of the major skeletal muscles?
4. What are some of the different types of progressive resistance exercises, and what are several methods for assessing each part of muscle fitness?

SELF-ASSESSMENT: **Muscle Fitness Testing**

Self-assessment of any part of fitness—including muscle fitness—is important because it allows you to establish your baseline level of fitness, determine your fitness needs, set goals, and determine whether you've met your goals. Certified personal trainers who know their stuff have their clients perform a baseline fitness test (a pretest) and, after they go through a fitness program, a follow-up fitness test (a post-test) to see if the program was effective. In this class, you are learning to become your own personal trainer.

Before performing these tests, perform a dynamic warm-up. If the 1RM test causes fatigue that keeps you from doing your best on the muscle fitness tests in parts 2 and 3 of this sequence, repeat those assessments on another day. Record your scores and ratings for the three parts of this self-assessment. If you're working with a partner, remember that self-assessment information is confidential and shouldn't be shared without the permission of the person being tested.

PART 1: Estimating Your 1RM

To review, 1RM means one-repetition maximum—the maximum weight a muscle or group of muscles can lift (or the maximum resistance they can overcome) one time. Because beginners should start gradually (without heavy lifting), a modified method has been developed that allows you to determine your 1RM without overexerting yourself. Your results indicate how strong you are.

The modified 1RM can be done with free weights or machines, but the instructions that follow are for machine use. Resistance machines are recommended for these assessments, especially for beginners, because they are safer. The two most common tests, which you will perform, are for your upper body (arm press) and your lower body (leg press).

Use the following directions for each of the two self-assessments.

- After a dynamic warm-up, choose a weight (resistance) that you think you can lift (move) 5 to 10 times. Do not use a weight that you can lift fewer than 5 times or more than 10 times.

- Using correct technique, lift the weight as many times as you possibly can. Count your lifts and write the total on your record sheet. If you were able to do more than 10 lifts, wait until another day before you try a heavier weight for that assessment. Go to the next muscle group assessment.

- If you can tell that you will not be able to lift the weight at least 5 times, stop and choose a lighter weight.

- If you were able to do 5 to 10 lifts (no fewer and no more), refer to table 10.1 and find the weight you lifted and your number of reps to determine your 1RM score.

- Divide each of your two 1RM scores (arm press and leg press) by your body weight to get your score for strength per pound of body weight. This is your relative strength. For example, a person who weighs 150 pounds and has a 1RM of 100 pounds on the arm press has a score of 0.67 pound lifted per pound of body weight. After figuring your relative strength score, use tables 10.2 and 10.3 to determine your fitness rating. Record your 1RM scores, relative strength scores, and ratings.

- Tables 10.2 and 10.3 do not show high performance ratings for the 1RM. For now, focus on getting into the good fitness zone. Athletes should consult coaches in their sport to get more information about appropriate 1RM scores.

Safety tip: *Proper form is essential for safety.* Before you do the 1RM test, read the descriptions of the exercises and the directions that follow. Before performing each assessment, practice the exercise and have a teacher check your form. Work with a partner to get feedback about proper lifting technique.

TABLE 10.1   Predicted 1RM Based on Reps to Fatigue

Weight (lb)	Repetitions						Weight (lb)	Repetitions					
	5	6	7	8	9	10		5	6	7	8	9	10
30	34	35	36	37	38	39	140	157	163	168	174	180	187
35	40	41	42	43	44	45	145	163	168	174	180	186	193
40	46	47	49	50	51	53	150	169	174	180	186	193	200
45	51	53	55	56	58	60	155	174	180	186	192	199	207
50	56	58	60	62	64	67	160	180	186	192	199	206	213
55	62	64	66	68	71	73	165	186	192	198	205	212	220
60	67	70	72	74	77	80	170	191	197	204	211	219	227
65	73	75	78	81	84	87	175	197	203	210	217	225	233
70	79	81	84	87	90	93	180	202	209	216	223	231	240
75	84	87	90	93	96	100	185	208	215	222	230	238	247
80	90	93	96	99	103	107	190	214	221	228	236	244	253
85	96	99	102	106	109	113	195	219	226	234	242	251	260
90	101	105	108	112	116	120	200	225	232	240	248	257	267
95	107	110	114	118	122	127	205	231	238	246	254	264	273
100	112	116	120	124	129	133	210	236	244	252	261	270	280
105	118	122	126	130	135	140	215	242	250	258	267	276	287
110	124	128	132	137	141	147	220	247	255	264	273	283	293
115	129	134	138	143	148	153	225	253	261	270	279	289	300
120	135	139	144	149	154	160	230	259	267	276	286	296	307
125	141	145	150	155	161	167	235	264	273	282	292	302	313
130	146	151	158	161	167	173	240	270	279	288	298	309	320
135	152	157	162	168	174	180	245	276	285	294	304	315	327

To convert from kilograms to pounds, divide by 0.45.

Adapted by permission from M. Brzycki, 1993, "Strength testing--predicting a one-rep max from reps-to-fatigue," *JOPERD* 64, no. 1 (1993): 89.

SEATED ARM PRESS

1. Sit on the stool of a seated press machine and position yourself so that the handles are even with your shoulders. Grasp the handles with your palms facing away from you. Tighten your abdominal muscles.

2. Push upward on the handles, extending your arms until your elbows are straight.
   Caution: Do not arch your back. Do not lock your elbows.

3. Lower the handles to the starting position.

4. If you have a bench press machine and do not have a seated press machine, you may substitute the bench press from Exercise Chart 1 at the end of this chapter.

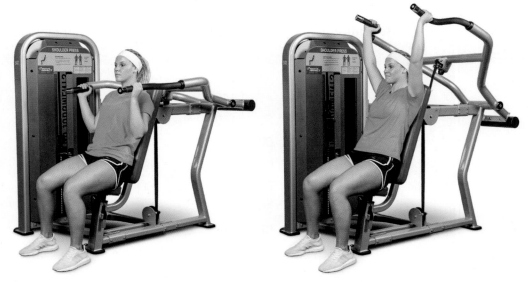

This test evaluates the strength of your arm and shoulder muscles.

TABLE 10.2   Rating Chart: Relative Strength for Arm Press

	15 years or younger		16–17 years old		18 years or older	
	Male	**Female**	**Male**	**Female**	**Male**	**Female**
Good fitness	≥0.80	≥0.60	≥1.00	≥0.70	≥1.10	≥0.85
Marginal fitness	0.67–0.79	0.50–0.59	0.75–0.99	0.60–0.69	0.80–1.09	0.67–0.84
Low fitness	≤0.66	≤0.49	≤0.74	≤0.59	≤0.79	≤0.66

Relative strength is calculated by dividing 1RM by body weight.

SEATED LEG PRESS

1. Adjust the seat position on a leg press machine for your leg length. Sit with your feet resting on the pedal.
2. Push the pedal until your legs are straight.
   Caution: Do not lock your knees.
3. Slowly return to the starting position.

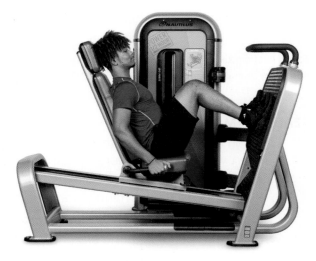

This test evaluates the strength of your quadriceps, gluteal, and calf muscles.

TABLE 10.3   Rating Chart: Relative Strength for Leg Press

	15 years or younger		16–17 years old		18 years or older	
	Male	**Female**	**Male**	**Female**	**Male**	**Female**
Good fitness	≥1.50	≥1.10	≥1.75	≥1.30	≥1.90	≥1.40
Marginal fitness	1.35–1.49	0.95–1.09	1.50–1.74	1.10–1.29	1.65–1.89	1.30–1.39
Low fitness	≤1.34	≤0.94	≤1.49	≤1.09	≤1.64	≤1.29

Relative strength is calculated by dividing 1RM by body weight.

PART 2: Muscular Endurance Tests

Many tests can help you evaluate muscular endurance, but the best ones assess your body's large muscles. In this self-assessment, you'll perform both isotonic and isometric tests. For each, record 1 point if you could do the test as long or as many times as indicated; do not record a point if you could not. Look up your rating in table 10.4. Record your results.

TABLE 10.4   Rating Chart: Muscular Endurance

Fitness rating	Number of tests passed
Good fitness	5
Marginal fitness	3–4
Low fitness	0–2

SIDE STAND (isometric)

1. Lie on your side.
2. Use both hands to get your body in position so that it is supported by your left hand and the side of your left foot. Keep your body stiff.
3. Raise your right arm and leg in the air. Hold this position. Record 1 point if you meet the standard (30 seconds if you are male, 20 seconds if you are female).
4. Return to the starting position and repeat the test on your right side.

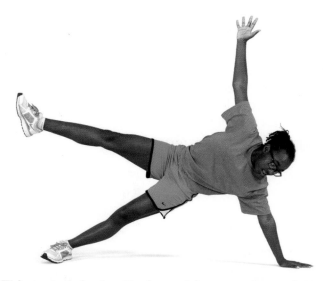

This test evaluates the isometric muscular endurance of some of your leg and arm muscles as well as your trunk-stabilizing muscles.

TRUNK EXTENSION (isotonic)

1. Lie facedown on a stable weight bench or the end of a bleacher that is 15 to 20 inches (38 to 51 centimeters) high. The top of your hips should be even with the end of the bench, and your upper body should hang off the end of the bench. If the surface is hard, cover it with a mat or a towel.

2. Have a partner hold your calves 12 inches (30 centimeters) above your ankles, using one hand on each leg. Overlap your hands and place them (palms away) in front of your chin.

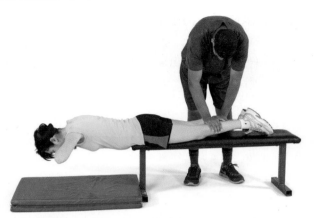

This test evaluates the isotonic muscular endurance of your upper back muscles.

3. Start with your upper body bent at the hip so that your chin is near the floor with the palm of your lower hand against the floor. Place a small mat on the floor below your hands and chin.

4. Keeping your head and neck in line with your upper body, slowly lift your head and upper body off the floor until your upper body is in line with your lower body.

   Caution: Do not to lift your upper trunk higher than horizontal (in line with your lower body).

5. Lower to the starting position so that the palm of your lower hand touches the floor.

6. Perform one lift every three seconds. You may want to have a partner say "up, down" to help you. Record 1 point if you can meet the standard (20 reps if you are male, 15 reps if you are female).

SITTING TUCK (isotonic)

1. Sit on the floor with your knees bent and your arms outstretched.

2. Lean back (to about a 45-degree angle) and balance on your buttocks. Keep your knees bent near your chest (feet off the floor).

3. Straighten your knees so your body forms a V. You may move your arms sideways for balance.

4. Bend your knees to your chest again. Repeat the exercise as many times as you can. Count each time you push your legs out. Record 1 point if you can meet the standard (25 reps if you are male, 20 reps if you are female).

Caution: Avoid arching your lower back repetitively.

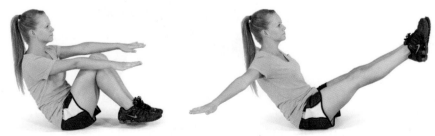

This test evaluates the isotonic muscular endurance of your abdominal muscles and some of your hip and leg muscles.

LEG CHANGE (isotonic)

1. Assume a push-up position with your weight on your hands and feet.
2. Pull your right knee under your chest, keeping your left leg straight.
3. Change legs by pulling your left leg forward and pushing your right leg back.
   Caution: Do not let your lower back sag.
4. Continue changing legs (about one change with each leg every 2 seconds).
5. Count the number of leg changes performed in 1 minute. Record 1 point if you can meet the standard (25 changes for both males and females).

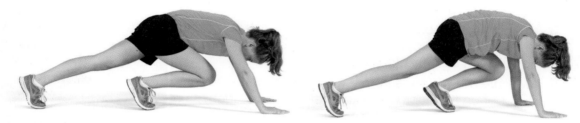

This test evaluates the isotonic muscular endurance of your hip and leg muscles.

FLEXED-ARM HANG (isometric)

1. Hang from a chinning bar with your palms facing away from your body.
2. Standing on a chair, or with help from a partner, lift your chin above the bar.
3. At the start signal, your partner lets go or removes the chair so you are hanging by your own power. Count how long you can hang. The time count begins when the support is removed and ends when your chin touches or goes below the bar or your head tilts backward. Record 1 point if you can meet the standard (16 seconds if you are male, 12 seconds if you are female).

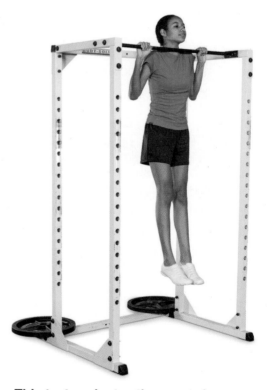

This test evaluates the muscular endurance of your arm, shoulder, and chest muscles (isometric).

223

PART 3: Muscular Power Tests

Two frequently used self-assessments for power are the standing long jump (lower body) and medicine ball throw (upper body). In this self-assessment, you'll perform the medicine ball throw. You already performed the standing long jump (see chapter 3).

MEDICINE BALL THROW

1. Sit on a chair positioned against a wall, with your back against the back of the chair.
2. Hold a 14-pound (about 6.5-kilogram) medicine ball with both hands so that it rests against the middle of your chest.
3. Keeping your back against the chair, push with both hands to throw the medicine ball as far as possible. Throw as you would in a basketball chest pass.
4. Measure the distance from the wall (behind the chair) to the spot on the floor where the ball landed in inches (or centimeters).
5. Measure your arm length in inches (or centimeters). Your score is the distance that the ball was thrown minus the length of your arm.
6. Perform the test two times and use the better of your two scores.

Based on your better score, use table 10.5 to determine your rating. As directed by your instructor, record your score and your rating.

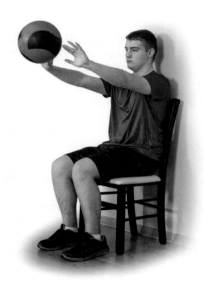

The medicine ball throw test evaluates power in your upper body.

TABLE 10.5   Rating Chart: Medicine Ball Throw (Inches)

	15 years or younger		16–17 years old		18 years or older	
	Male	**Female**	**Male**	**Female**	**Male**	**Female**
Good fitness	≥145	≥98	≥155	≥102	≥165	≥108
Marginal fitness	130–144	90–97	140–154	94–101	150–164	98–107
Low fitness	≤129	≤89	≤139	≤93	≤149	≤97

To convert centimeters to inches, divide by 2.54.

Building Muscle Fitness

Lesson Objectives

After reading this lesson, you should be able to

1. describe the FIT formula for building strength and muscular endurance using isotonic PRE and describe the advantages and disadvantages of resistance machine versus free weight exercises;

2. describe calisthenics, plyometrics, and isometric exercise;

3. describe basic guidelines for doing safe and effective PRE; and

4. describe some myths about muscle fitness and explain why they are myths.

Lesson Vocabulary

double progressive system
muscle bound
muscle dysmorphia

Do you want to increase your muscle fitness? Are you familiar with the types of resistance training and the FIT formula for each? In this lesson, you'll learn how to apply the FIT formula for the most popular methods of building muscle fitness, as well as recommended guidelines for properly performing progressive resistance exercise (PRE) and some common misconceptions concerning muscle fitness.

PRE for Strength: Resistance Machines and Free Weights

In this section, you'll learn about the FIT formula for isotonic PRE. Both the American College of Sports Medicine (ACSM) and the National Strength and Conditioning Association (NSCA) indicate that this formula will vary depending on whether a person is a beginning, intermediate, or advanced exerciser. Table 10.6 provides FIT formula information for teen exercisers of different levels using resistance machines and free weights. The same FIT formula can be used for isokinetic exercises. To make your workout more efficient, you can alternate arm and leg exercises. That way, when your arms are working, your legs are resting, and vice versa.

I thought resistance exercise was mostly for boys. It's not. I tried it and now my friends want to try it too.

Julia Sanchez

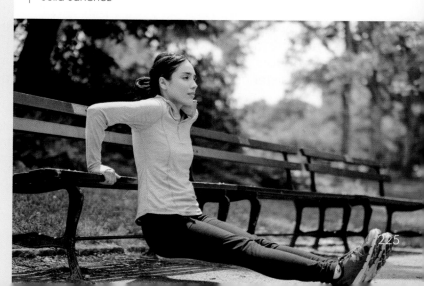

TABLE 10.6   **FIT Formula for Strength Development (Isotonic PRE)**

		Beginner		Intermediate		Advanced	
		Threshold	Target	Threshold	Target	Threshold	Target
Frequency (days per week)		2	2–3	2	2–3	3	3–5
Intensity (% of 1RM)		50	50–60	60	60–80	70	70–95
Time	Sets	1	1–2	2	2–3	3	3–5
	Reps	8	8–12	4	4–8	2	2–8
Rest intervals (minutes)		2	2	2	2–3	2	2–3

Adapted from Faigenbaum, Lloyd, and Oliver, *Essentials of Youth Fitness.*

The FIT formula for strength for teens, as shown in table 10.6, is different from the formula for adults. For adult strength development, the ACSM recommends PRE 2 or 3 days a week, beginning with an intensity of 40 and peaking at 80 percent of 1RM (advanced). The recommended range for sets is 2 to 3 and for reps is 8 to 12. Rest intervals between sets should range from 2 to 3 minutes.

SCIENCE IN ACTION: The Double Progressive System of PRE

You already know that in order to achieve optimal muscle fitness development, you need to progress gradually. The most commonly used method for applying the principle of progression to muscle fitness is the **double progressive system**. The first part of the system involves increasing repetitions (reps). For example, as shown in table 10.6, a beginner could start with 1 set of 10 reps at 50 percent of 1RM, then gradually increase the number of reps until they can easily perform 15 reps. The second part of the system involves increasing resistance or weight. The number of reps is dropped back to 10, and the resistance is increased by 5 to 10 percent of 1RM; for teens, this often means an increase of about 2 to 5 pounds (0.9 to 2.3 kilograms). This double progression—increasing reps, then resistance—continues until the person can do the maximum percent of 1RM in the beginner category. At that point, they can add a second set. It may be necessary to drop back to a lower number of reps and a lower percent of 1RM to perform 2 full sets of 10 to 15 reps.

When the person can perform 3 sets of 8 to 12 reps at 60 percent of 1RM or higher, the double progression sequence begins again (intermediate). The person follows the double progressive system until they can perform three sets of 8 to 12 reps at 70 percent of 1RM or higher. It may take a year or longer to progress to this point. At this point the FIT formula for advanced exercises can be used if desired. Some exercisers choose to stay at the intermediate level because many health benefits can be achieved using the FIT formula for this stage (moderate sets and reps and moderate resistance).

STUDENT ACTIVITY

Use your 1RM for one exercise (e.g., biceps curl). Select a level (beginner, intermediate, advanced). Try out the double progressive system using the information in table 10.6 to guide you.

PRE for Muscular Endurance: Resistance Machines and Free Weights

Teens interested in building muscular endurance can use resistance machines or perform free weight exercises. Table 10.7 shows the FIT formula for these exercises, based on ACSM recommendations.

TABLE 10.7   **FIT Formula for Muscular Endurance (Isotonic PRE)**

		Threshold	Target zone
Frequency (days per week)		2	2–3
Intensity (% of 1RM)		40	40–50
Time	**Sets**	1	1–2
	Reps	15	16–25
Rest intervals (minutes)		1	1–2

Resistance Machines Versus Free Weights

Resistance machine and free weight exercises require considerable equipment but are among the most popular and effective methods for building muscle fitness. They allow you to build both strength and muscular endurance and isolate most of the major muscle groups in your body with specific exercises. Some basic exercises using free weights and resistance machines are described at the end of this lesson; for each exercise, the muscles used are listed and illustrated. Their advantages and disadvantages are outlined in table 10.8.

TABLE 10.8   **Resistance Machines Versus Free Weights**

	Resistance machines	Free weights
Safety	Safer because weights cannot fall on lifter	Greater chance of injury from falling weights
	Spotter often not needed	Easy to lose control of; spotter needed
Cost	Very expensive to own	Relatively inexpensive
	If not owned, club membership required to use	
Versatility	Easy to isolate specific muscle groups	More balance, muscle coordination, and concentration required
		More muscles used, movements more like moving heavy loads in daily life
Convenience	Much floor space needed	Little space needed
	Must be used where installed	Some weights small enough to carry around
	Easy to change resistance	Easily scattered, lost, or stolen
		Takes time to change resistance

FIT FACT

An electromyograph (EMG) is a machine used by researchers to determine how hard a muscle contracts. In EMG results, smaller contractions (such as those used for muscular endurance) show a low muscle action wave, whereas harder contractions (such as those used for strength) show a larger muscle action wave.

FIT FACT

Some exercises, especially those done with free weights, require a spotter. A spotter is a person who monitors your exercise for safety.

Calisthenics

As you know, calisthenic exercises (e.g., push-ups, curl-ups) use all or part of your body weight to provide resistance and for this reason are often referred to as *body weight exercises*. The lower resistance makes this type of PRE better for building muscular endurance than for building strength and also means that you can do calisthenics more frequently. The FIT formula for isotonic calisthenics is shown in table 10.9. Calisthenics are good for both home use and travel because you can do them almost anywhere with little equipment. Specific descriptions for calisthenic exercises for the arms and legs are described in Exercise Chart 4 at the end of this lesson. Calisthenics for core muscles are described in chapter 11.

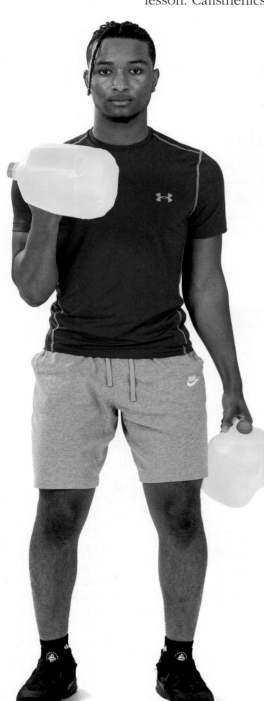

TABLE 10.9   FIT Formula for Calisthenics (Isotonic PRE)

		Threshold	Target zone
Frequency (days per week)		3	3–6
Intensity		Body weight*	Body weight*
Time	Sets	1	1–4
	Reps	10	15–25
Rest interval (minutes)		2	2–3

*The last rep in the last set should be difficult to perform (PRE rating of 7 or higher).

Other Types of Isotonic PRE

Additional PRE methods include exercises with elastic bands, homemade weights, or kettlebells. Each of these is described in the paragraphs that follow.

Isotonic PRE With Elastic Bands

Elastic bands can be used to provide resistance for PRE. The most common types of elastic bands include tube bands, strip bands, and loop bands and are available in different thicknesses to provide different amounts of resistance. Resistance can also be varied by using shorter or longer bands. Tube bands are typically available with handles that make gripping easier. Elastic band exercises can be performed for most of the major muscle groups and are especially good for beginners.

The FIT formulas for building muscle strength and muscular endurance apply when using elastic bands (see tables

Homemade weights, such as milk jugs filled with water, can provide resistance for building muscle fitness.

10.6 and 10.7). Intensity (resistance) is determined by the thickness and length of the band and is usually represented by different colors. With practice the best resistance can be determined.

Advantages of elastic band exercises include low cost, easy storage, light weight, ease in adjusting resistance, and low injury risk. However, elastic band exercises do not allow exact resistance determination and aren't as effective for advanced exercisers and athletes as resistance machines and free weights. Exercise Chart 3 at the end of the chapter illustrates some of the most effective elastic band exercises.

Isotonic PRE With Homemade Weights

Exercises with homemade weights are similar to resistance machine and free weight exercises but use other means to provide resistance, such as milk bottles filled with water or cans of food. They require no expensive equipment and can be easily performed at home but may be limited in benefitting those interested in preparing for high-level performance.

Isotonic PRE With Kettlebells

Kettlebells are a type of exercise equipment that look like metal balls with handles. It gets the name because it looks similar to a tea kettle without a spout. A variety of PRE exercises can be performed using kettlebells, but they require special skills for safe and effective use and are not generally recommended for beginners. Consult with your instructor for more information.

Plyometric PRE

Plyometric exercise involves a rapid eccentric contraction of a muscle followed by a concentric contraction of the muscle. For example, one common low-resistance form of plyometric exercise is jumping rope. Landing after a jump requires your calf muscle to do an eccentric, or lengthening, contraction, and the next jump into the air requires a concentric contraction of the calf muscle. Resistance is provided by body weight. Plyometrics often uses more vigorous jumping activities and often includes medicine ball exercises as well.

Plyometrics contributes to all parts of muscle fitness but is most often used as a method of developing muscle power. Like other forms of muscle fitness exercise, plyometrics was previously thought to be dangerous for teens. However, recent evidence suggests that when performed properly and progressively with good supervision, plyometrics can be safe for teens and improve

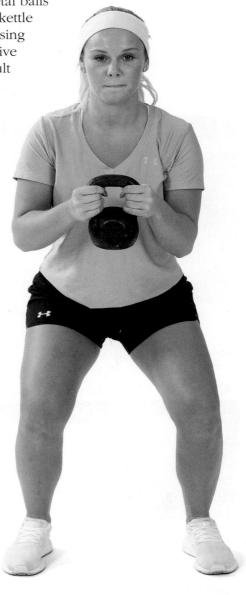

FIT FACT
Sand bells are synthetic rubber disks filled with sand. Like kettlebells, they can be used to provide resistance for building muscle fitness. The sand in the bell moves during exercise, resulting in the bell's weight shifting.

A squat is one type of exercise you can do with a kettlebell.

both power and speed. Exercise physiologists have shown that power is related to bone development in children and teens and offers health benefits similar to those provided by other parts of muscle fitness. It's also important for good performance in various sports, including track and field, baseball, and football. For this reason, athletes often want to improve their power.

Although this form of PRE can be effective at reducing athletic injury, plyometrics and other power-building techniques can also result in injury when performed excessively. The FIT formula for plyometrics is described in table 10.10; the formula, developed by experts, shows a progression based on current exercise status.

Isometric PRE

Isometric exercises can be done easily at home or when you travel because they require little or no equipment and can be done in a confined space—even a space as small as an airplane seat. A disadvantage of isometric PRE is that it's sometimes hard to tell when you're doing a maximum contraction, and this uncertainty can affect your motivation to work hard. In addition, experts do not consider isometric exercise to be as effective in building muscle fitness as isotonic PRE. As with all PRE, you should not hold your breath while performing isometric exercises. The FIT formula for isometric exercises is included in table 10.11.

Guidelines for Safe and Effective PRE

When performed correctly, PRE is safe and improves your muscle fitness while helping you feel and look your best. Stick to the guidelines created to help teens use PRE safely and effectively.

Before You Start

- *Make sure that your workout area is safe.* Use equipment in good working order. Keep free weights on weight racks rather

TABLE 10.10   **FIT Formula for Plyometric PRE**

	Beginner	**Intermediate**	**Advanced**
Frequency	2–3 days per week (nonconsecutive)	2–3 days per week (nonconsecutive)	2–3 days per week (nonconsecutive)
	2–4 exercises per session	4–6 exercises per session	6–8 exercises per session
Intensity	Low (jumps in place, low box, medicine ball)	Moderate (moving jumps and hops, box and obstacle jumps)	High (drop jumping, multiple jumps over distance)
Time	1–2 sets of 8–10 reps	2–3 sets of 4–8 reps	2–4 sets of 4–6 reps
	Rest for 1–2 min between sets	Rest for 1–3 min between sets	Rest for 2–3 min between sets

Pre- and early teen youth typically begin at the beginner level. However, youth who have been regularly active and have high fitness may move to more advanced levels with proper supervision by a qualified expert who has evaluated the maturational and fitness status of the exerciser.

Adapted from Faigenbaum, Lloyd, and Oliver (2020). *Essentials of Youth Fitness*, Human Kinetics.

TABLE 10.11   **FIT Formula for Isometric PRE**

	Threshold	**Target zone**
Frequency (days per week)	3	3–6
Intensity	Contracting muscle as tightly as possible or holding part or all of body weight	Contracting muscle as tightly as possible or holding part or all of body weight
Time	3 reps (1 rep = hold for 7 sec)	3–4 reps (1 rep = hold for 7–10 sec)

than scattered on the floor. Wipe machines with a towel before use, if necessary.

- *Warm up before your session.* Use a dynamic warm-up before strength and power exercises. A dynamic or general warm-up can be used before muscular endurance exercises.

- *Never use weights carelessly.* Concentrate on your technique. Use care when changing free weights and put them away properly when you're finished.

- *When working with free weights, use a spotter and weight rack.* Some exercises, especially those using barbells, require a spotter (person who assists you for safety) and a weight rack (see exercise descriptions). Practice spotting for each exercise using information in the illustrations.

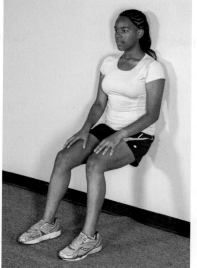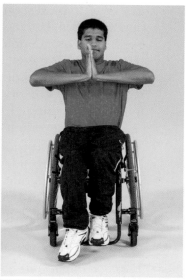

The hand push and the wall sit are examples of isometric exercises. Safety tip: Breathe normally while doing these exercises. Do not hold your breath. Holding your breath can cause dizziness and possibly a blackout.

- *Do not compete when you do PRE.* For example, do not have a contest to see who can lift the most weight. This leads to incorrect form and unsafe practices.

- *Progress gradually.* Young teens and those with little PRE experience should exercise with the FIT formula for beginners before moving to the intermediate level. Do not let the word *beginner* be a reason for violating the principle of progression. The advanced FIT formula is typically reserved for people with considerable PRE experience and for older teens who have reached physical maturity.

Performing Your PRE Workout
- *Get good instruction from an expert.* An expert includes someone like a physical education teacher or coach. Beware of taking advice from people in the gym or friends who are not experts.

- *Practice before performing your PRE plan.* Before you begin your PRE program, practice each exercise until you achieve mastery. Practice with no weight or very low weight (e.g., exercise wand or barbell without weights) and focus on technique. Follow the directions provided in the exercise charts and use the tips for good technique.

- *Breathe when you perform PRE.* Use a steady "breathe out" and "breathe in" count for all forms of PRE. Holding your breath can make you dizzy and, in the extreme, can cause you to pass out. Some resistance trainers recommend exhaling when applying resistance and inhaling on the return movement.

- *Use a full range of motion and moderate-velocity movements for both concentric and eccentric contractions.* The movement should not be too fast or

Mens sana in corpore sano (a sound mind in a sound body).

Juvenal, Roman poet

too slow (typically one to two seconds, depending on the range of motion for the exercise). For example, when doing the biceps curl, lift the weight all the way up (concentric contraction) and lower the weight all the way down (eccentric contraction), counting "1, 2" for the lift and "1, 2" when lowering.

- *Avoid sudden or quick movements.* Stop briefly at the beginning and end of each repetition. Use your muscles, not the movement of your body, to do the exercise (for example, don't rock forward and backward with the upper body during a biceps curl).

- *Use good biomechanics.* Avoid body positions and movements that cause your joints to move in ways for which they are not intended or that put your muscles at risk of injury. Use a wide base of support when performing standing exercises.

- *Master single-joint exercises before attempting multiple-joint exercises or sport movements.* A biceps curl is a single-joint exercise because the only joint it moves is the elbow. Most of the exercises needed to build good health, as shown in this book, are single-joint exercises. The clean and jerk in the sport of weightlifting is an example of a multiple-joint exercise. Multiple-joint exercises require a high level of fitness and special training to ensure good technique.

- *Select exercises for all major muscle groups.* The ACSM recommends 8 to 10 exercises from major muscle groups such as those identified in figure 10.7.

- *Follow the FIT formula and other PRE guidelines.* Each type of PRE uses a specific formula for frequency, intensity, and time. PRE guidelines also specify the appropriate rest intervals for each type of PRE.

- *Vary your program to keep it interesting.* The ACSM points out the importance of progression and volume when exercising. The double progressive method (see Science in Action) provides variety while helping you get optimal benefits.

You can also get variety by varying repetitions and resistance while keeping your volume constant (for example, many reps with low resistance can result in the same volume of exercise as fewer reps with higher resistance).

- *Monitor your performance.* Some experts use the phrase "feel is not real" to emphasize that just feeling as if you're doing an exercise properly does not necessarily mean that you really are. Have a partner give useful feedback or take a video of your performance so that you can evaluate your form. In many facilities mirrors are provided that also allow you to check your form.

After Your Workout

- *Restore the exercise area.* Put away free weights. Wipe down exercise machines with a towel so it is clean for the next user.

- *Cool down.* After a vigorous workout, taper off by performing light exercises or take a walk around the workout area.

Myths and Misconceptions

The amount of muscle fitness you need to stay healthy and perform activities depends on your personal situation and interests. For example,

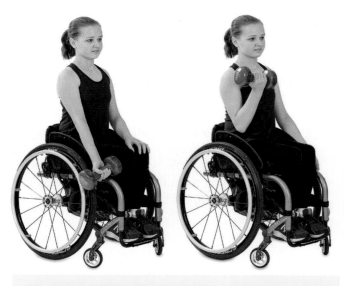

Moving a joint through the full range of motion is important for optimal functioning.

people who do jobs requiring a lot of lifting need more strength than people who work at a desk. Despite the fact that muscle fitness exercise offers many benefits, many people still hold misconceptions about them.

No Pain, No Gain

Some people still cling to the myth that exercise must hurt in order to be effective. Some of the worst offenders are people who are hooked on strength-building exercises. In reality, you should listen to your body. If you feel pain, your body is telling you something. When doing PRE, it's true that you'll become fatigued and sometimes feel a sensation called the *burn*, and you need to learn the difference between this feeling and pain. If in doubt, back off to avoid injury.

Muscle Bound

Some people think that strength training will cause them to be **muscle bound**—to have tight, bulky muscles that prevent them from moving freely. However, inflexibility is caused not by resistance training but by incorrect training, such as failing to stretch or training muscles on only one side of a joint. Recent research suggests that isotonic PRE can actually enhance flexibility when performed properly, through the full range of motion. For example, your elbow joint can bend to allow your hand to reach your shoulder and to let your arm straighten completely; therefore, when you do a biceps curl, bring the weight all the way to your shoulder, then fully straighten your elbow each time you lower the weight. *Caution:* Do not bend your elbow or any other joint backward beyond its full range of motion. You can damage a joint if you move it in a way in which it was not designed to move.

Muscle Fitness for Females

As noted earlier, some people think that females cannot build muscle fitness. Others think that building muscle fitness is not attractive. Both of these statements are false.

Muscle Tone

Advertisers often promise that a product or program can build something they call "muscle tone." However, *tone* in this usage does not refer to anything that can be measured in the same way as strength, muscular endurance, or power. Inspecting or feeling a muscle cannot objectively measure it; therefore, *tone* is not a good word to define muscle fitness and any claim based on it is suspect.

Muscle Dysmorphia

The term **muscle dysmorphia** refers to a condition in which a person becomes obsessed with building muscle. This body image disorder is sometimes referred to as *reverse anorexia* because it is defined not by how thin a person can get but how large and muscular a person can get. It often begins with a reasonable amount of exercise to build muscle fitness. At some point, however, a person with this problem gets carried away in wanting to build more and more muscle. This obsessive-compulsive disorder often requires treatment by a professional. In more than a few cases, people with this disorder resort to unhealthy behaviors, such as taking drugs and doing unhealthy exercises. People with this condition experience high injury rates. Doing reasonable PRE can enhance your health, but becoming obsessed with fitness can hurt it.

FIT FACT
Several groups of experts have now prepared statements indicating that resistance training can be safe for teens when performed properly. These groups include the National Strength and Conditioning Association, the American College of Sports Medicine, the American Academy of Pediatrics (medical doctors who specialize in treating children and youth), and the American Orthopaedic Society of Sports Medicine (medical doctors who specialize in bone problems associated with sport and activity). The self-assessments and muscle fitness exercises described in this book follow the guidelines of these organizations.

LESSON REVIEW

1. What are the FIT formulas for developing strength and muscular endurance using isotonic PRE, and what are the advantages and disadvantages of resistance machine and free weight exercises?
2. What are calisthenics, plyometrics, and isotonic exercise?
3. What are some of the guidelines for doing safe and effective PRE?
4. What are some myths about muscle fitness, and why are they wrong?

TAKING CHARGE: **Preventing Relapse**

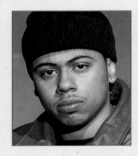

Anyone can begin a program to increase physical fitness, but just beginning a program is not enough. Some people are active for a while, then drop out. This behavior is called a *relapse*. Those who stay active all of their lives learn how to avoid relapses that can lead to becoming sedentary.

Luis missed his old school, especially his old friends. Now he usually came straight home after school instead of heading for the neighborhood court to play a little three-on-three basketball with his buddies. For the first month after he moved, Luis ate dinner, did his homework, and then clicked on the television to fill the time.

Early one evening, his mom said, "Luis, why are you lying around? You like to be active. Get up and get moving!"

Luis yawned and said, "Where am I going to go? Who am I going to go with? I don't have any friends here."

"What about that boy who lives down the hall? I saw him leave with a gym bag the other day. He must have been going somewhere you'd like to go."

"Well, maybe," Luis said. "But maybe he was going to do weight training or something like that—something I don't know how to do."

"Maybe it wouldn't kill you to learn more about weight training. It might help you be better at basketball, right?"

Luis smiled up at his mom. "Maybe. What's his apartment number?"

"3B—and while you're there, ask his mom whether she knows about any exercise classes around here for old people like me, okay?"

FOR DISCUSSION

What caused Luis to relapse into inactivity? What could he do if it turns out that the boy down the hall hates basketball? What are some other things that cause relapse? What can be done to avoid them? What other suggestions do you have to help Luis? Consider the guidelines in the following Self-Management feature as you answer these discussion questions.

SELF-MANAGEMENT: **Skills for Preventing Relapse**

A person who relapses stops doing something that they want to keep doing or should keep doing. For example, you might start a PRE program but then stop doing it because you feel you don't have time. Use the following guidelines to help you stick with something once you've started it.

- *Do a self-assessment.* It may help you see whether you're likely to stick with an activity, and it may give you ideas for how to stick with it if you've had relapse problems in the past.

- *Use your self-assessment information to determine areas in which you can improve.* Self-assessments help you learn about your current status (for fitness, activity, or nutrition, for example). If you are to improve, you first need to know where you need improvement.

- *Write down your goals for the activity.* Put them on the refrigerator or another place where you'll see them every day. You have good reasons to accomplish these goals or you would not have started to make a change in the first place. Stay focused on your goals.

- *Monitor your behavior by keeping a log or chart, then use it to reinforce or reward yourself.* Tell yourself that you've stuck with it so far and you can keep it up.

- *Tell other people what you're trying to accomplish.* Ask them to encourage you regularly.

- *Select a regular exercise time.* If you're trying to stick with exercise, select a time of day and try to work out at the same time every day.

- *Do not let one setback be a reason for a long-term relapse.* If you miss a day, tell yourself, "It's okay to take a day off once in a while."

- *Consider a variety of activities.* Consider trying different physical activities from time to time.

- *Select activities that you enjoy.* Research indicates that as the intensity of activity goes up, it reduces enjoyment for some people. For this reason, it is especially important to find vigorous activities that you enjoy. Building skills helps to improve enjoyment.

Taking Action: **Resistance Machine Exercises**

If you're just starting a muscle fitness program, you may want to begin by using resistance machines at your school or local recreation center. Developing muscle fitness through resistance training will build your muscle mass and bone density and can help you develop a healthy body composition. Muscle fitness can also help you look your best and make it easier for you to perform everyday tasks, as well as improve performance at your favorite sport and other physical activities.

Take action by trying some resistance machine exercises that you've learned in this chapter. Be sure to follow the guidelines for PRE described in the chapter.

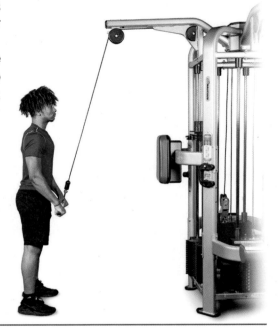
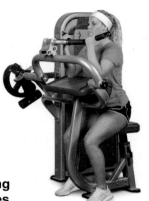

You can take action by doing PRE on resistance machines.

CHAPTER REVIEW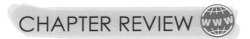

Reviewing Concepts and Vocabulary

Answer items 1 through 5 by correctly completing each sentence with a word or phrase.

1. _____ is the amount of force a muscle can exert.

2. _____ refers to an increase in muscle fiber size.

3. When you do calisthenics to develop strength, you use your body weight as the _____ .

4. _____ is a condition when a person becomes obsessed with building muscle.

5. The _____ system refers to altering reps, sets, and weight as muscle fitness improves.

For items 6 through 10, match each term in column 1 with the appropriate phrase in column 2.

6. isokinetic exercise

   a. the maximum weight or resistance that a person can overcome regardless of size

7. absolute strength

   b. the maximum weight that a person can lift once

8. 1RM

   c. exercise in which movement velocity is kept constant through the full range of motion

9. plyometrics

   d. exercise in which muscles exert force but do not cause movement

10. isometric exercise

   e. exercise that uses jumping and hopping to cause lengthening of a muscle followed by a contraction

For items 11 through 15, respond to each statement or question.

11. Describe several guidelines for safe and effective PRE for teens.

12. Describe several methods for testing muscle fitness discussed in this chapter.

13. Describe two myths about muscle fitness exercise.

14. Describe several guidelines for preventing relapse.

15. Identify and define several different types of PRE and explain the FIT formula for each.

Thinking Critically

Go to the web resource for this chapter and look for the URLs for PRE for Teens. Using the information provided there and in this chapter, write a short article about muscle fitness for high school students. You can find additional information on the websites of NSCA, ACSM, and the President's Council on Fitness, Sports, and Nutrition. Share your article with your class or submit it to the school newspaper for publication.

Project

Some schools provide wellness programs for teachers and other school employees. Typical offerings include exercise classes before and after school, fitness assessments, and classes in nutrition and stress reduction. Plan a special activity for teachers addressing one of these topics as it relates to muscle fitness. Prepare a written plan and work with other students to carry it out.

EXERCISE CHART 1: **Resistance Machine Exercises**

Seated Arm Press

1. Sit on the stool of a seated press machine and position yourself so that the handles are even with your shoulders. Grasp the handles with your palms facing away from you. Tighten your abdominal muscles.

2. Push upward on the handles, extending your arms until your elbows are straight.

   Caution: Do not arch your back. Do not lock your elbows.

3. Lower the handles to the starting position.

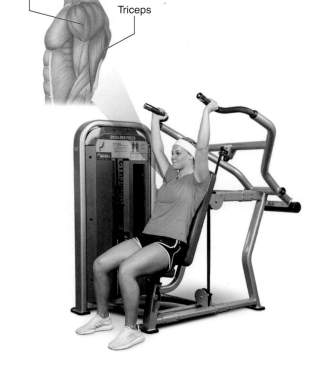

This exercise uses the muscles at the top of your shoulders, between your shoulder blades, and on the back of your arms.

Bench Press

1. Lie on your back on the bench with your feet flat on the floor. Grasp the handles with your palms facing away from your body. Flatten your back. If possible, place your feet on the floor to help flatten your back and avoid arching it. If your feet do not reach the floor easily, bend your knees and place your feet on the bench to accomplish the same purpose.

   Caution: Do not place your feet on the bench if it is so narrow that your feet might slip off the bench or if the bench is unstable.

2. Push upward on the handles, extending your arms completely.

   Caution: Do not lock your elbows. Do not arch your back.

3. Return to the starting position.

4. You may choose either this exercise or the seated arm press.

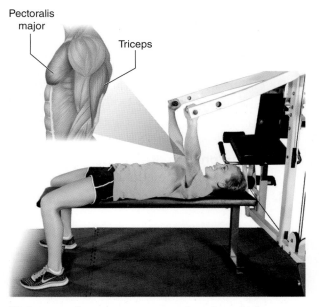

This exercise uses your pectoral and triceps muscles.

Seated Leg Press

1. Adjust the seat position on a leg press machine for your leg length. Sit with your feet resting on the resistance pad.
2. Push the pedal until your legs are straight.

   Caution: Do not lock your knees.
3. Slowly return to the starting position.

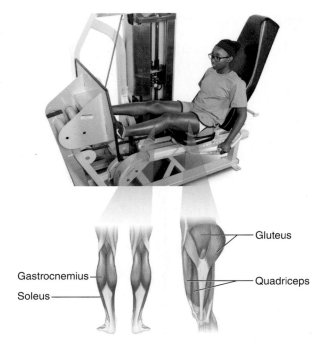

This exercise uses the quadriceps, gluteal, and calf muscles.

Knee Extension

1. Adjust the seat position on a leg exercise machine for your leg length. Sit with the front of the lower legs (just above the ankle) resting on the resistance pad.
2. Grasp the handles with your hands to stabilize your upper body.
3. Push against the pad until your legs are straight.

   Caution: Do not arch your back—keep it flat against the seat back.
4. Slowly return to the starting position.

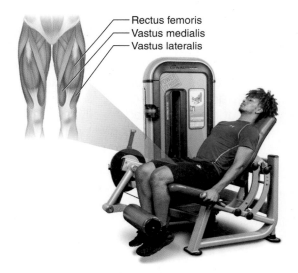

This exercise uses the muscles at the top of your thighs (quadriceps). The vastus intermedius, one of the four quadriceps muscles, lies beneath the rectus femoris and therefore is not shown in the illustration.

Seated Hamstring Curl

1. Adjust the seat position and the resistance pad (behind lower calf). Sit with the top pad over your thighs and your legs over the resistance pad.
2. Hold on to the handles to prevent upper body movement.
3. Push against the resistance pad until your legs are bent at a 90-degree angle.
4. Slowly return to the starting position.

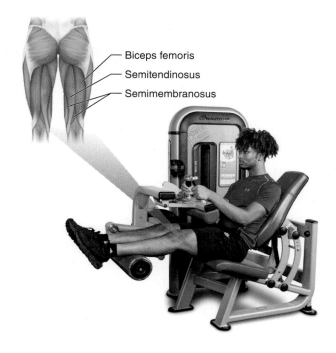

Biceps femoris
Semitendinosus
Semimembranosus

This exercise uses your hamstring muscles.

Biceps Curl

1. Stand in front of the station and grasp the handle with your palms up. Tighten your abdominal muscles and buttocks (gluteal muscles).
2. Pull the handle from thigh level to chest level. Bend your elbows but keep them close to your sides.

   Caution: Do not move other body parts.
3. Return to the starting position.

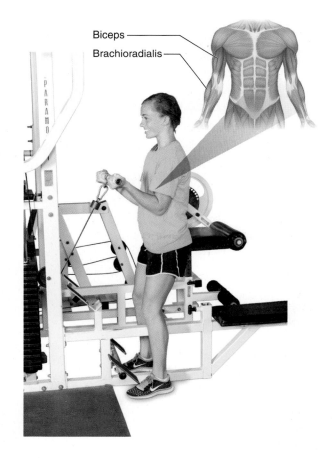

Biceps
Brachioradialis

This exercise uses your biceps and other elbow flexor muscles.

Heel Raise

1. Stand with the balls of your feet on an elevated platform (as shown) or on a 2-inch (5-centimeter) board. Keep the handles even with your shoulders.

2. Grasp the handles with your palms facing away from your body. Keep your hands and arms stationary during the lift.

3. Rise onto the balls of your feet, then lower to the starting position.

Beginners should stand with the feet on the ground and the toes turned slightly inward. Advanced lifters may perform the exercise with their toes pointing straight ahead (more difficult), with their toes turned outward (even more difficult), or with the balls of the feet elevated as illustrated (most difficult).

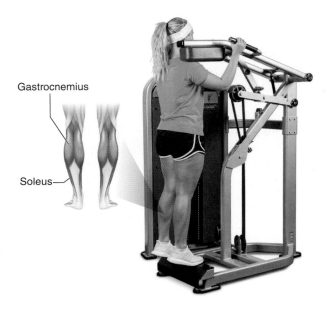

This exercise uses your calf muscles.

Lat Pull-Down

1. Sit on the bench (or floor, depending on the machine). Adjust the seat height so that your arms are fully extended when you grab the bar.

2. Grab the bar with your palms facing away from you. Your arms should be at least shoulder-width apart.

3. Pull the bar down to chest level.

4. Return to the starting position.

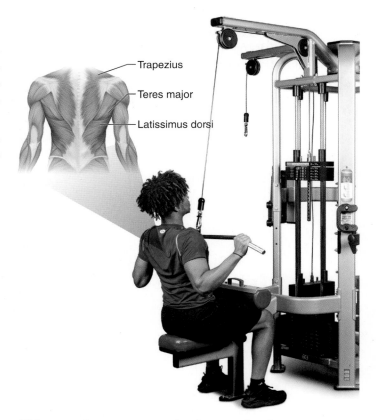

This exercise uses muscles in your back.

Triceps Press

1. With your palms facing away from you, grab the handles.

   Note: If performed while sitting, adjust the seat height so that your hands are on the handles just above shoulder height.

2. Keep your elbows by your sides and avoid leaning forward with your body.

3. Keeping your back straight, push down and forward with your arms until they are straight.

4. Return to the starting position.

This exercise uses the muscles on the back of your arms (triceps).

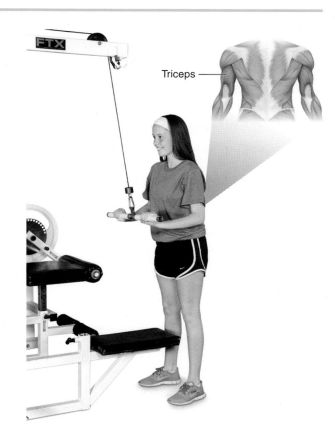

Seated Row

1. Adjust the machine so that your arms are almost fully extended and are parallel to the ground.

2. Grab the handles with your thumbs up.

3. Keeping your back straight, pull straight back toward your chest.

4. Return to the starting position.

This exercise uses the muscles of your back and shoulders.

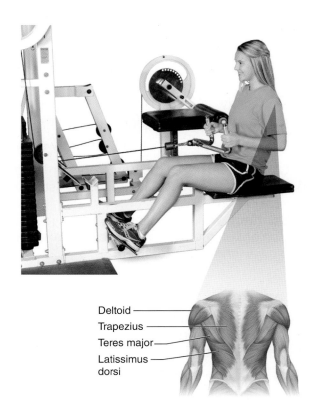

EXERCISE CHART 2: **Free Weight Exercises**

Many of these exercises can be done using either barbells (bar and weights) or dumbbells (small bar and weights or fixed weight dumbbells). For safety, a weight rack and a spotter should be used on certain exercises. If these are not available, alternate exercises should be substituted.

Standing Overhead Press

Weights: Barbell (bar or bar with weight)

This exercise is best performed with a weight rack and a spotter. If a weight rack is not available, dumbbells are recommended for this exercise.

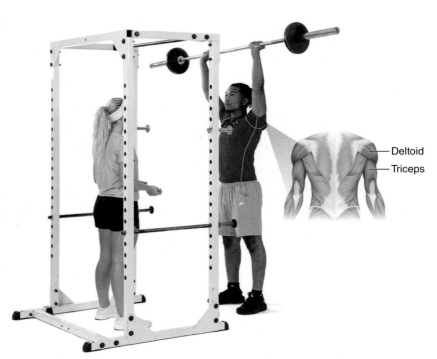

1. Place the weighted bar on a weight rack at shoulder height.

2. Face the bar with your hands at slightly more than shoulder-width apart, palms facing the bar. Grab the bar and hold it at shoulder height.

3. With your feet shoulder-width apart, take a half step back away from the weight rack.

4. Tighten your abdominal, back, and arm muscles. Tip your head back slightly.

This exercise uses the muscles at the top of your shoulders, between your shoulder blades, and on the back of your arms.

5. Keep your head facing forward. Press the bar upward until your arms are fully extended.

6. After the final repetition, step forward and place the bar on the weight rack.

Caution: Do not let the bar go forward or backward. Do not lock your elbows. Do not arch your back. If you lose control of the weight, step backward and let the bar and weights fall to the floor in front of you.

Spotting: While standing inside the rack facing the exerciser, the spotter can assist in moving the weight off the rack and placing the weight back on the rack. During the exercise, step back and away from the exerciser.

Bench Press

Weights: Bar or bar with weight

This exercise requires a weight rack and a spotter. If a weight rack is not available, dumbbells are recommended for this exercise.

1. Place the weight on a weight rack about a foot below your arm's length when fully extended.

2. Lie on your back on a bench with your feet on the floor and your lower back flat.

3. Grasp the bar, palms up, with your hands slightly more than shoulder-width apart, your elbows straight, and the bar approximately over your collarbones.

4. Lower the bar until it touches your chest just below your armpits. When the bar touches your chest, your forearms should be perpendicular to the floor and your elbows should point neither toward your feet nor out to the sides but halfway between (at 45 degrees).

5. Tighten your abdominal, back, and arm muscles. Tip your head back slightly.

6. Push the bar up to the starting position with your arms perpendicular to the floor. The bar follows a slightly curved path.

   Caution: Do not lock your elbows or bounce the bar off of your chest. Do not arch your back or lift your hips. If the weight gets in front of or behind your arms, you may lose control.

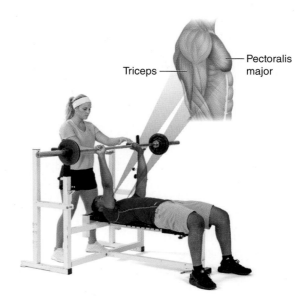

This exercise uses the muscles on the front of your chest (pectoral) and the back of your upper arms (triceps), as well as the muscles of the shoulder (deltoids).

Spotting: The spotter stands under the rack with both hands on the barbell (one hand under and the other over the bar). When the bar is above the lifter's chest, release the bar. Be prepared to assist with the bar if the lifter loses control. Use both hands to aid in replacing the bar on the rack after the last repetition.

Knee Extension

Weights: Weighted boot or ankle weight

One person can help the lifter put on the boot or ankle weight.

1. Put the weight on one foot or ankle. Sit on a bench with your lower leg hanging over the edge. Grasp the bench with your hands.

2. Lift the weighted boot by extending your knee until your leg is straight.

   Caution: Lift slowly. Do not lock your knee when you extend and do not kick your leg upward. Stay seated in an erect position and limit movement to the knee joint.

3. Repeat the exercise with your other leg.

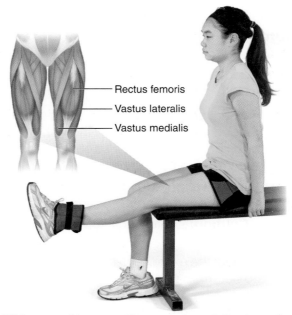

This exercise uses the muscles at the top of your thighs (quadriceps). The fourth quadriceps muscle, the vastus intermedius, lies beneath the rectus femoris and therefore is not shown in the illustration.

Half Squat

Weights: Dumbbells

1. Place a dumbbell on the floor outside and slightly to the front of each foot. Stand with your feet shoulder-width or slightly farther apart. Your toes should point straight ahead or be slightly turned out.

2. Squat low enough to pick up each dumbbell (palms facing the side of your legs). Straighten your legs until you are standing upright.

3. Squat until your knees are at a right angle, then rise. Keep your heels flat on the floor. Do not let your knees get in front of your toes. Focus on a spot on the wall slightly higher than your standing height for the duration of the lift. Keep your head up and your back straight.

4. After the last repetition, place the dumbbells back on the floor.

    Caution: Do not round your back. Do not lean too far forward at your hips or let your knees get in front of your toes. Do not squat too deeply.

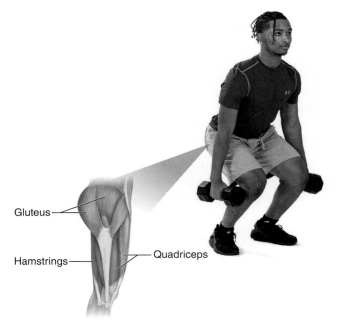

This exercise uses the muscles on the front of your thighs (quadriceps) and your buttock muscles (gluteal).

Hamstring Curl

Weights: Weighted boot or ankle weight
One person can help the lifter put on the boot or ankle weight.

1. Put the weight on one foot or ankle. Lie facedown on a bench, with your kneecaps hanging over the edge. Grasp the bench with your hands.

2. Lift the weighted boot by flexing your knee to a right angle.

    Caution: Do not lock your knee when you extend.

3. Repeat the exercise using your other leg. To determine your 1RM for this exercise, use the hamstring curl on the resistance machine.

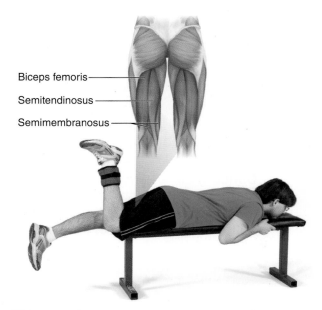

This exercise uses the muscles on the back of your thighs (hamstring).

Biceps Curl

Weights: Barbell

1. Stand behind a weighted bar placed on the floor in front of you, feet shoulder-width apart. Squat and grab the bar with your palms facing up, slightly more than shoulder-width apart.

2. Tighten your abdominal and back muscles. Keep your back straight and stand until you are upright.

3. Keep your elbows close to your sides and lift the weight by bending your elbows only. Raise the weight to near your chin, then return to the starting position.

4. Squat to return the weight to the floor after the last repetition.

    Caution: Do not move other joints, especially in your back.

5. You can also perform this exercise with your palms down.

Spotting: A spotter is not required but can be used to place the barbell in the lifter's palm-up hands.

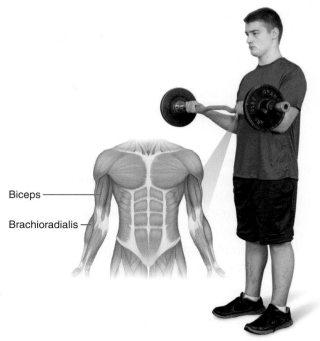

This exercise uses the muscles on the front of your upper arms (biceps) and other elbow flexor muscles.

Heel Raise

Weights: Dumbbells

1. Place a dumbbell on the floor outside and slightly to the front of each foot. Stand with your feet shoulder-width or slightly farther apart.

2. Squat low enough to pick up each dumbbell (palms facing the side of your legs). Straighten your legs until you are standing upright. Keep your head up and your back straight.

3. Rise onto your toes, then lower to the starting position.

4. After the last repetition place the dumbbells back on the floor.

Beginners should turn their toes slightly inward. Advanced lifters may perform the exercise with their toes pointing straight ahead (more difficult), with their toes turned outward (even more difficult), or with their toes on a 2-inch (5-centimeter) board (most difficult).

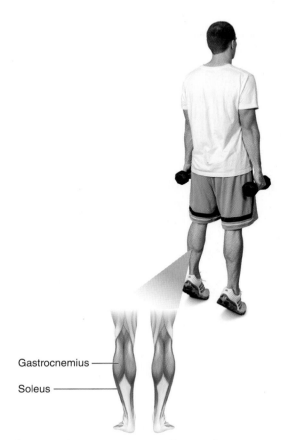

This exercise uses your calf muscles.

Seated French Curl

Weights: Dumbbell

1. Sit on the end of a bench with your elbows flexed at 90 degrees and your palms facing up.

2. Have a spotter hand you the dumbbell. Hold one end of a dumbbell in both hands. Tighten your abdominal and back muscles. Straighten your arms to lift the weight overhead. Return to the 90-degree starting position moving only your elbow joints. Keep your elbows high.

3. After the last repetition, allow the spotter to take the dumbbell from your hands.

Spotting: This exercise requires one spotter. The spotter stands behind the chair in a "ready" position to assist if necessary.

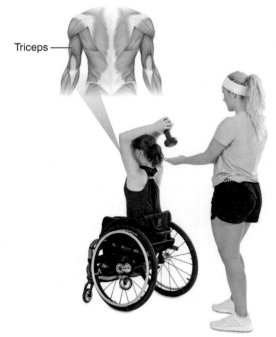

Triceps

This exercise uses the muscles on the back of your upper arms (triceps).

Bent-Over Dumbbell Row

Weights: Dumbbell

1. Begin standing beside an exercise bench.

2. Rest one hand (arm straight) and knee on a bench to support the weight of your trunk and protect your back. Hold the dumbbell in the other hand, with the same side leg straight beside the bench.

3. Pull the dumbbell upward until it touches the side of your chest near your armpit and your upper arm is parallel to the floor. Keep your back straight and parallel to the ground.

4. Slowly lower the weight.

5. Repeat the exercise with your other arm.

This exercise uses your back, shoulder, and arm muscles.

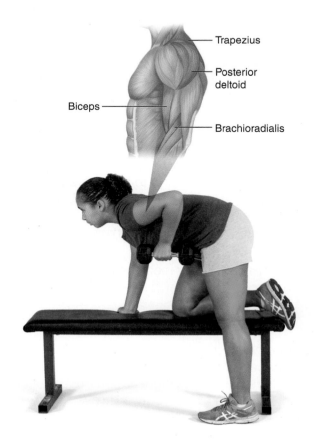

Trapezius

Posterior deltoid

Biceps

Brachioradialis

EXERCISE CHART 3: **Elastic Band Exercises**

Choose an exercise band that offers enough resistance so that you are fatigued after the last repetition in the last set. Band length should be adjusted to allow the exercise to be performed as described. Check your bands regularly for wear and tear. If a band breaks while you are exercising it can cause injury.

Arm Press

This exercise is best performed with a tube-type band with handles. The band length should be adjusted to allow the exercise to be performed as described.

1. Anchor the band at shoulder height or higher using a secure hook (avoid hooks that may damage the band). Stand close to the anchor so that the band is not tight.

2. Face away from the anchor. Hold a handle in each hand, palm facing down. With your hands and grips in front of your shoulders, walk forward until the band is tight. Stand with one foot about two feet in front of the other.

3. Press straight forward with your hands and arms until your arms are extended. Return slowly to the starting position.

   Caution: Keep the core muscles tight and limit movement to your arms.

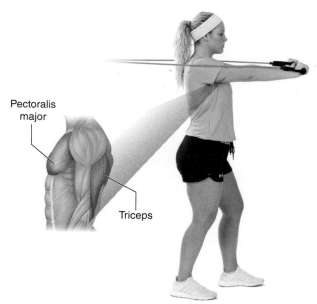

This exercise uses the muscles at the top of your shoulders, between your shoulder blades, and on the back of your arms.

Biceps Curl

This exercise is best performed with a tube-type band with handles.

1. Stand with both feet on the band with feet shoulder-width apart. Grab the handles with the arms extended and the palms facing up.

2. Flex the elbow until the handles are at shoulder level. Lower to the starting position.

3. You can also perform this exercise with your palms down.

   Caution: Do not move other joints, especially in your back.

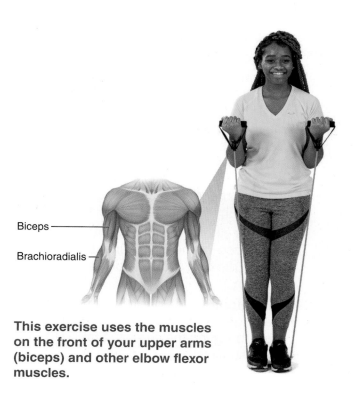

This exercise uses the muscles on the front of your upper arms (biceps) and other elbow flexor muscles.

French Curl

This exercise is best performed with a flat elastic band to allow easy adjustment of resistance.

1. Stand with your right foot about 18 inches in front of the left. Hold one handle of the band with the right hand (arm down to side with hand facing the right thigh).

2. Place the band under the left foot. Grab the other handle of the band with the left hand (elbow up beside the head and pointed forward). The forearm and band extend down behind the shoulder.

3. Extend the left elbow so that the hand moves upward until the arm is extended overhead. Lower the hand back to the starting position.

4. Repeat with the other arm.

   Caution: Keep the elbow pointed forward during the exercise. Stabilize the core muscles during movement.

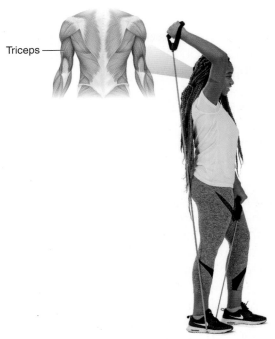

This exercise uses the muscles on the back of your upper arms (triceps).

Lat Pull-Down

This exercise is best performed with a tube band with handles. Door anchors are available to allow the band to be securely anchored at the top of a closed door. Standing closer or farther from the wall reduces or increases resistance.

1. Anchor the band on a hook above and in front of you (door anchors work well). While holding the handles (palms down), move away from the anchor until the bands are tight but not stretched. The arms should be fully extended. Kneel as shown in the illustration (a mat or carpet is recommended). Lean the upper trunk forward in line with the exercise bands.

2. Flex the elbows to pull down against the resistance of the band until the elbow is fully flexed. Return to the starting position.

   Caution: Keep your body in line with the angle of the bands and limit movement to flexing the elbows. Stabilize the core muscles.

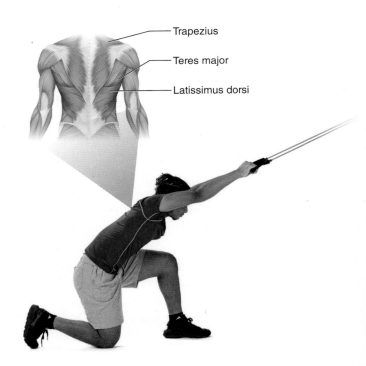

This exercise uses the muscles in your back.

Half Squat

This exercise is best performed with a flat exercise band to allow easy adjustment of resistance.

1. Stand with the band under both feet, slightly more than shoulder-width apart. Your toes should point straight ahead or be slightly turned out.

2. Squat until your thighs are parallel to the ground. With the arms fully extended to your sides, pick up the ends of the band with each hand (palms facing the body). Straighten your legs until you are standing upright.

3. Repeat the squat. Keep your heels flat on the floor. Do not let your knees get in front of your toes. Focus on a spot on the wall slightly higher than your standing height for the duration of the exercise. Keep your head up and your back straight.

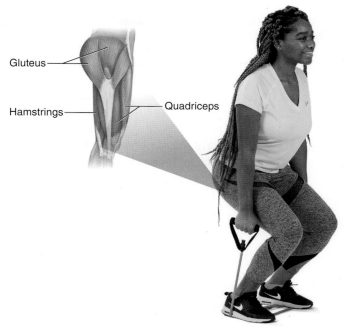

This exercise uses the muscles on the front of your thighs (quadriceps) and your buttock muscles (gluteal).

Knee Extension

This exercise is best performed with a flat exercise band to allow easy adjustment of resistance.

1. Sit on a straight-back chair. Loop one end of the band around your right ankle. Hold the other end of the exercise band against the floor with your left foot. Adjust the length of the band to provide optimal resistance.

2. Keep your back straight against the chair back and hold the side of the chair with each hand.

3. Extend the knee until the leg is straight. Return to the starting position.

4. Repeat with the left leg.

    Caution: Lift slowly. Do not lock your knee when you extend and do not kick your leg upward. Limit movement to the knee joint.

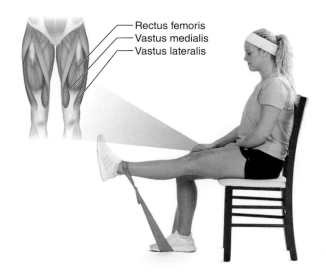

This exercise uses the muscles at the top of your thighs (quadriceps). The vastus intermedius, one of the four quadriceps muscles, lies beneath the rectus femoris and therefore is not shown in the illustration.

Side Leg Raise

This exercise is best performed with a flat loop band or a flat band tied to make a loop.

1. Lie on your left side on a mat or carpet. Place a looped exercise band around both legs just above the ankles (legs together). Place the left hand under your head and extend your flexed elbow in front of you. You may use a pillow under your head. Place your right hand on the floor in front of you (elbow bent at 90 degrees).

2. Lift your right leg upward as high as possible. Lower the leg to the starting position.

   Caution: Lift slowly. Stabilize the trunk muscles and avoid leaning your body forward during the lift.

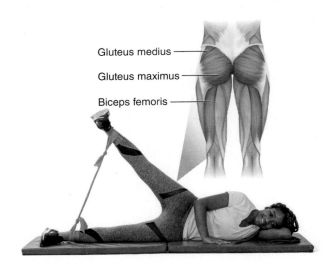

This exercise uses the gluteus maximus, medius, and minimus.

Hamstring Curl

This exercise is best performed with a flat loop band or a flat band tied to make a loop.

1. Stand so your hands can anchor on the back of a straight back chair. Loop the band under your right foot and behind your left ankle.

2. Flex the left knee until your lower leg is parallel to the floor. Return to the starting position.

3. Repeat with the right leg.

   Caution: Lift slowly. Stabilize the trunk muscles and avoid leaning your body.

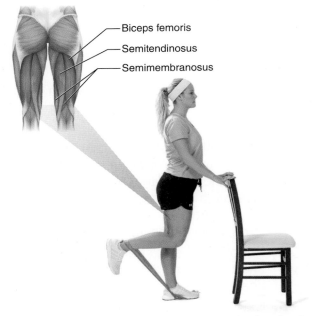

This exercise uses the muscles on the back of your thighs (hamstring).

EXERCISE CHART 4: **Calisthenic Exercises**

Push-Up

1. Lie facedown on a mat or carpet with your hands under your shoulders, your fingers spread, and your legs straight. Your legs should be slightly apart and your toes should be tucked under.

2. Push up until your arms are straight. Keep your legs and back straight. Your body should form a straight line.

3. Lower your body by bending your elbows until your upper arms are parallel to the floor (elbows bent at a 90-degree angle). Then push up until your arms are fully extended. Repeat, alternating between the fully extended and the 90-degree arm positions.

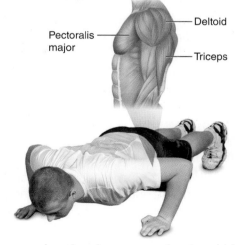

This exercise develops your chest muscles (pectorals) and the muscle (triceps) on the back of your upper arms.

Knee Push-Up

If you cannot complete 20 reps of the 90-degree push-up, try this modified version.

1. Begin in the same position as the regular push-up, but keep your knees on the floor.

2. Push up, keeping your body rigid, until your arms are straight.

3. Keep your body rigid and lower it until your chest touches the floor.

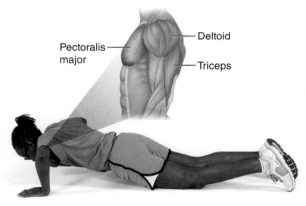

This exercise develops your chest muscles (pectorals) and the muscle (triceps) on the back of your upper arms.

Prone Arm Lift

1. Lie facedown on the floor with your arms extended and held against your ears.

2. Keep your forehead and chest on the floor and lift your arms so that your hands are 6 inches (15 centimeters) off the floor.

3. Lower your arms, then repeat the exercise. Keep your arms touching your ears and keep your elbows straight.

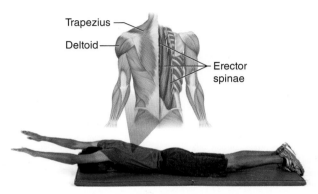

This exercise develops the muscles of your back and shoulders.

Stride Jump

1. Stand with your left leg forward and your right leg back. Hold your right arm at shoulder height straight in front of your body and your left arm straight behind you.

2. Jump and move your right foot forward and your left foot back. As your feet change places, your arms switch position. Keep your feet 18 to 24 inches (about 45 to 60 centimeters) apart.

3. Continue jumping, alternating your feet and arms. Count 1 rep each time your left foot moves forward.

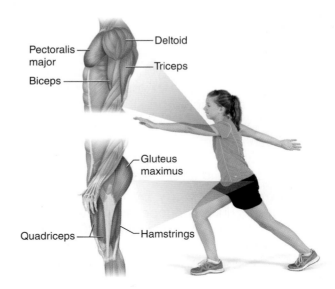

This exercise develops the muscles of your legs and arms as well as cardiorespiratory endurance and power.

Side Leg Lift

1. Lie on your right side. Use your arms for balance.

2. Lift your top (left) leg 45 degrees. Keep your kneecap pointing forward and your ankle pointing toward the ceiling. If your leg rotates so that your knee points upward, you will work the wrong muscles.

3. Lower your leg. Repeat the movement. To increase intensity, you can use an ankle weight.

4. Roll over and repeat the exercise with your right leg.

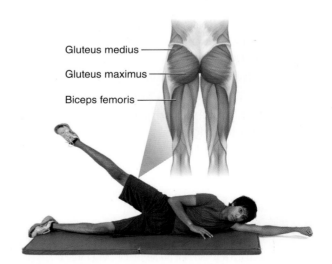

This exercise develops your hip and thigh muscles.

Knee-to-Nose

1. Kneel on all fours.
2. Pull your right knee toward your nose.
3. Extend your right leg until it is in line with the back and shoulders (parallel to the floor). Keep your head in line with the shoulders, back, and extended leg.

   Caution: Do not lift your leg higher than your hips. Do not hyperextend your neck or lower back.
4. Return to the starting position. Repeat the exercise with your left leg.

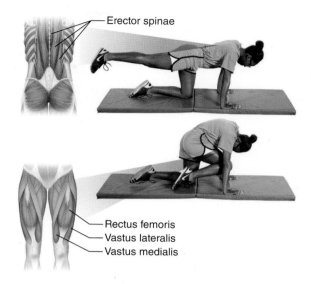

This exercise develops the gluteal, lower back, and quadriceps muscles. The vastus intermedius, one of the four quadriceps muscles, lies beneath the rectus femoris and therefore is not shown in the illustration.

High-Knee Jog

1. Jog in place. Try to lift each knee so that your thigh is parallel with the floor.
2. Count 1 rep each time your right foot touches the floor. Try to do one or two jog steps per second.

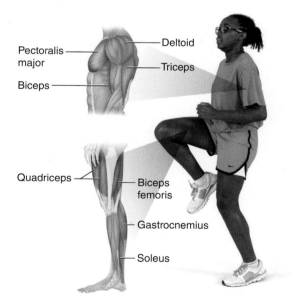

This exercise develops the muscles of your arms and legs and is also good for cardiorespiratory endurance.

Muscle Fitness Applications

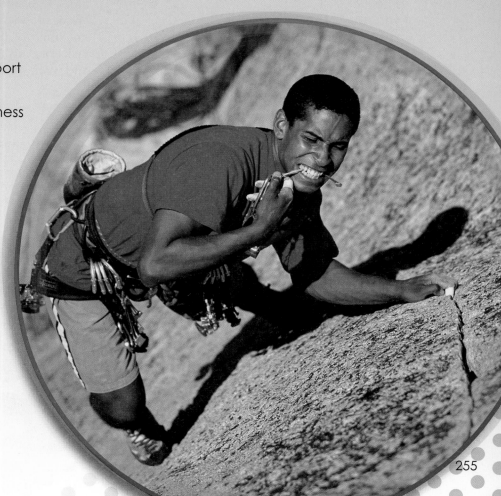

Lesson Objectives

After reading this lesson, you should be able to

1. name several core muscles and explain why they are important;

2. describe some common back and posture problems;

3. list some biomechanical principles and guidelines for the mechanics of lifting that can help you improve your posture and avoid back problems; and

4. describe the FIT formula for building core muscles and describe several methods of exercise for improving them.

Lesson Vocabulary

force
kyphosis
laws of motion
lordosis
Pilates
ptosis
scoliosis

Do you know what core fitness is? In this lesson, you'll learn about your core muscles and why they are important for good health and functioning. You'll also learn about exercises, including core muscle exercises, that you can perform to improve your posture and reduce your risk of back pain and other muscle injuries.

Core Muscles

Your core muscles support your spine, keep your rib cage and pelvis stable, and help you maintain a healthy posture while standing, sitting, and moving in a variety of body positions. They also are the muscles that connect the upper and lower parts of your body. They include the muscles of your back, hips and pelvis, and abdominal area (see figure 11.1).

It's not uncommon for people to neglect their core muscles and focus more on muscles in their arms, legs, and shoulders because these muscles are easily seen. But you need fit core muscles—not only for healthy living and performing the tasks of daily life, but also for performing sport and work-related activities and preventing injury.

> My dad started doing core exercises after he hurt his back. He helped me to get started doing core exercises and I was surprised that it improved my posture—I look better too.
>
> *Darla Wagner*

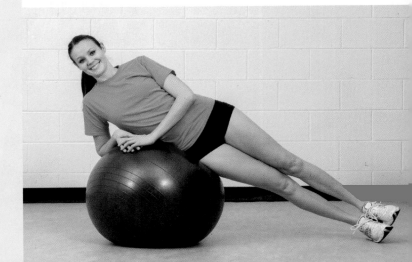

Core fitness allows you to keep your trunk stable while performing movements of all types. Some basic core exercises are presented at the end of this chapter.

Because core exercises are an important part of a total muscle fitness program, they are performed in addition to other progressive resistance exercises (PRE). As described later in this lesson, many core exercises can be done without special equipment or with inexpensive equipment.

Back and Posture Problems

Backache can be considered a hypokinetic condition because weak and short muscles are linked to some types of back problems. Poor posture is also associated with muscles that are not strong or long enough. By building fit muscles to improve your posture, you can help reduce your risk of back pain and look your best. Even if you never experience back pain, a healthy back and good posture help you function more efficiently in your daily activities.

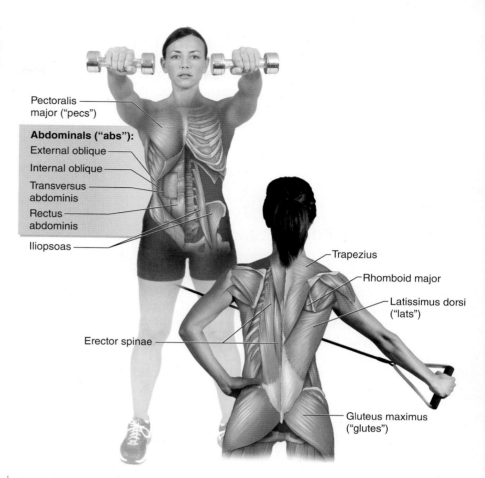

Figure 11.1   The core muscles.

Back Problems

Have you ever had a sore back after sitting for a long time or lifting a heavy object? Each year, as many as 25 million Americans seek a doctor's care for backache. According to some experts, back pain is second only to the common cold among leading medical complaints in the United States, and it will be experienced by 80 percent of all adults at some point in their lives. Back injuries are the number one source of work-related injury in the United States, and treatment of back pain costs billions of dollars each year.

Studies show that back problems often begin early in life. Approximately one-third of children in elementary school have had back pain, and by the age of 18 the incidence rate of back pain is near that of adults. There are many reasons why people have back problems. Some of the most common are injuries (e.g., sports, job related, home), disease, improper lifting, poor biomechanics, poor posture (e.g., standing, sitting, and lying), and lack of fitness of core muscles.

TECH TRENDS: **Exercise Machines With Memory**

Computer technology now allows exercise machines to store your information about resistance, reps, and sets, making it easy to quickly prepare for each exercise. You can also install fitness apps on a smartphone, tablet, or other personal computer to help you keep your own record of your exercises that do not require machines (for example, core exercises).

USING TECHNOLOGY

Identify and describe an exercise machine or app that can be used to self-monitor muscle fitness exercise.

Healthy Posture

Knowing what constitutes good posture can help you improve your own posture, which in turn helps you look good, helps prevent back problems, and helps you work and play more efficiently. When standing with a healthy posture, your body is aligned in a vertical column (see figure 11.2a). The head, shoulders and rib cage, spine, pelvis, and legs are lined up efficiently. Although the body parts are in line when standing with good posture, there are several normal curves at the neck, the shoulders (kyphotic curve), and the low back (lordotic curve) (see figure 11.2a).

The healthy spine relies on fit muscles to keep your body parts balanced (see figure 11.2b). If your muscles are not fit, posture problems can occur. One problem common among both teens and adults occurs when the normal curve of the lower back becomes exaggerated. This excessive low back curve is referred to as **lordosis** (see figure 11.2c). Lordosis is both a posture and a back problem that can lead to back pain. Weak back and abdominal muscles and short hip flexor and hamstring muscles can cause the pelvis to tip forward and cause lordosis (see figure 11.2d).

Other common posture problems are **kyphosis** and **ptosis**. Kyphosis refers to excessive kyphotic curve and is sometimes referred to as "rounded back" (see figure 11.2c). Weak upper back muscles and short chest muscles contribute to kyphosis (see figure 11.2d). It is not uncommon for the head to move forward

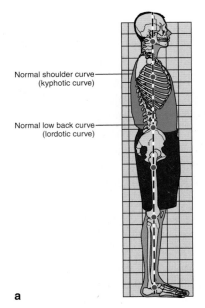
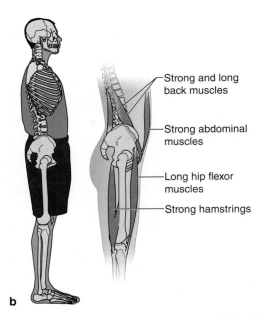

Figure 11.2 (a) Good posture; (b) core muscles for good posture; (c) posture problems; (d) unfit postural muscles.

SCIENCE IN ACTION: **PRE and Risk of Injury Among Teens**

Experts have now determined that PRE is safe for teens when performed properly and with good supervision. However, even when done properly, PRE and sports such as weightlifting carry a risk of injury, most frequently back injury, especially in the low back. The National Strength and Conditioning Association indicates, however, that "this risk is no greater than [the risk in] many other sports and recreational activities in which children and adolescents regularly participate." For example, studies show that the average injury rate in youth sports, especially contact sports, is much higher than for PRE. The risk of injury from PRE performed at home is also much higher than the risk of PRE done in schools, primarily because of better supervision, better equipment, and required use of spotters at school.

Some injuries associated with PRE are not immediately noticeable. As a result, when cautioned about improper lifting or using incorrect biomechanics, some people might say, "I've done that before and it didn't cause a problem." But we know that repeated small injuries (microtraumas) can lead to big problems later. Many people who ignore biomechanical guidelines eventually say, "I wish I hadn't done that."

STUDENT ACTIVITY

Investigate to determine what real-life activities, including sports and recreation, put you at risk of injury.

out of alignment when other posture problems occur. Ptosis refers to protruding abdomen. Weak abdominal muscles allow the abdomen to protrude and are one cause of ptosis (see figure 11.2, c and d).

Just as we all have normal forward and backward spinal curve, it is not uncommon to have some sideways curve of the spine. **Scoliosis** is a posture problem that occurs when the spine has too much sideways curve. It can be present at birth or develop during the growing years. Exercises can be helpful in treating scoliosis but the help of medical and health care professionals is often required.

FIT FACT

Many teens wear backpacks. To carry a backpack effectively, you need adequate strength and muscular endurance. In a typical year, the U.S. Consumer Product Safety Commission reports more than 6,000 backpack-related injuries, mostly among youth. Improving your muscle fitness can help you reduce your risk of injury from wearing a backpack.

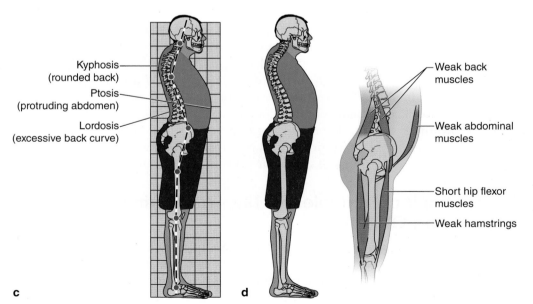

Kyphosis (rounded back)
Ptosis (protruding abdomen)
Lordosis (excessive back curve)

Weak back muscles
Weak abdominal muscles
Short hip flexor muscles
Weak hamstrings

c   d

Figure 11.2 *(continued)*

Preventing a back injury is much easier than repairing one.

U.S. Occupational Safety and Health Administration (OSHA)

You might recognize posture problems in your own posture or that of someone you know. Performing exercises to strengthen and stretch postural muscles helps prevent lordosis, kyphosis, and ptosis (figure 11.2c). Posture problems are most common among people who are inactive, who sit and stand for long periods of time with poor posture, and who do not follow the biomechanical principles described later in this lesson. However, even people who regularly participate in sports and games sometimes overdevelop some muscles and neglect others. As a result, it is not unusual for basketball players, gymnasts, band members, and other active people to have posture problems. The posture problems described here can cause the muscles to become fatigued and overstressed, causing pain. Over time poor posture can lead to more severe tissue problems that result in neck and back pain.

In the following sections you will learn about and perform the healthy back test (see Self-Assessment) to help you determine which of your muscles need to be strengthened and lengthened. You will also learn about various types of exercises that you can perform to prevent back problems and improve your posture. In addition, you will learn about methods of lifting and carrying objects to minimize risk of injury. In chapter 19 you will get a chance to do a posture self-assessment.

Back and Posture Improvement and Maintenance

You can take several steps to help yourself enjoy good back health. First, you can perform self-assessments to determine your current back health and posture status. You can then identify exercises that will help you develop or maintain the muscle fitness and flexibility necessary for good back health and good posture. You can also use key principles of biomechanics to prevent back pain and injury.

Healthy Back Test

In the Self-Assessment feature at the end of this lesson, you'll get the opportunity to take the healthy back test. This will help you determine what you can do to keep your back fit and healthy. Core exercises are especially good for back health and for maintaining good posture. Stretching exercises are also commonly recommended.

As shown in figure 11.2c, strong and long muscles help you avoid posture problems. The problems shown in figure 11.2c and 11.2d are not present in a healthy posture. In a healthy posture, the head is centered over the shoulders, the shoulders are back and balanced, the low back has a gentle curve, the abdomen does not protrude, and the knees do not bend backward. You can work with a partner to evaluate posture for problems and proper alignment. For more, see the Self-Assessment feature on assessing your posture in chapter 19.

Biomechanical Principles for Lifting, Carrying, and Moving Objects

Biomechanical principles and the **laws of motion** apply when you use your body's levers—the bones of your arms and legs—to apply **force** in lifting, carrying, and moving objects. The most frequent use of these levers occurs when you walk, run, or perform skills such as throwing, jumping, kicking, and striking. Using your body levers efficiently is also important in applying force when performing resistance exercises. Use the following biomechanical principles to help you avoid exercises that can lead to injury and back problems.

- *Use your large muscles when lifting.* Let your strong hip and leg muscles do the work.
- *Keep your weight (hips) low.* To make lifting safer, keep your weight low by squatting (bending your knees) with your back straight and your hips tucked.
- *Keep your core muscles firm when lifting.* Tighten your back and abdominal muscles to stabilize your body.
- *Use a wide base of support for balance.* Keep your feet spread about shoulder-width apart for stability when lifting.
- *Avoid a bent-over position when sitting, standing, or lifting.* Your body's levers, such as your spine, do not work efficiently when you are bent over. When sitting in a chair, sit back in the seat and lean against the backrest. Do not work for long periods of time in a bent-over position.
- *Divide a load to make it easier to carry.* For example, it is easier to carry a small suitcase in each hand than to carry one larger suitcase. Avoid overloading your backpack and use both straps rather than carrying it on one shoulder. If you must carry your books in your arms, carry some in each arm or change arms from time to time.
- *Avoid twisting while lifting.* If you have to turn while lifting, change the position of your feet. It's especially important to avoid twisting your spine as you are straightening or bending it.
- *Push or pull heavy objects.* Heavy lifting can cause injury. Pushing or pulling an object is more efficient than lifting it.

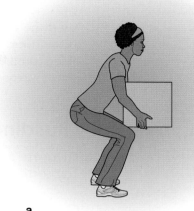

a

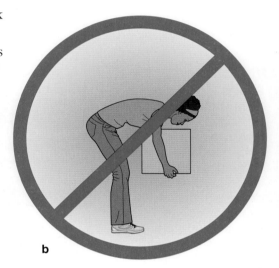

b

The Mechanics of Lifting and Carrying

The previous biomechanical principles can be applied to help you lift and carry objects efficiently and safely. Before considering the different methods of lifting, assess the object you need to move. If the object is large, heavy, or of an unusual shape, lifting and carrying by yourself is not the best option. Consider using a hand truck, getting the assistance of another person, or sliding the object. If you determine that the object is suitable for lifting, consider these guidelines. Keep the object close to the body (keep the levers short). Stabilize the trunk muscles. Use the muscles of the hips and legs to do the lifting.

- *Efficient lifting.* Squat with your legs on either side of the object. If it is too wide to fit between your legs, get help. Keep your head up and eyes forward. Contract your core muscles to stabilize the trunk. Straighten your legs to lift the object (see figure 11.3a). Avoid lifting with your legs straight and your trunk leaning forward (see figure 11.3b), which increases the force on the spine by 50 times compared to correct lifting. The longer lever magnifies the force required.

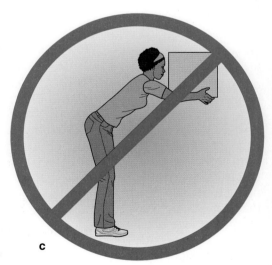

c

Figure 11.3 For efficiency, *(a)* lift with the weight close to the body. *(b)* Avoid bending forward at the waist or *(c)* reaching while lifting because the longer levers increase stress on the back.

• *Efficient carrying.* The guidelines for carrying are similar to those for lifting. Keep the object close to the body (see figure 11.3*a*). When lowering the object to the floor, use similar steps to lifting but in reverse. Avoid reaching to place the object on a counter or shelf (see figure 11.3*c*) because it lengthens the lever and places stress on the spine.

Building the Core Muscles

There are a variety of different exercises that can be used to build core muscles. The sections that follow describe some of these types of exercises.

Core Calisthenics

Calisthenics are often used to build the core muscles. The FIT formula for core calisthenics is shown in table 11.1. This formula is also appropriate for other core exercises. Illustrations and descriptions of nine core muscle exercises are provided in Exercise Chart 1 at the end of this chapter.

TABLE 11.1   **FIT Formula for Core Calisthenics**

		Threshold	Target zone
Frequency (days per week)		3	3–6
Intensity		Body weight	Body weight
Time	**Sets**	1	1–3
	Reps	10	10–25

Stability Ball Exercises

Stability balls (also called *exercise balls*) can be used with a number of different exercises to help you to improve fitness of specific core muscles (see figure 11.4). A link at the web resource provides illustrations and descriptions of a variety of stability ball exercises. If you choose to do this type of exercise, it is important to select a ball of the appropriate size. It is a good fit if your knees are at a 90-degree angle when you sit on the ball. You can use the FIT formula for calisthenics for this form of core exercise.

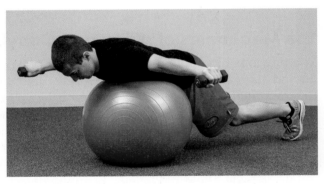

Figure 11.4   Stability ball exercises can help you build core fitness.

Stretching

Healthy back care and good posture also depend on flexibility. Stretching does not build core muscles, but it does lengthen muscles that are too short and that contribute to back pain and poor posture. You will learn more about stretching as well as activities such as yoga and tai chi in chapter 12.

LESSON REVIEW

1. What are some of the core muscles, and why they are important?
2. What are some common back and posture problems?
3. What are some biomechanical principles and guidelines for the mechanics of lifting that can help you improve your posture, avoid back problems, and lift efficiently?
4. What is the FIT formula, and what are some types of exercise for building core muscles?

SELF-ASSESSMENT: **Healthy Back Test**

Backache is often caused by muscles that are weak and too short. Test your back muscles by using the following self-assessment. Each part focuses on a certain muscle group. If you do well on this assessment, you're likely to have a healthy back. If not, it's especially important that you do exercises to improve your back health. Work with a partner to anchor your body for certain tests and help record scores. Add your scores for the individual test item to get your total score, then use table 11.2 to determine your risk of back problems. Record your results. Remember that self-assessment information is confidential and shouldn't be shared without the permission of the person being tested.

TABLE 11.2   Rating Chart: Healthy Back Test

Rating	Score
Good fitness	11–12
Marginal fitness (some risk)	9–10
Low fitness (greater risk)	6–8
High risk	≤5

SINGLE-LEG LIFT (SUPINE)

1. Lie on your back on the floor. Lift your left leg off the floor as high as possible without bending either knee.

2. Repeat using your right leg. Score 1 point if you can lift your left leg to a 90-degree angle with the floor. Score an additional point if you can lift your right leg to a 90-degree angle.

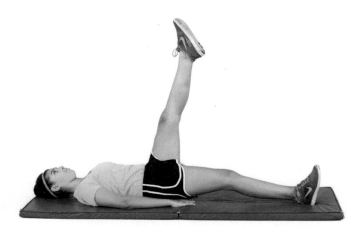

THIGH-TO-CHEST

1. Lie on your back on the floor. Make sure your lower back is flat on the floor.

2. Grasp the back of your thigh to bring your right knee up until you can hold it tightly against the bottom of your rib cage. Keep your left leg straight. The left leg may lift off the floor to allow the right thigh to make contact with your upper body.

3. Repeat using your left leg.

4. Score 1 point if you can keep your left leg touching the floor while holding your right thigh against your upper body. Score an additional point if you can keep your right leg touching the floor while holding your left thigh against your upper body.

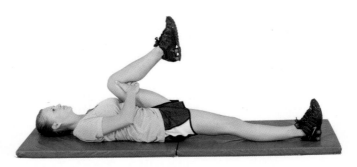

SINGLE-LEG LIFT (PRONE)

1. Lie facedown on the floor. Lift your right leg as high as possible (keep it straight). Hold the position for a count of 10. Then lower your leg.

2. Repeat using your left leg.

3. Score 1 point if you can hold your right leg 12 inches (30 centimeters) off the floor for a count of 10. Score an additional point if you can do the same with your left leg.

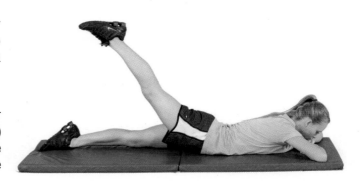

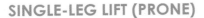

CURL-UP

1. Lie on your back with your knees bent at 90 degrees and your arms extended.

2. Curl up by rolling your head, shoulders, and upper back off the floor. Roll up only until your shoulder blades leave the floor.

3. Score 1 point if you can curl up with your arms held straight in front of you and hold the position for 10 seconds without having to lift your feet off the floor.

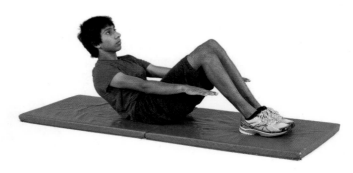

4. Score an additional point if you can curl up with your arms across your chest and hold the position for 10 seconds without your feet leaving the floor.

TRUNK LIFT AND HOLD

1. Lie facedown on a padded bench (or a bleacher with a towel on it) that is 16 to 18 inches (41 to 46 centimeters) high. Your upper body (from your waist up) should extend off the bench.

2. Have your partner hold your calves just below the knees.

3. Place one hand over the other on your forehead with your palms facing away and your elbows held to the side at the level of your ears.

4. Start with your upper body lowered. Lift slowly until your upper body is even with the bench. Hold the position for a count of 10.

5. Score 1 point if you can lift your trunk even with the bench. Score an additional point if you can hold your upper body even with the bench for a count of 10.

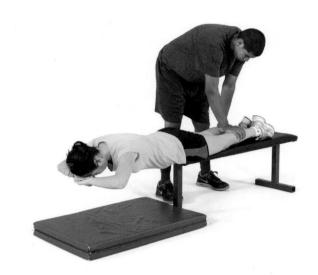

FRONT PLANK

1. On a mat or carpet, support your body with your forearms and toes.

2. Keep your head in line with your body and hold this position for 10 seconds.

3. Score 2 points if you can hold your body straight for the full 10 seconds.

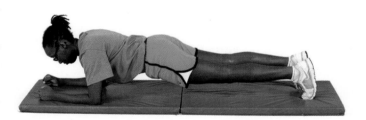

Muscle Fitness Exercise Planning and Ergogenic Aids

Lesson Objectives

After reading this lesson, you should be able to

1. describe the steps for preparing a personal muscle fitness exercise plan and explain how to use them to create your own personal plan;

2. identify and describe several food supplements used by people interested in building muscle fitness and describe guidelines for using the Internet to find health information;

3. describe several facts about supplements and their use; and

4. describe several other ergogenic aids (PEDs) and discuss the benefits and risks associated with their use.

Lesson Vocabulary

anabolic steroid
androgen
androstenedione
creatine
ergogenic aid
ergolytic
food supplement
human growth hormone (HGH)
PED
prohormones
rhabdomyolysis
T-booster

Are you among the nearly 50 percent of teens who does no regular muscle fitness exercise? Would you like to improve your muscle fitness? In this lesson you'll learn how to prepare a safe and effective personal muscle fitness exercise plan. Carrying out a good plan is the surest way to build your muscle fitness, which will help you meet national guidelines for physical activity both now and later in your life. You'll also learn about the benefits and problems associated with products advertised as muscle builders.

Planning a Muscle Fitness Exercise Program

Molly is 15 years old and has used the five steps of program planning to prepare a muscle fitness exercise program. Her program is described here.

> Planning a personal muscle fitness program worked for me. But some people try to take shortcuts by using performance enhancing drugs. To me that is cheating. Besides that, they have caused many athletes to be suspended.
>
> *Ray Alvarez*

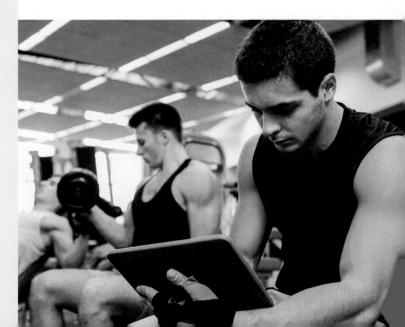

Step 1: Determine Your Personal Needs

To get started, Molly made a list of the muscle fitness exercises and activities she had performed over the last week, as well as her fitness test results that related to vigorous physical activity. Her results are shown in table 11.3.

Molly met the national activity guideline for muscle fitness (exercising two days a week). But when she was not in physical education class, she did no muscle fitness exercise. In addition, Molly's fitness test scores were mostly in the marginal zone, indicating that she needed improvement. Molly wanted to try out for the softball team, and she now knew that she needed to improve her fitness in order to be the best player she could be.

Step 2: Consider Your Program Options

Molly wanted to consider all of the various types of muscle fitness exercise, so she made a list of the types of PRE that she had to choose from. Her list is included here.

- Resistance machine exercises
- Free weight exercises
- Core exercises
- Calisthenics

TABLE 11.3   **Molly's Muscle Fitness Exercise (Physical Activity) and Fitness Profiles**

Physical fitness profile		
Fitness self-assessment	**Score**	**Rating**
1RM arm press (relative strength)	0.55 (strength per pound of body weight)	Marginal fitness
1RM leg press (relative strength)	1.10 (strength per pound of body weight)	Good fitness
Grip strength	105 lb	Marginal fitness
Muscle endurance test	4 points	Marginal fitness
Healthy back test	9 points	Marginal fitness
Standing long jump	59 in.	Marginal fitness
Medicine ball throw	95 in.	Marginal fitness
Physical activity profile		
Day	**Muscle fitness exercise(s)**	**Amount**
Mon.	Curl-up	1 set, 10 reps
	Knee push-up	1 set, 10 reps
Tues.	None	
Wed.	Curl-up	1 set, 10 reps
	Knee push-up	1 set, 10 reps
Thurs.	None	
Fri.	Curl-up	1 set, 10 reps
	Knee push-up	1 set, 10 reps
Sat.	None	None
Sun.	None	None

- Elastic band exercises
- Stability ball exercises
- Homemade weights
- Isometric exercises
- Isokinetic machine exercises
- Pilates
- Plyometric exercises

Step 3: Set Goals

For this muscle fitness plan, Molly set a time period of two weeks—too short for long-term goals—so she developed only short-term physical activity goals. Later, when she prepares a longer plan, she'll develop long-term goals, including some muscle fitness improvement goals. For now, she wanted to try some new exercises to get started and improve her chances of making the softball team.

Molly used the information she put together in step 2 to help develop her short-term goals

Varying your schedule for PRE can help keep it interesting.

for muscle fitness exercise (PRE). Out of the options, she decided on resistance machines, core exercises, and plyometrics (jump rope). Before writing down her goals, Molly made sure that she chose SMART goals.

- Continue to perform two calisthenics exercises in physical education class (1 set of 10 reps).
- Perform five resistance machine exercises two days a week (1 set of 10 reps at 50 percent of 1RM).
- Perform four core exercises three days a week (hold 10 seconds or do 1 set of 10 reps).
- Perform jump rope two days a week (5 minutes).

Step 4: Create a Written Program

Molly's fourth step was to write down her two-week muscle fitness plan (see table 11.4). Molly chose resistance machine exercises because she could use the school's exercise room on Tuesdays and Thursdays after school and she thought these exercises would be good to prepare for softball. She decided to do them two days a week because she was just beginning this type of exercise. She included her jump rope (plyometrics) on Tuesday and Thursday as well. She scheduled core exercises because they were good for back health and good posture and she could do them at home. She listed the exercises she did in physical education class because she expected to keep doing them for the two weeks of her plan. Molly's plan met the national guideline of performing muscle fitness exercises on at least two to three days a week.

Step 5: Keep a Log and Evaluate Your Program

Over the next two weeks, Molly will monitor her activities and place a checkmark beside each activity she performs. At the end of the two-week period, she'll evaluate her performance to see whether she met her goals, then use that evaluation to help her make another activity plan.

TABLE 11.4 **Molly's Two-Week Muscle Fitness Plan**

	Week 1			Week 2		
Day	**Exercises**	**Time, sets, reps**	✓	**Exercises**	**Time, sets, reps**	✓
Mon.	Curl-up*	1 set, 10 reps		Curl-up*	1 set, 10 reps	
	Knee push-up*	1 set, 10 reps		Knee push-up*	1 set, 10 reps	
	Core exercises			**Core exercises**		
	Front plank	Hold 10 sec		Front plank	Hold 10 sec	
	Side plank (left)	Hold 10 sec		Side plank (left)	Hold 10 sec	
	Side plank (right)	Hold 10 sec		Side plank (right)	Hold 10 sec	
	Reverse curl	1 set, 10 reps		Reverse curl	1 set, 10 reps	
Tues.	Jump rope	3:30–3:35 p.m.		Jump rope	3:30–3:35 p.m.	
	Resistance machine			**Resistance machine**		
	Arm press	3:35–4:30 p.m.		Arm press	3:35–4:30 p.m.	
	Knee extension	1 set		Knee extension	1 set	
	Hamstring curl	10 reps		Hamstring curl	10 reps	
	Biceps curl	50% 1RM for		Biceps curl	50% 1RM for	
	Heel raise	each exercise		Heel raise	each exercise	
Wed.	Curl-up*	1 set, 10 reps		Curl-up*	1 set, 10 reps	
	Knee push-up*	1 set, 10 reps		Knee push-up*	1 set, 10 reps	
	Core exercises			**Core exercises**		
	Front plank	Hold 10 sec		Front plank	Hold 10 sec	
	Side plank (left)	Hold 10 sec		Side plank (left)	Hold 10 sec	
	Side plank (right)	Hold 10 sec		Side plank (right)	Hold 10 sec	
	Reverse curl	1 set, 10 reps		Reverse curl	1 set, 10 reps	
Thurs.	Jump rope	3:30–3:35 p.m.		Jump rope	3:30–3:35 p.m.	
	Resistance machine			**Resistance machine**		
	Arm press	3:35–4:30 p.m.		Arm press	3:35–4:30 p.m.	
	Knee extension	1 set		Knee extension	1 set	
	Hamstring curl	10 reps		Hamstring curl	10 reps	
	Biceps curl	50% 1RM for		Biceps curl	50% 1RM for	
	Heel raise	each exercise		Heel raise	each exercise	
Fri.	Curl-up*	1 set, 10 reps		Curl-up*	1 set, 10 reps	
	Knee push-up*	1 set, 10 reps		Knee push-up*	1 set, 10 reps	
	Core exercises			**Core exercises**		
	Front plank	Hold 10 sec		Front plank	Hold 10 sec	
	Side plank (left)	Hold 10 sec		Side plank (left)	Hold 10 sec	
	Side plank (right)	Hold 10 sec		Side plank (right)	Hold 10 sec	
	Reverse curl	1 set, 10 reps		Reverse curl	1 set, 10 reps	
Sat.						
Sun.						

*Performed in physical education class

> Fitness—if it came in a bottle, everyone would have a great body.
>
> *Cher, singer and actress*

Ergogenic Aids: Supplements

For centuries, people have tried to find methods of enhancing performance—including methods other than or in addition to following a well-planned exercise program. An **ergogenic aid** is something that is designed to help you increase your ability to do work, including performing vigorous exercise. The word *ergogenic* is derived from the Greek word *ergo*, which means work, and *genic*, which means to cause or generate. Supplements are the most common products thought of as ergogenic aids, but some are classified as drugs and are commonly referred to as **PEDs** (performance-enhancing drugs). Various kinds of supplements are discussed in this lesson.

Supplement is a word that refers to "an extra amount" of something. For example, a **food supplement** is a substance that "adds to" a normal diet; it is not meant to be a substitute for healthy foods in your diet. Several supplements are commonly sold as ergogenic aids in health food and drugstores, as well as online. Food supplements thought to be ergogenic have been historically used by athletes and bodybuilders but are now often used by nonathletes with the hope of improving appearance. Because they are not classified as drugs, supplements are not regulated by the Food and Drug Administration (FDA), although the FDA does keep track of medical and safety complaints related to the use of supplements. Ephedra is one example of a supplement that was alleged to improve athletic performance and aid in weight loss but is now banned after complaints to the FDA showed that it causes irregular heart rate and has unhealthful effects on the heart and the nervous system.

Several studies suggest that teens who use supplements are at greater risk of using PEDs than those who do not use supplements. The ACSM source, Essentials of Youth Fitness, notes that the use of supplements is generally discouraged in youth.

Protein Supplements

Protein supplements are sold in grocery stores, specialty stores, and online and come in a variety of forms, including powders, pills, bars, and drinks (shakes). About 11 percent of adults buy and use protein supplements, including for athletic performance and to enhance appearance. Protein supplements are also used in rehabilitation programs and with older populations to maintain lean body mass.

Your body needs protein for growth and development of most tissues. However, most people eat more protein in their regular diet than they really need. The ACSM's Essentials of Youth Fitness indicates that teens should consume 0.39 to 0.50 grams of protein per pound of body weight per day, though active teens require more (0.45 to 0.91 grams per pound of body weight per day). The recommended maximum is 1.36 grams per pound of body weight per day. Dietary protein in excess of body needs is stored as fat, as are calories from extra dietary fat and carbohydrate.

The amount of protein that you need depends on your activity patterns and size. An active person requires more protein than an inactive person. An inactive 150-pound teen needs a minimum of 59 grams (236 calories) of protein a day, whereas a very active 150-pound teen needs a minimum of 68 grams (270 calories). A larger person (more than 150 pounds) would need more protein than a 150-pound person, whether active or inactive. However, the active person—especially one who does regular PRE—would need more protein than an inactive person of any weight.

FIT FACT

Protein supplements are very expensive, costing as much as 50 cents per gram of protein. In contrast, the protein in foods such as meat, poultry, fish, beans, and eggs is much cheaper, costing only a few cents per gram (figure 11.5).

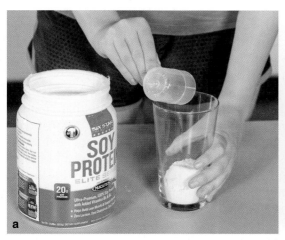
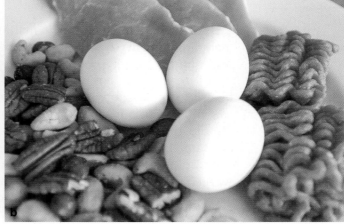

Figure 11.5 *(a)* Protein supplements can be expensive, but *(b)* foods with protein are generally less expensive than supplements.

Experts agree that the best way to obtain protein is through a healthy diet. Proteins are made up of 20 different amino acids, so it is important to consume a variety of foods to ensure sufficient intake. For optimal health and performance, the American Nutrition and Dietetics Academy (ANDA) and the ACSM recommend that active people space protein intake throughout the day.

SCIENCE IN ACTION: Before (Pre-) and After (Post-) Workout Supplements

In recent years, taking supplements before and after a workout has become common, especially among active adults. The most popular preworkout supplements typically contain a blend of caffeine, creatine, various amino acids (proteins), and a variety of other substances (e.g., herbs, nitrates). Because they have many ingredients, they are commonly referred to as *multi-ingredient preworkout supplements* (MIPS). Although adults may get some benefits from MIPS, they are not without risks. For example, the amounts of ingredients are often unknown and many supplements contain unwanted substances such as PEDs. MIPS are not recommended for teens. Studies done on MIPS are difficult because ingredients vary widely from one product to another.

Research done primarily on adult males has shown some benefits to taking caffeine supplements prior to a workout. However, the American Academy of Pediatrics recommends that teens consume no more than 100 milligrams of caffeine each day, and many MIPS contain double that amount. Eighty-six percent of MIPS contained some caffeine, but the exact amount is often unknown.

Research also indicates that eating enough protein, especially in the hours immediately after exercise, is important for building and maintaining muscle mass. For teens, consuming healthy food containing protein throughout the day, including before and after exercise, is recommended. The ACSM's Essentials of Youth Fitness indicates that low-fat milk, especially chocolate, is an excellent recovery drink for active youth. It contains a good source of fast-digesting protein, is dense in vitamins and minerals, and has a good ratio of carbohydrates to proteins.

STUDENT ACTIVITY

The Food and Drug Administration (FDA) monitors complaints about fraudulent (fake) supplements. These products look like supplements but they are not. Search FDA and fraudulent supplements. Write a brief summary of the problems created by fraudulent supplements and their dangers.

Creatine

Creatine is a natural substance manufactured in the bodies of meat-eating animals, including humans. It is needed for the body to perform anaerobic exercise, including many types of progressive resistance exercise. Creatine can also be taken as a food supplement, which allows your body to store more of it. Medical and kinesiology experts who have studied creatine use in adults indicate that creatine can be effective in improving performance when accompanied by appropriate muscle fitness or high-intensity aerobic or anaerobic exercise. Some evidence indicates that it allows for shorter rest intervals between high-intensity bouts of exercise. Short-term use of appropriate amounts of creatine has not been linked with serious health effects, but the safety of long-term use is not well established. There is also some concern about possible increased risk of dehydration among athletes who use creatine.

Less research is available on creatine use among children and teens and recommendations of experts are mixed. The ACSM and American Academy of Pediatrics recommends against use of creatine by those under 18. However, as many as 1 in 5 older teen male athletes report using creatine, leading some experts to suggest that it is better to oversee use of supplements rather than universally condemn them. They recommend parental and medical oversight, use of known high-quality creatine, a sound diet and training program, and monitoring of dosage and time period of use.

Testosterone Boosters (T-Boosters)

T-boosters are supplements marketed primarily to adult males. They promise a variety of benefits, including (but not limited to) increased energy, increased muscle mass, and improved sexual function. The supplements typically contain a variety of ingredients such as herbs, vitamins, and minerals. A discussion of T-boosters is included here because they are widely promoted online and on sports radio stations popular among teen athletes. As a result, some teens purchase or consider purchasing T-boosters with the hope of improving sport performance or building muscle mass to improve appearance.

Research conducted on the five most commonly purchased T-boosters sold on Amazon indicated that they had 19 different ingredients for the five products. Many of the products did not list quantities of the various ingredients, making it impossible for users to know what they are taking. Previous studies have shown that T-boosters sometimes contain banned substances, including steroids, and may cause adverse side effects. There was limited support for testosterone-producing benefits of the ingredients, with the majority of studies showing no benefit or undetermined effects. No research was found to support the claimed benefits of the products as advertised—however, the research did find evidence of faked reviews for the products. Once the fake reviews were filtered out, the claimed benefits disappeared. Products with the exact same ingredients are also sold as treatments for conditions other than low testosterone, suggesting that they are not promoted truthfully. For these reasons, T-boosters are not recommended for adults or teens.

▌Facts About Supplements

Many products sold as ergogenic aids are classified as food supplements. Although many people think that the FDA tests food supplements to make sure that they

FIT FACT

Over the past decade, the FDA has issued numerous warnings to supplement manufacturers. The most common offense is the inclusion of hazardous substances such as steroids or steroid precursors in over-the-counter supplements. Common terms in the names of these products include Xtreme, Tren, Mass, Hardcore, Testosterone Booster, and words ending in the letters "ol" (e.g., Beastdrol, Tren-Bol, Sterodol).

are safe, supplements are in fact unregulated by the government. Unlike medicines, which must be tested before they are approved for safe use, the law does *not* require that supplements be tested for effectiveness or safety before they are sold. And unlike foods, which must be labeled with nutrition information, food supplements are not required to carry a label. As a result, there is often great variation in the content of different products with the same name. Be aware of the following facts about food supplements.

- *Regulation.* The government does not regulate supplements to ensure their contents or safety. Some manufacturers regulate their products, but many do not.

- *Claims.* Manufacturers are not supposed to make unsubstantiated health claims for their products, but many do anyway. Although the FDA can investigate and take action against companies for false claims, there are few investigators and many false claims are not caught. Beware of health claims made for supplements.

- *Contents.* Many supplements do not contain what their makers claim they do. Some contain too little or too much of the key substance they are supposed to contain. Some have been shown to contain substances that they are *not* supposed to contain, including banned substances. These problems can lead to health risks or disqualification from competition. However, several independent companies now test supplements. They do not test to see if they are safe or effective, but they do test to see if supplements are what they claim to be. United States Pharmacopeia (USP) and NSF International are private nonprofit organizations and ConsumerLab (CL) and UL are for-profit groups that test supplements. A USP, NSF, CL, or UL label on a product indicates that it has been tested and is more likely than other products to be what it claims to be.

- *Side effects and interactions.* Supplements can have side effects that result in negative health consequences (e.g., fast heart rate,

CONSUMER CORNER: **Supplements and the Internet**

One of the important health goals of the Healthy People 2030 project is to increase access to high-quality health information. Thanks to technology, more health information is available than ever—however, increased use of the Internet for health information does not necessarily lead to high-quality health information.

Health information is the most common subject of web searches, and 75 percent of all teens and young adults seek health, fitness, and wellness information on the web. But many websites, including popular web encyclopedias, contain incorrect information about health, which can result in injury, illness, failure to get adequate care, and loss of money spent on products and treatments that don't work.

Of special concern is Internet searches for supplements. It is true that searches of reliable websites such as the FDA, the CDC, and the FTC can provide useful information, but hundreds of other websites provide false, misleading, and dangerous information. Be aware that Internet searches often lead you to websites that pay to appear at the top of the search list. These paid websites promote the sale of their product and may appear to be scientific sources. They are not!

One of the most important goals of *Fitness for Life* is to help you become a good consumer of fitness, health, and wellness information. Before searching the Internet for health or supplement information, read and consider the guidelines outlined in chapter 19, Making Good Consumer Choices.

STUDENT ACTIVITY

Search for terms such as "supplements," "ergogenic aids," or "steroids" on the CDC, FDA, or FTC website. Summarize what you learned, providing the URL from the source you accessed.

FIT FACT
The U.S. Anti-Doping Agency (USADA) and the World Anti-Doping Agency (WADA) keep a list of PEDs and other substances prohibited in sport. The goals of the organizations are to ensure fair competition and provide information to protect the health of athletes. Testing can detect the presence of banned substances in the body and many sport groups now do mandatory testing. Many high-profile athletes have destroyed their reputations and careers by using HGH and other substances described in this lesson. The organizations provide and regularly update their lists of banned substances.

headaches, nausea, kidney and liver problems). Some supplements interact with medicines by interfering with the medicine's effectiveness or causing negative side effects when taken together.

- *Dose or amount.* Because research is not required for supplements, as it is for medicines, very little is known about appropriate doses (amounts) for most supplements.
- *Recall.* Although the FDA does not regulate or test supplements, it does maintain a registry of side effects experienced from use of a supplement and user reports have resulted in FDA bans on several supplements. You can report side effects from supplement use to the FDA.

Ergogenic Aids: Performance Enhancing Drugs (PEDs)

Some supplements, such as those discussed earlier, may be beneficial to some but not to others. Others do not work at all. Some ergogenic aids, however, can be dangerous. Because they are detrimental to health or performance, they are better referred to as **ergolytic** (*ergo* meaning work and *lytic* meaning destruction). Examples of ergolytic substances include alcohol, tobacco, marijuana, and many PEDs. Several dangerous supplements and PEDs are discussed in the section that follows.

Androgens

Androgens are hormones primarily associated with male physical characteristics. For this reason, they are often called the "male hormone," although they also occur to a lesser extent in females. At puberty, the androgen testosterone becomes more prevalent, promoting facial hair, deeper voice, greater lean body mass, weight gain, and bone maturation in males. **Anabolic steroids** are synthetic drugs that resemble testosterone, which doctors prescribe in small doses to treat certain diseases. However, some people illegally buy and use anabolic steroids to increase

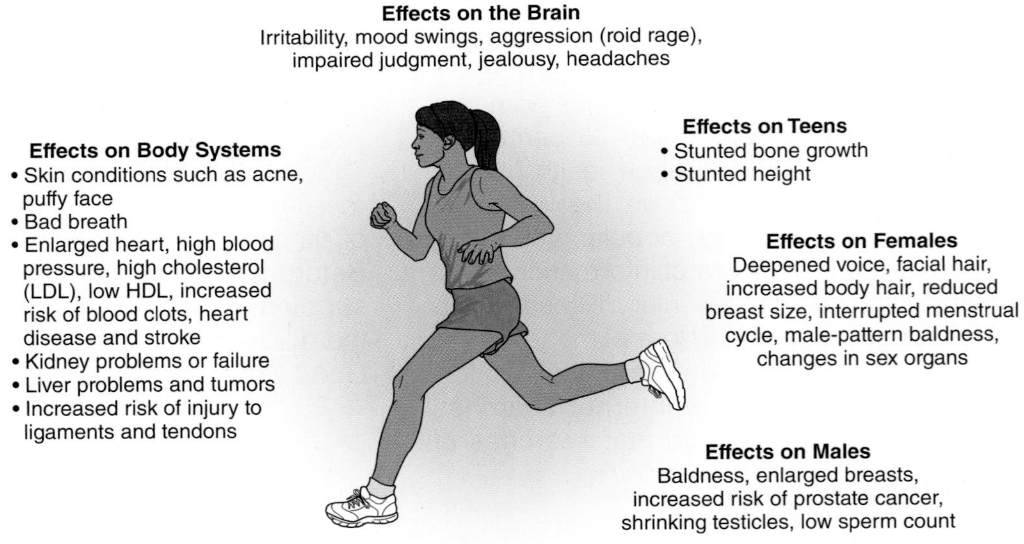
Effects on the Brain
Irritability, mood swings, aggression (roid rage), impaired judgment, jealousy, headaches
Effects on Body Systems
• Skin conditions such as acne, puffy face
• Bad breath
• Enlarged heart, high blood pressure, high cholesterol (LDL), low HDL, increased risk of blood clots, heart disease and stroke
• Kidney problems or failure
• Liver problems and tumors
• Increased risk of injury to ligaments and tendons
Effects on Teens
• Stunted bone growth
• Stunted height
Effects on Females
Deepened voice, facial hair, increased body hair, reduced breast size, interrupted menstrual cycle, male-pattern baldness, changes in sex organs
Effects on Males
Baldness, enlarged breasts, increased risk of prostate cancer, shrinking testicles, low sperm count

Figure 11.6 Potential dangers of using androgens.

muscle size and strength. Anabolic steroids are not only illegal when used without a doctor's prescription but also dangerous. Some of their harmful effects are illustrated in figure 11.6.

Teenagers are at high risk for harm from androgenic agents because their bodies are still growing. As shown in figure 11.6, anabolic steroids can damage the growth centers of bones, preventing a person from growing to their full height. Many side effects—including hair loss, acne, deepening voice, and dark facial hair growth in females—do not go away when use of the drug is discontinued. For athletes, another major problem is the increased risk of injury to tendons and ligaments, which become less elastic with steroid use. Because of these dangers, a variety of anabolic steroids are on the list of substances banned by the U.S. and World Anti-Doping Agencies and are prohibited by the United States Olympic Committee (USOC) and most other athletic associations.

Prohormones (Androgen Precursor)

A precursor is a substance from which another substance is formed; thus an androgen precursor (**prohormone**) is a nonsteroid substance that leads to the formation of a steroid. **Androstenedione**, often referred to as *andro*, is considered to be an androgen precursor because it is converted into anabolic steroids such as testosterone (male hormone) after it enters the body. In some countries, it is viewed as a food supplement. It was formerly considered to be a food supplement in the United States as well, but because manufacturers failed to meet marketing requirements, androstenedione and other prohormones, such as DHEA and androstenediol, are now classified as drugs and require a prescription. They are also banned by national and international anti-doping agencies.

Human Growth Hormone (HGH)

Human growth hormone (HGH) is a naturally occurring hormone important for the growth and development of bones and cartilage in children and teens, as well as protein production throughout life. HGH is available as a prescription drug and is used to treat several medical conditions. Taken improperly, it is exceptionally dangerous, especially for teens, because it can cause the bones to stop growing properly; the effects can be deforming and even life threatening. Like androgens and prohormones, HGH is banned by anti-doping agencies.

FIT FACT

Rhabdomyolysis is a condition in which muscle fibers break down and release proteins such as myoglobin into the bloodstream, which can be toxic to the kidneys. Symptoms include muscle weakness and aching, fatigue, joint pain, and, in severe cases, seizure. Causes of this condition include exercising in the heat, lack of water replacement, and severe exertion. In several reported instances, high school and college athletes have been hospitalized for rhabdomyolysis due to excessive calisthenics and training drills. Some athletes push beyond healthy limits after taking supplements that they think will give them the ability to do extreme training, which can result in this condition.

LESSON REVIEW

1. What are the steps for preparing a muscle fitness exercise plan, and how can you use them to create your own personal plan?

2. What are some of the supplements often considered by people interested in muscle fitness, and what are some guidelines for using the Internet to find health information?

3. What are some of the facts about supplements that you should consider before using them?

4. What are some ergogenic aids (PEDs), and what are some of the benefits and risks associated with their use?

TAKING CHARGE: **Finding Social Support**

Social support involves your family members, friends, teachers, and community members joining or encouraging your physical activities. You're more likely to begin or continue an activity if the people you associate with support you or join in.

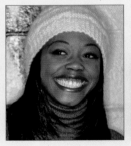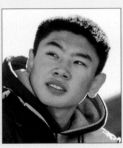

Shannon's family has always enjoyed bike riding. Every evening, the family would ride through the neighborhood. As a toddler, she would ride in the child's seat behind her mother. By the time she was in school, Shannon had her own two-wheeler. Now a teenager, Shannon still loves to ride, but school activities sometimes prevent her from riding with her family. She wants to continue riding but doesn't want to do it alone.

Jim's family has never been very active. Most of his friends tend to watch television, play video games, or just hang out. Sometimes, Jim watches while a group of his classmates plays a quick game of volleyball after school. They often invite him to join the game, but Jim has hesitated because he is not friends with any of the players. He has enjoyed the activities he has tried in the past but has never continued them for very long.

Both Shannon and Jim need social support. Shannon needs it to continue an activity she already enjoys. Jim needs it to begin an activity and then reinforce his participation.

FOR DISCUSSION

Who might Shannon ask to go riding with her? What could Jim do to become involved in physical activity? What groups might Shannon and Jim identify with to get social support? What other suggestions can you offer for finding social support? Consider the guidelines in the following Self-Management feature as you answer these discussion questions.

SELF-MANAGEMENT: **Skills for Finding Social Support**

Experts indicate that people who experience support from others are more likely to participate in regular physical activity, especially over the course of a lifetime. Social support is also helpful to people in losing weight, building muscle fitness, and improving their eating habits. Consider the following guidelines to help you gain others' support for your physical activity.

- *Do a self-assessment of your current level of social support.* Ask your teacher about the social support worksheet that can help you do this assessment. Use the assessment to determine areas in which you can improve your social support.

- *Birds of a feather flock together.* Find friends who are interested in the activities that interest you, or you can encourage your current friends to support you or join you in your participation.

- *Join a club or team.* If no club or team exists for your chosen activity, talk to a teacher, family member, or community recreation leader about starting one.

- *Discuss your interests with family and teachers.* Ask them to help you learn the activity and cheer you on.

- *If possible, get lessons.* In addition to formal lessons, you can also ask teachers and others to support you by helping you learn to perform an activity properly.

- *Family matters.* Encourage your family members to try the activity.

- *Get proper equipment.* Ask for equipment for your birthday or other special occasion.

Taking Action: **Performing Your Muscle Fitness Exercise Plan**

Prepare a muscle fitness exercise plan using the five steps described in the second lesson of this chapter. Like Molly, consider activities from a variety of types of PRE. The goal is to perform the exercises two or three days per week (depending on your fitness level). Carry out your written plan over a two-week period. Your teacher may give you time in class to do some of the activities included in your plan. Consider the following suggestions for **taking action**.

- Before your PRE, perform a dynamic warm-up.
- Follow the tips for safe PRE.
- Progress gradually—don't try to do too much too soon.
- After your workout, perform a cool-down.

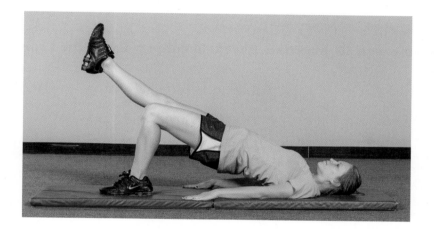

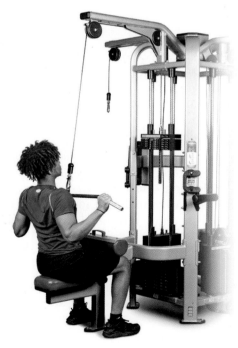

Take action by performing your muscle fitness plan.

CHAPTER REVIEW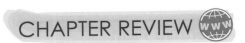

Reviewing Concepts and Vocabulary

Answer items 1 through 5 by correctly completing each sentence with a word or phrase.

1. The muscles that support your spine and keep your rib cage and spine stable are referred to as your _____ muscles.

2. About _____ percent of adults experience back pain at some point.

3. The bones act as _____ that help you apply force when lifting, carrying, and moving objects.

4. _____ is the real name of the supplement sometimes called *andro*.

5. The full name for the substance called HGH is _____.

For items 6 through 10, match each term in column 1 with the appropriate phrase in column 2.

6. rhabdomyolysis   a. too much lower-back curve

7. ergolytic   b. rounded shoulders

8. lordosis   c. condition caused by breakdown of muscle fiber

9. kyphosis   d. substance that is detrimental to performance

10. ptosis   e. protruding abdomen

For items 11 through 15, respond to each statement or question.

11. Define ergogenic aids and PEDs and describe some of them.

12. What are some of the best exercises for building your core muscles?

13. Describe three guidelines for properly lifting, carrying, and moving objects.

14. What self-assessments can you do to determine whether you are at risk for back pain?

15. What are some good strategies for finding social support?

Thinking Critically

Write a paragraph to answer the following question.

A friend of yours is excited about an advertisement in a muscle magazine. The ad describes a pill that is "guaranteed to add size to your muscles in two weeks without exercise." What advice would you give your friend?

Project

Assume that you've been hired as a reporter for your local newspaper. Write an article about preventing back pain or injury. Interview relevant people, such as a physical therapist, a physical education teacher, an athletic trainer, or a person who has experienced back pain or injury. Present your article in class or submit it to a newspaper for publication.

EXERCISE CHART 1: Core Muscle Fitness Exercises

Curl-Up

The curl-up is considered to be among the best abdominal exercises because it isn't risky like some abdominal exercises. The curl-up is sometimes referred to as the *crunch*, and it's a good substitute for the straight-leg sit-up and hands-behind-the-head sit-up.

1. Lie on your back with your knees bent at 90 degrees and your arms extended.
2. Curl up by rolling your head, shoulders, and upper back off the floor. Roll up only until your shoulder blades leave the floor.

    Caution: Do not hold your feet while doing a curl-up. Do not clench your hands behind the head or neck. Do not perform a full sit-up.

3. Slowly roll back to the starting position.

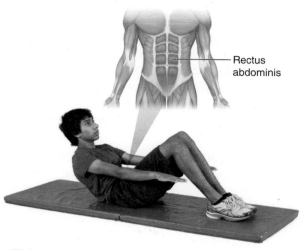

Rectus abdominis

This exercise uses your abdominal muscles.

VARIATIONS

- *Arms across chest or hands by face (more difficult):* Fold your hands across your chest rather than keeping them straight, or place your hands on your face by your cheeks (not behind your head or neck).
- *Twist curl (builds oblique muscles):* Fold your arms across your chest, turn your trunk to the left, and touch your right elbow to your left hip. Repeat to the opposite side.

Trunk Lift (bench)

1. Lie facedown on a padded bench (or a bleacher with a towel on it) that is 16 to 18 inches (41 to 46 centimeters) high. Your upper body (from your waist up) should extend off the bench.
2. Have your partner hold your calves just below the knees.
3. Place one hand over the other on your forehead with your palms facing away and your elbows held to the side at the level of your ears.
4. Start with your upper body lowered. Lift slowly until your upper body is even with the bench (in line with your legs).

    Caution: Do not lift the trunk higher than horizontal.

5. Lower to the beginning position.

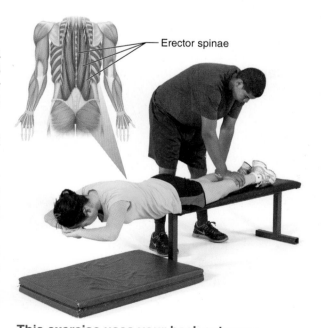

Erector spinae

This exercise uses your back extensor muscles.

Safety tip: As you do these exercises, lift slowly and move only as far as specified in the directions. This exercise is appropriate when performed properly, but, as noted earlier, using the trunk muscles for lifting or carrying is not recommended.

Trunk Lift (floor)

1. Lie facedown with your hands clasped behind your neck.
2. Pull your shoulder blades together, raise your elbows off the floor, and then lift your head and chest off the floor. Arch your upper back until your breastbone (sternum) clears the floor. You may need to hook your feet under a bar or have someone hold your feet down.

   Caution: Do not lift your chin more than 12 inches (30 centimeters) off the floor. This exercise is appropriate when performed properly but, as noted earlier, using the trunk muscles for lifting or carrying is not recommended.
3. Lower your trunk and repeat the exercise.

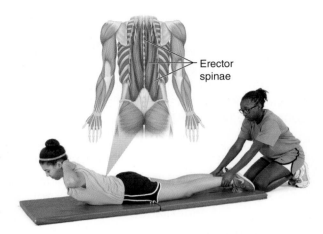

This exercise develops the muscles of your upper back and helps prevent "humpback."

Arm-and-Leg Lift

1. Lie facedown with your arms stretched in front of you.
2. Raise your right arm, then lower it. Raise your left arm, then lower it. Finally, raise both arms, then lower them.
3. Raise you right leg, then lower it. Raise your left leg, then lower it.
4. Raise your right arm and right leg, then lower them. Raise your left arm and left leg, then lower them.
5. Raise your left arm and right leg, then lower them. Raise your right arm and left leg, then lower them.

Caution: Do not arch your back during this exercise.

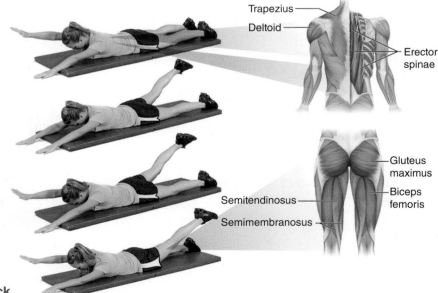

This exercise helps prevent rounded shoulders, sunken chest, and rounded upper back.

Bridging

1. Lie on your back with your knees bent and your feet close to your buttocks.
2. Contract your gluteal muscles. Lift your buttocks and raise your back off the floor until your hip joint has no bend.

   Caution: Do not overarch your lower back.
3. Lower your hips to the floor and repeat the exercise.

This exercise develops the muscles of your buttocks (gluteal) and the muscles on the back of your thighs (hamstrings).

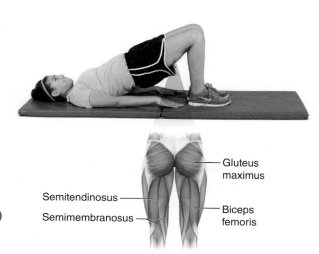

Side Plank

1. From a right-facing, side-lying position on a mat or carpet, lift your body into a side support position, supporting your body weight on your right forearm and your feet. Your left arm is bent and on your left hip. Tighten your abdominal and back muscles.
2. Keep your hips in line with your body. Hold this position for 7 to 10 seconds.
3. Repeat facing to the left.

This exercise develops the abdominals and back muscles.

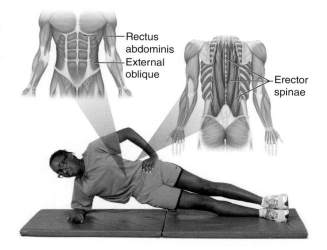

Reverse Curl

1. Lie on your back. Bend your knees, placing your feet flat on the floor. Place your arms at your sides.
2. Lift your knees to your chest, raising your hips off the floor.
3. Return to the starting position. Repeat the exercise up to 10 times.

This exercise develops your abdominal muscles.

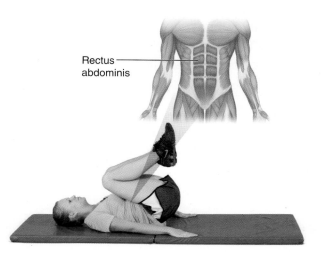

Front Plank

1. Lying facedown on a mat or carpet, support your body with your forearms and toes.

2. Keep your head in line with your body. Hold this position for 7 to 10 seconds.

VARIATIONS

- *Less difficult:* Support your body with your knees rather than your feet.
- *More difficult:* Perform the same exercise in the full push-up position.

This exercise develops the abdominals, buttocks, and back muscles.

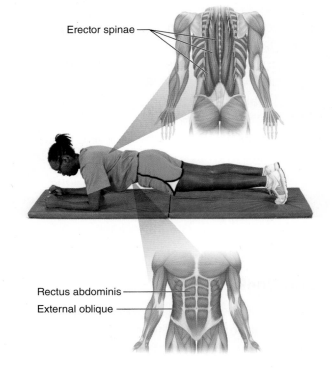

Erector spinae

Rectus abdominis

External oblique

Double-Leg Lift (bench or table)

1. Lie face down on a table (or bench) with your legs extending off the end. With a partner holding your upper body, lower your legs to the ground. If you have no partner, grasp under the edge of the table.

2. Lift your legs slowly until they are even with the top of the table.

   Caution: Do not lift any higher than the table. If necessary, lift one leg at a time until you are able to lift both legs at once.

3. Lower to the starting position.

This exercise strengthens your gluteus and lower back muscles.

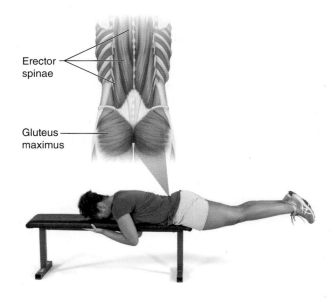

Erector spinae

Gluteus maximus

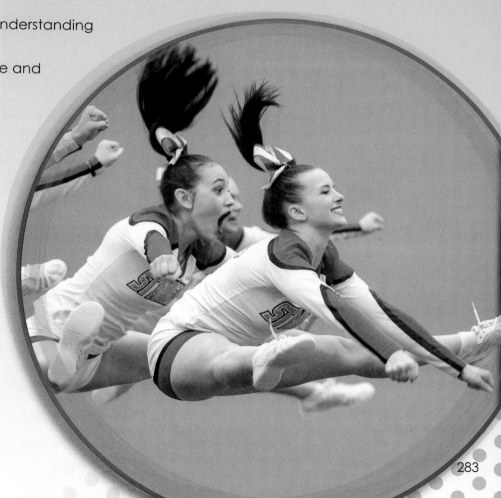

Flexibility

Lesson Objectives

After reading this lesson, you should be able to

1. define flexibility terms and explain why flexibility is important;
2. describe some of the factors that influence flexibility;
3. explain the benefits of good flexibility; and
4. describe types of flexibility exercise, the FIT formula for each, and several of the specific exercises for building flexibility.

Lesson Vocabulary

active stretch
antagonist
ballistic stretching
CRAC
dynamic movement exercise
dynamic stretching
hypermobility
muscle–tendon unit (MTU)
passive stretch
PNF stretching
range of motion (ROM)
range-of-motion (ROM) exercise
static stretch

Do you have good flexibility? Do you do any regular stretching to improve your flexibility? In this lesson, you'll learn about the importance of being flexible and how to improve your flexibility by applying fitness principles. You'll also learn to evaluate your flexibility.

What Is Flexibility?

Flexibility is the ability to move your joints through a full **range of motion (ROM)**, or the full amount of movement you can make in a joint (figure 12.1). A joint is a place in your body where bones come together, such as the knees, ankles, elbows, wrists, and the joints between the vertebrae in the spine. Some joints, such as your knees and elbows, work like a hinge, permitting movement in only two directions. Other joints, such as your hips and shoulders, work like a ball and socket, allowing movement in all directions.

Your bones are connected at your joints by inelastic bands called ligaments. In figure 12.1,

> I watched the dancers and said, "How do they do that? I have a hard time touching my toes." I decided I needed to work on my flexibility.
>
> *Caleb Young*

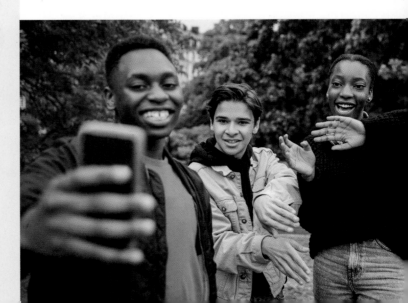

the ligament that connects the bones of the upper and lower leg is illustrated. Ligaments should not be stretched. Your bones are connected to your muscles by tendons. In figure 12.1, a tendon connecting a lower leg bone with the hamstring muscle is shown. When your muscles contract, they pull on your tendons, causing your bones to move. Muscles often work as **antagonists**—meaning they perform opposite functions—to allow multiple movements and full range of motion. For example, if you're lying down and contract the quadriceps muscles on the front of your thigh, they lift your leg off the floor. At the same time, the muscles on the back of your thigh, the antagonists, relax to allow the quadriceps to lift your leg.

Together, muscles and tendons are called a **muscle–tendon unit (MTU)** (figure 12.1). Unlike ligaments, muscles and tendons need to be stretched in order to maintain a healthy length. Both parts of the MTU are stretched when performing flexibility exercises, but we frequently refer only to "stretching the muscle" for simplicity. If your muscles and tendons are too short, they restrict a joint's ROM.

Sometimes people confuse a warm-up with a flexibility workout, but they are two different things. A warm-up is done to get ready for a specific workout, whereas a flexibility workout is exercise done to build flexibility. Stretching exercises are now used less frequently in warm-ups than in the past, especially when preparing for workouts involving strength, speed, and power. But this does not mean that flexibility exercises, including stretching, are not important. Flexibility is a key component of health-related physical fitness.

Benefits of Good Flexibility

Flexibility is sometimes considered the forgotten part of health-related fitness because many people focus exclusively on the other parts. However, good flexibility provides many health and wellness benefits, especially when you grow older.

Improved Function

Everyone needs at least some flexibility in order to maintain health and mobility. The exact amount of flexibility needed for normal daily function depends on the demands of the activities that you perform. For example, plumbers, painters, dentists, and window washers (see figure 12.2a) often need to bend and stretch, and some musicians need very flexible fingers and wrists. As people grow older, their flexibility tends to decrease, which can limit simple movements such as looking over the shoulder while driving. Therefore, it's especially important for older people to do exercises that build and maintain a full range of motion.

Flexibility is also important to many athletes (see figure 12.2b). Dancers and gymnasts must be very flexible to perform their routines. Swimmers need good flexibility to get maximum performance, as do kickers in football. Good flexibility also allows a longer backswing—and therefore a faster forward swing—in the throwing and striking movements that are crucial in golf, tennis, and baseball pitching. Although

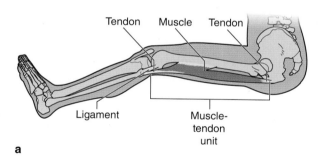

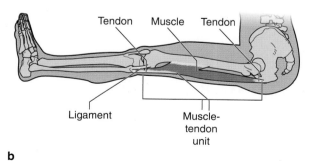

Figure 12.1 Range of motion in the knee joint: (a) Poor—the knee does not fully extend because of short hamstring muscles; (b) good—the knee fully extends because of long hamstring muscles.

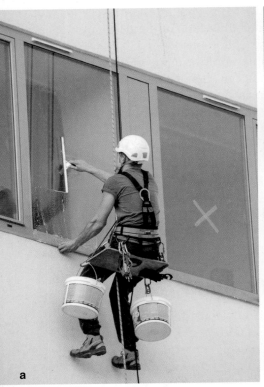

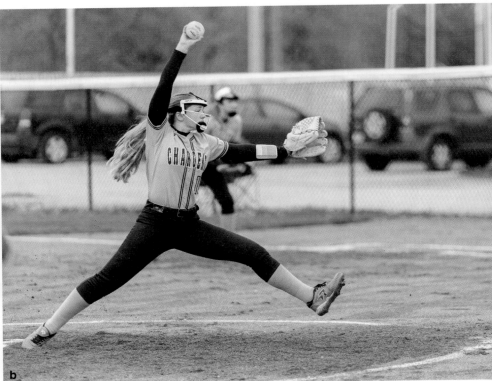

Figure 12.2   Good flexibility is needed *(a)* for some jobs and *(b)* by most athletes.

some research has questioned the value of stretching right before a competition or performance, muscles of adequate length can be beneficial even in such activities as weightlifting and the shot put.

Improved Health and Wellness

Good flexibility is important for your back health and posture. For example, back pain and poor posture are associated with short hamstring and hip flexor muscles. More generally, very short muscles are at risk of being overstretched and injured. Stretching exercises also have a beneficial effect on a number of conditions and can help you manage stress. Flexible musicians are less likely to have pain in their joints. Stretching exercises can often alleviate menstrual cramps in females and prevent or provide relief from leg cramps and shin splints. Stretching a muscle can also help it relax.

Rehabilitation From Injury and Medical Problems

Flexibility exercises are used for rehabilitation from a variety of injuries and medical problems. Both physical therapists (PTs) and athletic trainers (ATs) use a variety of techniques, including stretching and muscle fitness exercises, in their work. PTs treat patients after surgery and patients with medical conditions such as arthritis, back pain, stroke, and osteoporosis. ATs help athletes train to prevent injury and help them recover when injury does occur.

I want to get old gracefully. I want to have good posture, I want to be healthy and be an example to my children.

Sting, musician

Factors Influencing Flexibility

You already know that short muscles and tendons reduce flexibility and that they can be stretched to improve flexibility. Your flexibility is also influenced by the following factors.

Heredity

Inherited anatomical differences in our bodies help determine what we can and cannot do. Some people inherit joints that do not favor a large a range of motion. These people will have to exercise regularly in order to develop a healthy range of motion. Some people have an unusually large range of motion in certain joints, a condition sometimes referred to as being *double jointed*. However, experts note that there is no such thing; **hypermobility** is the correct term to use. People with hypermobility score better on flexibility tests and can extend the knee, elbow, thumb, or wrist joint past the typical ROM. Some people who have hypermobile joints are prone to joint injury and may be more likely to develop arthritis, a disease in which the joints become inflamed. For the most part, however, those with hypermobile joints do not have problems, other than a slight disadvantage in some sports. For example, when doing push-ups, the elbows of a hypermobile person might lock when the arms straighten, making it difficult to unlock the elbows to begin the downward movement.

Body Type

Can short people touch their toes more easily than tall people? In most cases, no, because a shorter person tends to have not only shorter legs and trunk but also shorter arms (though there are exceptions). In contrast, a taller person tends to have longer arms, in addition to longer legs and trunk. However, some people do have exceptionally long arms or legs, and these characteristics may affect their score on flexibility tests.

Sex and Age

Generally, females tend to be more flexible than males. About twice as many females as males are hypermobile, and at most ages more females than males meet minimum fitness standards for flexibility. Younger people also tend to be more flexible than older people. As people age, their muscles typically shorten from lack of use, and their joints tend to stiffen due to conditions such as arthritis. With this in mind, it is important to do regular flexibility exercises when you're young to reduce your risk of joint problems when you're older. Good flexibility also enhances performance in a variety of tasks for people of all ages.

Different Types of Flexibility Exercises

The following discussion presents methods of building and maintaining flexibility. For best results, perform exercises especially designed to improve your flexibility (see step 5 of the Physical Activity Pyramid in figure 12.3). The four major types of exercise for building flexibility are range-of-motion exercise, static stretching, ballistic stretching, and dynamic stretching.

FIT FACT
Physical therapists (PTs) are health care professionals who help patients manage pain and improve their mobility. They also help people perform regular exercises to prevent muscle-related problems and to maintain or regain their ability to function normally. PTs have many years of advanced education and, in the United States, must be licensed in the state in which they practice. They work in many settings, including private practices, hospitals, nursing homes, outpatient clinics, schools, and sport and fitness facilities. More than 100,000 PTs belong to the American Physical Therapy Association, a professional group whose goal is to help people improve their health and quality of life.

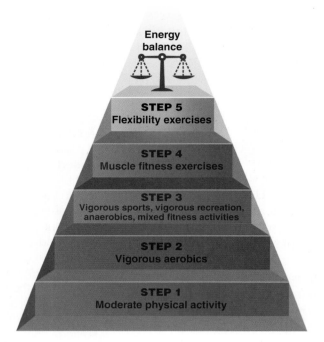

Figure 12.3 Exercises for building flexibility are represented by step 5 of the Physical Activity Pyramid.

Range-of-Motion (ROM) Exercise

Technically, all flexibility exercises are range-of-motion exercises because they are all designed to help allow a healthy ROM in the joints. More specifically, the term **range-of-motion (ROM) exercise** refers to exercise that requires a joint to move through a full ROM, powered either by the body's own muscles or by assistance from a partner or therapist. Such exercises are commonly used in physical therapy for people to regain or retain ROM associated with an injury or medical problem. The exercise movement is typically continuous and performed at a slow to moderate pace.

Each joint has its own normal or healthy ROM. The shoulder and the hip (ball and socket joints) have greater ROM than the elbow and knee (hinge joints). Because of these differences, exercises should be designed specifically for each joint, such as shoulder rotation exercises for people with shoulder injuries (for example, baseball pitchers) and knee flexion and finger extension for people with arthritis. The weight of the body part and the momentum of the movement do cause some stretch in the muscles and connective tissues, but these exercises are typically not as intense as those described in the next section; therefore, ROM exercises are not as good as stretching exercises for improving flexibility.

Static Stretching

A **static stretch** involves slowly stretching as far as you can, until you feel a sense of pulling or tension (not pain). A static stretch requires an assist from an external source, such as gravity, a partner, or some other source. For best results, static stretches are held for 10 to 30 seconds. The FIT formula for static stretching is described in table 12.1. Done correctly, static stretching increases your flexibility and can help you relax. Some experts think that static stretching exercises are safer than ballistic stretching exercises because you're less likely to stretch too far and injure yourself.

Static stretching can be performed using either **active stretch** or **passive stretch**. Active static stretch uses your own antagonist muscles—for

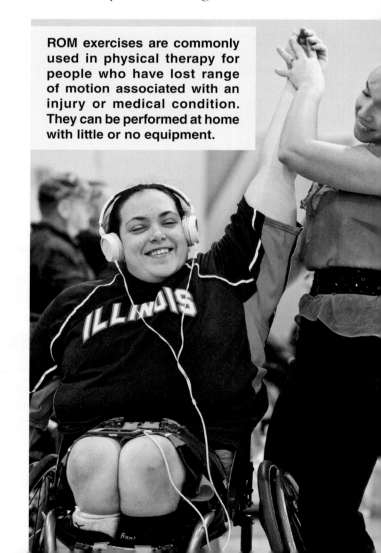

ROM exercises are commonly used in physical therapy for people who have lost range of motion associated with an injury or medical condition. They can be performed at home with little or no equipment.

TABLE 12.1   **FIT Formula and Fitness Target Zones for Stretching Exercise**

	Static and PNF*	Ballistic
Frequency	**Threshold of training:** Stretch each muscle group 2–3 days each week. **Target zone:** Stretch each muscle group 2–7 days each week.	**Threshold of training:** Stretch each muscle group 2–3 days each week. **Target zone:** Stretch each muscle group 2–7 days each week.
Intensity	**Threshold of training:** Stretch the muscle beyond its normal length until you feel tension, then hold. **Target zone:** Stretch the muscle beyond its normal length, from first point of tension to point of mild discomfort (not pain), then hold.	**Threshold of training:** Stretch the muscle beyond its normal length until you feel tension. Use slow, gentle bounces or bobs. Use the motion of your body part to stretch the specific muscle. **Target zone:** Stretch the muscle beyond its normal length, from first point of tension to point of mild discomfort (not pain). Use the same gentle bouncing stretch as for threshold. *Caution:* No stretch should cause pain, especially sharp pain. Be especially careful when doing ballistic stretching.
Time	**Threshold of training:** Do 2 stretches of 10–30 sec for each muscle group. **Target zone:** Do 2–4 stretches with a goal of 60 sec (total) of stretching for each muscle group (6 × 10, 4 × 15, or 2 × 30 sec). Rest for 15 sec between stretches.	**Threshold of training:** For each muscle group, perform 2 sets. Bounce against the muscle slowly and gently. Perform 15 reps. Rest for 10 sec between sets. **Target zone:** For each muscle group, perform 2–4 sets of 15 reps. Rest for 10 sec between sets. Start with 2 sets and progress to 4.

*Before stretch, contract antagonist muscle at 20%–75% of maximal contraction for 3–6 sec.

example, contracting your shin muscle to move your toes upward, thus causing a stretch in your calf muscles (figure 12.4*a*). Passive static stretch is achieved without use of an antagonist muscle—for example, by having a partner push gently on your foot or by using your own arms to pull your foot upward to stretch your calf (figure 12.4*b*).

Some experts consider active static stretch to be safer than other types of stretch because you don't have to worry about the external force overstretching your muscle (for example, if a partner pushes too hard). The advantage of passive static stretch is that makes it easier to create adequate stretch in order to improve the length of the muscle.

The FIT formula for static stretch is described in table 12.1. The table also includes FIT formulas for PNF and ballistic stretch, which are described in later sections of this lesson.

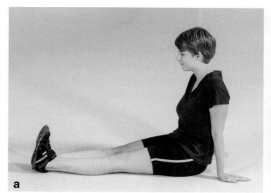
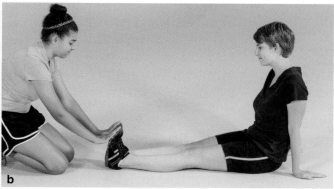

Figure 12.4   Stretching the calf: *(a)* active stretch; *(b)* passive stretch (with a partner assisting).

PNF Stretching

PNF stretching (or proprioceptive neuromuscular facilitation) is a stretching technique originally used by physical and occupational therapists to help injured soldiers. It is now widely used by those interested in improving their flexibility, including athletes. PNF stretching is a variation of static stretching that involves contracting the muscle to help it relax so that it can then be more easily stretched. One popular form of PNF is called **CRAC** (contract-relax-antagonist-contract). After you contract a muscle that you want to stretch, the muscle automatically relaxes. Contracting the opposing (antagonist) muscles during the stretch also relaxes the muscle you're stretching. A passive assist adds to the stretch. Because CRAC helps relax the muscle to be stretched, it is considered to be more effective than other forms of stretching. The FIT formula for PNF is shown in table 12.1.

Most static stretching exercises can be converted to CRAC PNF exercises by pre-stretching the muscle and adding an active stretch to the regular passive stretch. Figure 12.5 illustrates the three steps in the calf stretcher exercise. First, contract the calf muscles to help them relax by pushing your toes against resistance. In this case, the resistance is the pressure from the hands of a partner (figure 12.5*a*). After the contraction, pull your toes and foot forward to flex the ankle and actively stretch the calf muscles (figure 12.5*b*). Finally, passively stretch the calf muscle by having a partner push against your toes and foot (figure 12.5*c*). If a partner is not available, you can loop a rope or towel behind the ball of your foot and push against it to contract the calf muscles. You then actively stretch the calf muscles and pull on the rope to statically stretch them.

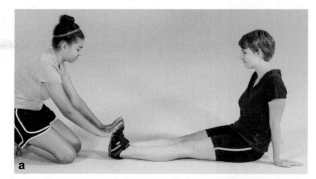
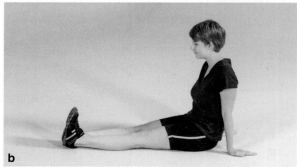
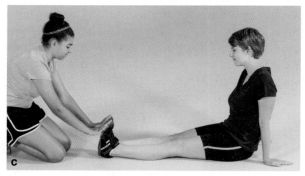

Figure 12.5   PNF stretch: *(a)* contract the calf muscles (push toes and foot against partner resistance); *(b)* active stretch (contract shin muscles to pull toes toward knees), *(c)* passive stretch (partner pushes to stretch calf muscle).

Ballistic Stretching

Ballistic stretching involves a series of gentle bouncing or bobbing motions that are not held for a long time. The FIT formula for ballistic stretching is described in table 12.1. Like static and PNF stretching, ballistic stretching exercises are designed

TECH TRENDS: **Goniometers**

When you perform flexibility self-assessments, you use low-tech aids such as a yardstick or ruler. In some cases, you may use a flexibility box that includes a built-in measuring stick. When experts do research on flexibility, they use more sophisticated instruments, such as a goniometer, which measures joint angles. Your school may have an inexpensive goniometer, such as the one shown, that you can use to assess the range of motion in your joints.

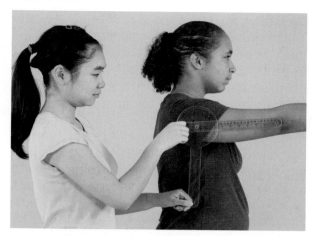

A goniometer can be used to assess range of motion and flexibility.

USING TECHNOLOGY

Do some investigation to learn more about goniometers and other devices for measuring flexibility.

to use the joints through a full range of movement and cause the muscles and tendons to stretch beyond their normal length. Most of the static stretching exercises shown in this chapter can be made into ballistic stretching exercises. For example, the hamstring stretch can be made into an active ballistic stretch by using the thigh muscles to bob the upper leg forward. It can be made into a passive ballistic stretch by having a partner alternately push forward and pull backward to produce a bobbing movement of the upper leg.

Sport movement stretching (also referred to as *sport-specific ballistic stretching*) uses sport-specific movements that cause the muscles to be used beyond their normal ROM—for example, baseball hitters who swing a weighted bat and golfers who take several practice swings with the club. Consult with your instructor or coach to find out about recommended exercises for a given sport.

Some teachers and coaches have concerns about ballistic stretching because of the possibility for overstretching and injury. However, studies show that, if performed properly, ballistic stretching can be safe and does not cause as much muscular soreness as static stretching. Therapists do caution against ballistic stretching

after a muscle or tendon injury, and they recommend consulting an expert to determine the best method of stretch for rehabilitation.

Flexibility Exercises

Experts recommend doing exercises to build flexibility for all of your major muscle groups. Stretching exercises are included in Exercise Chart 1 at the end of this chapter. Use the descriptions and illustrations to perform the exercises properly. Muscle illustrations are also provided to show which muscles and tendons are stretched by each exercise. The exercises can be done using static stretch or PNF.

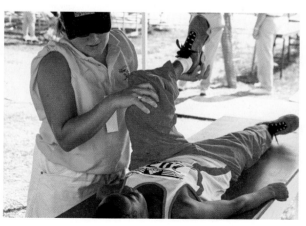

SCIENCE IN ACTION: **Dynamic Movement Exercise**

Dynamic movement exercises include jumping, skipping, and calisthenics such as those used in a warm-up. They move the joints beyond normal resting ROM and cause the muscles and tendons to stretch. The stretch caused by dynamic movement exercise is followed by a contraction of the stretched muscle. For example, jumping stretches the calf muscle; after the stretch caused by landing, the muscle contracts again to provide the force for the next jump. This type of exercise is also referred to as *dynamic calisthenics*. Dynamic movement exercises should not be confused with dynamic stretching exercises (see the Fit Fact on dynamic stretching).

Experts who pioneered the use of dynamic movement exercises point out that they are not the same as ballistic stretching exercises because they do not involve bobbing or bouncing against the muscle. Dynamic movement exercise routines use many kinds of movement, including muscle fitness calisthenics (such as push-ups, curl-ups, and half squats) and some other types of muscle fitness exercise (such as elastic band exercise).

Whereas dynamic *stretching* exercises are done primarily to build flexibility, that is not the primary intent of dynamic *movement* exercises (calisthenics). For this reason, a specific FIT formula is not provided for this type of exercise. However, it is often included in

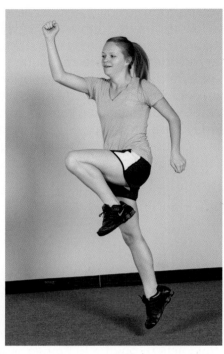

Dynamic movement exercises are often used in exercise circuits or as a warm-up.

a warm-up and as part of other exercise circuits, and it does provide flexibility benefits and improve muscle fitness and power. Typically, when dynamic movement exercises are included in a warm-up, exercises are chosen for different muscle groups, and the total time for the exercise is 5 to 10 minutes.

STUDENT ACTIVITY

Prepare a brochure explaining dynamic movement exercise and the reasons for doing it.

LESSON REVIEW

1. What are some flexibility terms, and why is flexibility important?
2. What are some of the factors that influence flexibility?
3. What are the benefits of good flexibility?
4. What are some types of flexibility exercise, the FIT formula for each, and several of the specific exercises for building flexibility?

SELF-ASSESSMENT: **Arm, Leg, and Trunk Flexibility**

In this self-assessment, you'll evaluate the flexibility in several areas of your body. Use these general directions for the tests that follow, then score yourself using table 12.2.

- After a warm-up, perform each exercise as described and illustrated here.
- Stretch and hold the position for two seconds while a partner checks your performance.
- Score one point for each test for which you meet the standard. Total your score for all tests.
- Determine your rating using table 12.2. Record your results as directed by your instructor.

You are expected to do these tests in class only once, unless your instructor tells you otherwise. However, you may want to retest yourself periodically. A retest helps you to see progress and can also be used to help set new goals. If you're working with a partner, remember that self-assessment information is confidential and shouldn't be shared without the permission of the person being tested.

Safety tip: Before taking a flexibility test, do a general warm-up and try each movement two or three times.

TABLE 12.2   Rating Chart: Flexibility

Fitness rating	Score (items passed)
Good fitness	8–11
Marginal fitness	5–7
Low fitness	0–4

ARM LIFT

1. Lie facedown. Hold a ruler or stick in both hands. Keep your fists tight and your palms facing down.
2. Raise your arms and the stick as high as possible. Keep your forehead on the floor and your arms and wrists straight.
3. Hold this position while your partner uses a ruler to check the distance of the stick from the floor.
4. Record one point if you meet the standard of 10 inches (25 centimeters) or more.

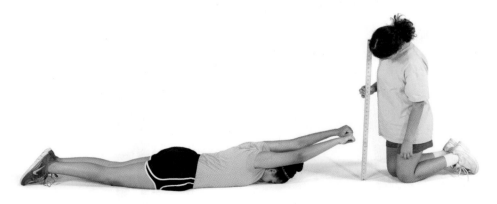

This test evaluates your chest and shoulder flexibility.

ZIPPER

1. Reach your left arm and hand over your left shoulder and down your spine, as if you were going to pull up a zipper.
2. Hold this position while you reach your right arm and hand behind your back and up your spine to try to touch or overlap the fingers of your left hand.
3. Hold the position while your partner checks it.
4. Repeat, this time reaching your right arm and hand over your right shoulder and your left arm and hand up your spine.
5. Record one point for each side on which you meet the standard of touching or overlapping fingers.

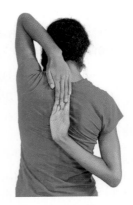

This test evaluates your shoulder, arm, and chest flexibility.

TRUNK ROTATION

1. Stand with your toes on a designated line. Your left shoulder should be an arm's length (with fist closed) from the wall. Place your fist on a target spot on the wall marked directly above the tape line on the floor.
2. Extend your right arm to your side at shoulder height. Make a fist with your palm down.
3. Without moving your feet, rotate your trunk to the right as far as possible. Your knees may bend slightly to permit more turn, but don't move your feet. Try to touch the target spot or beyond with a palm-down right fist.
4. Hold the position while your partner checks it.
5. Repeat, rotating to the left.
6. Record one point for each side on which you meet the standard of touching the *center* of the target.

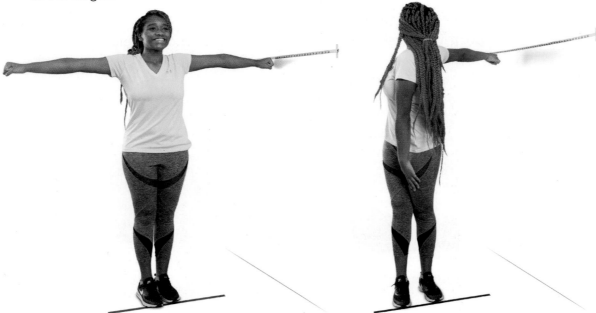

This test evaluates your spine, shoulder, and hip flexibility.

WRAP-AROUND

1. Raise your right arm and reach behind your head. Try touch the left corner of your mouth. You may turn your hea and neck to the left.
2. Hold the position while your partner checks it.
3. Repeat with your left arm.
4. Record one point for each side on which you meet th standard of touching the corner of the mouth.

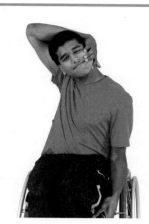

This test evaluates your shoulder and neck flexibility.

THIGH-TO-CHEST

1. Lie on your back and extend your right leg. Place your hands on the back of your left thigh and pull toward you to draw your upper thigh against your lower ribs. Do not place your hands on top of the knee.
2. Keep your right leg straight and on the floor if possible. Keep your lower back flat on the floor.

This test evaluates the flexibility of your hamstrings, lower back, and hip flexors.

3. Hold the position. Have your partner check to see if your upper left thigh is held against the lower ribs while your right leg is straight and on the floor.
4. Repeat with the opposite leg.
5. Record one point for each side on which you meet the standard of holding the thigh against the lower ribs and calf on the floor.

ANKLE FLEX

1. Sit erect on the floor with your legs straight and together. You may lean backward slightly on your hands if necessary.
2. Start with the soles of your shoes at 90 degrees (perpendicular) to the floor.
3. Flex your ankles by pulling your toes toward your shins as far as possible. Hold this position while your partner checks whether the angle that the sole of each foot makes with the floor is 75 degrees. (You can use a protractor to make a 75-degree angle on a sheet of paper.)

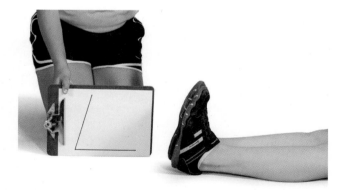

This test evaluates the flexibility of your calf muscles and your range of ankle movement.

4. Record one point for each ankle for which you meet the standard of soles angled 75 degrees or more.

Preparing a Flexibility Exercise Plan

Lesson Objectives

After reading this lesson, you should be able to

1. describe several basic flexibility exercises;
2. describe other forms of activity that build flexibility;
3. describe and explain how to apply basic guidelines for stretching; and
4. select flexibility exercises and prepare a written flexibility exercise plan.

Lesson Vocabulary

neuromotor exercise
tai chi
yoga

Do you know which specific exercises and stretches are best for developing flexibility? Do you know how to safely perform flexibility exercise? In the previous lesson, you learned about several types of flexibility exercise. In this lesson, you'll learn some of the most common exercises used to build flexibility and how to plan a personal flexibility exercise program.

Alternative Methods for Building Flexibility

In addition to the static, PNF, and ballistic stretching exercises described in the previous lesson, other popular activities can also be good for building flexibility. ACSM refers to these types of activities as *functional fitness training* because they help people (especially older people) perform tasks of daily living effectively. If you're considering any of these alternative methods, you should seek qualified instruction and follow the guidelines outlined in this chapter for building flexibility.

> I started doing yoga in my physical education class. Now I do it three days a week on my own. It helps me to relax and makes me feel good.
>
> *Zoe Jensen*

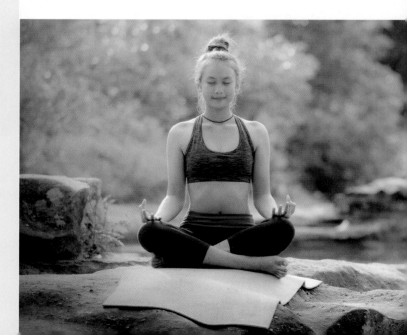

Yoga

Yoga, which blends exercise poses, breathing techniques, and sometimes meditation, was developed centuries ago in India. Yoga poses, called *asanas*, are similar to many flexibility exercises and can contribute to improved flexibility and other health benefits. Yoga is practiced by millions as a method of relaxing and training, and many schools now have yoga clubs. However, yoga should be undertaken with care. Physical therapists and other health experts caution against performing certain yoga poses because they are considered to be risky exercises. In addition, beginners are cautioned to progress gradually; it can be more harmful than helpful to try advanced poses without weeks or even months of practice.

Tai Chi

Tai chi is an ancient martial art that originated in China. Tai chi is now practiced worldwide as a form of exercise rather than a martial art, and its basic movements have been shown to increase flexibility and reduce symptoms of arthritis in some people. When practiced regularly, it can help develop muscle fitness, prevent back pain, and improve posture and balance. It is especially good for helping older people who are at risk of falling, but research has shown benefits for teens and adults of all ages.

Pilates

Pilates was originally developed as a form of therapy but is now practiced as a method of building core muscle fitness and flexibility. When practiced properly, it helps prevent back pain, improves posture, and aids functional capacity in daily life.

Neuromotor Exercise

The ACSM describes **neuromotor exercise** as a method of training that involves balance, coordination, and agility as well as resistance and flexibility exercise. It has been shown to be effective with older adults but may have benefits for younger people as well. This type of training is also called *functional fitness training* because it helps people perform the functions of normal daily living. No specific neuromotor exercise program has been designed specifically for teens. However, yoga and tai chi are considered to be neuromotor exercise and can be used by teens with proper instruction. Sessions of at least 20 minutes in length at least 2 to 3 days per week are recommended.

Appropriate Use of Flexibility Exercise

To ensure that stretching is effective in building flexibility, it is important to do exercises that meet your specific needs and that balance muscle fitness and flexibility.

FIT FACT

Research studies show that tai chi and yoga can provide a variety of benefits, including improved bone health, improved functional fitness, better quality of life, and reduced risk of falls among older people.

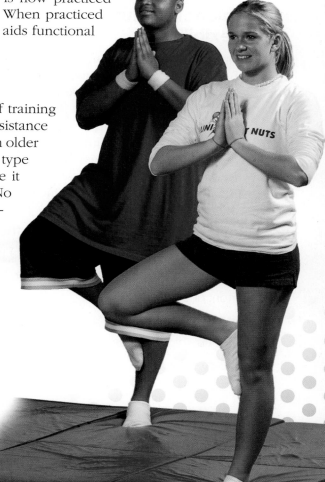

Specificity of Stretching

You have learned about the many exercises for building flexibility—but are there any muscles that do *not* need stretching? For many people, the answer is yes. For example, some people eventually begin to develop a hunched-over posture (often called *humpback*) when the upper back muscles become overstretched. These people should avoid further stretching of the upper back muscles. Experts recommend that abdominal stretching be avoided. If they're stretched, they begin to sag and the abdomen protrudes, leading to poor posture.

Each person must evaluate their own needs to avoid stretching overstretched muscles and avoid strengthening muscles that are already so strong that they are out of balance with their opposing muscles. Keeping muscles on opposites sides of a joint in balance helps them pull with equal force in all directions. This balance helps align your body parts properly, ensuring good posture.

Balancing Muscle Fitness and Flexibility

You should do muscle fitness and flexibility exercises together. We now know that muscle fitness exercises, when properly performed, need not limit flexibility. In fact, when done through a full range of motion, they can even help you build flexibility. But muscle fitness exercises are best for building muscle fitness, and flexibility exercises are best for building flexibility; therefore, a balanced exercise program includes both.

People commonly use the flexors (muscles on the front of the body) a great deal because many daily activities emphasize the use of those muscles. For example, the majority of people have strong biceps (front of the arms), pectorals (front of the chest), and quadriceps (front of the thighs). The pull of these strong muscles results in the body hunching forward. To avoid becoming permanently hunched over, you need to stretch these strong, short muscles on the front of your body and strengthen the weak, relatively unused muscles on the back of your body. Table 12.3 lists the muscles for which most people need the most flexibility exercise.

Flexibility Exercise Guidelines

To benefit the most from your exercise program, perform the exercises correctly and exercise caution to avoid injury. Before you begin stretching, follow these guidelines to help you safely achieve and maintain flexibility.

- *Before stretching, do a general warm-up.* Warm muscles respond better than cold ones. ACSM recommends doing a general warm-up of 5 to 10 minutes before performing stretching exercise.
- *Make flexibility exercises part of your workout.* Don't rely on warm-up exercises to build flexibility. Select an appropriate type of exercise and follow the FIT formula for that type.

TABLE 12.3 **Muscles That Need the Most Stretching**

Muscle(s)	Reason for stretching
Chest	Prevent poor posture
Front of shoulders	Prevent poor posture
Front of hip joints	Prevent swayback posture, backache, pulled muscle
Back of thighs (hamstrings)	Prevent swayback posture, backache, pulled muscle
Inside of thighs	Prevent back, leg, and foot strain
Calf	Avoid soreness and Achilles tendon injury (may result from running and jumping)
Lower back	Prevent soreness, pain, back injury

- *Choose exercises for all major muscle groups.* Ten different exercises for all muscle groups are described in Exercise Chart 1 at the end of this chapter.
- *When beginning (or for general health), use static stretching or PNF.* Consider ballistic stretching after achieving the good fitness zone. Dynamic and developmental stretching may also be beneficial.
- *Progress gradually.* Regardless of the type of flexibility exercise you choose, progress gradually. Some flexibility exercises may seem easy, but, as with muscular endurance exercise, it does not take much to make your muscles sore. Gradually increase the time and number of repetitions and sets.
- *Avoid risky exercises.* Exercises that hyperflex or hyperextend a joint should be avoided, as should exercises that cause joint twisting and compression.
- *Do not stretch joints that are hypermobile, unstable, swollen, or infected.* People with these conditions or symptoms are at risk of injury from over-stretching.
- *Do not stretch to the point of feeling pain.* The old saying "no pain, no gain" is wrong. Stretch only until your muscle feels tight and a little uncomfortable.
- *Avoid stretching muscles that are already overstretched from poor posture.* The abdominal muscles, for example, typically do not need to be stretched.
- *Avoid stretches that last 30 seconds or more before performing strength and power activities.* Research suggests that stretches lasting longer than 30 seconds may have a negative effect on performances involving strength and power. As a result, some experts recommend doing dynamic movement exercises rather than stretching before these activities.

I never struggled with injury problems because of my preparation—in particular my stretching.

Edwin Moses, Olympic gold medalist

FIT FACT
Once you've reached an acceptable level of muscle flexibility, you must continue to move all of your joints and muscles through this new and improved range of motion on a regular basis. If you don't, your muscles will begin to shorten again, and you'll lose that flexibility. All types of exercise described in this lesson help maintain flexibility.

Planning a Flexibility Exercise Program

Elijah is a 16-year-old who used the five steps of program planning to prepare a flexibility exercise program. His program is described here.

Step 1: Determine Your Personal Needs

To get started, Elijah prepared a table summarizing his flexibility activity (or lack thereof) over the past two weeks, as well as his flexibility scores (table 12.4). As you can see, he did no flexibility exercise during that period. Because it was

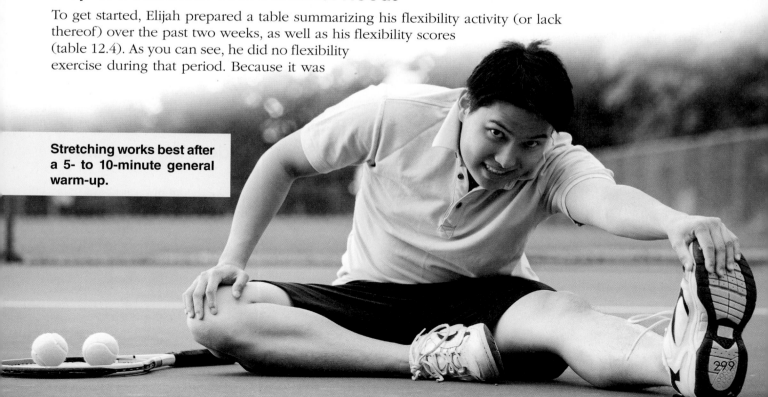

Stretching works best after a 5- to 10-minute general warm-up.

299

TABLE 12.4   **Elijah's Flexibility Fitness and Physical Activity Profiles**

Physical fitness profile		
Fitness self-assessment	**Score**	**Rating**
Arm lift	8 in. (20 cm)	Needs improvement
Zipper		
Right	Fingers touch	Met standard
Left	Fingers do not touch	Needs improvement
Trunk rotation		
Right	Reached target	Met standard
Left	Did not reach target	Needs improvement
Wrap-around		
Right	Touched mouth	Met standard
Left	Touched mouth	Met standard
Knee-to-chest		
Right	Calf lifted >1 in. (2.5 cm)	Needs improvement
Left	Calf lifted >1 in. (2.5 cm)	Needs improvement
Ankle flex		
Right	75 degrees	Met standard
Left	80 degrees	Needs improvement
Total score	6 items passed	Marginal fitness
Back-saver sit-and-reach	5 in. (13 cm)	Low fitness
Physical activity profile		
Day	**Flexibility exercises**	**Amount**
Mon.	None	None
Tues.	None	None
Wed.	None	None
Thurs.	None	None
Fri.	None	None
Sat.	None	None
Sun.	None	None

summer and he was not in school, he also had not done any recent flexibility tests, but he did have scores from tests he had done the previous semester.

Elijah obviously did not meet the ACSM recommendation of performing flexibility exercise for the major muscle groups at least two days a week. Even so, he had passed several of his recent flexibility tests (and he had been doing some flexibility exercises at that time).

Step 2: Consider Your Program Options

Elijah listed seven types of flexibility exercise that he wanted to consider. He reviewed many types of exercises before preparing a list of exercises that he thought would be good for him and that he would be most likely to perform.

- Static stretching exercises
- PNF exercises

- Ballistic stretching exercises
- Yoga
- Tai chi
- Pilates
- Dynamic movement exercises (for warm-up)

Step 3: Set Goals

Elijah chose a time period of two weeks for his flexibility exercise plan. Because this is too short for setting long-term goals, he developed only short-term physical activity goals for this plan. Later, when he prepares a longer plan, he'll develop long-term goals, including some flexibility improvement goals. For now, he just wanted to get started by trying some new exercises. Besides, it was summer, and he didn't have access to school facilities, nor was he a member of a fitness club. Elijah chose the following SMART goals.

- Perform one set of eight static stretching exercises on three days a week, including back-saver sit-and-reach, knee-to-chest, side stretch, sitting stretch, zipper, hip stretch, chest stretch, and calf stretch.
- Perform a dynamic movement exercise warm-up for 10 minutes, including nine basic exercises, before playing sports.
- Perform yoga for 30 minutes on one day a week.

Step 4: Create a Written Program

Elijah's next step was to write down his two-week flexibility exercise plan (see table 12.5). He chose static stretching that he could do at home three days a week. Because he played soccer two days a week, he also decided to do a dynamic movement exercise warm-up prior to his matches. He didn't expect the warm-up to be his main source of flexibility development, but he thought it would supplement his other flexibility exercise. He also agreed to go to yoga class with his sister Nicole, who was allowed to bring a guest for two free sessions.

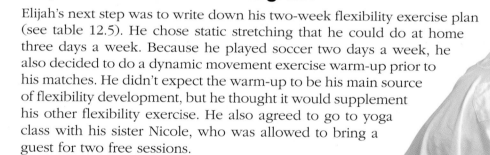

TABLE 12.5   **Elijah's Two-Week Flexibility Exercise Plan**

Day	Exercises	✓	Time, sets, reps
Mon.	**Static Stretch** Back-saver sit-and-reach Knee-to-chest Side stretch Sitting stretch Zipper Hip stretch Chest stretch Calf stretch		3:00 p.m. after daily jog All: 1 set, 2 reps each (hold 15 sec)
Tues.	**Dynamic Movement Exercise Warm-Up** High-knee march Standing flutter Quarter-turn cha-cha Shutter Grapevine Frankenstein Knee-high skip Jump-and-tuck Slow jog, fast sprint		1:00 p.m. before soccer All: 5 reps each Exercises followed by a slow jog for 30 sec and a fast sprint for 10 sec (×3)
Wed.	**Static Stretch** Back-saver sit-and-reach Knee-to-chest Side stretch Sitting stretch Zipper Hip stretch Chest stretch Calf stretch		3:00 p.m. after daily jog All: 1 set, 2 reps each (hold 15 sec)
Thurs.	**Dynamic Movement Exercise Warm-Up** High-knee march Standing flutter Quarter-turn cha-cha Shutter Grapevine Frankenstein Knee-high skip Jump-and-tuck Slow jog, fast sprint		1:00 p.m. before soccer All: 5 reps each Exercises followed by a slow jog for 30 sec and a fast sprint for 10 sec (×3)

Day	Exercises	✓	Time, sets, reps
Fri.	**Static Stretch**		3:00 p.m. after daily jog
	Back-saver sit-and-reach		All: 1 set, 2 reps each (hold 15 sec)
	Knee-to-chest		
	Side stretch		
	Sitting stretch		
	Zipper		
	Hip stretch		
	Chest stretch		
	Calf stretch		
Sat.	Yoga class		10:00–10:30 a.m.
Sun.	None		None

Step 5: Keep a Log and Evaluate Your Program

Over the next two weeks, Elijah will monitor his activities and place a checkmark beside each activity he performs. At the end of the two weeks, Elijah will evaluate his activity to see whether he met his goals, then use the evaluation to help him write a future activity plan.

LESSON REVIEW

1. Describe several basic flexibility exercises.
2. What are some other forms of activity that build flexibility?
3. What are the basic guidelines for stretching?
4. What flexibility exercises should you include in your written flexibility exercise plan?

TAKING CHARGE: **Building Knowledge and Understanding**

Anish's mother, Mrs. Bhalla, made a New Year's resolution to be more active. She did not know a lot about how to exercise, so she searched the web for information about fitness programs. She found a website that claimed: "Get fit in five minutes a day without getting sweaty!" Anish was concerned because he had learned in class that it takes weeks of regular exercise to improve fitness.

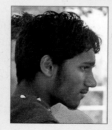

Anish told his mom, "I think you need to learn more about fitness and physical activity before you get started." But his mother decided to try the plan.

Months later, her fitness had not improved, and she felt discouraged.

At this point, she talked with Anish about the fitness and activity strategies he was learning at school. They both decided that it was important for her to learn about fitness before trying a new program. Anish wanted to help his mother answer some questions to help her

>continued

>continued

get the best results. Why should I exercise (what are the benefits)? Why is this plan best for me (what are my personal needs)?

Anish and his mother agreed that she would learn along with him as he studied fitness and physical activity at school so that she could do things right the next time she tried.

FOR DISCUSSION

Mrs. Bhalla made one good decision and one bad decision. How can someone who wants to make a healthy New Year's resolution avoid making a bad decision about fitness and physical activity? Why do you think people choose programs such as the one Mrs. Bhalla

tried? Is it possible to get fit in five minutes a day? How might Anish help his mother in the future? Consider the guidelines in the following Self-Management feature as you answer these discussion questions.

SELF-MANAGEMENT: Skills for Building Knowledge and Understanding

Knowledge based on sound information can help you make good decisions. But knowledge alone does not always lead to good decisions—you must understand the information you take in. A person with knowledge knows facts, but a person with understanding comprehends the significance of the facts and can use that understanding to make good decisions.

The following guidelines will help you use this book to build both your knowledge and your understanding about health and fitness.

- *Learn the facts first.* Learning the facts is a necessary first step toward building higher-level understanding.

- *Use the scientific method.* Collect as much information as possible to help you analyze and test hypotheses. For example, you might have a hypothesis that you can get fit in five minutes a day. After getting the facts and analyzing them, you would learn your hypothesis is false. The scientific method helps you understand the information you learn and make sound decisions.

- *Ask why.* When studying healthy lifestyle choices, ask yourself "why" questions: Why do I need this? Why should I believe this information? Why will this information be beneficial?

- *Consult reliable sources.* Whether you're consulting a website, magazine article, or book, check with trusted people to help you find good sources. Your knowledge and understanding are only as good as the sources you use. Chapter 19, Making Good Consumer Choices, provides more information about how to find reliable source material.

- *Try to apply.* When learning new information, ask: How can I apply this? Applying new information to real situations helps you understand it, which in turn helps you apply it more effectively. For example, regarding the dangers of fat in your diet, ask yourself: What else do I need to know? How much fat is too much? What changes can I make in my diet to reduce my fat intake?

- *Put it all together.* When you learn about something new, you often find many pieces of information. Taking time to fit the pieces together will help you make sense of what you've learned. Another word for putting all the facts together is *synthesizing.* For example, if you feel stressed out, and you know that there are several reasons for the stress, how do you use all of the information together—synthesize it—to make a good decision about how to reduce stress?

Taking Action: **Performing Your Flexibility Exercise Plan**

Prepare a flexibility exercise plan using the five steps of program planning described in this chapter. Try out your program over two weeks and see if you can meet your goal to perform flexibility exercises three days a week. Your teacher may give you time in class to do some of the activities in your plan. Consider the following suggestions for **taking action**.

- Before performing stretching exercises, do a general warm-up.
- Consider the guidelines for flexibility exercise presented in this chapter.
- If you're already participating in organized sport or physical activity, consider doing your flexibility exercise during the cool-down portion of your workout.

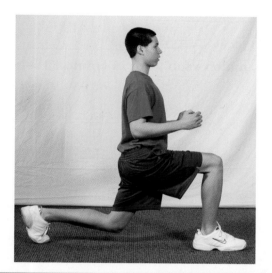

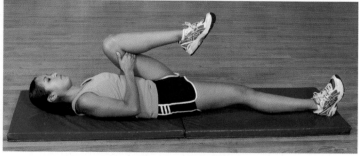

Take action by performing your flexibility exercise plan.

CHAPTER REVIEW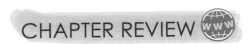

Reviewing Concepts and Vocabulary

Answer items 1 through 5 by correctly completing each sentence with a word or phrase.

1. The amount of movement you can make in a joint is called your _____.

2. Exercises including jumping, skipping, and calisthenics (such as those used in a warm-up) are called _____ exercises.

3. Being able to move beyond a typical healthy range of motion is called _____.

4. _____ is an ancient form of exercise that originated in China.

5. Gentle bouncing motions are part of _____ stretching.

For items 6 through 10, match each term in column 1 with the appropriate phrase in column 2.

6. zipper   a. stretch created by outside force without antagonist muscle

7. passive stretch   b. exercise poses originating from India

8. active stretch   c. stretch created by an antagonist muscle

9. PNF   d. stretch after muscle contraction

10. yoga   e. arm stretching exercise

For items 11 through 15, respond to each statement or question.

11. What are some benefits of good flexibility?

12. What are some factors that influence flexibility other than stretching?

13. What are some good tests of flexibility described in this chapter?

14. List and describe three different stretching exercises that you would include in your personal flexibility plan.

15. What are some guidelines for building knowledge and understanding?

Thinking Critically

Write a paragraph to answer the following question.

Sean's father went to a physical therapist to get treatment after a hip injury. The therapist recommended static stretching with a passive assist. Sean's dad asked him to help with the exercises. What safety concerns should Sean have while helping his father?

Project

Young people typically have better flexibility than older people. For this reason, your parents and grandparents are likely to be less flexible than you are. Prepare a list of five questions related to current flexibility, past flexibility, steps taken to maintain flexibility, and future plans for flexibility exercise and interview a parent or grandparent. Prepare a report presenting your findings.

EXERCISE CHART 1: **Flexibility Exercises**

The back-saver sit-and-reach and zipper exercises are similar to the self-assessments of the same names. The exercises are performed to improve flexibility whereas the self-assessments are performed to assess flexibility.

Back-Saver Sit-and-Reach (PNF or static)

1. Assume the back-saver sit-and-reach position with your right knee bent and your left leg straight. Keep your head up.

2. Bend your left knee slightly and push your heel into the floor as you contract your hamstrings hard for 3 seconds. Relax.

   Note: For static stretch, omit step 2.

3. Immediately grasp your ankle with both hands and gently pull your chest toward your knee. Hold the position for 15 seconds.

4. Repeat the exercise with the other leg.

   This exercise stretches the lower back and hamstring muscles.

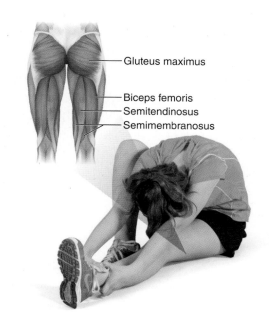

Gluteus maximus

Biceps femoris
Semitendinosus
Semimembranosus

Thigh-to-Chest

1. Lie on your back on a table with your right leg extended over the end of the table. Place your hands on the back of your left thigh and pull your upper thigh against your lower ribs. Do not place your hands on top of the knee.

2. Keep your right leg straight and your lower back flat against the table. To stretch the right hip flexor muscles, lower the right leg as low as possible without moving your left thigh away from your chest or arching your back.

3. Hold the position for 15 seconds.

4. Repeat with the opposite leg.

   Note: If you cannot lower your right leg to a level even with the height of the table, you can perform this exercise while lying on a mat on the floor.

   This exercise stretches your hip flexor muscles.

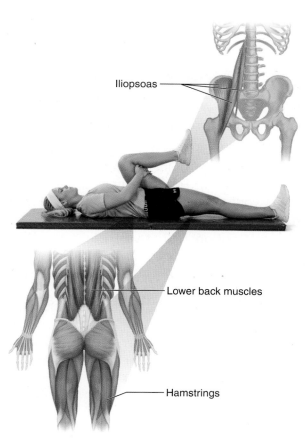

Iliopsoas

Lower back muscles

Hamstrings

Back and Hip Stretch (PNF or static)

1. Lie on your back with your knees bent and your arms at your sides.

2. Lift your hips until there is no bend at the hip joint. Squeeze the buttocks muscles hard for 3 seconds. Relax by lowering your hips to the floor.

    Note: For a static stretch, omit step 2.

3. Immediately place your hands under your knees and gently pull them to your chest. Hold the position for 15 seconds or more.

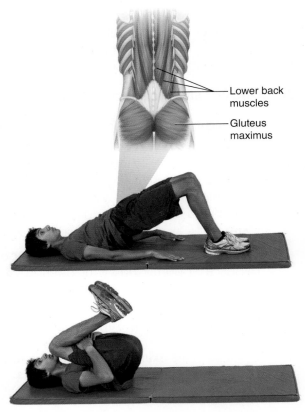

Lower back muscles

Gluteus maximus

This exercise stretches your lower back and gluteal muscles.

Side Stretch (static or ballistic)

1. Stand with your feet slightly wider than shoulder-width apart.

2. Lean to your left.

3. Reach down to your left foot with your left hand. Reach over your head with your right arm. Hold for a count of 10 to 30 seconds.

    Caution: Do not twist or lean your body forward.

4. Repeat the exercise on your right side.

    Note: For a ballistic stretch, do a gentle bouncing stretch.

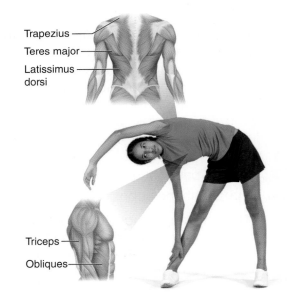

Trapezius

Teres major

Latissimus dorsi

Triceps

Obliques

This exercise stretches the muscles of your arms and shoulders and the sides of your body.

Trunk and Hip Stretch (static)

1. Lie on your back with your knees bent and your arms extended at shoulder level.
2. Slowly lean your bent legs to the right until your right leg is in contact with the ground.
3. Keep your shoulders and arms on the floor. Turn your head slightly to the left. Hold the position for 10 to 30 seconds.
4. Return to the starting position and repeat to the left side.

This exercise stretches the hip and lower back muscles.

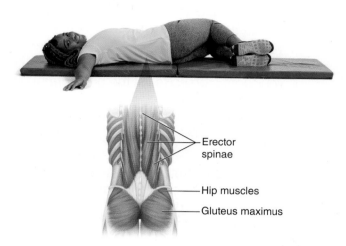

Erector spinae

Hip muscles

Gluteus maximus

Sitting Stretch (PNF or static)

1. Sit with the soles of your feet together and your elbows or hands resting on your knees.
2. Contract the muscles on the inside of your thighs, pulling up as you resist with your arms pushing down. Hold the position for 3 seconds. Relax your legs.

    Note: For a static stretch, omit step 2.

3. Immediately lean your trunk forward and push down on your knees with your arms to stretch your thighs. Hold the position for 10 to 30 seconds.

This exercise stretches the muscles of the inside of your thighs.

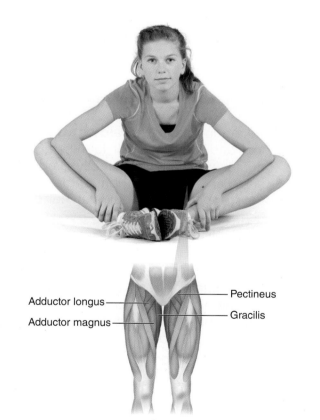

Adductor longus

Adductor magnus

Pectineus

Gracilis

Zipper (PNF or static)

1. Stand or sit. Lift your right arm over your right shoulder and reach down your spine.
2. With your left hand, press down on your right elbow. Resist the pressure by trying to raise that elbow, contracting the opposing muscles. Hold the position for 3 seconds. Relax.

   Note: For a static stretch, omit step 2.
3. Immediately stretch by reaching down your spine with your right arm as your left arm assists by pressing on your elbow. Hold the position for 10 to 30 seconds.
4. Repeat the exercise with your other arm.

This exercise stretches your triceps and latissimus muscles.

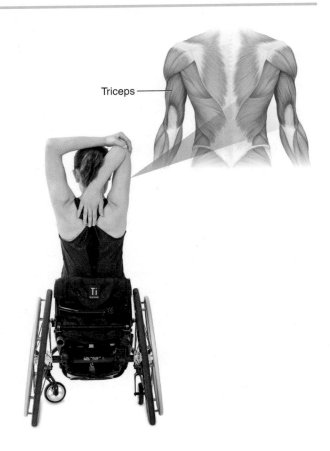

Triceps

Hip Stretch (static or ballistic)

1. Take a long step forward on your right foot and kneel on your left knee. Your right knee should be directly over your ankle and bent at a right angle. Keep your upper body erect (vertical position). Place your hands on your knee for stability.
2. Stretch by shifting your weight forward as you tilt your pelvis and trunk backward slightly. Keep your back knee in the same spot. You should feel a stretch across the front of your left hip joint and in the front of your thigh muscles.
3. Hold the position for 10 to 30 seconds.
4. Repeat the exercise with your other leg.

   Note: For a ballistic stretch, do a gentle bouncing motion forward as you tilt the top of your pelvis back.

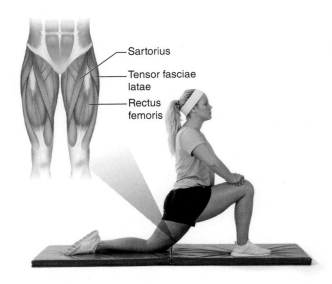

Sartorius

Tensor fasciae latae

Rectus femoris

This exercise stretches the quadriceps muscles on the front of your thighs and the muscles on the front of your hips.

Chest Stretch (PNF, static, or ballistic)

1. Stand in a forward stride position in a doorway. Raise your arms slightly above shoulder height. Place your hands on either side of the doorway.

2. Lean your body into the doorway. Resist by contracting your arm and chest muscles. Hold the position for 3 seconds. Relax.

3. Immediately lean further forward, letting your body weight stretch your muscles. Hold the position for 10 to 30 seconds.

4. For a ballistic stretch, gently bounce your body forward.

   Note: For a static stretch, omit steps 2 and 4.

This exercise stretches your chest and shoulder muscles.

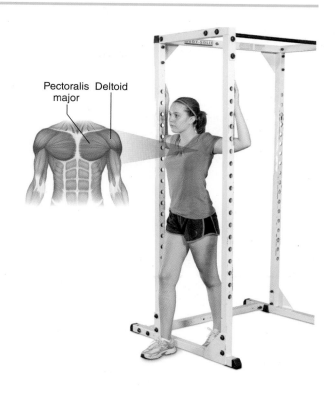

Calf Stretch (static or ballistic)

1. Step forward with your right leg in a lunge position. Keep both feet pointed straight ahead and your right knee directly over your right foot. Place your hands on your right leg for balance.

2. Keep your left leg straight and the heel on the floor. Adjust the length of your lunge until you feel a good stretch in your left calf and Achilles tendon. Hold the position for 10 to 30 seconds.

3. Repeat the exercise with your other leg.

   Note: For a ballistic stretch, gently bounce your heel toward the floor.

This exercise stretches your calf muscles and Achilles tendons.

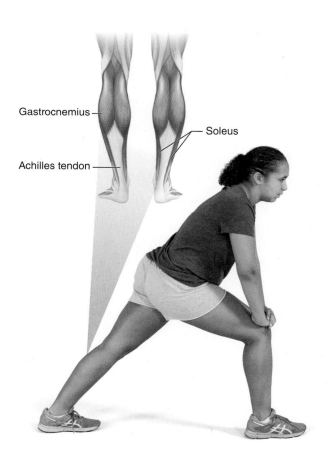

UNIT V

Skills, Skill-Related Fitness, Body Composition, and Program Planning

CHAPTER 13   Skill-Related Fitness, Skills, Tactics, and Strategy
CHAPTER 14   Body Composition and Energy Balance
CHAPTER 15   Planning and Maintaining Active Lifestyles

Healthy People 2030 Objectives

Overarching Goals

- Attain healthy, thriving lives and well-being, free of preventable disease, disability, injury, and premature death.
- Eliminate health disparities, achieve health equity, and attain health literacy to improve the health and well-being of all.

Objectives

- Increase the proportion of teens who play sports.
- Reduce the proportion of teens with obesity.
- Reduce consumption of added sugars and saturated fat among teens.
- Increase the proportion of schools that don't sell less healthy foods and drinks.
- Increase the proportion of adolescents and adults who do enough aerobic and muscle fitness physical activity for health benefits.
- Increase the proportion of teens who walk or bike to get places.
- Reduce the proportion of people who do no physical activity in their free time.
- Increase the proportion of teens who participate in daily school physical education.
- Increase health literacy of the population.

Self-Assessment Features in This Unit

- Assessing Skill-Related Physical Fitness
- Body Measurements
- Your Personal Fitness Test Battery

Taking Charge and Self-Management Features in This Unit

- Developing Tactics
- Improving Physical Self-Perception
- Changing Attitudes

Taking Action Features in This Unit

- Skill Learning Experiment
- Elastic Band Workout
- Performing Your Physical Activity Plan

Skill-Related Fitness, Skills, Tactics, and Strategy

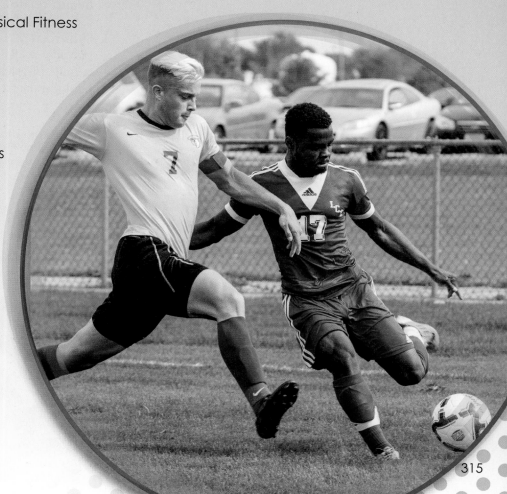

Skill-Related Physical Fitness and Skills

Lesson Objectives

After reading this lesson, you should be able to

1. describe some factors that influence skill-related fitness;

2. describe a skill-related fitness profile and explain some of its uses;

3. define *motor skills* and describe the factors that influence them; and

4. describe the three stages of skill learning.

Lesson Vocabulary

associative stage
autonomous stage
cognitive stage
feedback
motor unit
skill

Do you have good skill-related physical fitness? Do you have good skills? Do you know the difference? Learning about your own skill-related fitness will help you determine which sports and lifetime activities will be easiest for you to learn and enjoy. Because people differ in their levels of skill-related fitness, different people find success in different activities. In this lesson, you'll learn how to assess your skill-related fitness so that you can choose activities that match your abilities, learn to improve your abilities, and find activities that you can enjoy for a lifetime. You'll also learn about skills and how to acquire them.

Skill-Related Fitness

You already know that physical fitness is divided into two categories: health-related fitness and skill-related fitness. All parts of fitness have health and performance benefits. However, health-related fitness, as the name implies, focuses on helping you maintain good health. Skill-related fitness focuses on helping you perform well in sports and activities requiring certain physical skills. These are the five parts of skill-related fitness:

> I started playing volleyball because my friends played it. I wasn't very good, but I practiced hard. Now I really enjoy it. Practice pays off.
>
> *Briella Banks*

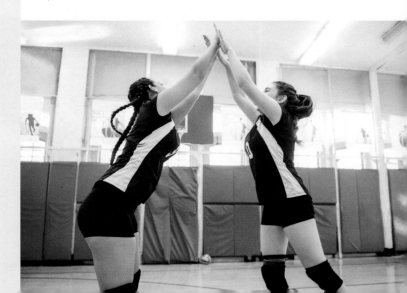

- *Agility:* The ability to change the position of your body quickly and control your body's movements
- *Balance:* The ability to keep an upright posture while standing still or moving
- *Coordination:* The ability to use your senses together with your body parts or to use two or more body parts together
- *Reaction time:* The amount of time it takes you to move once you recognize the need to act
- *Speed:* The ability to perform a movement or cover a distance in a short time

Several factors affect skill-related fitness, including heredity, age, maturation, sex, and training. Together the factors help determine your skill-related fitness (see figure 13.1). Each is described in the paragraphs that follow.

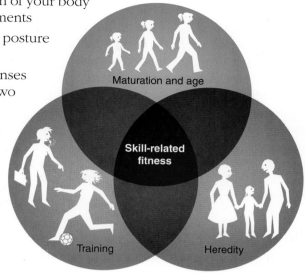

Figure 13.1 Various factors influence skill-related fitness.

SCIENCE IN ACTION: Improving Speed and Agility

Speed is important for sports performance. Sprinting, as in running a 100-meter dash, is an example of an activity that requires speed. To improve speed in sprinting, a person can learn sprinting skills. Instruction and technical drills with assistance of a coach help you learn the skills of sprinting. The most common training techniques appropriate for teens interested in improving speed include resisted speed drills (e.g., sled pushing or pulling, parachute sprinting, uphill running) and assisted sprint drills (e.g., downhill running). Muscle fitness training, as outlined in the chapters on muscle fitness, is also important for improving speed. Speed training is also important for swimming sprints and requires special skills and training techniques.

Agility is also important to sports performance, particularly high-speed agility, or the ability to change directions at high speed. Like speed, improvement in agility requires improved skills (e.g., coordinating upper- and lower-body movements) and specialized training (e.g., agility course drills, step pattern drills). Deceleration drills are also important for improving the ability to stop quickly.

The FIT formula for speed and agility training varies depending on the type of activity being performed. Experts from the ACSM indicate that speed and agility training is appropriate for teens when the FIT guidelines are followed and when performed with the proper progression under the supervision of qualified instructors. It is important to establish a solid muscle fitness foundation prior to high-intensity speed and agility training. Experts also note that it is *always* better to undertrain than overtrain.

STUDENT ACTIVITY

Interview one of your school's athletic coaches about speed and agility training. Ask them how important speed and agility are to the sport that they coach and what activities they recommend for training them.

Heredity

Skill-related fitness abilities are influenced by heredity. Some people are able to run fast or react quickly because they inherited these traits from their parents. A person who did not inherit these tendencies may have more difficulty performing well on skill-related fitness tests. However, it is possible to improve skill-related fitness with techniques such as speed and agility training (see Science in Action). In addition, lack of inherited ability can sometimes be made up for by desire and motivation.

Maturation and Age

In general, teens who mature early perform better on skill-related fitness tests than those who mature later. Because older teens are typically more mature, they often have an advantage over younger classmates or teammates. However, late-maturing teens typically catch up as they grow older.

Training

It has long been thought that changing one's skill-related fitness is hard to do. However, recent research has shown that with the right kind of training, considerable effort, and strong motivation, you can improve your skill-related fitness.

Building a Skill-Related Fitness Profile

In previous chapters you learned how to build several health-related fitness profiles. You can do the same for skill-related fitness. Building a profile can help you choose activities that can improve your skill-related fitness and that can help you match your abilities to activities in which you have the greatest chance of success. A good first step is to assess your skill-related fitness abilities to determine your strengths and weaknesses (see Self-Assessment later in this chapter).

Remember that skill-related fitness has many subparts; you may be good in one area but not as good in another. For example, coordination is a skill-related ability that includes both eye–hand coordination (e.g., hitting a ball) and eye–foot coordination (e.g., kicking a ball). In addition to working on the areas that need improvement, you should consider selecting activities for your program that match your strengths.

One student, Sue, did all of the skill-related physical fitness assessments presented in this chapter, then developed a profile for her skill-related fitness (see table 13.1). Sue's profile helped her identify her strengths and weaknesses.

Sue's profile helped her determine her areas of need. She then used table 13.2 to choose activities that provided the most benefit for areas she wanted to improve. For example, Sue didn't do well in agility and balance, so she decided to

TABLE 13.1   **Sue's Skill-Related Fitness Profile**

Part of fitness	Skill-related performance rating			
	Low	**Marginal**	**Good**	**High**
Agility	✓			
Balance		✓		
Coordination				✓
Speed		✓		
Reaction time		✓		

TABLE 13.2   **Skill-Related Benefits of Sports and Other Activities**

Activity	Balance	Coordination	Reaction time	Agility	Speed
Badminton	Fair	Excellent	Good	Good	Good
Baseball	Good	Excellent	Excellent	Good	Good
Basketball	Good	Excellent	Excellent	Excellent	Good
Bicycling	Excellent	Fair	Fair	Fair	Fair
Bowling	Good	Excellent	Poor	Fair	Fair
Circuit training	Fair	Fair	Poor	Fair	Fair
Dance (aerobic or social)	Fair	Good	Fair	Good	Poor
Dance (ballet or modern)	Excellent	Excellent	Fair	Excellent	Poor
Extreme sports	Good	Good	Excellent	Excellent	Good
Fitness calisthenics	Fair	Fair	Poor	Good	Poor
Football	Good	Good	Excellent	Excellent	Excellent
Golf (walking)	Fair	Excellent	Poor	Fair	Poor
Gymnastics	Excellent	Excellent	Good	Excellent	Fair
Interval training	Fair	Fair	Poor	Poor	Fair
Jogging or walking	Poor	Poor	Poor	Poor	Poor
Martial arts	Good	Excellent	Excellent	Excellent	Excellent
Racquetball or handball	Fair	Excellent	Good	Excellent	Good
Rope jumping	Fair	Good	Fair	Good	Poor
Skating (ice or roller)	Excellent	Good	Fair	Good	Good
Skiing (cross-country)	Fair	Excellent	Poor	Good	Fair
Skiing (downhill)	Excellent	Excellent	Good	Excellent	Poor
Soccer	Fair	Excellent	Good	Excellent	Good
Softball (fastpitch)	Fair	Excellent	Excellent	Good	Good
Swimming (laps)	Poor	Good	Poor	Good	Poor
Tai chi	Excellent	Good	Fair	Excellent	Good
Tennis	Fair	Excellent	Good	Good	Good
Volleyball	Fair	Excellent	Good	Good	Fair
Weight training	Fair	Fair	Poor	Poor	Poor

take tai chi lessons to help her improve these parts of fitness. She also didn't do well in reaction time and speed, and she thought that tai chi might also help her improve these abilities to some degree. However, she also decided not to worry that she does not perform as well as some other people in these parts of fitness. She was willing to try to improve but because of her heredity she felt that she would never be a really fast person with good reaction time.

You can build your own skill-related fitness profile similar to the one Sue developed in table 13.1. Use your profile as well as table 13.2 to determine which activities can help you improve where you need to and which activities you can most easily learn and enjoy.

Physical or Motor Skills

A **skill** is the ability to perform a task that is acquired through knowledge and practice. Examples of physical skills used in sports and games include catching, throwing, swimming, batting, and dancing. As you can see, skill-related fitness abilities and physical skills are not the same thing, although having skill-related fitness can help you learn particular skills. For example, if you have good speed and agility, you'll be able to learn running skills used in football more easily. Similarly, if you have good balance, you'll be able to learn gymnastics skills more easily. You'll learn more about skills later in this lesson.

Physical skills are often referred to as *motor skills*, because learning a skill requires your body to use motor units. A **motor unit** is made up of the muscle fibers that contract to cause movement, along with the nerves that stimulate them (figure 13.2). If motor units are used over and over again (as when you practice a skill), you learn to use the nerves and muscles to move more efficiently and thus improve your skills.

Skill Learning

The five parts of skill-related fitness are abilities that help you learn physical skills. For this reason, factors that affect your skill-related fitness, such as heredity, maturation, and age, also affect your skill learning (see figure 13.1). However, the two factors that affect skill learning the most are knowledge and practice.

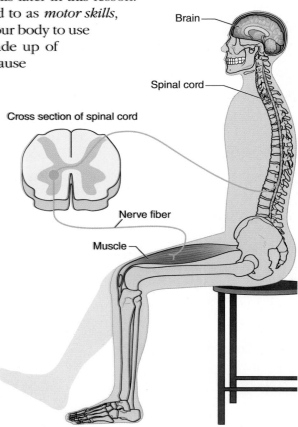

Figure 13.2 A motor unit consists of nerves that stimulate and muscles that contract to cause movement.

Knowledge

Practice helps you learn skills, but first you have to have basic information about how to perform skills and how best to practice them. You have learned about biomechanical principles that are important for skill learning in previous chapters. Later, you will also learn how to practice properly.

> The more I practice, the luckier I get.
>
> *Common sports adage*

Practice

Everyone can learn skills with practice. However, it takes some people longer than others to learn skills, and some people will be better at performing skills than others. Not everyone can become an Olympic athlete, but with practice everyone can learn the basic skills necessary to enjoy some sports and to perform physical tasks efficiently. Considerable evidence shows that people who are dedicated and willing to work hard can even overcome hereditary disadvantages and outperform people who have a hereditary advantage. The key is practice.

Practice involves repeating a skill over and over again. If you correctly repeat a skill, such as a tennis serve, you will become better at that skill. You'll learn more about skill development later in this chapter.

Feedback

One key to motor or skill learning is **feedback**. Feedback refers to information (also called knowledge of results) you receive about your performance that helps you make changes in order to perform better. It helps you use practice effectively. One of the best forms of feedback comes from experts such as teachers and coaches. After watching your performance, they can give you specific comments about how to improve. Another way to receive feedback is to watch a video recording of your performance to see what mistakes you may be making and what you are doing well. Motor learning experts suggest that you use one piece of feedback at a time.

Guidelines for Learning Skills

Experts in sport pedagogy and motor learning have studied the best ways to learn sport skills and developed guidelines that can help you as you work to improve your skills. Several guidelines for improving skills were presented in the Self-Management feature of chapter 9. It would be good to review these guidelines at this time.

Three Stages of Skill Learning

When learning to perform a motor skill, you typically move through three stages (figure 13.3). The first stage is called the **cognitive stage** because you have to think about how to apply knowledge to help you perform the skill. During this stage, movements are inefficient and typically slow. Verbal feedback helps you perform the skill properly. The second stage is called the **associative stage** because you begin to associate the knowledge of the skill with the actual movements. You still have to think about what you're doing, but skills start to become more automatic and your performance becomes more efficient and consistent. The final stage of skill learning is called the **autonomous stage** because you perform the movements automatically, accurately, and efficiently. (*Autonomous* is a word that refers to performing independently, without outside control.)

FIT FACT

Too much feedback can cause "analysis paralysis," a state of mind in which you can't focus on the few things that are really important. For example, if a softball batter is trying to remember "keep your eyes level, keep your elbows up, stride straight forward, lead with your hips, and keep your eye on the ball," she may swing and miss the ball entirely. Too much feedback all at once can be more harmful than helpful.

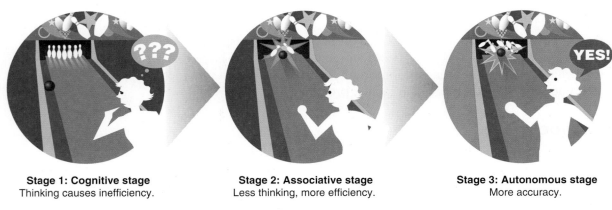

Stage 1: Cognitive stage
Thinking causes inefficiency.

Stage 2: Associative stage
Less thinking, more efficiency.

Stage 3: Autonomous stage
More accuracy.

Figure 13.3   The three stages of skill learning.

Talent is something you are born with and skill is something that you develop.

Tiger Woods, professional golfer

Practice is the most important factor in skill learning, but practicing a skill incorrectly can be harmful to your learning because it may cause you to perform the skill incorrectly. Practice doesn't make perfect—*perfect practice* makes perfect. Therefore, it is crucial that you know both what to practice and how to practice it correctly. When first learning a skill (cognitive stage), you gain knowledge about the skill. As you begin to practice, you rely on cognitive information, including feedback from instructors. In the associative stage, you continue to improve and refine your skills using the knowledge, but focus more on repeating the skill rather than thinking about it. Even highly skilled athletes, who typically perform at the autonomous stage, practice regularly to keep their skills sharp and to make their performances more consistent and reliable.

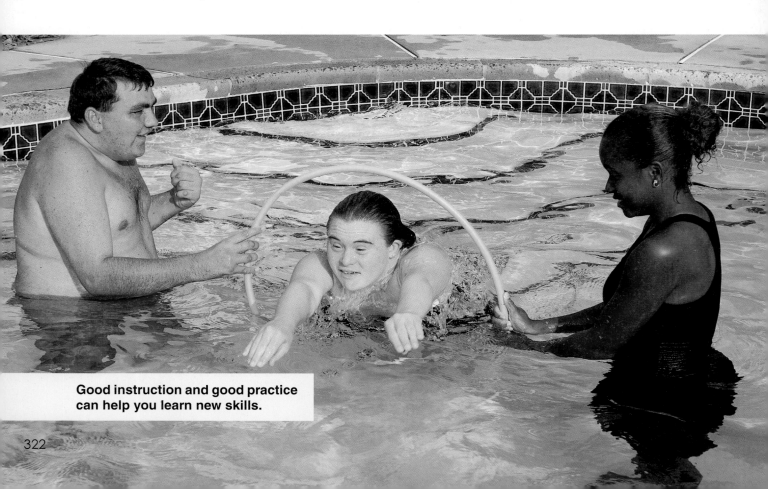

Good instruction and good practice can help you learn new skills.

TECH TRENDS: Motion Analysis Systems

Before the invention of video recording, scientists depended on live observation of sport and recreational skill performance to determine the most efficient and effective ways for people to perform motor skills. The invention of the first motion pictures allowed this technology to be used for analyzing work skills during the early 1900s. As sport became more popular in the United States after World War II, moving pictures were also used to analyze the performance of baseball players to improve their mechanics in batting and pitching. Researchers such as John Cooper at Indiana University and Richard Nelson at Pennsylvania State University used special high-speed cameras to perform slow-motion analysis of very fast movements recorded on film.

In the early 1950s, the magnetic video tape recorder replaced film as the most popular method of recording and analyzing movements in physical activity. Digital photography was used by the U.S. National Aeronautics and Space Administration for space exploration in the 1960s, but digital cameras did not become commonly used by the public until the 1990s. Now, digital cameras are paired with computer software to analyze movement. The software was originally developed for use in research laboratories and by professional sports teams but is now available for leisure sports and recreational activities. For example, many golf stores use special cameras and software to offer motion analysis of a player's golf swing. Programs are also available to help individuals analyze their own sport performance on a home computer.

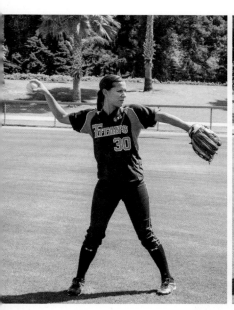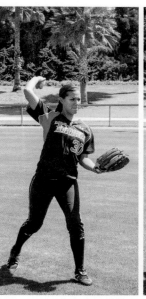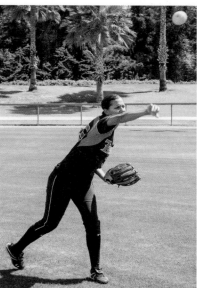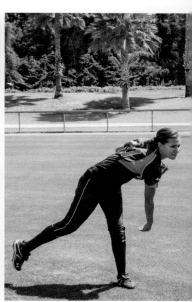

Movement sequences can be studied to provide feedback for improved performance.

STUDENT ACTIVITY

If your school has a motion analysis system for student athletes, ask for a demonstration. If not, check with a local golf or tennis store to get a demonstration, or investigate the motion analysis apps found in the web resource. Write a brief report summarizing your investigation.

LESSON REVIEW

1. What are some of the factors that influence skill-related fitness?
2. What is a skill-related fitness profile, and what are some of its uses?
3. What is the definition of *motor skills,* and what are some of the factors that influence them?
4. How is each stage of skill learning best described, and how does each contribute to skill learning?

SELF-ASSESSMENT: **Assessing Skill-Related Physical Fitness**

You can assess your skill-related fitness abilities by using the following tests. Use tables 13.3 and 13.4 to get your ratings. Record your scores and ratings as directed by your teacher. Keep the following points in mind, especially if you do not score well.

- You can improve all parts of your skill-related fitness, particularly with dedication and consistent effort.
- Due to the principle of specificity, you may excel in some and do less well in others.
- Some activities, such as jogging, do not require a high level of skill-related fitness.
- You do not need to excel in skill-related fitness in order to enjoy physical activity.

PART 1: Side Shuttle (agility)

Use masking tape or another material to make five parallel lines on the floor 2 to 3 feet (61 to 91 centimeters) long on the floor, spaced 3 feet apart. Have a partner count while you do the side shuttle, then switch.

1. Stand with the first line to your right. When your partner says "go," step to the right with the right foot, and then slide the left foot over to the right foot. Continue to step-slide until your right foot steps over the last line. Then reverse direction, stepping with the left foot and sliding with the right until your left foot steps over the first line.

    Caution: Do not cross your feet.

2. Move from side to side as many times as possible in 10 seconds. Only one foot must cross the last line.

3. When your partner says "stop," freeze in place until they determine your score. Score 1 point for each line you crossed in 10 seconds. Subtract 1 point for each time you crossed your feet.

4. Do the side shuttle twice and record the better of your two scores. Use table 13.3 to determine your rating. Record your rating.

The side shuttle assesses agility.

PART 2: Stick Balance (balance)

You may take one practice try before doing each test for a score.

TEST 1

1. Use a square stick 1.5 inches (about 4 centimeters) by 1.5 inches that is 1 foot long (30 centimeters). Stand with the balls of both feet across the stick so that your heels are on the floor.

2. Lift your heels off the floor and maintain your balance on the stick for 15 seconds. Hold your arms out in front of you for balance. Once you begin, do not allow your heels to touch the floor or your feet to move on the stick.

   Hint: Focus your eyes on a stationary object in front of you.

3. Try the test twice. Give yourself 2 points if you succeed on the first try but fail on the second, 1 point if you fail on the first try but succeed on the second, and 3 points if you succeed on both tries. Record your score.

TEST 2

1. Stand on the stick with your dominant foot (the one you use to kick a ball). Your foot should run the length of the stick.

2. Lift your other foot off the floor. First, balance for 10 seconds with your base foot flat. Then rise onto the ball of your foot (with your heel off the stick) and continue balancing for 10 seconds.

3. Try the test twice. Give yourself 1 point if you balance flat-footed for 10 seconds, 1 point if you balance on the ball of your foot for 10 seconds, and 1 point if you successfully performed both trials. Your maximum score is 3 points.

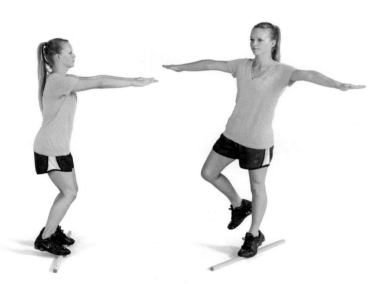

The two stick balance tests assess balance.

4. Add the scores from both stick tests. Use table 13.3 to determine your rating. Record your scores and rating.

PART 3: Wand Juggling (coordination)

You may take three practice tries before doing this test for a score.

1. Hold a stick in each hand. Have a partner place a third stick across the sticks held in your hands.

2. Using the two sticks you're holding, toss the third stick into the air so that it makes a half turn. Catch it with the sticks you're holding. The tossed stick should not hit your hands.

3. Do this test five times by tossing the stick to the right, then five times by tossing the stick to the left. Score 1 point for each successful catch.

   Hint: Absorb the shock of the catch by giving with the held sticks, as you might do when catching an egg or something breakable.

4. Record your results and use table 13.3 to determine your rating. Record your rating.

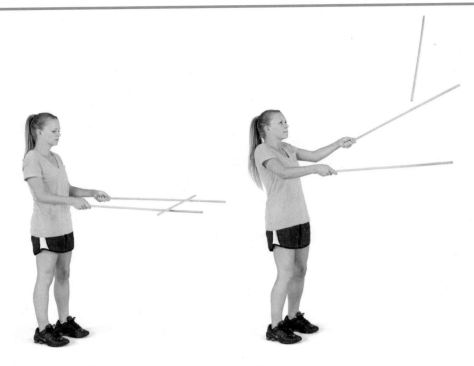

The wand juggling test assesses coordination.

TABLE 13.3   Rating Chart: Agility, Balance, and Coordination

	Side shuttle		Stick balance	Wand juggling
	Male	**Female**	**Male or female**	**Male or female**
Excellent	≥31	≥28	6	9–10
Good	26–30	24–27	5	7–8
Fair	19–25	15–23	3–4	4–6
Poor	≤18	≤14	≤2	≤3

PART 4: Stick Drop (reaction time)

1. Have a partner hold the top of a yardstick (or meter stick) with their thumb and index finger between the 1-inch (2.5-centimeter) mark and the end of the stick.

2. Position the 24-inch (61-centimeter) mark on the stick between your thumb and fingers. Do not touch or grip the stick. Your arm should rest on the edge of a table with only your fingers over the edge.

3. When your partner drops the stick, catch it as quickly as possible between your thumb and fingers. Your partner should not give a warning before dropping the stick.

   Hint: Focus on the stick, not your partner, and be very alert.

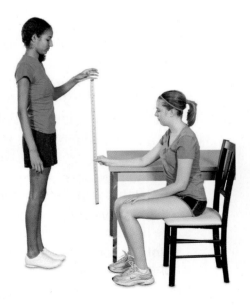

The stick drop test assesses reaction time.

4. Try this test three times. Your partner should be careful not to drop the stick after the same waiting period each time—in other words, you should not be able to guess when the stick will drop. Your score for each try is the number on the stick at the place where you catch it. Record your scores.

5. Use table 13.4 to determine your rating based on your middle score (the one between your lowest and highest scores). Record your rating.

PART 5: Short Sprint (speed)

Use masking tape to mark 10 lines on the floor that are 2 to 3 feet long (61 to 91 centimeters). The first line is a starting line; the second is 10 yards (9.1 meters) from the starting line, and the remaining lines are 2 yards (1.8 meters) apart beginning after the 10-yard line, for a total distance of 26 yards (23.8 meters). Work with a partner who will time you and blow a whistle to signal you to stop.

Try the test once for practice without being timed, then do it for a score.

1. Stand two or three steps behind the starting line.

2. When your partner says "go," run as far and as fast as you can. Your partner will start a stopwatch when you cross the starting line. Three seconds later, your partner will blow the whistle. When the whistle sounds, do not try to stop immediately, but do begin to slow down.

3. Your partner should mark where you were when the whistle blew and measure the distance to the nearest line. If you were more than halfway to a line, count that line when scoring. Your score is the distance you covered in the three seconds after crossing the starting line. For example, if you cross five lines after the starting line plus 1 foot, your score is 18 yards because 1 foot is less than half the distance to the next line.

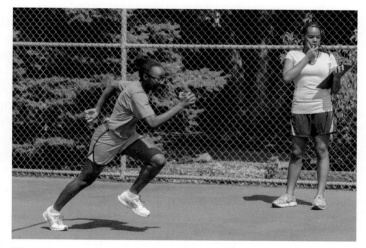

The short sprint test assesses speed.

4. Record your score and use table 13.4 to determine your rating. Record your rating.

TABLE 13.4   Rating Chart: Reaction Time and Speed

	Stick drop (inches)	Short sprint (yards)	
	Male or female	Male	Female
Excellent	≥22	≥24	≥22
Good	19–21	21–23	19–21
Fair	14–18	16–20	15–18
Poor	≤13	≤15	≤14

To convert centimeters to inches, divide by 2.54. To convert meters to yards, divide by 0.91.

The rating categories for skill-related physical fitness describe levels of performance ability, not health or wellness.

Strategy and Tactics

Lesson Objectives

After reading this lesson, you should be able to

1. define *strategy* and provide examples that relate to physical activity and healthy lifestyle choices;
2. define *tactic* and explain its role in implementing a strategy;
3. explain the five steps for planning strategy and tactics; and
4. describe some ways that you can use strategy and tactics in daily activities other than sports and physical activities.

Lesson Vocabulary

strategy
tactic

Success in sport and other physical activities requires certain abilities, including good fitness and motor skills. You can achieve fitness and master skills with proper training and good practice. But physical abilities are not the only requirements for success—you also need a good strategy and sound tactics.

Strategy

A **strategy** is a master plan for achieving a goal. The word *strategy* comes from the Greek word *strategos*, which refers to the general or leader of an army and is still often used in military contexts. However, it is also used in business and organizational contexts; for example, companies use marketing to develop strategies for selling their products. Strategies are also useful in sport and other physical activities: Coaches develop strategies or master plans for winning games, and players use strategies to be effective team members.

> I played an old guy in a local tennis tournament. I was much better than him, but I lost. He kept dinking the ball and made me run all over the place. Now I see how strategy and tactics are important.
>
> *Gamal Morcos*

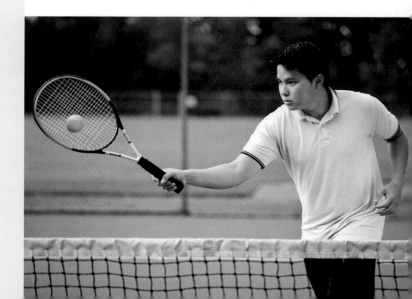

Tactics

A **tactic** is a specific method for carrying out a strategy. The word *tactic* derives from the Greek *taktikos*, which refers to arranging forces in a battle formation. As with strategy, tactics were first used in the military to carry out the strategy or battle plan.

Companies similarly use specific tactics to carry out their marketing strategy. For example, a food manufacturer that sells sugary cereals might have a strategy to convince children that they want the cereal. Even though adults buy the cereal, children have a big influence on what adults buy, so specific tactics might include running ads for the cereal with children's TV shows or placing toys in cereal boxes (figure 13.4). Children see the ad or want the toy and beg a parent to buy the cereal.

> A strategy lays out a plan for reaching your goals; tactics help you carry out your strategy.
>
> *Phil Abbadessa, teacher and coach*

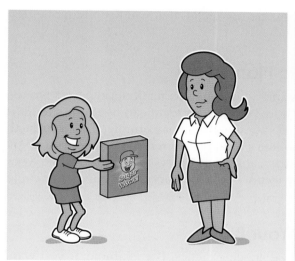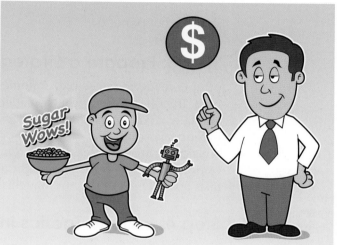

Figure 13.4 A marketing strategy could include tactics such as a food manufacturer including toys in their breakfast cereal.

In team sports, a coach or team captain develops the strategy. For example, a basketball team might decide to adopt a defensive strategy—that is, emphasize defense in order to force the other team to make errors. One specific defensive tactic would be to use a full-court press, in which players guard their opponents at both ends of the court. Another defensive tactic might be to double-team (have two players guard) the other team's best shooter.

FIT FACT
The game of chess requires both strategy and specific tactics. In fact, many coaches and military leaders use the game to sharpen their ability to use tactics to carry out a strategy.

Planning a Strategy and Developing Tactics

Using strategies and tactics can help you be successful in sports and games. But how do you develop them? You can use steps similar to those in the scientific method and those used in program planning. Because tactics are used to implement a strategy, the strategy is planned first.

Step 1: Use Existing Information

There are already many successful strategies for various sports and activities. Therefore, a good first step is to read books and articles about your chosen sport

> Even the best strategy will not be effective unless you implement good tactics to carry it out.
>
> *Anonymous*

or activity. You can also consult with experts and others who have succeeded in the sport or activity, as well as track your own successful strategies. Keeping notes about successful strategies can help you carry out steps 2 through 5.

Step 2: Collect New Information

One way to decide which strategy will work best for you is to conduct a self-assessment of your strengths and weaknesses. It is also helpful to assess your opponent's strengths and weaknesses. Coaches do this by means of scouting reports that describe other teams' strengths and weaknesses and identify strategies and tactics they have been known to use. Even the pros collect information. For example, professional basketball player LeBron James, who has excellent physical abilities and skills, also studies video and reads the full scouting report of other teams in order to implement a strategy and use tactics that will keep him one step ahead of opponents.

Step 3: Prepare a Strategic Plan

After considering possible strategies and collecting information, prepare a written plan. In competitive sport, consider how you or your team can use your strengths and take advantages of your opponent's weaknesses. For example, if your strength in tennis is your serve and your opponent's weakness is return of serve, you might consider an offensive strategy. On the other hand, if you're quite fit and your opponent is not so fit, you might try to tire out your opponent so that you could take advantage later in the match.

FIT FACT
Preparing a written plan is a commitment to action. People who make a formal commitment are more likely to act than those who do not.

Step 4: Include Tactics in Your Plan

To carry out your strategy, plan to use specific tactics. For example, if you want to implement an offensive strategy in tennis, you might consider coming to the net after each of your serves to take advantage of your opponent's poor service return. If your opponent is out of shape, you might make them move around a lot

TECH TRENDS: **Computers Keep Getting Smarter**

Continually evolving technology allows computers to store and process more information more quickly than ever. In this light, perhaps it's no surprise that in 2011 a computer named Watson—developed by researchers at IBM and named after the company's founder, Thomas Watson—used its artificial intelligence to beat two human competitors on the TV game show *Jeopardy*. Competing against the biggest winners in the show's history, Ken Jennings and Brad Rutter, Watson won the million-dollar prize by quickly retrieving and analyzing information stored in its computer memory in ways similar to those of the human brain. Watson also performed some physical tasks in ways similar to or better than those of humans—it had better reaction time and thus was able to respond to the buzzer more quickly than the human contestants. However, Watson did have some problems interpreting clues provided by the show's host and was unable to play the game strategically, occasionally making errors in common sense a human would not have made.

USING TECHNOLOGY

Prepare a report explaining some ways that computers can be used to help people who have physical disabilities.

by hitting the ball first to one side of the court and then to the other.

When deciding on tactics, you can use the same steps as in planning a strategy. First, become familiar with existing information (study known tactics), then collect information, and then make a list of the tactics to consider and decide which ones are best for implementing your strategy.

Step 5: Practice

When most people think of practice, they think of practicing skills to get better at performance, but practicing your strategy and tactics is also important. For the tennis player in our example, this practice would involve serving, coming to the net, and volleying. It would also include hitting the ball from side to side to make the opponent move.

As with any plan, you should also evaluate the success of the strategy and tactics you implement. What you learn will become part of step 1 when you plan your next strategy.

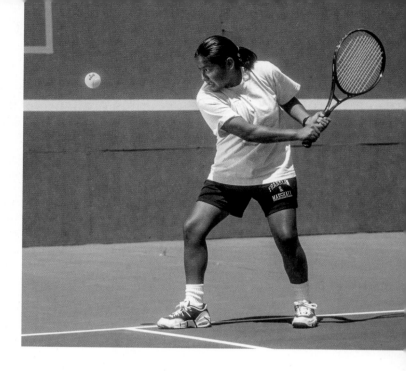

Using Strategies and Tactics in Daily Life

Strategy and tactics are useful in many different daily activities. Some examples are provided in table 13.5.

TABLE 13.5 **Examples of Strategies and Tactics**

Situation	Strategy	Tactics
Playing a team sport Your intramural team wants to do well in the soccer league.	Focus on defense.	Assign more players to defense. Use zone defense because some players lack skills. Use long defensive kicks to clear ball and reduce shots on goal.
Physical activity You do not meet national activity guidelines.	Prepare a written physical activity plan.	Follow the five steps for writing a plan. Log daily activity.
Healthy eating You consume more calories than you expend each day.	Eat less food with empty calories.	Remove food with empty calories from house. Learn to say no. Eat healthy snacks. Avoid buying food from vending machines.
Managing stress You have too many things to do and not enough time to do them.	Reduce commitments and spend more time on important things.	Self-assess current time use. Rank current commitments from high to low importance. Focus on important commitments. Say no to unimportant commitments.
Preventing back pain You want to reduce risk of back pain.	Focus on good posture in standing, sitting, and moving.	Assess current posture and core fitness. Perform core exercises. Practice good posture.

CONSUMER CORNER: **TV Strategies and Tactics**

As you know, companies develop strategies and tactics—however, sometimes their strategies help them but are not good for you. For example, a company's strategy may be to get you to buy something you don't really want or need. Their tactics may include advertising on television, the web, and the radio as well as in magazines and newspapers. The money these companies pay for advertisements is what allows media outlets to survive, so both the companies that sell the products and the media outlets who sell the ads are trying to influence your consumer behavior in order to make money. In fact, marketers create media messages that flood our senses every day. Of course, not all advertisements are deceptive, but many are. It takes a very critical eye to detect the messages being conveyed in ads and to distinguish between good and bad information.

Today, teens represent one of the largest groups of consumers in the United States. Using the "merchants of cool" strategy is one way companies target the teen market. In this approach, companies (merchants) try to make their products seem cool to teens. One specific tactic is to feature movie stars and entertainers promoting a brand. This strategy is used to sell, among other things, clothing, electronics, energy drinks, sport drinks, and soda. Another tactic used in the strategy to increase sales, especially to teens, is for companies to track web searches or "likes" on social media so that they can send you specific advertisements for things you like. Nutrition scientists and dietitians want to make you aware of these strategies and tactics so you can make informed decisions when you choose foods and drinks.

STUDENT ACTIVITY

As you're exposed to media advertisements, try to determine the strategy and tactics being used. Answer the following questions: What is this ad trying to get me to do? Is the product they're selling something I really need? Is the product likely to work as advertised?

LESSON REVIEW

1. How do you define *strategy,* and what are some examples that relate to physical activity and healthy lifestyle choices?

2. How do you define *tactics,* and what is their role in implementing a strategy?

3. What are the five steps for planning strategy and tactics, and how can you use them effectively?

4. What are some ways that you can use strategy and tactics in daily activities other than in sports and physical activities?

TAKING CHARGE: **Developing Tactics**

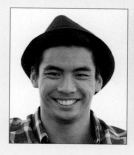 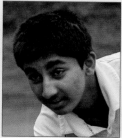 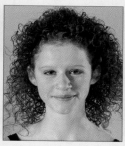 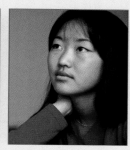

Jason, Ali, Lucy, and Katie have been friends since elementary school. When Ali's mother was diagnosed with breast cancer, the friends wanted to do something to show Ali and his family how much they cared. Jason, Lucy, and Katie got together to plan a strategy. First, they considered what they already knew. They knew the dangers of breast cancer. They also knew that they were not qualified to help medically. After collecting information and considering all options, the group decided on a strategy: They would raise money for breast cancer by planning a special event.

The American Cancer Society (ACS) provides creative opportunities to raise money for the fight against cancer and invites people to raise funds in a variety of ways. The friends went to the ACS website and signed up to do a Bowl-a-thon for Breast Cancer event. After discussing it with their parents, they met with the bowling alley owner, who agreed to help with their plan. To raise money, they asked family, friends, and community members to participate by entering a team. Teams then solicited pledges of money for every pin that they knocked down during the event. The friends needed to find team members, ask supporters for pledges, and take care of other details such as publicizing the event. The funds raised from the Bowl-a-thon were used to make a difference in the fight against cancer.

FOR DISCUSSION

Is the friends' strategy a good one? What other strategies might they have considered? What tactics should they consider to carry out their strategy? How can they best recruit other team members, get pledges, and arrange for the details of the event? Consider the guidelines in the following Self-Management feature as you answer these discussion questions.

SELF-MANAGEMENT: **Skills for Developing Tactics**

You will have opportunities to use strategies and tactics in the future. Use the following guidelines to help you succeed.

- *Plan your strategy.* Use the five steps described in this lesson. Plan tactics after you adopt a strategy.

- *Learn about and list available tactics.* Read, consult with others who have expertise, and observe. Make a list and rate tactics in terms of their likely effect on your strategy's success.

- *Collect information about yourself (or your team or group).* Choose tactics that emphasize your strengths and minimize your weaknesses.

- *Collect information about others who are involved.* If you're competing against another team or individual, collect information about your opponent. If you're planning an event, collect information from others who've been successful and find out as much as you can about the event.

>continued

>*continued*

- *Choose the best tactics.* If you're working with others, consult with your group when making decisions about which tactics to use. If a coach or team leader decides the tactics, provide input.

- *Commit.* Once you've decided, commit to your strategy and tactics.

Taking Action: **Skill Learning Experiment**

In lesson 13.1, you learned that practice and feedback are important for learning skills. **Take action** by conducting a skill learning experiment. Identify a motor skill that you would like to improve or attempt a skill that you have not tried before. For example, you might want to improve your free throw shooting or putting a golf ball, or you might try a new skill such as wand juggling (see Self-Assessment) or pitching pennies into a coffee can.

Have a friend or a coach observe your performance. Perform the skill 10 times (one set). Repeat the skill two more times (2 more sets of 10). Keep a record of each of your performances. Then have your friend or coach offer feedback about how to improve your skill performance. Practice the skill for 3 more sets of 10. Record and analyze your results. Did the practice improve your performance? Did the feedback help? How important is it for the feedback to come from an expert in the skill you are performing? If possible, try the experiment again using a different skill and finding an expert to provide feedback.

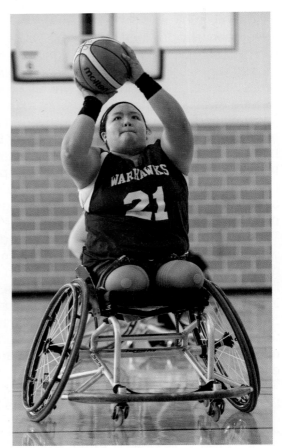

Take action by trying to improve or attempt a skill that you have not tried before.

CHAPTER REVIEW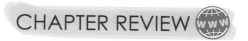

Reviewing Concepts and Vocabulary

Answer items 1 through 5 by correctly completing each sentence with a word or phrase.

1. _____ refers to a group of basic abilities that help you perform physical skills.

2. A _____ is made up of nerves and muscle fibers.

3. Information you receive about your performance that helps you improve is called _____.

4. A _____ is a master plan for achieving a goal.

5. The first step in planning a strategy is to _____.

For items 6 through 10, match each term in column 1 with the appropriate phrase in column 2.

6. marketing   a. first stage of skill learning

7. cognitive stage   b. repetition of a skill to aid improvement

8. Watson   c. a business strategy created to sell a product

9. tactics   d. a supercomputer created by IBM

10. practice   e. methods of implementing a strategy

For items 11 through 15, respond to each statement or question.

11. What are some ways to self-assess your skill-related physical fitness?

12. What is the difference between skills and skill-related physical fitness?

13. Describe the five steps in preparing a strategy and developing tactics.

14. What are some examples of using strategy and tactics in daily life?

15. Describe several guidelines for effective skill learning.

Thinking Critically

Write a paragraph to answer the following question.

How can you use feedback to improve your skill in a specific activity?

Project

You and several friends have started a club for people interested in participating in a sport or other activity. Name the club and develop a marketing strategy for promoting the club. Prepare a report, including details about tactics that will be used to carry out your marketing strategy.

Body Composition and Energy Balance

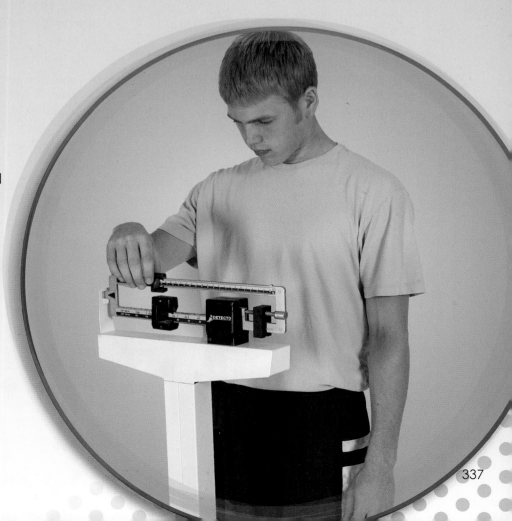

Body Composition Facts

Lesson Objectives

After reading this lesson, you should be able to

1. describe body composition and list some factors that influence body composition;

2. explain how body composition and body fat level are related to good health and describe several eating disorders and their effect on health;

3. describe several laboratory tests for measuring body composition; and

4. describe several nonlaboratory tests for measuring body composition.

Lesson Vocabulary

anorexia athletica
anorexia nervosa
basal metabolism
bioelectrical impedance analysis (BIA)
bulimia
essential body fat
lean body tissue
obesity
overweight
skinfold
underweight

Previously you learned about body composition and how it is defined. But do you know how to assess body composition? In this lesson you will learn about the basics of body composition including information about factors that affect it, methods of self-assessing it, and how to determine whether it is optimal for good health and wellness.

Body Composition Basics

As you know, body composition is a part of health-related physical fitness. In the paragraphs that follow, you'll learn about the types of tissue that make up your body and factors that influence body composition.

Body Composition Definitions

Your body is made up of two major types of tissue. In a healthy person, the great majority of the body consists of **lean body tissue**, including

> I exercise because it is fun—I enjoy it. A bonus is that it helps me to maintain a healthy body composition.
>
> *Presley Olsen*

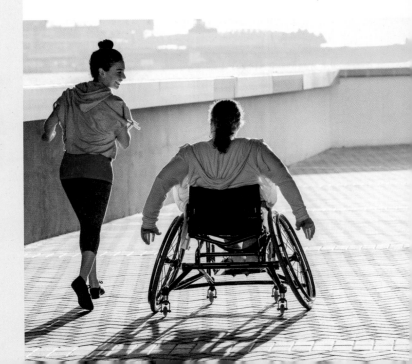

muscle, bone, skin, and organs such as the heart, liver, kidneys, and lungs (figure 14.1). All of the types of physical activity included in the Physical Activity Pyramid build lean body tissue, but muscle fitness exercises are especially important because they both build muscle and enhance bone development.

The other major type of body tissue is fat. Your *body fat level* refers to the percentage of your body that is fat tissue. About half of your body fat is located deep within your body (referred to as central fat). The remaining fat is located between your skin and your muscles.

A fit person has the right amount of body fat—neither too much nor too little. People who do regular physical activity typically have a larger percentage of lean body weight (especially from muscle and bone) and less body fat than people who do not do such activity. Fat should account for a relatively low percentage of your total body weight. However, you do need some body fat for good health. Determining your body fatness requires special equipment and expertise. In the Self-Assessment feature for this chapter, you'll learn how to measure the fat between your skin and muscles to estimate your total body fatness.

The terms **underweight** and **overweight** are commonly used to describe a body weight that is above or below the healthy weight range. However, these terms have limitations because weight does not always accurately reflect the amount of fat and lean tissue in the body. You'll learn more about underweight and overweight later in this chapter.

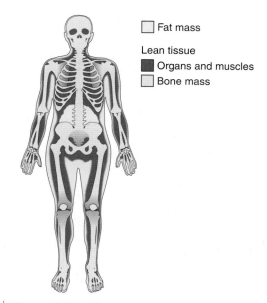

Fat mass

Lean tissue
Organs and muscles
Bone mass

Figure 14.1   Body composition includes body fat and lean body tissue.

Factors Influencing Body Fatness

Many factors influence a person's level of body fat. The most obvious are diet and physical activity. These two factors will be discussed in detail later in this chapter. However, some other factors also determine body composition.

For example, some people are born with a tendency to be lean, or muscular, or heavy. Inherited tendencies make it easier for some people and harder for others to keep their body fat level in the good fitness zone. You can't control your heredity, but you can be aware of tendencies in your family.

Age and sex also influence body composition. Most young people have a high metabolism because their bodies are growing and building muscle. As you grow older and lose muscle mass, your metabolism typically slows, which means that most people need to reduce the number of calories in their diet in order to avoid gaining fat. Keeping your body fat level within the good fitness zone during your childhood and teen years will also help you keep it in check throughout life, because children who are too fat develop extra fat cells that make it more difficult to control their fat level later. Adult females have higher relative body fat levels than males and, as described later, have a different pattern of distributing it.

Maturation is another factor—as you mature, your hormone and body fat levels begin to change. During the teen years, the different female and male hormones are a principal reason why female teens develop more body fat than male teens and why male teens have a relatively higher muscle mass than female teens.

FIT FACT
The term **obesity** refers to the condition of being especially overweight or high in body fat. More than 70 percent of all American adults are considered overweight or obese. About 21 percent of all youth and teens (12 to 19 years of age) are considered obese— more than three times the rate of 30 years ago. This percentage varies by age, sex, and ethnic group. Obesity is especially high among Hispanic, African American, and Native American youth.

Your body composition is also influenced by your **basal metabolism**, or the amount of energy (calories) your body uses just to keep you living. Your basal metabolism does not include the calories you burn while working, studying, or even sitting and watching television. Some people have a higher basal metabolism than others. This means that their bodies, at complete rest, burn more calories than the bodies of people with a lower metabolism. This also means that they can consume more calories than others can without increasing their level of body fat. People with more muscle mass typically have a higher metabolism than people with less muscle mass.

Body Fatness, Health, and Wellness

For good health and normal functioning, your body must maintain a certain amount of body fat, called **essential body fat**. This fat

- helps your body adapt to heat and cold,
- acts as a shock absorber, protecting your organs and bones from injury,
- helps your body use vitamins effectively,
- is stored energy that is available when your body needs it, and
- in reasonable amounts, helps you look your best, thus increasing your feelings of well-being.

High Body Fat Levels

Having too much fat can be unhealthy. Scientists report that people who are high in body fat have a higher risk of heart disease, high blood pressure, diabetes, cancer, and other diseases. Until recently, type 2 diabetes was considered to be an adult disease, but it has become more common among children and teens primarily because of increases in body fat levels among youth. High levels of body fat are also associated with a condition called *metabolic syndrome*. It occurs when a person has a combination of specific health risks, such as high blood pressure, high blood cholesterol, large waist size, and high blood sugar.

In addition, health costs for obese people total thousands of dollars a year more than for people with healthy levels of body fat, and high body fat levels reduce a person's chances of successful surgery. A person with too much body fat also tires more quickly and easily than a lean person and therefore might be less efficient in both work and recreation. Many experts believe that one of the reasons so many adults have too much body fat is that they try to achieve an unrealistic weight or fat level. Instead, experts recommend setting less extreme goals that are achievable, which helps people maintain a healthy level of body fat throughout life.

We have to make sure that our kids still feel good about themselves no matter what their weight, no matter how they feel. We need to make sure that our kids know that we love them no matter who they are, what they look like.

Michelle Obama, former First Lady of the United States

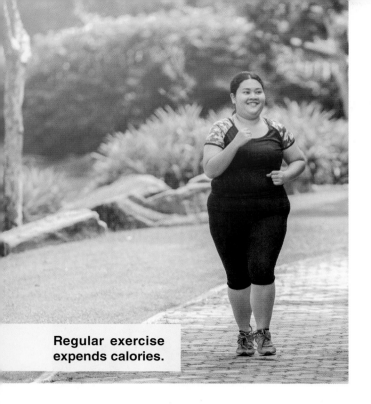

Regular exercise expends calories.

Low Body Fat Levels

Having too little body fat is also a health risk that can cause abnormal functioning of various organs. Females with especially low body fat experience health problems related to their reproductive system and risk losing bone density. Low body fat and low body weight are often associated with eating disorders such as anorexia nervosa, anorexia athletica, and sometimes bulimia. It is extremely important to identify the symptoms of an eating disorder as early as possible. Some eating disorders were mentioned in an earlier chapter but are discussed in more detail here.

Anorexia Nervosa

Anorexia nervosa is a serious eating disorder. A person who has this disorder severely restricts the amount of food that they eat in an attempt to be exceptionally low in body fat. In addition, many people with anorexia do extensive physical activity, thus further lowering their body fat to extremely dangerous levels.

Anorexia is most common among teenage females, but it is becoming increasingly common among teenage males. People with this disorder are usually very hard workers and high achievers. They have a distorted view of their body and see themselves as being too fat even when they are extremely thin. Persons with this disorder

often fear maturity and the weight gain associated with adulthood. They often try to hide their condition by wearing baggy clothing, pretending to eat, and exercising in private. Anorexia is a life-threatening condition, and people who have it need immediate professional help.

Anorexia Athletica

Anorexia athletica typically has symptoms similar to those of anorexia nervosa. It is most common among athletes involved in sports—such as gymnastics, wrestling, and cheerleading—in which low body weight is desirable. It is thought to be related to the pressure to maintain low weight and an excessive preoccupation with dieting and exercising for weight loss. This disorder can lead to anorexia nervosa.

Bulimia

Bulimia is an eating disorder in which a person engages in binge eating (eating a very large amount of food in a short time) followed by purging, either by vomiting or by the use of laxatives to rid the body of food and prevent its digestion. Bulimia can result in severe digestive problems and other health problems such as tooth loss and gum disease. Bulimia is sometimes, but not always, associated with low body fat levels.

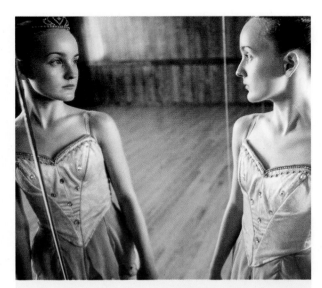

People with eating disorders may be obsessed with their body weight even if they're already thin.

SCIENCE IN ACTION: **Media Misrepresentation**

Over the years, both exercise psychologists and nutrition scientists have conducted research about physical self-perceptions and found that people of all ages are self-conscious about the way they look. In fact, most people are far more critical of their own body than other people are. One reason is that we often compare ourselves with movie stars and other celebrities whose pictures have been designed specifically to make them look as glamorous as possible and are touched up to enhance appearance. For example, a female movie star's waist can be digitally altered to look smaller and a male star's muscles larger. Some magazines have promised to limit changes in photos, but there are no regulations, and each magazine can do as it pleases.

Websites also use fake or altered pictures. Advertisements frequently show supposed before-and-after pictures to promote a product. The "before" photos are taken with bad lighting and in unflattering conditions, with the "after" photos taken in better lighting and conditions. "After" photos may also be altered as well. Video games also present unrealistic images of the human body, often using proportions that are literally impossible for real-life people to attain.

Many experts believe that the misrepresentation of the human body in the media has resulted in an obsession with leanness. Studies show that the number of teens who think they are overweight is four to five times the number who really are. At the same time, interviews with teens who actually are overweight show that 44 percent either have been

or currently are being teased or bullied about their body weight, or "body shamed." This can result in low physical self-perception. For this reason, experts point out the importance of not making critical comments about others. You'll learn more about self-perceptions in the Taking Charge feature in the next lesson of this chapter.

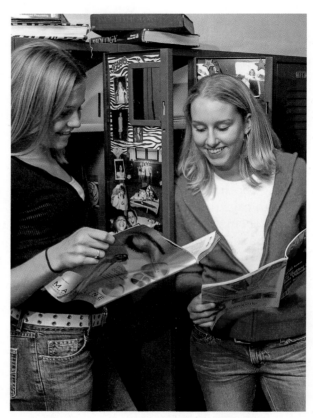

Magazines and websites often alter photos of models and celebrities to make their bodies look unrealistically thin.

STUDENT ACTIVITY

Explore a variety of media sources to find examples of misrepresentation of the human body.

Laboratory Measurements for Assessing Body Composition

The most accurate methods for measuring body composition are typically done in a laboratory and require special equipment and training. Three of the best methods are dual-energy X-ray absorptiometry (DXA), underwater weighing, and air displacement chambers (figure 14.2). All three are useful in determining how much of the body weight is fat and how much is lean tissue.

Dual-Energy X-Ray Absorptiometry

Dual-energy X-ray absorptiometry (DXA) is now considered the best method of assessing body composition (figure 14.2a) because it can accurately detect body fat, bone, muscle, and other body tissues. First, a high-tech X-ray machine takes a three-dimensional picture of the entire body. Then a computer analyzes the picture to determine the amounts of different kinds of tissue, including fat, bone, and muscle.

Underwater Weighing

Until recently, underwater weighing was considered the best way to assess body fat level, and it is still a very good laboratory method. With this technique, you are weighed on land, then immersed in a tank of water and weighed again (figure 14.2b). Measurements of your lung capacity are also taken because the amount of air in your lungs influences your weight in water. A formula is then applied to determine your body fat level based on your land weight, your underwater weight, and your lung capacity.

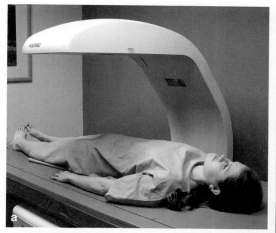

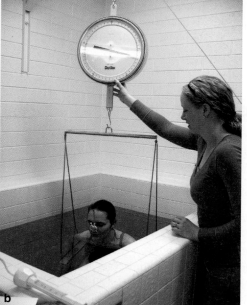

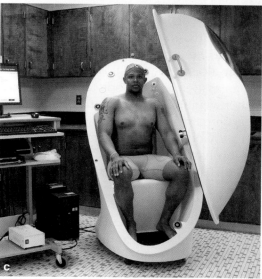

Figure 14.2 Laboratory methods for assessing body composition: *(a)* DXA; *(b)* underwater weighing; *(c)* the Bod Pod Air Displacement Chamber.

FIT FACT

Body shaming or bullying a person about their body is common among teens, especially on social media. Athletes (e.g., Prince Fielder), musicians (e.g., Taylor Swift, Rihanna, Miley Cyrus), and other celebrities (e.g., Jennifer Lawrence, Tyra Banks) have spoken out against body shaming. Teens are encouraged to reject body shaming and embrace positive statements such as "Don't let your mind bully your body" and "Your weight does not define who you are."

Today you are you! That is truer than true! There is no one alive who is you-er than you!

Dr. Seuss, children's author

343

Air Displacement Chambers

A third type of laboratory assessment of body composition uses an air displacement chamber and computer. The most well known is the Bod Pod. In this method, the person being tested sits in an egg-shaped chamber or pod (figure 14.2c), which displaces air from the pod. Information gained from changes in the air in the chamber is then entered into a computer to determine the person's body composition.

Nonlaboratory Measures

Because laboratory measures require special equipment and training, they are rarely used in schools. For school and home use, there are several practical methods of assessment. However, not all of these measures accurately predict the amount of fat and lean body tissue; for this reason, they are typically referred to as *body measurements*. Because you will probably encounter all of these measures at some time in your life, you should try each one of them.

Skinfold Measurements

Your body fat level can also be determined by measuring **skinfold** thickness (the amount of fat under your skin). Skinfold thickness is measured by means of a special instrument called a *caliper* (see figure 14.3). Skinfold measurements can be used to provide an estimate of the total amount of fat in the body. As noted earlier, a high level of body fat is associated with a variety of health problems, including diabetes, heart disease, and other chronic diseases. You'll learn to do skinfold measurements in this chapter's Self-Assessment feature.

Height–Weight and BMI

Height and weight are commonly used in two ways. One method uses height–weight tables that show "normal" weight ranges for people according to age, height, and sex. These tables indicate what the average person of a given sex weighs at a given height. However, because nearly two-thirds of adults in the United States are overweight or obese, many people who are classified as "normal" or "average" are still over-

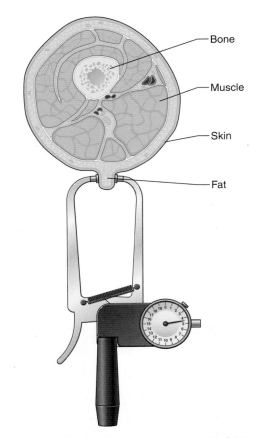

Figure 14.3   A caliper measures skinfolds.

weight or obese. For this reason, height–weight tables are considered less useful than some other methods. Because they are not especially accurate, height–weight tables are not included in this book.

Height and weight are used to calculate a person's body mass index (BMI). This index is considered to be a better measure than height and weight alone, but it still does not give as accurate an assessment of body fatness as DXA, underwater weighing, Bod Pod analysis, or skinfold measurement. Like height–weight charts, BMI can provide inaccurate measurements for people who have a lot of muscle (athletes, for example) because muscle weighs a lot more than fat. As a result, a very muscular person could be high in weight but not too fat. Similarly, a person who appears normal according to BMI charts could actually have an unhealthy level of body fat. This is why skinfolds and laboratory techniques are often considered to be better measures.

In spite of the BMI index's limitations, however, high BMI has been associated with a variety of health problems among both teens and adults. In addition, BMI is often used because it's easy to measure, especially in large groups.

Waist-to-Hip Ratio

The waist-to-hip ratio is used not to determine body fatness but to assess health risk. Scientists now know that people who carry more weight in the middle of the body have a higher risk of disease than people who carry more weight in the lower body (legs and hips). People who carry too much weight in their midsection are said to have an "apple" body type, whereas people who carry more weight in their hips are said to have a "pear" body type. In general, females are more likely to be the pear type, and males are more likely to be the apple type.

The waist-to-hip ratio is a simple method for assessing the risk associated with body type. This ratio is determined by using a tape to measure your waist circumference and your hip circumference. It is desirable to have a waist circumference smaller than your hip circumference. You will measure your waist-to-hip ratio in the Self-Assessment feature.

Waist Girth (Circumference)

Waist girth (also called *waist circumference*) can be used by itself as an indicator of health risk.

Evidence indicates that people with a very large waist are at risk for health problems. As people grow older, their waist size often increases, thus exposing them to greater health risk. Thus, waist girth is a useful health risk indicator that you can use throughout your life.

Bioelectrical Impedance Analysis (BIA)

Bioelectrical impedance analysis (BIA) requires a special machine and was once considered to be a lab measure of body composition. However, in recent years BIA machines have become more common in schools because of lower prices and improved ease of use. Used properly, they can provide reliable and accurate estimates of body fatness. It is important to use the same machine and to be sure that the machine is properly calibrated (tested for accuracy). In addition, it is important to not be dehydrated when tested.

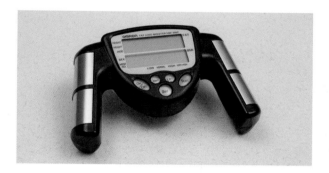

TECH TRENDS: Smart Scales

Many modern scales now have options to provide information other than body weight. Some, called *body fat scales*, measure body fat using built-in BIA. Others can also calculate your BMI. However, *Consumer Reports* found that none of the scales tested were accurate for testing body fat levels. The value of the BMI feature is also questionable, because you must input your height and BMI is easy to calculate yourself.

The most important features of a scale are accuracy (giving your correct weight) and reliability (giving accurate results every time you weigh). *Consumer Reports* found accuracy and reliability to range from fair to excellent for various scales. The most accurate and reliable scales were relatively low in cost—and the most expensive scale tested was the least accurate. Consult current ratings before buying a scale.

USING TECHNOLOGY

Consult an authoritative source, such as *Consumer Reports*, to determine which smart scales give the most accurate and reliable measurement. Write a report indicating which scale you would recommend.

What Is My Ideal Body Weight?

Even after learning about the various forms of assessment, many people wonder what their ideal body weight is. Experts agree that there is no such thing as one ideal body weight for all people. The best advice is to set a long-term goal of achieving a body fat level in the good fitness zone. Once you have achieved this goal (see Self-Assessment), weigh yourself and maintain that weight (this is sometimes referred to as *target weight*). It's a desirable lifetime goal to maintain this weight and a fat level in the good fitness zone.

If you're in the marginal or low fitness zone, develop a plan that will gradually move you to the next zone. Trying to achieve the good fitness zone when you're too far from it is unrealistic. Instead, people in the low fitness zone should try to move to the marginal zone. Those in the marginal zone should try to move to the good fitness zone. If you're already in the good fitness zone, a reasonable goal for you is simply to stay there.

Some athletes and people in careers that require high levels of fitness may be in the very lean zone, and some people can be very lean because of hereditary factors. Though it is possible to be fit and healthy and be in the very lean zone, exceptional leanness is not necessarily a sign of good health and may not be a realistic goal for all people. As noted earlier in this chapter, your body needs a certain amount of essential body fat, and having too little can cause health problems. It is important for all people to eat well, especially people who want to be athletes or perform jobs that require high levels of fitness.

As part of a lifelong self-assessment plan, you may choose to monitor your waist-to-hip ratio and your waist girth, especially if you find it difficult to get a good assessment of your body fat level. These measurements are good indicators of health risk. You may also choose to track your BMI over time because physicians often use this measure. High BMI is associated with health risks, but as noted earlier, BMI does not estimate body fat levels or lean body mass.

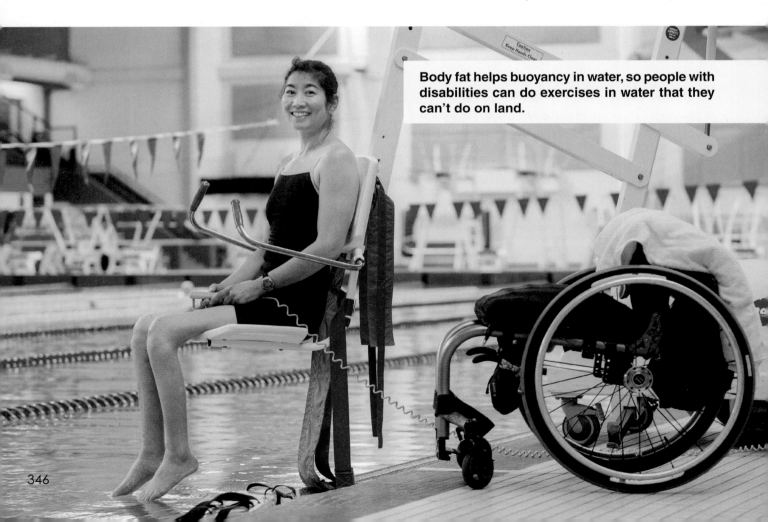

Body fat helps buoyancy in water, so people with disabilities can do exercises in water that they can't do on land.

For this reason, it may misclassify some people as overweight or obese when they are not. Similarly, BMI may classify a person as "normal" in weight when the person has a higher than healthy level of body fat. The same is true for height–weight charts.

Assessment Confidentiality

Self-assessments are done to gain information that will help the person build an accurate personal profile and plan for healthy active living. As noted throughout this book, the results of self-assessments are personal information. Body composition measurements are especially sensitive. For this reason, it is especially important that care be taken to ensure that results of self-assessments remain confidential. When you work with a partner, you and your partner must agree to keep test results private. Information may be submitted to an instructor or a parent or guardian but always with the expectation that the information is private. Assessment-related information should not be shared with others without permission from the person being tested.

LESSON REVIEW

1. What is body composition, and what are some factors that influence body composition?
2. How do body composition and body fat levels relate to good health? What are eating disorders and how do they affect health?
3. What are some laboratory tests for measuring body composition?
4. What are some nonlaboratory tests for measuring body composition?

SELF-ASSESSMENT: Body Measurements

Earlier in this chapter, you learned about ways to determine body composition. Laboratory measures are the most accurate, but they require expensive equipment and trained professionals. BMI is the most commonly used nonlaboratory measure because it can be determined easily using height and weight and does not require a lot of equipment.

In addition, body measurements (such as waist-to-hip ratio and waist girth) can be used to determine health risks, and skinfold measurements can be used both to estimate body fat and to assess health risk. Your fitness scores are your personal information and should be kept confidential. You should also be sensitive to the feelings of others when body fat measurements are being taken; it may be appropriate to take measurements privately. Record your results as directed by your instructor.

BODY MASS INDEX (BMI)

In chapter 4 you completed height and weight measurements and determined your BMI. For this reason, it is not described here.

WAIST-TO-HIP RATIO (MALE AND FEMALE)

1. Measure your hips at the largest point (the largest circumference of your buttocks). Make sure that the tape is parallel to the ground all the way around. The tape should be snug but not so tight as to cause indentations in your skin. Do not use an elastic tape. Stand with your feet together when making the measurement.
2. Measure your waist at the smallest circumference (called the natural waist). If there is no natural waist, measure at the level of the navel. Measure just after a normal in-breath.

Do not suck in to make your waist smaller. This measurement is slightly different from the one used to measure waist girth by itself.

3. To calculate your waist-to-hip ratio, divide your waist girth by your hip girth.

4. Find your ratio in table 14.1 to determine your rating.

5. Record your hip and waist measurements and rating.

To determine your waist-to-hip ratio, measure (a) your hips and (b) your waist.

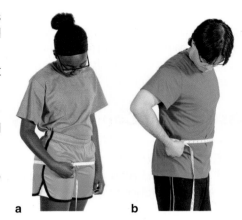

TABLE 14.1   Rating Chart: Waist-to-Hip Ratio

	Male	Female
Good fitness	≤0.90	≤0.79
Marginal fitness	0.91–1.0	0.80–0.85
Low fitness	≥1.1	≥0.86

WAIST GIRTH (CIRCUMFERENCE)

1. Measure your waist at a level just above the top of your hipbones. Mark the top of your hipbone on each side and hold the tape just above the marks.

2. Measure at the end of a normal in-breath. Do not suck in to make your waist smaller. Keep the tape horizontal to the ground when making the measurement.

3. Use table 14.2 to determine your rating.

4. Record your waist girth and rating.

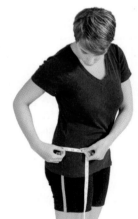

Waist girth is determined by measuring your waist above the hipbone.

TABLE 14.2   Rating Chart: Waist Girth (Inches)

Age (years)	12	13	14	15	16	17	≥18
Male							
Good fitness	≤28.9	≤29.9	≤30.9	≤31.9	≤32.9	≤33.9	≤34.9
Marginal fitness	29.0–33.4	30.0–34.4	31.0–35.9	32.0–37.4	33.0–38.4	34.0–39.9	35.0–41.4
Low fitness	≥33.5	≥34.5	≥36.0	≥37.5	≥38.5	≥40.0	≥41.5
Female							
Good fitness	≤28.9	≤29.9	≤30.9	≤31.9	≤32.4	≤33.4	≤34.4
Marginal fitness	29.0–32.4	30.0–33.9	31.0–34.9	32.0–35.9	32.5–38.4	33.5–38.4	34.5–39.9
Low fitness	≥32.5	≥34.0	≥35.0	≥36.0	≥38.5	≥38.5	≥40.0

To convert centimeters to inches, divide by 2.54 (1 ft = 12 in.).

SKINFOLD MEASUREMENTS

Skinfolds are measured with a caliper, and using a caliper effectively requires special training (learning correct technique and practicing on many people). But when done properly by a trained expert, skinfold measurements can provide a good estimate of body fatness. For best results, an expensive caliper is used, but research has shown that an inexpensive plastic caliper can also be quite accurate if used properly. Various measurements can be used; in this book, the calf and triceps are used because of their ease of measurement.

Use the following procedures to complete the measurements and determine your ratings for each measurement. You can use skinfold measurements to estimate your body fat percentage. For teenagers, upper arm (triceps) and calf measurements provide a good estimate. Work with a partner to take each other's measurements. With practice, you and your partner will improve your measurement skills. If possible, also have measurements done by an expert. Comparing your measurements to those done by an expert will help you determine the accuracy of the measurements. Remember that self-assessment information is confidential and shouldn't be shared with others without the permission of the person being tested.

For the triceps skinfold, use a skinfold on the middle of the back of the right arm, halfway between the elbow and the shoulder. The arm should hang loose and relaxed at the side.

For the calf skinfold, the person being tested should stand and place their right foot on a chair. Measure a skinfold on the inside of the right calf, halfway between the shin and the back of the calf, where the calf is largest.

1. Use your left thumb and index finger to hold the skinfold. Do not pinch or squeeze the skinfold.

2. Hold the skinfold with your left hand while you pick up and use the caliper with your right hand to get a reading.

3. Place the caliper over the skinfold about 0.5 inch (1.3 centimeters) below your finger and thumb. Hold the caliper on the skinfold for 3 seconds, then note the measurement. If possible, read the caliper measurement to the nearest half-millimeter.

4. Make three measurements each for the triceps and the calf skinfolds. Allow at least 10 seconds between measurements. Use the middle of the three measures as the score. If your three measurements differ by more than 2 millimeters, take a second, or even third, set of three measurements.

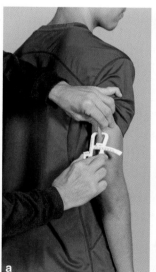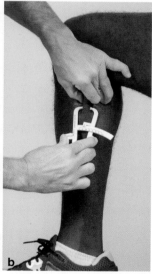

Skinfold measurements: *(a)* triceps; *(b)* calf.

5. Now determine your body fat percentage and your body fatness rating. Add your triceps and calf scores to get your sum in millimeters, then use table 14.3 to estimate your body fat percentage based on your sum. Use the appropriate table for your sex and find your skinfold sum. Your body fat percentage is the number just to the right. For example, if you're male and your skinfold sum is 26, your body fat percentage is 21.

6. Once you have determined your percent body fat, use table 14.4 to determine your body fatness rating.

TABLE 14.3   Body Fat Percentage From Skinfolds

Sum (mm)	% fat	Sum (mm)	% fat	Sum (mm)	% fat	Sum (mm)	% fat	Sum (mm)	% fat	Sum (mm)	% fat
Male											
5	6	15	13	25	20	35	28	45	35	55	42
6	7	16	14	26	21	36	28.5	46	36	56	43
7	7.5	17	14.5	27	21.5	37	29	47	36.5	57	43.5
8	8	18	15	28	22	38	30	48	37	58	44
9	9	19	16	29	23	39	30.5	49	37.5	59	44.5
10	10	20	17	30	24	40	31	50	38	60	45
11	10.5	21	17.5	31	25	41	32	51	39		
12	11	22	18	32	26	42	33	52	39.5		
13	11.5	23	18.5	33	26.5	43	33.5	53	40		
14	12	24	19	34	27	44	34	54	41		
Female											
5	7	15	14	25	21	35	29	45	36	55	43
6	8	16	15	26	22	36	29.5	46	37	56	44
7	8.5	17	15.5	27	22.5	37	30	47	37.5	57	44.5
8	9	18	16	28	23	38	30.5	48	38	58	45
9	10	19	17	29	24	39	31	49	38.5	59	45.5
10	11	20	18	30	24.5	40	32	50	39	60	46
11	12	21	18.5	31	25	41	33	51	40		
12	12.5	22	19	32	26	42	34	52	40.5		
13	13	23	19.5	33	27	43	34.5	53	41		
14	13.5	24	20	34	28	44	35	54	42		

Reprinted by permission, from Dr. Tim G. Lohman, Department of Exercise and Sport Sciences, University of Arizona.

TABLE 14.4   Rating Chart: Body Fatness (Percentage)

	Age (years)					
Rating	**13**	**14**	**15**	**16**	**17**	**18 or older**
Male						
Very lean	≤7.7	≤7.0	≤6.5	≤6.4	≤6.6	≤6.9
Good fitness	7.8–22.8	7.1–21.3	6.6–20.1	6.5–20.1	6.7–20.9	7.0–22.2
Marginal fitness	22.9–34.9	21.4–33.1	20.2–31.4	20.2–31.5	21.0–32.9	22.3–35.0
Low fitness	≥35.0	≥33.2	≥31.5	≥31.6	≥33.0	≥35.1
Female						
Very lean	≤13.3	≤13.9	≤14.5	≤15.2	≤15.8	≤16.5
Good fitness	13.4–27.7	14.0–28.5	14.6–29.1	15.3–29.7	15.9–30.4	16.6–31.3
Marginal fitness	27.8–36.2	28.6–36.7	29.2–37.0	29.8–37.3	30.5–37.8	31.4–38.5
Low fitness	≥36.3	≥36.8	≥37.1	≥37.4	≥37.9	≥38.6

Lesson Objectives

After reading this lesson, you should be able to

1. define *energy balance* and describe the FIT formula for fat control;

2. describe how many calories are expended doing various physical activities;

3. explain how physical activity helps a person maintain a healthy body fat level; and

4. describe some common myths about fat control.

Lesson Vocabulary

calorie
calorie expenditure
calorie intake
energy balance

Do you know what *energy balance* means? Do you know how many calories you consume and expend in a typical day? One major health goal is to achieve and maintain an acceptable level of body fat throughout your life. To do this, you must balance the calories you consume and the calories you expend. In this lesson, you'll learn the FIT formula for fat control and appropriate activities for gaining weight and losing body fat.

Energy Balance Basics

The term **calorie** is commonly used to describe the amount of energy in a food. The true term is *kilocalorie* (a unit of energy or heat), but when talking about diet and nutrition, *calorie* is typically used. **Energy balance** refers to balancing calorie intake and calorie expenditure (figure 14.4). **Calorie intake** is the number of calories (or total energy) in the foods you eat. **Calorie expenditure** is the number of calories (energy) you burn by doing physical activity. If you take in

> I accept and love my body for what it is, but I still give effort to make it better. That's why I stay active and eat a healthy diet.
>
> *Mateo Esquibel*

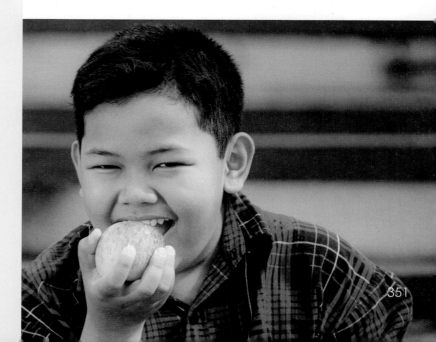

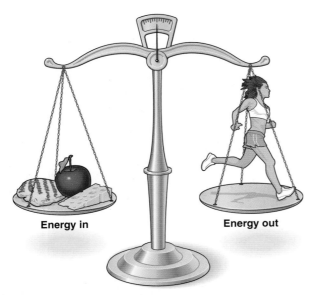

Figure 14.4 Balancing energy intake with energy output is essential for healthy weight maintenance.

(eat) more calories than you expend (in activity), you will gain weight because extra energy is stored in the body as fat. If you expend more calories than you take in, you will lose weight. If you balance the calories you consume and expend, you will maintain your current weight.

Table 14.5 provides the FIT formula for diet and physical activity. The information will help you determine the optimal frequency of activity and eating, the calories you need to expend and consume for energy balance, and appropriate time lines for maintaining a healthy body composition.

Calories In and Calories Out

Earlier in this lesson, you learned about the importance of balancing calories in your diet

TABLE 14.5 **FIT Formula for Maintaining a Healthy Body Composition**

	Diet*	Physical activity**
Frequency	Eat three regular meals or four or five small meals daily. Regular, controlled eating is best. Skipping meals and snacking is usually not effective for fat loss. Extra healthy meals or snacks are necessary for highly active people.	Participate in physical activity daily. Regular physical activity is best for losing fat. Muscle fitness exercise is necessary for gaining muscle mass.
Intensity	To lose 1 pound (about 0.5 kg) of fat, you must eat 3,500 fewer calories than normal over a given span of time. To gain 1 pound (0.5 kg) of fat, you must eat 3,500 more calories than normal over a given span of time. To maintain your weight, you must maintain energy balance.	To lose 1 pound (0.5 kg) of fat, you must use 3,500 more calories than normal over a given span of time. To gain 1 pound (0.5 kg) of fat, you must use 3,500 fewer calories than normal over a given span of time. Building muscle with muscle fitness exercise expends calories that must be replaced with healthy calorie intake.
Time	Neither dietary change nor physical activity results in quick fat loss. Medical experts recommend that a person lose no more than 2 pounds (1 kg) per week without medical supervision.	Together, diet and physical activity can be used to safely lose 1–2 pounds (0.5–1.0 kg) per week. Together, diet and muscle fitness exercises can result in muscle gain but should be done gradually because it takes time for exercise to build muscle mass.

*Assumes that physical activity is constant

**Assumes that diet is constant

and calories expended in your physical activities. In the paragraphs that follow you will learn more about typical teen calorie intake and the number of calories expended in various activities.

Calories in the Food You Eat

According to the national dietary guidelines, the number of calories consumed by teens varies depending on age, sex, and activity level. For males, daily calorie intake should range from 2,000 to 2,400 for inactive teens, 2,400 to 2,800 for somewhat active teens, and 2,800 to 3,200 for very active teens. For females, daily calorie intake ranges from 1,800 to 2,000 for inactive teens, 2,000 to 2,400 for somewhat active teens, and 2,400 to 2,800 for very active teens.

Physical Activity and Calories

To maintain a healthy weight, you must balance the calories that you take in with the calories that you expend. As you learned earlier, you expend calories even at rest (basal metabolism). The majority of calories are expended in various forms of physical activity, including activities from all steps of the Physical Activity Pyramid (figure 14.5). Even light activities, such as playing computer games or practicing a musical instrument, expend calories above resting levels. All calories count.

The more intense the activity, the greater the number of calories expended. Moderate activity (step 1) expends more calories than resting or light activity. Vigorous activities (steps 2 through 4) expend more calories than moderate activities. On the other hand, moderate activities can be performed for long periods of time, so they can be equally effective in expending calories as vigorous activities—it just takes more time.

Muscle fitness exercises (step 4) build muscle tissue and expend calories. Additionally, muscle expends more energy at rest, so building muscle helps you expend more calories over time. Flexibility exercises typically do not expend as many calories as vigorous activities but are similar in intensity to moderate activity.

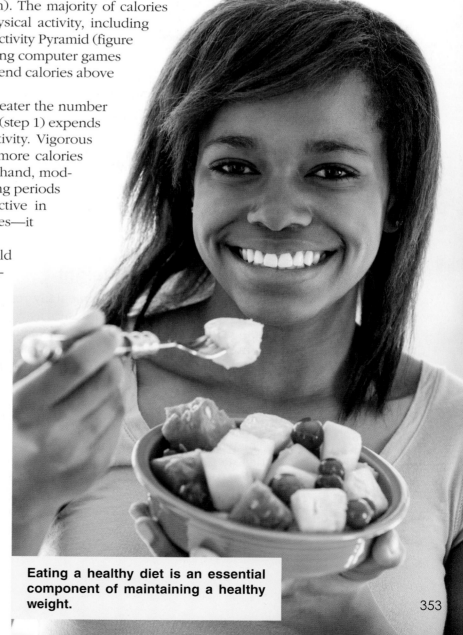

Eating a healthy diet is an essential component of maintaining a healthy weight.

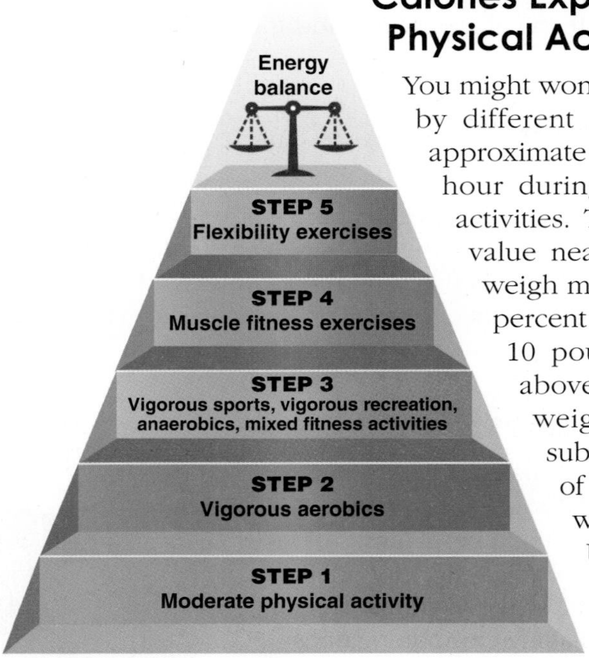

Calories Expended in Specific Physical Activities

Figure 14.5 All activities in the Physical Activity Pyramid result in calorie expenditure and aid in energy balance.

You might wonder how many calories are burned by different activities. Table 14.6 shows the approximate number of calories burned each hour during selected vigorous recreational activities. To use the table, find the weight value nearest to your own weight. If you weigh more than the nearest weight, add 5 percent to the number of calories for each 10 pounds (4.5 kilograms) you weigh above the listed weight value. If you weigh less than the nearest weight, subtract 5 percent from the number of calories for each 10 pounds you weigh below the listed weight value. Use this table to determine which physical activities are best for burning calories, then see which activities appeal to you.

Choice, not chance, determines your destiny.

Aristotle, Greek philosopher

FIT FACT

A distance runner burns 100 to 150 calories per mile depending on factors such as sex, body size, and speed and efficiency of running. For a full marathon (26.2 miles), that amounts to 2,620 to 3,930 calories expended.

Gaining and Losing Weight

As you have learned, to lose weight, you must expend more energy than you take in (3,500 calories = 1 pound). To gain weight, you must take in more calories than you expend. In the paragraphs that follow you will learn more about healthy ways to lose and gain body weight and fat.

Gaining Muscle Weight

Regular physical activity, particularly resistance exercise, is the best way to gain muscle. Remember that all physical activity burns calories, so you need to increase your calorie intake in order to gain weight and sometimes to maintain weight when you increase your activity. Most people do not need to eat a special diet or take supplements to gain muscle; you need only eat a well-balanced diet that contains more calories and adequate amounts of all important nutrients (see chapter 16).

Physical Activity and Weight Loss

The best way to lose weight is to combine regular physical activity with a healthy diet. Research shows that a person who reduces calorie intake without increasing activity will lose both fat and muscle tissue, whereas a person who increases physical activity and reduces calorie consumption loses mostly body fat.

Selecting a variety of activities that you enjoy improves your chances of sticking with your activity plan. As indicated earlier in this lesson, moderate activities expend fewer calories per minute than vigorous activities but are often equally effective

TABLE 14.6 **Energy Expenditure in Physical Activities**

	Calories used per hour based on weight				
	100 lb (45 kg)	120 lb (54 kg)	150 lb (68 kg)	180 lb (82 kg)	200 lb (91 kg)
Backpacking/Hiking	307	348	410	472	513
Badminton	255	289	340	391	425
Baseball	210	238	280	322	350
Basketball (half-court)	225	240	300	345	375
Bicycling (normal speed)	157	178	210	242	263
Bowling	155	176	208	240	261
Canoeing (4 mph [6.5 kph])	276	344	414	504	558
Circuit training	247	280	330	380	413
Dance (ballet/modern)	240	300	360	432	480
Dance (aerobic)	300	360	450	540	600
Dance (social)	174	222	264	318	348
Fitness calisthenics	232	263	310	357	388
Football	225	255	300	345	375
Golf (walking)	187	212	250	288	313
Gymnastics	232	263	310	357	388
Horseback riding	180	204	240	276	300
Interval training	487	552	650	748	833
Jogging (5.5 mph [9 kph])	487	552	650	748	833
Judo/Karate	232	263	310	357	388
Jumping rope (continuous)	525	595	700	805	875
Racquetball/Handball	450	510	600	690	750
Running (10 mph [16 kph])	625	765	900	1,035	1,125
Skating (ice or roller)	262	297	350	403	438
Skiing (cross-country)	525	595	700	805	875
Skiing (downhill)	450	510	600	690	750
Soccer	405	459	540	575	621
Softball (fastpitch)	210	238	280	322	350
Swimming (slow laps)	240	272	320	368	400
Swimming (fast laps)	420	530	630	768	846
Tennis	315	357	420	483	525
Volleyball	262	297	350	403	483
Walking	204	258	318	372	426
Weight training	352	399	470	541	558

ACADEMIC CONNECTION: **Calculating Your Calorie Expenditure in Physical Activity**

Tools are now available that help you to determine how much energy (how many calories) you expend when you perform physical activity. One tool is an energy expenditure table such as table 14.6. But energy expenditure tables often do not include every activity that you perform. To find calorie expenditures for additional activities, an activity calculator from a reliable organization such as the American Council on Exercise (search "ACE physical activity calorie counter") can be used.

Consider this example. Roger kept an activity log and made calculations for a two-hour period during one weekend day. He used table 14.6 and his weight (180 pounds) to determine calories expended in jogging and basketball (half court). To determine calories expended in watching TV and talking on the phone, he use the ACE online physical activity calculator. He entered his weight (180 pounds) and the time spent in each activity to get the calorie values. His activity log is shown in table 14.7.

TABLE 14.7   Roger's Calories Expended for a Two-Hour Time Period

Time of day	Activity	Minutes	Calories expended
9:00–9:30	Morning jog	30	374
9:30–10:10	Watch TV	40	48
10:10–10:40	Basketball (half-court)	30	173
10:40–11:00	Talking on phone (sitting)	20	24
	Total	**120**	**619**

STUDENT ACTIVITY

Record your activities for a two-hour period in which you participate in moderate or vigorous activity for at least half of the time. Prepare a table and calculate your calorie expenditure using steps similar to Roger's.

FIT FACT

If you maintain your normal calorie intake and increase your activity by playing 30 minutes of tennis daily, you will lose 16 pounds (about 7 kilograms) in a year. If you walk briskly for 15 minutes a day instead of watching TV, you will lose 5 or 6 pounds (about 2.5 kilograms) in a year. On the other hand, if you sit for 15 minutes instead of taking a regular 15-minute walk each day, you will gain 5 to 6 pounds in a year.

because they can be performed for longer periods of time. Research shows that for many people, vigorous activity is considered less enjoyable than moderate activity. If this is true of you, consider moderate activity.

Eating a healthy diet and limiting calorie intake are equally important. As long as you are meeting activity guidelines, excessive calorie restriction is counterproductive. More information on nutrition is presented in chapter 15.

Myths About Fat Loss

Table 14.8 identifies some common myths and mistakes about fat loss, as well as the facts about losing body fat. No matter what your body is like now, regular physical activity and proper diet will help you control body fat. When you're fit, you look better, feel better, and have fewer health problems than unfit people who have a high level of body fat.

TABLE 14.8 **Myths and Facts About Fat Loss**

Myth	Fact
Exercise cannot be effective for fat loss because it takes many hours of exercise to lose even 1 pound (0.5 kg) of fat.	You can lose body fat over time with regular physical activity if your calorie intake remains the same. Fat lost through physical activity tends to stay off longer than fat lost through dieting alone.
Exercise does not help you lose fat because it increases your hunger and encourages you to overeat.	If you are moderately active instead of inactive, your hunger should not increase. Even moderate to vigorous activity will not cause hunger to increase so much that you overeat. People who overeat usually do so for other reasons (habit, anxiousness, presence of empty calories, large portion sizes, and so on).
Most people with too much body fat have glandular problems.	Some people do have glandular problems, but most people who are high in body fat eat too much, do too little physical activity, or both.
You can spot-reduce by exercising a specific body part to lose fat in that area.	Any exercise that burns calories will cause the body's general fat deposits to decrease. A given exercise does not cause one area of fat to decrease more than another.

LESSON REVIEW

1. What is energy balance, and what is the FIT formula for fat control?
2. How many calories are expended while doing various physical activities?
3. How does physical activity help a person maintain a healthy weight and body fat level?
4. What are some common myths about fat control?

TAKING CHARGE: **Improving Physical Self-Perception**

Everyone has their own self-perception, or mental picture of themselves. If you think you will do well in a certain activity, you'll probably take part. If you feel embarrassed about your appearance or ability level while doing an activity, you'll probably avoid it. Here are two very different examples of physical self-perception.

Michael was not sure that he wanted to go back

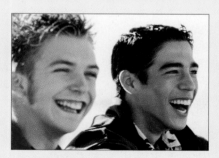

to school after the summer break. It seemed as if all of his friends had grown taller in the last few months, but he had stayed the same height.

Michael felt embarrassed and a little jealous, even though none of his friends seemed to notice. His height certainly did not alter his ability to play tennis. In fact, his friends still called him "King of the Court" because he usually won.

Michael's friend Raul was one of the shortest people in his class, but his height did not stop him from being involved in activities. He

>continued

>continued

knew that he had never been a great basketball player, but he still liked to play with his friends from school. He also knew that height had nothing to do with his ability to go hiking, nor did it prevent him from being a good wrestler.

FOR DISCUSSION

Michael had a negative self-perception because of his height. What can he do to change his negative self-perception? How does Raul keep a positive self-perception? What else can a person do to develop a positive self-perception? Consider the guidelines in the following Self-Management feature as you answer these discussion questions.

SELF-MANAGEMENT: Skills for Improving Physical Self-Perception

A self-perception is an idea you have about your own thoughts, actions, or appearance. It is influenced by how you think other people view you. Some of the many kinds of self-perception are academic, social, and artistic. In this book, the focus is on physical self-perception—the way you view your physical self.

Four aspects of physical self-perception are strength, fitness, skill, and physical attractiveness. People with good physical self-perceptions are happy with their current strength and fitness levels; they also feel that their skills are adequate to meet their needs, and they like the way they look. We know that people who have positive physical self-perceptions are more likely to be physically active than those who do not. The following list provides guidelines you can use to maintain or improve your physical self-perceptions.

- *Assess your physical self-perceptions.* You may use the worksheet provided by your teacher to determine whether you have any areas in which your physical self-perceptions are especially low (strength, fitness, skill, or physical attractiveness).

- *Work to improve your physical fitness and skills.* Regular physical activity can help you look your best, and learning and practicing skills can help you perform your best.

- *Consider a new way of thinking about yourself.* People often set unrealistic standards for themselves, such as looking like someone they see on television or in the movies. Understand that in real life these people do not look the way they look on the screen. Their appearance is enhanced by makeup, lighting, and even special cameras and computer graphics. You also do not know whether a movie star has an eating disorder or practices healthy habits. Consider your heredity and set realistic standards for yourself.

- *Think positively.* Almost all people have a physical characteristic that they would like to change. But studies show that the things people don't like about themselves are rarely seen as problems by other people. You're often your own worst critic, and thinking positively can help you present yourself in a positive way.

- *Do not let the actions of a few insensitive people cause you to feel negatively about yourself.* There will always be some people who are insensitive to others' feelings. These people often have low self-perceptions and try to build themselves up by tearing other people down. Recognize that criticism from these people is their problem, not yours.

- *Consider how your behavior and actions influence the way other people view you.* Acting cheerful and friendly has as much to do with how others perceive you as your physical characteristics.

- *Realize that all people have some imperfections.* Try to build on your strengths and improve your areas of weakness.

- *Find a realistic role model and be a role model for others.* Instead of trying to be like someone who is totally unlike you, find someone you admire who has characteristics you can realistically achieve. And, just as you look to others, remember that others may look to you as a role model. Providing a positive model for others can help you think positively about yourself.

Taking Action: **Elastic Band Workout**

Muscle fitness exercises provide a triple benefit in helping you to maintain a healthy body composition. First, they build muscles that help you look your best. Second, they expend energy, thus helping you to achieve a good energy balance. Finally, the extra muscle that you build through resistance exercise causes you to burn extra calories even at rest.

You can **take action** by completing an elastic band resistance circuit. Elastic bands are useful because they are affordable, travel well, and allow you to easily exercise many muscles. They are appropriate for people of all fitness levels, and they will help you improve your overall coordination and your muscular fitness. Consider the following guidelines for performing elastic resistance band exercises.

- When choosing bands, make sure they are the right length for you and that they do not have cracks or other signs of wear.
- Choose a band that provides the proper resistance for you to perform the recommended number of sets and reps.
- You can also do resistance exercises that use your body weight to add variation and create a good workout circuit.

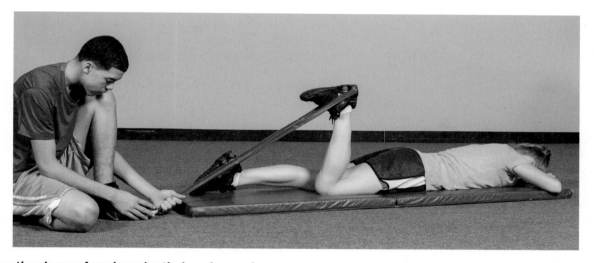

Take action by performing elastic band exercises.

CHAPTER REVIEW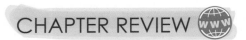

Reviewing Concepts and Vocabulary

Answer items 1 through 5 by correctly completing each sentence with a word or phrase.

1. The majority of the body consists of _____ such as muscle, bone, and body organs.

2. An eating disorder characterized by bingeing and purging is called _____.

3. The minimum amount of body fat needed for good health is called _____.

4. The amount of energy necessary to keep your body living is called _____.

5. Keeping your calories consumed equal to your calories expended is called _____.

For items 6 through 10, match each term in column 1 with the appropriate phrase in column 2.

6. metabolic syndrome   a. best laboratory measure of body composition

7. caliper   b. device used to measure skinfolds

8. DXA   c. condition associated with multiple health risk factors, such as high blood pressure and cholesterol

9. anorexia athletica   d. energy your body uses just to keep you living

10. basal metabolism   e. eating disorder characterized by excessive exercise

For items 11 through 15, as directed by your teacher, respond to each statement or question.

11. Explain why 3,500 calories is an important number for maintaining a healthy body composition.

12. Why is confidentiality so important when making body composition assessments?

13. Why is it important to maintain essential body fat?

14. Describe one myth about fat loss and explain how it is incorrect or misleading.

15. What are some guidelines for improving physical self-perceptions?

Thinking Critically

Write a paragraph to answer the following question.

Each year, people spend billions of dollars on weight loss and muscle building products that do not work. Look at a newspaper, popular magazine, or website and find an advertisement for a weight loss product. Read the ad and make a list of its claims. Which claims are consistent with the information presented in this chapter? Which claims appear to be false or questionable?

Project

The U.S. government provides annual ratings of obesity for each state and for some cities. Prepare a poster showing how your city or state compares with the U.S. average. List five factors that you think may cause your state to rank as it does.

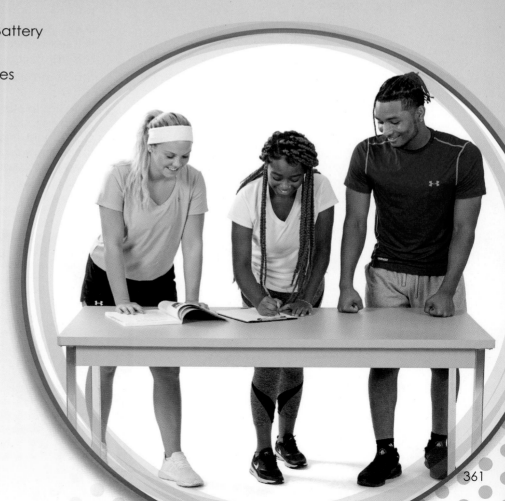

Planning and Maintaining Active Lifestyles

15

In This Chapter

Preparing a Comprehensive Physical Activity Plan

Lesson Objectives

After reading this lesson, you should be able to

1. explain how to use a personal fitness profile to establish personal needs;

2. describe how you prepare a list of physical activity options;

3. describe how you prepare a list of short-term and long-term program goals; and

4. describe what you should include in a written plan and how you evaluate its success.

Lesson Vocabulary

cognitive skills
fitness profile

Do you have a personal fitness and physical activity plan? In other chapters, you've been introduced to the five steps of program planning, learned which types of activity are most appropriate for building each part of health-related physical fitness, and planned a program for each of the five types of activity included in the Physical Activity Pyramid. In this lesson, you'll read about the comprehensive program that Alicia developed, then use the plans you've previously developed to create your own comprehensive personal physical activity program.

Step 1: Determine Your Personal Needs

As you know from your previous program planning, collecting information is the first step toward making good decisions and preparing a good plan. In this case, you will use the many self-assessments that you've performed throughout this class to construct a comprehensive fitness profile.

> By failing to plan, you are planning to fail. That's what Coach said. I have found that the saying works for me in more ways than playing sports.
>
> *Cayden Perkins*

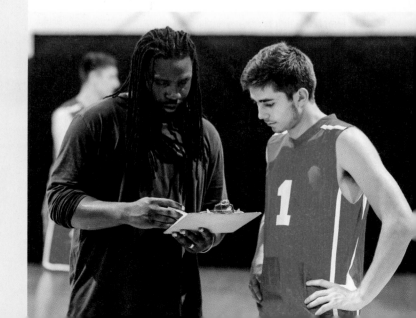

A **fitness profile** is a brief summary of self-assessment results that helps you determine your areas of personal need. You can see a sample fitness profile for 15-year-old Alicia in table 15.1. To create a fitness profile, make a list of all of the fitness self-assessments that you have performed and your scores and ratings for each. Your profile should look similar to the one that Alicia prepared.

Alicia also prepared a physical activity profile (see table 15.2). Walking to school, jogging, tennis, and aerobic dance accounted for 60 minutes of moderate to vigorous activity on five days a week, so she was close to meeting the national guidelines for these activities. Alicia did not do any exercises for muscle fitness and flexibility on a regular basis and did none for the last week, so she did not meet those national goals.

Prepare a written activity profile similar to the one prepared by Alicia.

Step 2: Consider Your Program Options

Alicia prepared a list of several activities to consider for her activity plan. She was already doing some walking and jogging, but she was not

TABLE 15.1   **Alicia's Fitness Profile**

Self-assessment	Rating
Cardiorespiratory endurance	
PACER	Good fitness
Step test	Good fitness
Walking test	Good fitness
One-mile run	Marginal fitness
Muscle fitness	
Curl-up	Good fitness
Push-up	Marginal fitness
1RM arm press (per lb of body weight)	Good fitness
1RM leg press (per lb of body weight)	Marginal fitness
Muscular endurance	
Grip strength (left)	Marginal fitness
Grip strength (right)	Good fitness
Standing long jump	Marginal fitness
Medicine ball throw	Good fitness
Body composition	
Body mass index (BMI)	Good fitness
Skinfold measures	Good fitness
Waist-to-hip ratio	Good fitness
Waist girth	Good fitness
Flexibility	
Back-saver sit-and-reach	Low fitness
Trunk lift	Marginal fitness
Arm, leg, and trunk flexibility	Marginal fitness

TABLE 15.2 **Alicia's Physical Activity Profile**

Physical activities	Mon.	Tues.	Wed.	Thurs.	Fri.	Sat.	Sun.
Moderate activities Walking	30 min		30 min		30 min	60 min	
Vigorous aerobic activities Jogging		30 min		30 min			
Vigorous sport, recreation, anaer- obic, and mixed fitness activities Aerobic dance Tennis	30 min		30 min		30 min		60 min
Moderate/Vigorous total	60 min	30 min	60 min	30 min	60 min	60 min	60 min
Muscle fitness exercises None	0	0	0	0	0	0	0
Flexibility exercises None	0	0	0	0	0	0	0
Muscle fitness/flexibility totals	0	0	0	0	0	0	0

doing any muscle fitness or flexibility exercise. She included her current activities and additional activities from the Physical Activity Pyramid that she thought she might enjoy and was likely to perform regularly.

Moderate Physical Activity
- Walking to and from school
- Additional walking
- Yardwork
- Biking

Vigorous Aerobics
- Jogging
- Aerobic dance

Vigorous Sport, Recreation, Anaerobic, and Mixed Fitness Activities
- Volleyball club
- Tennis

Muscle Fitness Exercises
- Elastic band exercises
- Jumping rope

Flexibility Exercises
- Static stretching exercises
- Yoga

Make a list similar to the one that Alicia made. Consider activities that you currently perform, as well as other types of moderate activity, vigorous activity (including vigorous aerobics, sports, recreation, anaerobic, and mixed fitness activities), muscle fitness exercise, and flexibility exercise. As you choose activities, consider the benefits provided by each.

Step 3: Set Goals

Setting SMART goals can help you build a complete fitness and physical activity program that meets your personal needs. First, consider the reasons for doing your program—for example, are you primarily interested in improving your health and wellness, or in building a higher level of fitness necessary for playing a sport or doing a specific job?

Alicia is interested in health but also wants to try out for the volleyball team. First, however, she's going to participate in the volleyball club to develop skills that will help her make the team when volleyball season comes.

Next, consider your fitness and activity profiles. If you're low in one part of physical fitness, you may want to work on it. If you did not meet national activity guidelines for one type of physical activity, you might want to do more of that type. Alicia had marginal ratings in flexibility and muscle fitness and did not meet the national guidelines for muscle fitness and flexibility exercise.

In your earlier plans, you've focused only on short-term physical activity goals. Now that you're more experienced in planning, you can build a plan that addresses long-term goals, including physical fitness goals.

In earlier chapters, Alicia planned programs for different types of activities. She limited the number of goals because she was just beginning, and she wanted to be realistic. Now, Alicia expanded the number of goals because she had experience in successfully meeting them and because she wanted to build a comprehensive program with multiple activities.

Alicia did not use all of the activities from her list of possible activities because she wanted to be realistic. As you can see in table 15.3, Alicia

TABLE 15.3 **Alicia's Activity and Fitness Goals**

Physical activity goals	Days	Amount	Weeks
Long-term goals			
1. Brisk walk to and from school	5	30 minutes a day (15 minutes each way)	18
2. Tennis	1	60 minutes a day	18
Short-term goals			
1. Jump rope warm-up	3	5 minutes, alternate jumping 30 seconds, walking 15 seconds	3
2. Volleyball club	2	60 minutes after school	3
3. Stretching exercises (see table 15.5)	2	2 sets of 2 reps of each exercise, hold stretch 30 seconds (performed after volleyball club when the muscles are warm)	3
4. Resistance machine exercises (see table 15.5)	3	2 sets of 10 reps, 60% of 1RM	3
5. Cool-down	3	5-minute walk	3
6. Jump rope warm-up	1	5 minutes, alternate jumping 30 seconds, walking 30 seconds	3
7. Cool-down	1	5-minute walk	3
Long-term goals			

Physical fitness component	Goal	Completion date
1. Improve push-up score.	8 reps	Oct. 15 (8 weeks)
2. Improve leg press score.	1.75 lb (0.8 kg) per lb (kg) of body weight	Oct. 15 (8 weeks)
3. Improve back-saver sit-and-reach score.	12 in. (30 cm)	Oct. 15 (8 weeks)
4. Improve arm, leg, and trunk flexibility score.	Score of 8 points	Oct. 15 (8 weeks)

chose both long-term and short-term physical activity (process) goals. She included walking and tennis as long-term activity goals. She has performed these a long time and knows she can easily continue them, so she set a goal of doing these activities for 18 weeks (the entire fall semester). For her new activities, she set a short-term goal of performing them for 3 weeks. She would see how things went for her volleyball club and her new muscle fitness and flexibility exercises and reset her goals after 3 weeks.

Alicia set only long-term fitness goals because she knew that improving fitness takes time to achieve. Her goal was to improve her results in two muscle fitness self-assessments and two flexibility self-assessments. She hoped to achieve these fitness goals in 8 weeks, but her first priority was achieving her short-term goal of performing the exercises for muscle fitness and flexibility. Using a table similar to Alicia's (table 15.3), prepare your own SMART physical activity and physical fitness goals, including both short-term and long-term goals.

TABLE 15.4   Alicia's Schedule for Her Physical Activity Plan

Day	Activity	Time of day	How long?
Mon.	Walk to school	7:15–7:30 a.m.	15 min
	Jump rope warm-up	3:35–3:40 p.m.	5 min
	Muscle fitness exercises	3:40–4:10 p.m.	30 min
	Walking cool-down	4:10–4:15 p.m.	5 min
	Walk home	4:15–4:30 p.m.	15 min
Tues.	Walk to school	7:15–7:30 a.m.	15 min
	Volleyball club	3:45–4:45 p.m.	60 min
	Cool-down and flexibility exercises	4:45–5:00 p.m.	15 min
	Walk home	5:00–5:15 p.m.	15 min
Wed.	Walk to school	7:15–7:30 a.m.	15 min
	Jump rope warm-up	3:35–3:40 p.m.	5 min
	Muscle fitness exercises	3:40–4:10 p.m.	30 min
	Walking cool-down	4:10–4:15 p.m.	5 min
	Walk home	4:15–4:30 p.m.	15 min
Thurs.	Walk to school	7:15–7:30 a.m.	15 min
	Volleyball club	3:45–4:45 p.m.	60 min
	Cool-down and flexibility exercises	4:45–5:00 p.m.	15 min
	Walk home	5:00–5:15 p.m.	15 min
Fri.	Walk to school	7:15–7:30 a.m.	15 min
	Jump rope warm-up	3:35–3:40 p.m.	5 min
	Muscle fitness exercises	3:40–4:10 p.m.	30 min
	Walking cool-down	4:10–4:15 p.m.	5 min
	Walk home	4:15–4:30 p.m.	15 min
Sat.	Jump rope warm-up	9:00–9:05 a.m.	5 min
	Tennis	9:05–10:05 a.m.	60 min
	Walking cool-down	10:05–10:10 a.m.	5 min
Sun.	None		

Steps 4 and 5: Create a Written Program and Evaluate Your Progress

Once Alicia had established her goals, she prepared a weekly schedule of the activities that she listed as goals in step 3 at times the exercise was most convenient for her (table 15.4). She chose Monday, Wednesday, and Friday for her jump rope and muscle fitness exercise because the school fitness center was open after school on those days. Volleyball club met on Tuesdays and Thursdays and she planned to do her flexibility exercises after volleyball club when the muscles were warm; the exercises would also serve as a good cool-down. She chose to do tennis on Saturday morning and planned no activities on Sunday. She decided to stop aerobic dance for now because her schedule was quite busy with her other new activities.

In a separate chart, she listed her flexibility and muscle fitness exercises (see table 15.5). Because they were the same exercises each time, she needed to list them only once to help her remember them.

The Taking Action feature in this chapter allows you to begin your plan, but you won't have time to complete your entire plan in this class. Therefore, you'll need to put your program into action on your own. In the weeks ahead, use a log to keep a record of your activities to see if you met your goals.

After you've tried your program for some time (the specific time depends on your goals), evaluate it. List the activities in your plan that you did and did not complete. For the part of your plan that you didn't complete, list your reasons (for example, bad weather or homework). Perform tests of fitness to see if you met your fitness goals. Prepare a written evaluation, and after answering the following questions, prepare a new (revised) plan.

> A good plan is like a road map: it shows the final destination and usually the best way to get there.
>
> *H. Stanley Judd, author*

FIT FACT
Walking or biking to school increases the amount of activity that teens accumulate by an average of 16 minutes a day. According to a report by the Surgeon General of the United States, approximately 200,000 lives could be saved each year if adults were more physically active.

TABLE 15.5 **Alicia's Muscle Fitness and Flexibility Exercises**

Cool-down and flexibility exercises	Repetitions	Time
Back-saver sit-and-reach	2 sets of 2 reps	15 sec
Knee-to-chest	2 sets of 2 reps	15 sec
Sitting stretch	2 sets of 2 reps	15 sec
Zipper	2 sets of 2 reps	15 sec
Hip stretch	2 sets of 2 reps	15 sec
Calf stretch	2 sets of 2 reps	15 sec
Muscle fitness exercises	**Repetitions**	**Resistance**
Bench press	2 sets of 2 reps	60% of 1RM
Knee extension	2 sets of 2 reps	60% of 1RM
Hamstring curl	2 sets of 2 reps	60% of 1RM
Biceps curl	2 sets of 2 reps	60% of 1RM
Triceps press	2 sets of 2 reps	60% of 1RM

SCIENCE IN ACTION: **Exercise and Academics**

The U.S. Centers for Disease Control and Prevention (CDC) is a government agency created to help people and communities "protect their health through health promotion; prevention of disease, injury, and disability; and preparedness for new health threats." The CDC recognizes the importance of regular physical activity as one means of achieving its goal of good health for all. CDC scientists reviewed more than 400 studies and found that in addition to providing health benefits, regular physical activity can "help improve academic achievement, including grades and standardized test scores." The CDC also concluded that physical activity improves **cognitive skills** such as concentration and attention, as well as academic and classroom behavior.

The conclusion that physical activity helps students concentrate on academic tasks is supported by studies from kinesiology researchers. They found, for example, that walking stimulates brain areas that increase concentration and attention in the classroom. The image on the left shows brain activation after 20 minutes of sitting. The image on the right shows brain activation after 20 minutes of walking. The red and yellow areas (after exercise) indicate activation of the brain.

The CDC report suggests that classroom-based physical activity, including exercise breaks, can help students perform well both on tests and in academics in general.

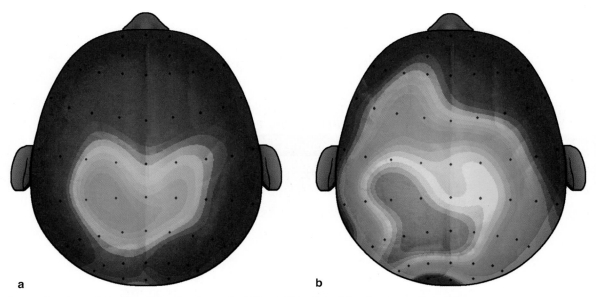

a b

Brain activation: *(a)* **after 20 minutes of sitting;** *(b)* **after 20 minutes of walking.**

Reprinted from *Neuroscience*, Vol. 159, C.H. Hillman et al., "The Effect of acute treadmill walking on cognitive control and academic achievement in preadolescent children," pgs. 1044-1054, copyright 2009, with permission of Elsevier.

STUDENT ACTIVITY

Given the evidence concerning physical activity and academic achievement, create a plan for introducing physical activity in high school classes that are not typically active, such as math, language arts, and science.

TECH TRENDS: **Swim Watches**

One good option for your personal physical activity program is swimming, which is an excellent total body activity. It can also be done by most people, including those who have joint problems, who are recovering from an injury, or who are high in body fat and have a hard time with other forms of exercise. To help you self-monitor your swimming activity, consider using a swim watch. These waterproof devices are worn on the wrist and have a built-in accelerometer similar to those used in activity watches to monitor steps. Most swim watches provide information about total time for a swim session, laps completed, pace and total time per lap, total distance covered, stroke type, and stroke length. You can download the information to your computer and store or print

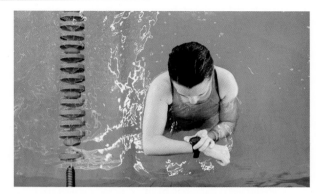

A waterproof swim watch can help you self-monitor swimming activity.

records of each workout. The watch can also estimate the number of calories you expend in a swim session.

USING TECHNOLOGY

Investigate different types of swim watches and prepare a review. Submit your review to the school newspaper or a school blog.

LESSON REVIEW

1. How do you prepare and use a personal fitness profile to establish personal needs?
2. How do you prepare and use a list of physical activity options?
3. How do you prepare and use a list of short-term and long-term program goals?
4. What should you include in a written plan, and how do you evaluate its success?

SELF-ASSESSMENT: **Your Personal Fitness Test Battery**

As you've worked your way through this book, you've had the opportunity to take many physical fitness tests. After you finish this class, you would be wise to continue assessing your fitness, but it's not reasonable to use all the tests you've done here. You can prepare your own fitness test battery that includes tests from each of the four categories (cardiorespiratory endurance, body composition, muscle fitness, and flexibility) listed in table 15.6. As you know, a test battery refers to several tests designed to measure all parts of fitness. Use the following guidelines in choosing tests for your test battery.

- For cardiorespiratory endurance, choose at least one test.
- For flexibility, choose at least two tests.
- For body composition, choose at least one test.
- For muscle fitness, choose at least one test for the arms and upper body, one test for

the trunk and abdominals, and one test for the lower body. Consider including tests for different parts of muscle fitness (muscular endurance, strength, and power).

- Choose tests for which you have adequate equipment.
- Choose tests that you think you're likely to actually do.
- Use a chart similar to table 15.6 to select tests for your battery.

Perform the tests in class, then retest yourself from time to time to see how you're doing and to help you set future fitness and physical activity goals. If you're working with a partner, remember that self-assessment information is confidential and shouldn't be shared without the permission of the person being tested.

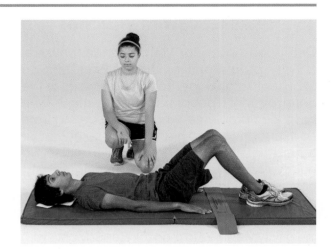

Create your own fitness test battery to track your fitness over time and help you prepare future personal plans.

TABLE 15.6   Choices for Your Personal Fitness Test Battery

Self-assessment	Place a ✓ to select a test	Self-assessment	Place a ✓ to select a test
Cardiorespiratory endurance			
PACER		Walking test	
Step test		One-mile run	
Muscle fitness			
Curl-up		Leg press 1RM (per lb of body weight)	
Push-up		Grip strength (right)	
Side stand		Grip strength (left)	
Sitting tuck		Standing long jump	
Arm press 1RM (per lb of body weight)		Medicine ball throw	
Body composition			
BMI		Waist-to-hip ratio	
Skinfold measures		Waist girth	
Flexibility			
Back-saver sit-and-reach		Arm, leg, and trunk flexibility tests	
Trunk lift			

Maintaining Active Lifestyles

Lesson Objectives

After reading this lesson, you should be able to

1. describe the five stages of change and discuss how carrying out your plan helps you move toward maintenance;

2. list and describe several self-management skills that help you maintain physical activity throughout life;

3. define *attitude* and describe several positive attitudes about physical activity; and

4. describe some negative attitudes about physical activity and some ways to change them to positive attitudes.

Lesson Vocabulary

attitude

Now that you have learned how to plan your comprehensive physical activity program, do you think you will be able to perform your plan on a regular basis? Consider the following information to help you stick with your plan.

Stages of Change

As you learned earlier, people go through five stages of change when modifying their behavior, such as becoming active. By now, you have probably moved well past the first three stages of change (see figure 15.1) and are either at the stage of action or maintenance. You have learned about the benefits of physical activity, including the enjoyment that you get from being active. By preparing and then trying your plan, you have moved to the action stage. Ultimately, the goal is to stick with your plan (reach the maintenance stage and stay there).

> My sister likes to run. She jogs all the time. I like to hike because it's fun and I can do it with other people. I like that.
>
> *Jerry Burdine*

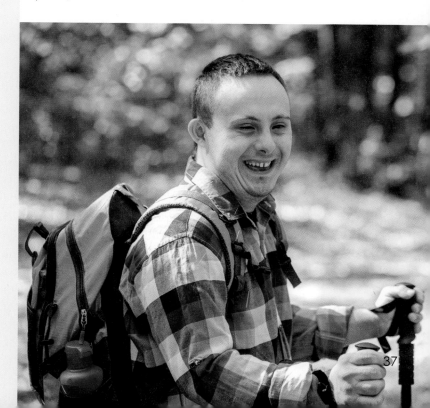

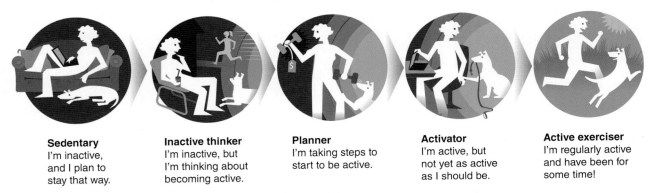

Sedentary
I'm inactive, and I plan to stay that way.

Inactive thinker
I'm inactive, but I'm thinking about becoming active.

Planner
I'm taking steps to start to be active.

Activator
I'm active, but not yet as active as I should be.

Active exerciser
I'm regularly active and have been for some time!

Figure 15.1   Five stages of change for physical activity.

Using Self-Management Skills

In each chapter of this book you have learned a self-management skill that can help you reach and stay at the maintenance stage for being active. Research shows that people who use self-management skills are likely to be active throughout life. Table 15.7 provides an overview of the different self-management skills. Review the list to remind yourself how you can use the different skills as you implement your personal program.

Building Positive Attitudes

A physical activity plan is worthwhile only if you carry it out, and that is determined in large part by your attitude. The word **attitude** refers to your feelings about something. We all have attitudes about food, subjects of study, music, clothing, and many other topics—including physical activity. Active people have more positive attitudes toward physical activity than negative ones. Here's a list of reasons that people like to be physically active. Think about these attitudes and how you might make some of them your own.

- *"Physical activities are a great way to meet people."* Many activities provide opportunities to meet people and strengthen friendships. Aerobic dance and team sports, for example, are good social activities.

- *"I think physical activity is really fun."* Many teenagers do activities simply because they're fun. Participating in activities you enjoy also helps you reduce stress.

- *"I enjoy the challenge."* When the famous mountain climber George Mallory was asked why he climbed Mount Everest, he replied, "Because it's there." Helen Keller was deaf and blind but became a famous author. She said in one of her books that "life is either a daring adventure or nothing at all." Some people just enjoy a challenge. Are you one of them?

- *"I like the rigor of training."* Some people enjoy intense training. For these people, competition and winning can be secondary to training.

- *"I like competition."* If you enjoy competition, sport and other physical activities provide ways to test yourself against others. You can even compete against yourself by trying to improve your score or time in an activity.

- *"Physical activity is my way of relaxing."* Physical activity can help you relax mentally and emotionally after a difficult day.

FIT FACT
Active teens have more positive attitudes than negative attitudes. This state of mind is called a *positive balance of attitudes.*

TABLE 15.7 **Self-Management Skills for Fitness, Health, and Wellness**

Skill	Description
Effective communication	This skill helps you effectively receive information and pass it on to others.
Self-assessment	This skill helps you see where you are and what to change in order to get where you want to be.
Setting goals	This skill creates a foundation for developing your personal plan by helping you set goals that are SMART (specific, measurable, attainable, realistic, and timely).
Overcoming barriers	This skill helps you find ways to overcome barriers to making healthy lifestyle choices, such as lack of time, temporary injury, lack of safe places to be active, inclement weather, and difficulty in selecting healthy foods.
Resolving conflicts	This skill helps you adapt when confronted with problems with other people.
Self-monitoring	This skill involves keeping records or logs to see whether you are in fact doing what you think you're doing.
Managing time	This skill helps you be efficient so that you have time for the important things in your life.
Building self-confidence	This skill helps you build the feeling that you're capable of making healthy lifestyle changes.
Improving performance	This skill helps you enjoy and stay interested in being physically active for a lifetime.
Preventing relapse	This skill helps you stick with healthy behaviors even when you have problems getting motivated.
Finding social support	This skill enables you to get help and support from others (such as your friends and family) as you adopt healthy behaviors and try to stick with them.
Building knowledge and understanding	This skill helps you solve problems—such as how to make healthy changes in your life—using a modified form of the scientific method.
Developing tactics	This skill helps you focus on a specific plan of action and successfully execute the plan.
Improving self-perception	This skill helps you think positively about yourself so that you're more likely to make healthy lifestyle choices and feel that they will make a difference in your life.
Building positive attitudes	This skill helps position you to succeed in adopting healthy lifestyles.
Saying no	This skill helps keep you from doing things you don't want to do, especially when you're under pressure from friends or other people.
Managing competitive stress	This skill involves preventing or coping with the stresses of competition.
Thinking success	This skill helps you adapt your way of thinking to help you believe that you can achieve success.
Thinking critically	This skill enables you to find and interpret information that helps you make good decisions and solve problems.
Positive self-talk	This skill helps you perform your best and make healthy lifestyle choices by thinking positive thoughts rather than negative ones that detract from success.
Choosing good activities	This skill involves selecting the activities that are best for you personally so that you will enjoy and benefit from doing them.

- *"I think physical activity improves my appearance."* Physical activity can help you build muscle and control body fat. (Remember, however, that regular activity cannot completely change your appearance.)

- *"Physical activity is a good way to improve my health and wellness."* As you are learning from this book, regular physical activity helps you resist illness and improves your general sense of well-being.

- *"Physical activity just makes me feel good."* Many people just feel better when they exercise, and many have a sense of loss or discomfort when they don't exercise.

Changing Negative Attitudes

Negative attitudes can be a reason why people fail to carry out their physical activity plan. The following list shows you some negative attitudes along with suggestions for turning them into positive ones. Read the negative statement and then give some thought to the suggested alternative.

Negative: "I don't have the time."

Positive: "I will plan a time for physical activity." If you plan time for physical activity, you will feel better, function more efficiently, and have more time to do other things that you want to do.

Negative: "I don't want to get all sweaty."

Positive: "I'll allow time to clean up afterward." Sweating is a natural by-product of a good workout. Allow yourself time to change before exercising and to shower and change afterward. Focus on how good you will feel.

Negative: "People might laugh at me."

Positive: "When they see how fit I get, they'll wish they were exercising too." Find friends who are interested in getting fit. Anyone who does laugh may simply be jealous of your efforts and results.

Negative: "None of my friends work out, so neither do I."

Positive: "I'll ask my friends to join me, and maybe we'll work out together." Talk with your friends. Some of them may be interested in working out or doing physical activities together.

Negative: "I get nervous and feel tense when I play sports."

Positive: "Everyone gets nervous. I'll stay as calm as I can and do the best I can." Many athletes learn techniques to reduce their stress levels. You can learn them too.

The greatest discovery of my generation is that human beings can alter their lives by altering their attitudes.

William James, American philosopher

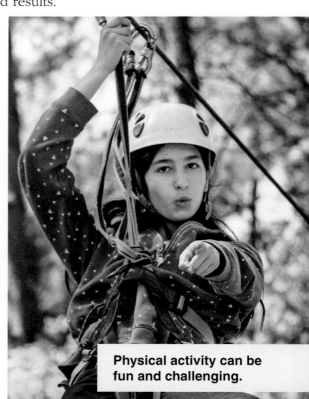

Physical activity can be fun and challenging.

Negative: "I'm already in good condition."

Positive: "Physical activity will help me stay in good condition." Use the self-assessments in this book, then take an honest look at yourself. Are you as fit as you thought? Physical activity can help you get in shape and stay in shape.

Negative: "I'm too tired."

Positive: "I'll just do a little to get started, then as I get more fit I'll do more." You'll probably find that once you get started, physical exertion gives you *more* energy. Begin realistically, then gradually increase the amount of activity you do.

LESSON REVIEW

1. What are the five stages of change, and how can carrying out your plan help you move toward maintenance?
2. What are some self-management skills that help you maintain physical activity throughout life?
3. What are some positive attitudes that can help you commit to physical activity?
4. What are some negative attitudes about physical activity, and how can you change them to positive attitudes?

TAKING CHARGE: **Changing Attitudes**

Allen and Matt are friends who often do things together, including sport activities. Sometimes they play tennis together on the weekend. Lately, Allen has been winning most of their matches.

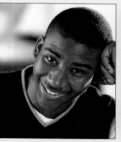

"You ready to hit the court?" Allen asked Matt as he grabbed his tennis racket.

"I don't feel like playing today," Matt said. "Anyway, there's a good show on TV." He walked into the family room and sat on the couch.

Allen followed him. "I think you just don't want to lose again."

"You're right," Matt admitted. "I hate losing."

"You win sometimes, Matt. The competition is what makes tennis fun."

"Not when I lose," Matt replied.

Allen thought for a minute. "How about taking a jog around the block?" he asked. "There'll be no winner or loser that way."

"I don't want to get all sweaty," Matt replied. "I'd rather relax watching TV."

"Oh, come on, Matt. Jogging will help you relax. We need to stay in shape."

Matt looked at Allen and said, "I'm thinking about it."

FOR DISCUSSION

What does Allen like about being physically active? What does Matt like—and not like—about physical activity? How could Matt change his negative attitudes and become more active? What are some other negative attitudes that keep people from being active, and how can they be changed? What are some positive attitudes that help people stay active? Consider the guidelines in the following Self-Management feature as you answer these discussion questions.

SELF-MANAGEMENT: **Skills for Building Positive Attitudes**

Most of us have had both positive and negative attitudes about physical activity at one time or another. Experts have shown that people with more positive attitudes toward physical activity than negative ones are likely to be active. Use the following guidelines to build positive attitudes and get rid of negative ones.

- *Assess your attitudes.* Make a list of your positive and negative attitudes. You can use the attitudes listed in this lesson to help you.

- *Identify your reasons for any negative attitudes.* Ask yourself why you feel negative about physical activity. If you can find the reason, it may help you change. For example, you may not have liked playing a sport when you were young because you didn't like a particular coach or player. Maybe you can now find a situation that will make an activity more fun. Consider the alternatives to negative attitudes described earlier in this chapter.

- *Find activities that bring out fewer negative attitudes.* For example, maybe you don't like team sports but you do enjoy recreational activities. List your negative attitudes, then ask yourself whether there are activities you don't dislike. If so, consider trying them.

- *Choose activities that accentuate the positive.* If you really like certain activities and feel good about them, focus on these activities rather than ones you don't like as much.

- *Change the situation.* You may feel negatively about an activity because of things unrelated to the activity. For example, if you hated playing basketball because you had too little time to get dressed and groomed after participating, maybe you can make changes so you have more time to shower and dress.

- *Be active with friends.* Activities are often more fun when you do them with friends. Sometimes participating with other people you like is enough to change your feelings about an activity.

- *Discuss your attitudes.* Just talking about your attitudes can sometimes help. People sometimes think they're the only ones who have problems in certain situations. Talking about it with others can help you change the situation to make it more fun for everyone concerned.

- *Help others build positive attitudes.* The ways in which others react can affect a person's feelings about physical activity. Consider the following suggestions when you interact with others in physical activity.

- *Instead of laughing, provide encouragement.* Do you remember how difficult it is to start something new or different? You can encourage others by making statements such as, "Good to see you exercising. Way to go!"

- *Make new friends through participation in physical activities.* Introduce yourself to others and offer to help when appropriate. Consider starting or joining a sport or exercise club at school. An activity club can be a great way for you and your friends to combine socializing with physical activity. If you're thinking about starting a club, check with your school's activity coordinator first.

- *Be sensitive to people with special needs.* Some people need certain accommodations or modifications when performing physical activity. Others can help by joining those who have special challenges and by being sensitive to their needs.

- *Be considerate of differences.* The popularity of physical activities varies from culture to culture. For example, field hockey and curling are not popular in the United States but are very popular in other countries. Similarly, what one person enjoys may not be so enjoyable to another. Learning to accept cultural and personal differences helps everyone enjoy activity and contributes to better interpersonal understanding.

Taking Action: **Performing Your Physical Activity Plan**

In previous chapters, you learned how to prepare a physical activity plan for each type of activity included in the Physical Activity Pyramid. Now you'll prepare a comprehensive written plan that includes many types of physical activity. **Take action** by performing one day of your personal physical activity plan in class. Choose a day from your program that includes enough activities to fill a full class period. If no single day's activities last as long as one class period, supplement your program for that day with activity planned for another day. If needed equipment is not available for your chosen activity, select a different activity that offers similar benefits and is one that you're likely to enjoy.

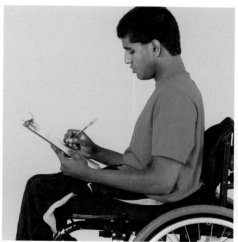

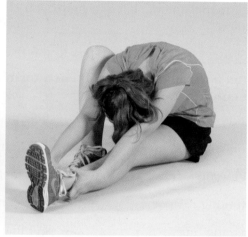

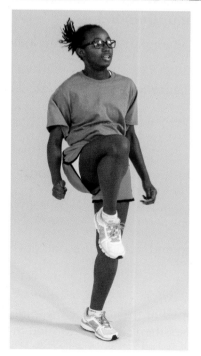

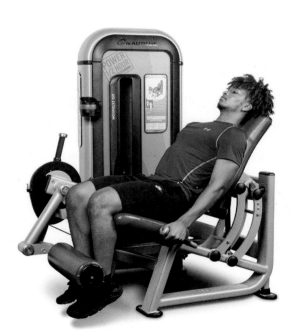

Take action by performing your physical activity plan.

CHAPTER REVIEW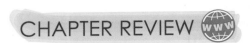

Reviewing Concepts and Vocabulary

Answer items 1 through 5 by correctly completing each sentence with a word or phrase.

1. A _____ is a brief summary of your fitness self-assessment results.

2. The _____ is a government agency created to help people and communities protect their health.

3. A device that can be used in the water to monitor physical activity is called a _____.

4. A self-management skill that helps you see where you are and what you need to change is called _____.

5. _____ refers to the five steps for modifying your behavior.

For items 6 through 10, match each term in column 1 with the appropriate word or phrase in column 2.

6. attitude   a. skills that help you to be efficient

7. cognitive skills   b. skill that helps you focus on a plan of action

8. developing tactics   c. your feelings about something

9. preventing relapse   d. your concentration and attention

10. managing time   e. skill that helps you stick with healthy behaviors

For items 11 through 15, respond to each statement or question.

11. Explain why constructing a fitness profile is an important part of collecting information for program planning.

12. Describe the relationship between academic performance and regular physical activity.

13. Describe the steps in preparing a personal physical fitness test battery.

14. Describe some of the most common positive attitudes about physical activity.

15. Describe several guidelines for turning negative attitudes into positive attitudes.

Thinking Critically

Write a paragraph to answer the following question.

Why is it important to develop your own fitness program and not just use one developed for someone else?

Project

FitnessGram is a national youth fitness test battery developed at the Cooper Institute in Dallas, Texas, by an advisory board of experts. Many of the self-assessments you performed in this book are derived from FitnessGram.

Build a FitnessGram profile by summarizing your results on all of the FitnessGram self-assessments. Create your own profile summary sheet or use a worksheet provided by your teacher. If available, you can enter your results on a computer as directed by your teacher and print a computer summary. If you choose, you can share your fitness profile with your parents or guardians. You may also want to encourage them to perform health-related fitness assessments of their own.

UNIT VI

Living Well: Making Healthy Choices

CHAPTER 16   **Choosing Nutritious Food**

CHAPTER 17   **Stress Management**

CHAPTER 18   **Making Healthy Choices and Planning for Health and Wellness**

Healthy People 2030 Goals and Objectives

Overarching Goals

- Attain healthy, thriving lives and well-being, free of preventable disease, disability, injury, and premature death.
- Eliminate health disparities, achieve health equity, and attain health literacy to improve the health and well-being of all.

Objectives

- Increase consumption of fruits, vegetables, and whole grains.
- Reduce intake of foods high in saturated fat, added sugars, and sodium.
- Increase consumption of foods containing calcium, potassium, and vitamin D.
- Reduce the percentage of teens with iron deficiency.
- Increase the proportion of schools that don't sell less healthy foods and drinks.
- Increase the percentage of people who follow safe food practices.
- Reduce the proportion of teens with obesity.
- Increase the proportion of teens who have an adult that they can talk to about serious problems and who can communicate positively with parents.
- Increase preventive mental health care in schools and mental health visits by teens.
- Increase the proportion of teens with depression and trauma who get treatment.
- Increase health literacy of the population.
- Reduce suicide rate and attempted suicide among teens.
- Reduce suicidal thoughts among teens especially among lesbian, gay, bisexual, and transgender teens.
- Reduce bullying among teens especially among lesbian, gay, bisexual, and transgender teens.
- Increase the proportion of schools with policies and practices that promote health and safety.
- Increase use of CPR and AEDs by bystanders.
- Increase the percentage of teens who get sufficient sleep.
- Reduce incidence of destructive habits (e.g., tobacco use, alcohol and drug misuse).
- Reduce the percentage of teens who report sunburn.

- Achieve high-quality, longer lives by reducing preventable disease, injury, and early death.
- Increase the percentage of teens who have preventive medical exams every year.
- Reduce the percentage of people exposed to unhealthy air and unsafe water.
- Increase prevention check-ups.

Self-Assessment Features in This Unit
- Energy Balance
- Identifying Signs of Stress
- Healthy Lifestyle Questionnaire

Taking Charge and Self-Management Features in This Unit
- Saying No
- Managing Competitive Stress
- Thinking Success

Taking Action Features in This Unit
- Burn It Up Workout
- Performing Relaxation Exercises
- Your Healthy Lifestyle Plan

Choosing Nutritious Food

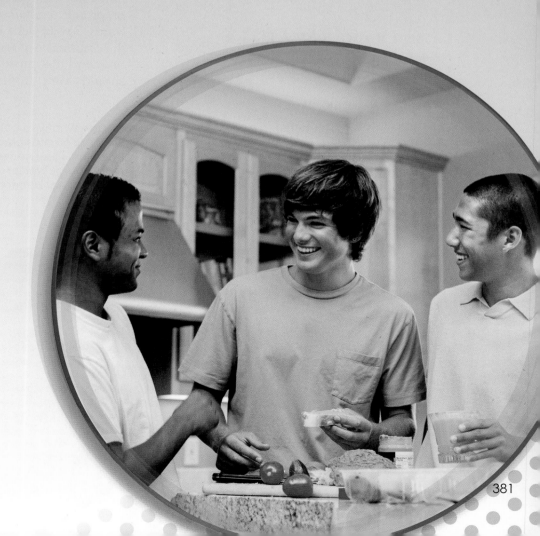

A Healthy Diet

Lesson Objectives

After reading this lesson, you should be able to

1. describe the three types of nutrients that provide energy and provide examples of foods for each type of nutrient;

2. describe the three types of nutrients that do not provide energy and provide examples of foods for each type of nutrient;

3. describe the six groups from which foods are chosen for healthy eating and foods that should be limited in the diet; and

4. discuss the importance of limiting the number and size of servings for healthy eating.

Lesson Vocabulary

Adequate Intake (AI)
amino acids
carbohydrate
complete protein
Dietary Reference Intake (DRI)
empty calories
fat
fiber
incomplete protein
macronutrient
micronutrient
protein
Recommended Dietary Allowance (RDA)
resting metabolism
saturated fat
Tolerable Upper Intake Level (UL)
trans-fatty acid
unsaturated fat

What kinds of food are important to your health? How much food do you need to eat? In this lesson, you'll learn about healthful foods and how to select foods for a balanced diet. Scientists have identified 45 to 50 nutrients—food substances required for the growth and maintenance of your cells. These nutrients have been divided into six groups—carbohydrate, protein, fat, vitamin, mineral, and water—each of which is discussed in this chapter.

Nutrients That Provide Energy

Three types of nutrients supply the energy that your body needs to perform its daily tasks: fat, carbohydrate, and protein. These are referred to as **macronutrients**. One gram of fat contains nine calories, whereas one gram of carbohydrate or protein contains four calories. The United States Department of Agriculture (USDA) and the National Academy of Medicine (NAM) recommend that most of the calories in your diet should come from carbohydrate. Figure 16.1

You are what you eat! That's what my gramps always said. He's right. I feel better and have more energy when I avoid junk food and eat better.

Keiko Tanaka

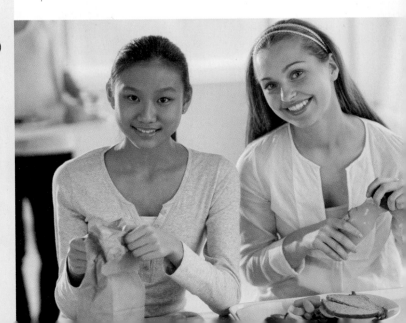

somewhat active teens, and 2,400 to 2,800 for very active teens.

Carbohydrate

Carbohydrate is your main source of energy and comes in two types: simple and complex. Simple carbohydrate includes sugars such as table sugar, fructose, and sucrose. They are commonly referred to as *added sugars*. For example, fructose and sucrose are added sugars found in soft drinks and other sweetened foods. Simple carbohydrates provide a quick source of energy but contain few nutrients (figure 16.2*a*). You should minimize your intake of simple carbohydrate to no more than 10 percent of your recommended daily calorie intake. Some simple carbohydrate sources are better than others. For example, bananas and oranges contain simple carbohydrate but also contain essential nutrients such as vitamins, minerals, and fiber. Foods such as candy, pastries, and sugared soft drinks are said to contain **empty calories**, which provide energy but few if any other nutrients such as vitamins and minerals.

Most of your carbohydrate calories should come from complex carbohydrate. They have a more complex chemical structure than simple carbohydrates and take longer to digest (figure 16.2*b*). Complex carbohydrates supply no energy but contain more nutrients than simple carbohydrates. They are often rich in **fiber**, a type of complex carbohydrate that your body cannot digest. Fiber sources (figure 16.2, *b* and *c*) include beans, leaves, stems, roots, and seed

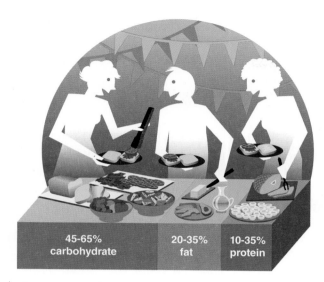

Figure 16.1 Percentage of calories recommended by the National Academy of Medicine's Food and Nutrition Board for carbohydrate, fat, and protein.

45-65% carbohydrate
20-35% fat
10-35% protein

shows the recommended percentage of calories from each of the three types of macronutrient.

Calories

As noted in chapter 14, the number of calories needed by teens varies depending on age, sex, and activity level. For males, daily calorie intake should range from 2,000 to 2,400 for inactive teens, 2,400 to 2,800 for somewhat active teens, and 2,800 to 3,200 for very active teens. For females, daily calorie intake ranges from 1,800 to 2,000 for inactive teens, 2,000 to 2,400 for

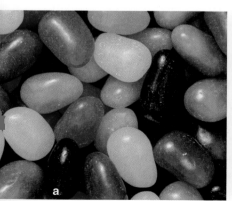
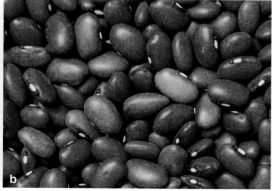
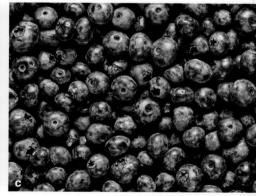

Figure 16.2 Types of carbohydrate: *(a)* Simple carbohydrate (such as in candy) contains empty calories, but (*b* and *c*) complex carbohydrate (such as in vegetables and fruit) contains more nutrients and fiber.

coverings of fruits, vegetables, and grains (figure 16.2c). Examples of foods high in fiber include whole-grain bread and cereal, the skin of fresh fruits, raw vegetables, nuts, and seeds. Fiber helps you avoid intestinal problems and may reduce your chances of developing some forms of cancer.

Protein

Protein is the group of nutrients that builds, repairs, and maintains body cells; they are the building blocks of your body. Protein is contained in animal products (such as milk, eggs, meat, and fish) and in some plants (such as beans and grains). Protein provides energy but doesn't contain as many calories as fat. If you consume more protein than is needed to build your body tissue, the additional calories will be either used to produce energy for daily activity or stored as body fat.

During digestion, your body breaks protein down into simpler substances called **amino acids**, which your small intestine can absorb. Your body can manufacture 11 of the 20 known amino acids; you need to get the other 9—known as the *essential amino acids*—from food.

Foods containing all nine essential amino acids are said to provide **complete protein**. Animal sources such as meat, milk products, and fish provide complete protein. A grain called quinoa (pronounced keen' wah) and some forms of soy provide complete protein as well. Quinoa can be served hot, like rice, or cold in a salad.

Foods that have some, but not all, the essential amino acids are said to contain **incomplete protein**. Examples include beans, nuts, rice, and certain other plants. You can usually get enough essential amino acids from a daily diet that includes some foods with complete protein and some with incomplete protein. People who do not eat meat need to eat a variety of foods that contain incomplete protein and, taken together, provide all the essential amino acids.

Fat

Fat is contained in animal products as well as some plant products, such as nuts and vegetable oils. Fat is necessary to grow and repair your cells; it dissolves certain vitamins and carries them to your cells. In addition, fat enhances the flavor and texture of many foods. Fat is classified as either saturated or unsaturated. In general, **saturated fat** is solid at room temperature, and **unsaturated fat** is liquid. Saturated fat comes mostly from animal products, such as lard, butter, milk, and meat fat. Unsaturated fat comes mostly from plants, such as sunflower, corn, soybean, olive, almond, and peanut. In addition, fish produce unsaturated fat in their cells.

At most, fewer than 35 percent of the total calories you consume should come from fat, and many experts recommend a level closer to 20 percent. The bulk of the fat in your diet should come from unsaturated fats, including fish oils. The Dietary Guidelines for Americans 2020–2025 recommend that calories from saturated fat should be less than 10 percent of your daily calorie intake. Some kinds of fat, such as fish oil, are considered to be healthier than others.

As you know, cholesterol is a waxy, fatlike substance found in the saturated fat of animal cells, meaning that you produce your own and also consume it in foods that are high in saturated fat, such as meat. Trans-fatty acids also affect cholesterol, which was the primary reason they were banned in foods. Medical experts recommend eating foods that are low in cholesterol and saturated fat to help prevent atherosclerosis and other heart diseases.

Nutrients That Do Not Provide Energy

Minerals, vitamins, and water have no calories and provide no energy, but they all play a vital role in staying fit and healthy. Minerals and vitamins are called **micronutrients** because the body needs them in relatively small amounts compared to carbohydrate, protein, and fat.

The **Dietary Reference Intake (DRI)** is a system used by the Food and Nutrition Board of the National Academy of Medicine to describe recommended amounts of each micronutrient. Three types of DRI help you know how much of each vitamin or mineral you should consume. The first, **Recommended Dietary Allowance (RDA)**, is the minimum amount of a nutrient necessary to meet the health needs of most people. The second, **Adequate Intake (AI)**, is used when there is not sufficient evidence to establish an RDA for a given micronutrient. The third, the **Tolerable Upper Intake Level (UL)**, refers to the maximum amount of a vitamin or mineral that can be consumed without posing a health risk.

Minerals

Minerals are essential nutrients that help regulate the activity of your cells. They come from elements in the earth's crust and are present in all plants and animals. You need 25 minerals in varying amounts. Table 16.1 shows major functions and food sources of the most important minerals.

Some minerals are especially important for young people—for example, calcium. During your teen years, your body needs calcium to build your bones. During young adulthood, your bones become less efficient at getting calcium from food and begin to lose calcium. Later, typically around age 55, females experience a change in hormones that leads them to experience much more bone loss than men do. In fact, a large percentage of older females develop osteoporosis, a condition in which their bones become porous and break easily. Males can also have this disease, but they get it less often and much later in life. You can reduce your risk for osteoporosis by getting enough calcium and doing weight-bearing exercise (such as walking and jogging) and resistance exercise throughout your life.

Another important mineral is iron, which is needed for proper formation and functioning of your red blood cells. Red blood cells carry oxygen to your muscles and other body tissues. Iron deficiency is especially common among females. If your body has insufficient iron, you

TABLE 16.1   **Functions and Sources of Minerals**

Mineral	Function in the body	Food sources
Calcium	Builds and maintains teeth and bones; helps blood clot; helps nerves and muscles function	Cheese, milk, dark green vegetables, sardines, legumes
Iron	Helps transfer oxygen in red blood cells and other cells	Liver, red meat, dark green vegetables, shellfish, whole-grain cereals
Magnesium	Aids breakdown of glucose and proteins; regulates body fluids	Green vegetables, grains, nuts, beans, yeast
Phosphorus	Builds and maintains teeth and bones; helps release energy from nutrients	Meat, poultry, fish, eggs, legumes, milk products
Potassium	Regulates fluid balance in cells; helps nerves function	Oranges, bananas, meat, bran, potatoes, dried beans
Sodium	Regulates internal water balance; helps nerves function	Most foods, table salt
Zinc	Aids transport of carbon dioxide; aids healing of wounds	Meat, shellfish, whole grains, milk, legumes

have a condition called *iron-deficiency anemia*, which causes you to feel tired all the time. Iron from animal foods is more easily absorbed than iron from plants. The best sources of iron are meat (especially red meat), poultry, and fish. You can also help your body absorb iron by getting an adequate amount of vitamin C.

Sodium is a mineral that helps your body cells function properly. It's present in many foods and is especially high in snack foods, processed foods, fast foods, and cured meats (for example, ham). For many people, dietary sodium comes primarily from table salt (sodium chloride). Most people eat more sodium than they need. U.S. nutrition guidelines recommend limiting the amount of sodium in your diet. People with high blood pressure need to be especially careful to limit sodium because it can cause their body to retain water, thus keeping their blood pressure high.

Vitamins

You need vitamins for the growth and repair of your cells. Vitamin C and the B vitamins dissolve in your blood and are carried to cells throughout your body. Because your body cannot store excess B and C vitamins, you need to eat foods containing these vitamins every day. In contrast, vitamins A, D, E, and K dissolve in fat, and excess amounts of these vitamins are stored in fat cells in your liver and other body parts. Folacin, or folic acid, is especially important for teen and young adult females. Research shows that children born to women low in folacin are at risk of birth defects. Table 16.2 gives you more information about specific vitamins.

TABLE 16.2   **Functions and Sources of Vitamins**

Vitamin	Function in the body	Food sources
A (retinol)	Helps produce normal mucus; part of the chemical necessary for vision	Butter, margarine, liver, eggs, green or yellow vegetables
B_1 (thiamin)	Helps release energy from carbohydrate	Pork, organ meat, legumes, greens
B_2 (riboflavin)	Helps break down carbohydrate and protein	Meat, milk products, eggs, green and yellow vegetables
B_6 (pyridoxine)	Helps break down protein and glucose	Yeast, nuts, beans, liver, fish, rice
B_{12} (cobalamin)	Aids formation of nucleic and amino acids	Meat, milk products, eggs, fish
Biotin	Aids formation of amino, nucleic, and fatty acids and glycogen	Eggs, liver, yeast
C (ascorbic acid)	Aids formation of hormones, bone tissue, and collagen	Fruits, tomatoes, potatoes, green leafy vegetables
D	Aids absorption of calcium and phosphorus	Liver, fortified milk, fatty fish
E (tocopherol)	Prevents damage to cell membranes and vitamin A	Vegetable oils
Folacin	Helps build DNA and protein	Yeast, wheat germ, liver, greens
K	Aids blood clotting	Leafy vegetables
Niacin	Helps release energy from protein and carbohydrate	Milk, meat, whole-grain or enriched cereals, legumes
Pantothenic acid	Converts food fuel for producing energy and helps nervous system function properly	Most unprocessed foods

SCIENCE IN ACTION: **Vitamin and Mineral Supplements**

Scientists who study nutrition and medicine have researched the value of vitamin and mineral supplements. The most common type of supplement is taken daily and contains the full amount of vitamins and minerals recommended for daily intake. If you eat a balanced diet, however, you will most likely get the proper amounts without a supplement. Some medical and nutrition experts recommend a multivitamin for people who do not eat regular meals and thus may not get the vitamins and minerals they need. Other experts, including scientists from the U.S. Centers for Disease Control and Prevention, say there is not enough evidence to indicate that a daily supplement is beneficial for most people.

With all this in mind, the decision to take a vitamin or mineral supplement should be made only with the advice of a nutrition or medical expert based on your medical history and personal nutrition habits. Unless advised otherwise by an expert, a supplement should contain no more than the RDA or AI value for each mineral and vitamin. Excessive amounts can lead to health problems.

STUDENT ACTIVITY

Investigate a multivitamin supplement. Determine whether it contains more than 100 percent of the recommended amount of each vitamin.

Water

Many dietitians suggest that water is the single most important nutrient. It carries the other nutrients to your cells, carries away waste, and helps regulate your body temperature. Most foods contain water. In fact, 50 to 60 percent of your own body weight comes from water. Your body loses 2 to 3 quarts (1.9 to 2.8 liters) of water a day through breathing, perspiring, and eliminating waste from your bowels and bladder. You lose even more water than usual in very hot weather and when you exercise vigorously. As a result, you need to drink plenty of extra fluid in those conditions.

The best beverages for this purpose are water, fruit juice, and milk. The type of juice or milk makes a difference. Pure fruit juices contain vitamins and minerals, and some contain fiber (for example, orange juice pulp), but others contain small amounts of real juice and are supplemented with simple sugar. Skim milk provides the same basic nutrients as whole milk but without the fat. Soft drinks that contain caffeine are not as effective as water and contain added sugar and empty calories. Sport drinks usually contain sodium and other ingredients that you don't need unless you exercise for several hours.

Healthy Eating Patterns

The Dietary Guidelines for Americans 2020–2025 recommend following healthy eating patterns across the life span. This includes a variety of nutrient-rich foods and limits saturated fats, sugar, and sodium (see figure 16.3). Some foods are richer in nutrients than others. The goal is to eat more foods that are high in nutritional value and fewer unhealthy foods. For example, when choosing grains, look for the whole-grain label on bread, cereal, and other grain products.

Together, vegetables and fruits should constitute approximately half of your total diet. There are five vegetable groups: dark green (e.g., broccoli, spinach),

FIT FACT
The Dietary Guidelines for Americans 2020–2025 and the Healthy People 2030 objectives emphasize the importance of limiting added sugars, saturated fats, and sodium in the diet. Both documents recommend cutting back on foods and beverages that are high in these components.

A healthy eating pattern includes:

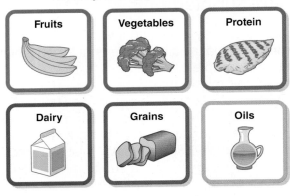

A healthy eating pattern limits:

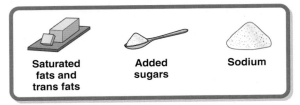

Figure 16.3   Foods for healthy eating and foods that should be limited in the diet.

From USDHHS and USDA.

red/orange (e.g., carrots, tomatoes), legumes (e.g., peas and beans), starchy (e.g., lima beans, white potatoes), and other (iceberg lettuce, cucumbers). In figure 16.3, the red area represents fruits and the green area represents vegetables. The guidelines emphasize getting most of your vegetable servings from dark green and red/orange vegetables. Fruits can be fresh, canned, frozen, or dried. Fruit juices that are 100 percent juice are a legitimate source of fruit consumption, but too much juice is not recommended because of its high simple-sugar content. In general, the public is low in consumption in these groups and can benefit from a shift toward more vegetables and fruits in the diet.

The purple area represents the protein group. As noted earlier, this group includes meats (such as beef, poultry, and pork), seafood (fresh and canned), beans and peas, and nuts and seeds. Most Americans consume adequate protein, but some types of proteins are overabundant in the typical diet and others are underrepresented. You should limit your intake of processed meats such as hot dogs and some lunch meats, which contain very high levels of salt. Recommended foods in the protein group include lean meat cuts, poultry (without skin), and fish high in omega-3 fatty acids (such as salmon and trout). You should also use cooking methods that do not add fat to your food. For example, broiling lets fat drip away, whereas frying adds extra fat and calories.

The blue area represents the dairy group. The group includes milk, cheese, milk-based desserts, and yogurt. These foods are good sources of calcium. When choosing foods from this group, consider low-fat and fat-free options. Research indicates that, as a group, teens are low in consumption of foods rich in calcium. Low-fat dairy products (e.g., yogurt, milk), dark leafy greens (e.g., spinach, kale), and fortified cereals are good sources.

The brown area represents the grains group. Grains, especially whole grains, are a source of fiber, vitamins (e.g., niacin, folacin), and minerals (e.g., iron, magnesium). The most common grains are found in bread, cereal, and pasta and include wheat, rice, corn, and oats. At least half of the grains in your diet should be whole grains.

Oil (yellow area) is fat that is liquid at room temperature (unsaturated fat). Oils do not constitute a separate food group, but they are included in figure 16.3 because they are a source of important nutrients. Dietary guidelines suggest that oils replace solid fats in the diet. When considering oils, choose monounsaturated oils (such as canola, sunflower, or olive oil) or polyunsaturated oils (such as corn or safflower oil). Polyunsaturated oils from some types of fish (e.g., salmon, tuna, trout) are a source of omega-3 fatty acids considered to be a healthy part of your diet. Nuts and seeds also are a source of healthy oils. Some fats made from plants (for example, coconut and palm oils) are not included in the oils category because they are high in saturated fat and therefore are not considered to be healthy diet options. Because oils are fats, they are part of the total amount of fat to be included in your diet (see figure 16.1).

An apple a day keeps the doctor away.

Proverb

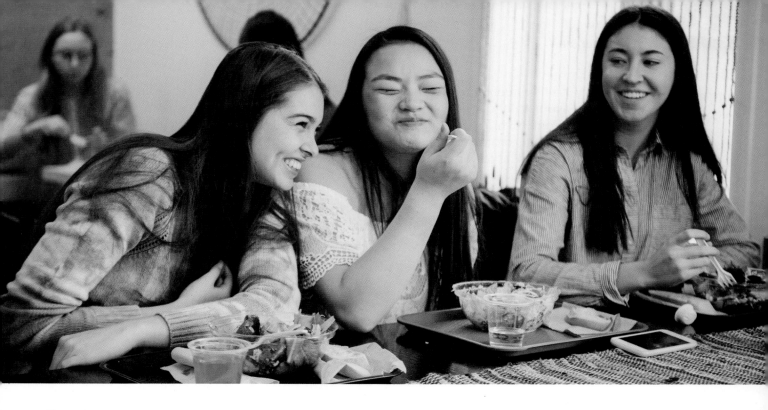

▍Servings and Serving Sizes

A healthy eating pattern includes appropriate amounts of macro- and micronutrients from the various food groups. The FDA requires that food labels contain the size of a serving and the number of servings in a food package. Size of servings are shown in common measurements (e.g., cup, tablespoon, piece, slice). The size of serving on a food container is not a recommendation of how much to eat or drink. Rather, a serving size is based on the amount of food people typically consume rather than how much they *should* consume. The size of serving is provided so that you know the nutrition value of food in a serving of the size noted on the package.

CONSUMER CORNER: **MyPlate**

The Dietary Guidelines for Americans 2020–2025 provide easy-to-use information about eating for good health. Earlier you learned about the food groups from which you can choose to eat well (see figure 16.3). The guidelines also recommend the use of MyPlate (see figure 16.4) to encourage you to fill your plate with a variety of foods at each meal. As noted earlier, oils do not constitute a separate food group, so they are not included in MyPlate.

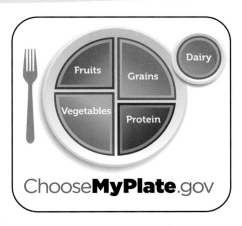

Figure 16.4 MyPlate: A USDA food graphic.
FROM USDHHS and USDA.

STUDENT ACTIVITY

Explore the MyPlate website to learn more about the different food choices that contribute to healthy eating patterns.

FIT FACT
No single diet is best for all people. The exact amount of food that should be consumed from each food group depends on factors such as age, sex, and activity level. Alternative guidelines for eating have been developed by groups such as the American Heart Association and the American Diabetes Association for people with specific medical needs. Ethnic food pyramids are also available.

The recommended number of servings from a given food group depends on your daily calorie intake. Table 16.3 shows the recommended number of servings from each food group from MyPlate, as well as serving sizes. In general, boys require more servings than girls because they are larger and have more muscle mass. The lower calorie amounts are appropriate for more sedentary teens, and the higher amounts are appropriate for active teens. Sedentary adults need fewer calories (2,000 or below).

Dietitians often use common objects to help you to better understand the size of a recommended serving. The following list provides some examples of single servings:

- Baked potato: Computer mouse
- Bagel: Can of tuna
- Apple: Baseball
- Hard cheese: Three game dice
- Lean beef: Deck of cards

TABLE 16.3   **Recommended Number and Size of Servings**

Food group	Calorie range			Serving size examples
	<2,200	**2,200–2,800**	**>2,800**	
Grain	6 servings	9 servings	11 servings	1 slice bread; 1/2 cup cooked cereal, rice, or pasta; 1 cup cold cereal; 1/4 cup wheat germ; 1 6-in. (15-cm) tortilla
Vegetable	3 servings	4 servings	5 servings	1 cup raw leafy vegetables, 1/2 cup other vegetables (chopped or cooked), 3/4 cup vegetable juice, 1/2 cup cooked vegetables
Fruit	2 servings	2 or 3 servings	3 or 4 servings	1 orange, 3/4 cup fruit juice, 1 cup cooked fruit
Dairy	2 or 3 servings	2 or 3 servings	2 or 3 servings	1 cup milk or yogurt, 1 1/2 cups ice cream, 1 1/2 oz. (43 g) cheese
Protein foods	2 servings	3 servings	3 servings	2–3 oz. (57–85 g) cooked meat, poultry, or fish; 1/2 cup cooked dried beans; 2 tbsp peanut butter; 1/4 cup nuts or seeds; 1 whole egg

LESSON REVIEW

1. What are the three types of nutrients that provide energy, and what are some examples of foods for each type of nutrient?

2. What are the three types of nutrients that do not provide energy, and what are some examples of foods for each type of nutrient?

3. What are the six groups from which foods are chosen for healthy eating, and what foods should be limited in the diet?

4. What is the importance of limiting the number and size of servings for healthy eating?

SELF-ASSESSMENT: **Energy Balance**

This self-assessment helps determine how many calories you take in and expend each day. As directed, record the required information on worksheets provided by your instructor. Remember that self-assessment information is confidential.

STEP 1: Determine Your Calorie Intake

Prepare a log of the foods, food groups, and amounts you consumed in one day. Table 16.4 shows a sample food log prepared by Sandy, a 15-year-old male in the ninth grade. He recorded the number of servings for each food and made a check by the food group it came from to help him see if he was eating from each group. To help him determine serving sizes, he used table 16.3. Then he used a food calculator to determine the number of calories in each food. Finally, he added the calories and the number of servings of each food to determine his total calorie intake and see if he had met the recommended guidelines for each food group. Sandy's total calorie intake for Wednesday was 2,551, which falls in the recommended range for a male teen.

Prepare a one-day food log similar to Sandy's. Check to see if all food groups were represented. Use a food calculator to determine the number of calories in the foods you ate (see the web resource for this chapter).

TABLE 16.4   Sandy's Food Log for Wednesday

Food	Servings	Calories	Grain	Vegetables	Fruit	Protein	Milk	Other
Breakfast								
Scrambled egg	1	104				✓		
Fried ham slice	1	82				✓		
Whole-wheat toast slice	2	138 (69 × 2)	✓					
8 oz. glass of orange juice	1	112			✓			
Breakfast total		436						

>continued

TABLE 16.4 >continued

Food	Servings	Calories	Grain	Vegetables	Fruit	Protein	Milk	Other
Lunch								
Cheese pizza slice	3	693 (231 × 3)	✓			✓	✓	
Small salad	1	33		✓				
Salad dressing	1	71						✓
12 oz. soda	1	150						✓
Lunch total		947						
Dinner								
Green beans	2	88 (44 × 2)		✓				
Baked potato	2	242 (121 × 2)		✓				
Sour cream for potato	1	62					✓	
Broiled chicken breast	2	282 (141 × 2)				✓		
16 oz. glass of fat-free milk	2	166 (83 × 2)					✓	
Salad	1	33		✓				
Salad dressing	1	71						✓
Dinner total		944						
Snack								
Bag of chips	1	152		✓				✓
Apple	1	72			✓			
Snack total		224						
Daily total		2,551						

STEP 2: Estimate Your Calorie Expenditure

First, determine your **resting metabolism**—the number of calories expended by your body for its basic functions and the typical light activities done during the day. Resting metabolism includes your basal metabolism (the calories required for sleeping, digesting food, and other sedentary behavior) plus the calories you use for light daily activities such as teeth brushing, eating, reading, and typing. Sandy used table 16.5 to determine his resting metabolism based on his sex, age (15 years), weight (150 pounds, or 68 kilograms), and height (70 inches, or 1.8 meters). The chart indicated a resting metabolism of 1,800 calories each day. Sandy recorded this figure in his activity log.

Determine your resting metabolism using the appropriate table. For males, use table 16.5 (ages 12 through 15) or table 16.6 (age 16 or older). For females, use table 16.7 (ages 12 through 15) or table 16.8 (age 16 or older). Record your resting metabolism.

Next, Sandy prepared a log of his physical activity for one day, including each activity and its length (table 16.9). Here are Sandy's calculations.

TABLE 16.5   Resting Metabolism (Calories) for Males Aged 12 to 15

Height (in.)	Weight (lb)					
	100	120	150	180	200	≥220
<60–64	1,380	1,500	1,700	1,900	2,000	2,100
65–68	1,430	1,550	1,750	1,950	2,050	2,200
69–72	1,480	1,600	1,800	2,000	2,100	2,230
≥73	1,500	1,630	1,820	2,010	2,130	2,240

To convert centimeters to inches, divide by 2.54. To convert kilograms to pounds, divide by 0.45.

TABLE 16.6   Resting Metabolism (Calories) for Males Aged 16 or Older

Height (in.)	Weight (lb)					
	100	120	150	180	200	≥220
<60–64	1,360	1,480	1,670	1,860	1,980	2,110
65–68	1,410	1,540	1,720	1,910	2,035	2,160
69–72	1,460	1,590	1,770	1,960	2,085	2,210
≥73	1,490	1,610	1,800	1,985	2,110	2,235

To convert centimeters to inches, divide by 2.54. To convert kilograms to pounds, divide by 0.45.

TABLE 16.7   Resting Metabolism (Calories) for Females Aged 12 to 15

Height (in.)	Weight (lb)					
	90	100	120	150	180	≥200
<60–64	1,275	1,320	1,410	1,540	1,670	1,755
65–68	1,295	1,340	1,425	1,560	1,690	1,775
69–72	1,315	1,360	1,445	1,575	1,705	1,795
≥73	1,325	1,370	1,455	1,585	1,715	1,800

To convert centimeters to inches, divide by 2.54. To convert kilograms to pounds, divide by 0.45.

TABLE 16.8   Resting Metabolism (Calories) for Females Aged 16 or Older

Height (in.)	Weight (lb)					
	90	100	120	150	180	≥200
<60–64	1,260	1,300	1,390	1,520	1,650	1,740
65–68	1,275	1,320	1,405	1,540	1,670	1,755
69–72	1,295	1,340	1,425	1,555	1,685	1,775
≥73	1,305	1,350	1,440	1,565	1,700	1,785

To convert centimeters to inches, divide by 2.54. To convert kilograms to pounds, divide by 0.45.

- Sandy looked at a physical activity compendium (see the web resource for this chapter) and found that a person weighing 150 pounds (68 kilograms) expends 318 calories in one hour of walking, or 5.3 calories per minute (318 calories ÷ 60 minutes = 5.3 calories per minute). Therefore, he expends 53 calories in a 10-minute walk (5.3 × 10 = 53).

- Sandy also did 30 minutes of the Burn It Up workout in physical education class (see the Taking Action feature at the end of this chapter). This activity causes a 150-pound person to expend 340 calories per hour, or 5.7 calories per minute (340 ÷ 60 = 5.7). Therefore, in 30 minutes, Sandy expended about 170 calories (5. × 30 = 170).

- Mowing the lawn expends 316 calories per hour for a person of Sandy's size, or about 5.25 calories per minute (316 ÷ 60 = about 5.25). He therefore expended about 79 calories mowing the lawn for 15 minutes (5.25 × 15 = 79).

Sandy recorded his calories expended in his activity log (see table 16.9). His calories expended in physical activity totaled 355. He added this number to his resting metabolism of 1,800 to determine that his total energy expenditure for the day was 2,155 calories (355 + 1,800 = 2,155).

Prepare an activity log similar to Sandy's, including each activity you performed during the day. Use the physical activity compendium or a physical activity calculator to determine the number of calories you expended for each activity, then add this calorie total to your resting metabolism calories to determine your total calories expended for the day.

TABLE 16.9   Sandy's Activities for Wednesday

Activity	Minutes	Calories per hour	Calories
Morning			
Physical education: Burn It Up workout	30	340	170
Walk to and from classes	10	318	53
Afternoon			
Walk to and from classes	10	318	53
Evening			
Mow lawn	15	316	79
Daily activity total	65		355
Resting metabolism			1,800
Total daily calories expended			2,155

STEP 3: Evaluate Your Calorie Balance

Compare your calorie expenditure to your calorie intake to see if your calories balance for the day. Sandy expended 2,155 calories for the day but consumed 2,551, so he consumed 396 calories more than he expended (2,551 − 2,155 = 396). It's not unusual to consume more calories than expended on one day, then consume less on another. However, if Sandy regularly consumed 396 calories a day more than he expended, he would gain body fat over time.

Determine if you have energy balance by subtracting the smaller number (whether calorie intake or calorie expenditure) from the larger number.

Making Healthy Food Choices

Lesson Objectives

After reading this lesson, you should be able to

1. describe the FIT formula for meeting nutritional needs;

2. explain the difference between a food serving and a food portion;

3. identify several important elements of food labels and describe the difference between an FDA label and the food label of the manufacturer; and

4. describe some common nutrition myths and the guidelines for eating before physical activity.

Lesson Vocabulary

calorimeter
food label

Do you know how to read a nutrition label? Have you ever wondered if your portion sizes are the same as the serving size listed on a nutrition label? In the previous lesson, you learned how to choose healthy foods to build a nutritious diet. You also learned how dietary guidelines can help you attain and maintain good health. In this lesson, you'll learn more about being an informed nutrition consumer.

The FIT Formula and Nutrition

Just as there is a FIT formula for each type of physical activity in the Physical Activity Pyramid, there is a FIT formula for nutrition. Table 16.10 shows how you can use the FIT formula as a guide to healthy eating.

Teens in particular often violate the FIT formula. For example, they may skip breakfast or lunch, which can lead them to overeat later in the day. Skipping meals can make you feel tired and make it difficult to concentrate, contributing to poor school performance. If you play on a sports team, skipping meals can also negatively affect your performance.

I always thought that the calories listed on a box of candy was for the whole box. I was surprised to learn that most boxes of candy have several servings.

Jasmine Brady

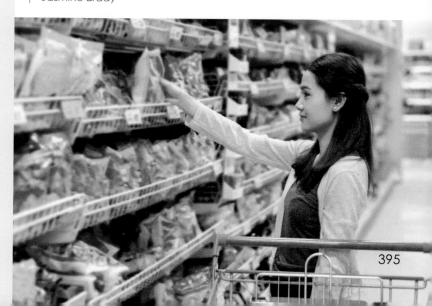

TABLE 16.10   **FIT Formula for Healthy Eating**

	Nutrition target zone
Frequency	Eat three healthy meals a day. You may choose more meals per day (four or five) with similar total calories. Healthy planned snacks can be part of a healthy diet.
Intensity	The number of calories you consume should be equal to the calories you expend each day. Calories should come from recommended servings for each food group.
Time	Eat meals at regular intervals, such as morning, noon, and evening.

As shown in table 16.10, frequency refers to how often you eat. The calories in all of the foods you eat each day can be used to describe the "intensity" of your diet. The calories in your diet should be similar to the calories you expend based on your metabolism and your daily activities. Your metabolism depends on your age, sex, height, and weight (see Self-Assessment). Young people who are going through puberty or are still growing have special nutritional needs; specifically, they need to eat foods high in minerals that aid in the development of bones and blood (potassium, calcium, iron). The time when you eat meals is also important—dietitians recommend eating at regular intervals during the day. If you eat the recommended number of servings from each of the food groups, you're well on your way to meeting your nutritional needs.

Portions

In the previous lesson you learned about the number of servings of each type of food necessary for a nutritious diet. As you know, a serving is a specific measured amount of food. However, it is not necessarily the same as a portion of food. A portion is the amount of food you put on your plate or that is served at a restaurant. It can also be the amount of food that you eat from a package (e.g., box of candy, bag of chips). A large portion can contain much more than a recommended serving, and a small portion can contain less.

The United States Department of Health and Human Services indicates that the size of portions in restaurants and on store shelves has increased considerably over the last 20 years, referred to as "portion distortion." As shown in figure 16.5, a typical soda has tripled in size and a box of popcorn has more than doubled in size. One reason for Americans' increase in portion sizes is the marketing of larger meals—for example, the original size of most French fry orders contained 450 calories, but the size of a large order currently promoted by many fast food outlets contains more than 600 calories. Another example is all-you-can-eat buffets offered at a set price, which can motivate people to eat large portions in order to get their money's worth. The following guidelines can help you control portion size.

- Know the size of a recommended serving.
- Choose portions equal to recommended servings.
- Eat only part of large portions; save extra food for another meal.
- Read food labels carefully to determine the size of servings in a package or container (see next section). Calorie totals listed on food labels (see figure 16.6) typically show the number of calories in one serving, but a package often contains several servings. To consume the number of calories on the label, choose only an amount from the package that is equal to a recommended serving.

FIT FACT

The Dietary Guidelines for Americans 2020–2025 encourage people to "customize and enjoy" nutrient-dense foods and beverages to reflect personal preferences, cultural traditions, and budgetary considerations. You can "make every bite count" by making shifts in eating patterns to nutrient-dense foods that you enjoy.

Portion distortion

	Bagel	Cheeseburger	Popcorn (medium bag)	Soda
20 years ago	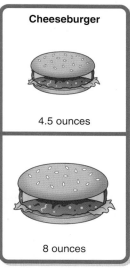 3 inches (diameter)	4.5 ounces	5 cups	6.5 ounces
Today	6 inches (diameter)	8 ounces	11 cups	20 ounces

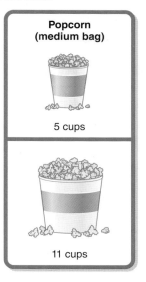
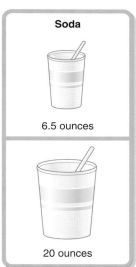

Source: *National Heart, Lung, and Blood Institute*

Figure 16.5 Increased portion size over last 20 years.

Food Labels

Many teenagers do not shop for groceries, plan meals, or cook for a family, but these are important skills you can start learning now. You also need to know the ingredients of snacks and other foods that you buy personally. Reading and understanding **food labels** can help you plan your diet and shop for healthy foods. By law, manufacturers must now use a standard format for FDA-approved food labels.

FDA-Approved Labels

The FDA requires food manufacturers to provide food labels on their products. Typically these labels are included on the side or occasionally the back of the food package. You've probably already used nutrition labels at one time or another, but you may not know how to use them most effectively. When reading an FDA-approved food label, start at the top and use the six steps in the following paragraphs. Food labels are typically all white, but colors are used in figure 16.6 to help you easily find each area on the label.

Reading FDA food labels will help you select healthy foods.

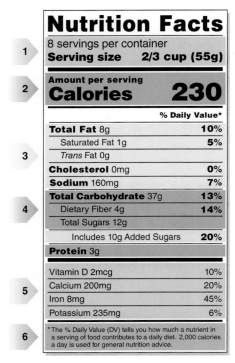

Figure 16.6   Sample food label.

From USDA.

Step 1: Servings

The number of servings in the container is shown in the green area of figure 16.6. In this case, eight servings are listed, and the size of each serving is 2/3 of a cup, thus making a total of 5 1/3 cups (8 × 2/3 = 5 1/3) in the package.

Step 2: Calories

The red area shows the number of calories per serving—in this case, 230 calories. Therefore, the total calorie content of the food package is 1,840 (230 calories × 8 servings = 1,840 calories).

Step 3: Percentage of Daily Requirement: Fats and Salts

The yellow area presents information about some nutrients that should be limited in your diet, including total fat, saturated fat, trans fat, cholesterol, and salt. The number beside each nutrient indicates the amount in grams (g) or milligrams (mg) and the percentage of that nutrient's daily calorie amount provided by one serving. In this case, one serving provides 10 percent of the total fat and 7 percent of the salt you should consume each day. If you eat two servings, you need to double the listed numbers to know how much fat and salt you're consuming. Trans fat amounts are shown in figure 16.6, although they are no longer allowed in processed food. Until the FDA ban is fully implemented, the grams of trans fat in foods must still be included on food labels.

Step 4: Percentage of Daily Requirement: Carbohydrate and Protein

Carbohydrate and protein are two of the three macronutrients that provide your body with energy. Two types of carbohydrate are listed on the label: dietary fiber and sugars (total and added). As shown in the blue box, one serving of this food provides 13 percent of the daily requirement of carbohydrate (37 grams). Dietary fiber, a type of carbohydrate, is desirable in the diet—one serving of this food provides 14 percent of the daily fiber requirement (4 grams). Added sugars (shaded in yellow) should be limited in the diet like fat and sodium. This food is high in added sugars, providing 20 percent of the daily requirement (10 grams). This food also provides 3 grams of protein. The label does not provide a percentage of the daily requirement. However, the FDA recommends a minimum of 0.3 grams of protein per pound of body weight each day (45 grams for a person weighing 150 pounds), so one serving provides about 7 percent (3 ÷ 45 = 6.7 g) of the daily protein requirement for a 150-pound person. This may be adjusted based on your body weight.

Step 5: Percentage of Daily Requirement: Micronutrients

Micronutrients, such as vitamins and minerals, are especially important to your diet. Four types of micronutrients, two vitamins and two minerals, are highlighted in orange on the label. As you can see, one serving of this food provides 10 percent of vitamin D, 20 percent of calcium, 45 percent of iron, and 6 percent of potassium required each day.

Step 6: Footnote

The information in the purple area at the bottom of the label is designed to inform you that the percentages in the label are based on a diet of 2,000 calories a day. The total number of calories needed each day varies from person to person depending on factors described in the Self-Assessment for this chapter. People who require more or fewer calories need to adjust the nutrient amounts accordingly. For example, a person requiring 2,500 calories per day consumes 500 calories more than a person consuming 2,000 calories per day. So this person's daily requirements for nutrients is 25 percent higher ($500 \div 2000 = 0.25$) than a person consuming only 2,000 calories a day.

Other Food Labels

Be aware that the food labels required by the FDA are not the same as the food labels sometimes provided by manufacturers on the front of food packages. Front-of-box labels are not regulated and may not be accurate. In fact, the FDA has sent warning letters to companies that make false claims on front-of-the-box labels. Front-of-the-box labels may include unauthorized health or nutrition claims or unauthorized use of terms such as *healthy*. Nutrition experts criticize manufacturer labels not only because they are deceptive but also because they are part of a strategy to sell the food rather than provide nutrition information. Rather than the front-of-box label, you should check the regulated FDA label for scientifically sound information.

You've learned that approved labels provide useful information and that some front-of-box labels can be deceiving. But there are also other food labels you should know about. One type of label refers to a food's fat content. In the United States, labels such as "fat free" can be displayed on food containers only if the food meets legal standards set by the government. The terms, presented in table 16.11, were developed to prevent false advertising. Even with these standardized terms, however, you can still be fooled by advertisements relating to a food's fat content. Some foods, such as milk and packaged meats, are advertised as 2 percent fat—that is, 98 percent fat free. This is true if fat is measured by the product's weight, but it is not true if fat is measured by the total number of calories in the food. For example, only 2 percent of the weight of a glass of 2 percent milk is fat, but more than 30 percent of the calories come from fat.

You also might see health claims such as "good for heart health" on some food labels. Manufacturers must comply with government regulations regarding

FIT FACT

Calories from soda add up fast. Most soft drinks contain about 150 calories in a 12-ounce (about 0.4-liter) can, and many teens drink multiple cans per day. A 64-ounce (about 1.8-liter) drink, such as those sold at many fast food and convenience stores, contains almost 800 calories. Not surprisingly, studies show that excessive consumption of soft drinks may be one reason for the high incidence of overweight in developed countries. In fact, if all other aspects of your diet stayed the same, adding one soft drink a day would cause you to gain 15 pounds (about 7 kilograms) of fat in a year. The solution? Water quenches your thirst and contains zero calories.

TABLE 16.11 **Key Words on Food Labels and What They Mean**

Key words	What they mean
Fat free	Equal to or less than 0.5 g of fat
Low fat	Equal to or less than 3 g of fat per serving
Lean	Equal to or less than 10 g of fat, 4 g of saturated fat, and 95 mg of cholesterol
Light (or "lite")	1/3 fewer calories or no more than 1/2 the fat of the higher-calorie or higher-fat version; or no more than 1/2 the sodium of the higher-sodium version
Cholesterol free	Equal to or less than 2 mg of cholesterol and 2 or less g of saturated fat per serving

TECH TRENDS: **What's in Your Food?**

A **calorimeter** is an apparatus designed to determine the amount of heat generated by a chemical reaction. (In Latin, *calor* means heat and *metron* means measure; thus a calorimeter measures heat.) A special type of calorimeter is used to determine the amount of heat created when different types of food are burned. In this way, nutrition scientists have determined the calorie counts of various foods.

The web has also made it easy for you to find other information about food content. For example, some nutrition websites list the specific nutrient content (carbohydrate, protein, fat, vitamins, and minerals) of various foods. Some address foods of all kinds, and others provide information specifically about fast food. You can find these amounts using an online nutrition calculator.

USING TECHNOLOGY

Search the web for nutrition calculators. Try one of the calculators and write an evaluation explaining how the tool would or would not be useful.

such labeling. For example, if a product is advertised as "good for your heart," the product must be low in fat, saturated fat, and cholesterol. Fruits, vegetables, and grain products for which such claims are made must not only be low in fat, saturated fat, and cholesterol but also contain at least the minimum amount of fiber per serving. Foods that display health claims related to blood pressure must be low in sodium.

▌Common Food Myths

Many myths exist about what to eat and when to eat. There is also confusion about patterns of eating prior to physical activity. This is at least partly because people share incorrect information in conversation and on social media. In this section some common myths are discussed and guidelines for eating prior to physical activity are presented.

ACADEMIC CONNECTION: **Calculating Fat Content in Food**

To calculate the calories of fat in a product, use the label to determine the fat content in grams for one serving. Multiply the number of grams of fat by 9 (the number of calories in a gram of fat) to determine the calories of fat in one serving. Then divide the calories of fat per serving by the total calories per serving to find what percent of the calories are from fat. The following is a sample calculation for one serving of macaroni and cheese.

Fat content in one food serving

Calories in one gram of fat = 9

Grams of fat in one serving = 12

Calories of fat in one serving = $9 \times 12 = 108$

Total calories in one serving = 250

Percent of fat in one serving = 108/250 = 43%

STUDENT ACTIVITY

You can do your own calculation to determine the true percentage of fat calories in a food. Choose a food for which you have a food label. Use the information from the label and the method of calculation above to determine the percentage of fat in the food.

TABLE 16.12 **Myths and Facts About Nutrition**

Myth	Fact
Skipping meals is a good way to lose weight.	Studies show that people who skip meals often eat more than those who eat regular meals. Skipping meals stimulates the appetite, so eating fewer meals can lead to eating more food at each meal, whereas eating more meals usually means eating less at each meal. Skipping breakfast or lunch is common but is ineffective for weight loss and results in lower work and school performance.
A food supplement is tested to ensure that it is safe and that it meets the claims advertised by the seller.	Since 1994, food supplements have not been regulated in the United States. This means that they are not tested by the government for safety or effectiveness. Beware of supplements that make claims that are too good to be true.
As long as you limit the amount of fat in your food, you do not need to be concerned with how many calories a food contains.	It's the total number of calories you consume that makes a difference in weight maintenance. Fat does contain more calories per gram (9) than carbohydrate (4) and protein (4), but many foods advertised as low in fat actually contain more calories than foods higher in fat.
Diets very low in calories are effective for weight loss.	Your body needs calories in order to function. Eating too few calories in a day (800 or less) causes the body to conserve calories to keep the body functioning, which means your body uses fewer calories than it normally would. Eating too few calories is not an effective way to reduce body fat and in fact can be dangerous because very low calorie diets typically do not provide the basic nutrients that your body needs.
You should avoid eating before exercise.	Most people can do moderate activity after a meal if they wait about 30 minutes to an hour. People who have problems doing activity after eating may have to wait longer or modify when and what they eat. You may also have to modify your eating pattern if you plan to do vigorous physical activity or participate in a highly competitive athletic event.

Food Myths

You may have heard a number of incorrect or misleading statements about nutrition. Some common nutrition myths are exposed in table 16.12.

Because health and nutrition quackery is so common, many other myths also exist. When making choices about your nutrition, follow the Dietary Guidelines for Americans. Use information that comes from reliable sources, such as the USDA, the U.S. Food and Drug Administration (FDA), the American Dietetic Association, the American Medical Association, the American Heart Association, the American Cancer Society, and the Center for Science in the Public Interest.

Eating Before Physical Activity

Use the following guidelines for eating before vigorous or competitive physical activity.

- *A special diet is usually not necessary before an athletic competition.* Some athletes think they need a steak before they compete. Steak, however, is high in protein and fat, both of which are digested slowly. As a result, eating steak within two hours of the event might interfere with your performance. In general, you can eat what you like as long as it doesn't disagree with you.

- *Allow extra time between eating and a vigorous competitive event.* Eat one to three hours before competing. Allow more time if you're eating food that's difficult to digest (for example, large servings of meat, spicy foods, and high-fiber foods).

- *Before competition, reduce meal size.* Small meals are easier to digest than large ones. If you get very nervous or often have an upset stomach before competition, limiting meal size can be helpful.

- *Before competition, avoid snacks that are high in simple carbohydrate (simple sugar).* Some people think that having a candy bar or drink that's high in simple carbohydrate before competition will provide quick energy. In fact, taking a big dose of simple carbohydrate right before an event causes blood sugar to go up, but a drop in blood sugar level often follows after exertion. This can cause lack of energy and even dizziness, and it may negatively affect performance and increase risk of injury.

- *Drink before, during, and after activity.* Whether you're competing or not, it's important to drink water. You don't usually need added salt or sugar, except for during especially long events and events occurring in high heat and humidity. Using drinks with too much sugar can even detract from your performance. Drinking too much before activity can cause a side stitch in some people; these people should drink fluids well before the activity in several small amounts.

Snacks with friends can be all right if they are low in empty calories and included as part of a total dietary plan.

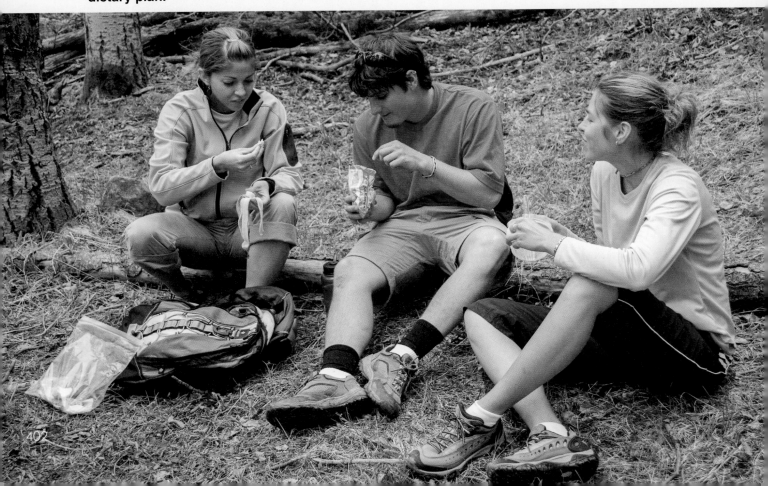

LESSON REVIEW

1. How can the FIT formula help people meet their nutritional needs?
2. What are some differences between a food serving and a food portion?
3. What are several of the important elements of food labels, and what is the difference between an FDA label and a manufacturer food label?
4. What are some common nutrition myths, and what are the guidelines for eating before physical activity?

TAKING CHARGE: **Saying No**

Sometimes the simple act of saying no is the best way to avoid a potentially harmful situation. However, while it may seem easy, saying no can actually be very difficult to carry out successfully. Here's an example.

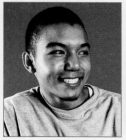 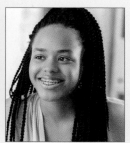

Many cultures celebrate special occasions with special meals and foods. On one such occasion, Manny was invited to celebrate his girlfriend's quinceañera with her family. Plans were made to spend the afternoon waterskiing at a nearby lake, then have a big party. Manny's girlfriend Rita warned him that her mother always prepared huge amounts of food for this special day. The family did not normally eat so much, but on this special day it was their tradition to feast on traditional foods. She told him to make sure he came with a big appetite. Unfortunately, Manny's doctor had just instructed him to restrict his intake of salt, fat, and calories.

Manny arrived at the party just as Rita's mother was setting out the food. The table was loaded with tortilla chips, guacamole, beef and bean burritos, chiles rellenos, and fresh corn, as well as cakes, pies, and cookies. Manny knew that he faced a difficult situation as Rita came forward with a plate piled with high cookies.

"Manny, you're just in time," she said. "The food is great!" Manny was concerned about the salt and fat in the food and wanted to avoid consuming too many calories, but he did not want to hurt Rita's feelings, so he replied, "Everything looks good, but I have to watch my diet."

Rita offered him a cookie, knowing they were Manny's favorite. "But you've got to try my mother's cookies. Everyone says they're the best. You'll hurt my mother's feelings if you don't eat one." Manny felt pressured to eat something he didn't really want.

FOR DISCUSSION

In what way does the party put Manny in a difficult situation? How can Manny say no to Rita without embarrassing her or hurting her feelings? What can he do so that his refusal won't hurt Rita's mother's feelings? What could he have done to prepare for the situation before going to the party? What are some other situations in which saying no would be the best response? Consider the guidelines in the following Self-Management feature as you answer these discussion questions.

SELF-MANAGEMENT: **Skills for Saying No**

Most of us try to eat well, do regular physical activity, and live a healthy lifestyle. But sometimes the situation we're in or the people we're around make it difficult to stick with healthy behaviors. You can take steps to make it easier to say no when you're in situations that encourage you to engage in behaviors you know are not best for you. The following guidelines will help you say no to eating food that you don't want or need. You may also be able to use these strategies to help you say no in other situations involving choices about health-related behavior.

- *Say no to food offered on special occasions.* Eat a light meal before a holiday event so that you don't arrive hungry. Practice ways to refuse food so that you don't hurt the host's feelings. For example, talk to the host or hostess ahead of time to explain why you may limit your food intake. Prepare statements ahead of time that you can use if you're pressured to eat.

- *Use strategies to avoid temptation.* Avoid standing near food. If you feel the urge to eat, talk to someone or find something else to do.

- *Plan in advance when eating out.* Resist ordering foods that are advertised or that others eat. Avoid big orders such as large burgers and fries. Say no to special deals that include foods you don't want; instead, order single items you do want. Say no to extra sauces, toppings, and condiments such as mayonnaise.

- *Shop with a strategy.* Prepare a list ahead of time and stick with it to help you say no to foods that are high in empty calories. Use food labels and avoid foods that are high in calories per serving. Look for better choices. Eat before you shop so that you're not hungry while making choices.

- *Consume healthy snacks.* Eating vegetables and fruits for snacks can help you say no to snacks that are high in empty calories, such as potato chips, cookies, and candy. Avoid sugared soft drinks and sport drinks; instead, carry a water bottle.

- *Eat healthy foods at school.* Prepare your own lunch and snacks for school to help you say no to unhealthy food offered in snack machines. If you have free time, find a way to be active to avoid thinking about eating things you don't really want or need. If you eat school food, ask for small servings to avoid eating too much. If you have free time with friends, bring healthy snacks to share.

- *Say no to large servings and seconds.* Tell family members and friends not to offer seconds. Limit dessert servings.

- *Eat slowly and avoid eating while studying or watching television.* Some experts recommend that you limit your eating to the kitchen or dining room to help you say no to unwanted food.

Taking Action: **Burn It Up Workout**

All types of activity included in the Physical Activity Pyramid use calories and therefore help you balance your calorie expenditure with your calorie intake. Moderate and vigorous activity can both be beneficial—moderate activity can be performed over a longer span of time, whereas vigorous activity burns more calories in the same amount of time. For example, a 120-pound (54-kilogram) person burns about 85 calories by walking for 20 minutes (a moderate activity) but 125 calories by jogging for 20 minutes (a vigorous activity). You can also boost your energy expenditure fairly easily by adding bursts of higher-intensity effort to your exercise routine. Muscle fitness exercises also expend calories, as well as build muscle mass that causes you to expend more calories even at rest.

Take action with a "Burn It Up" workout by selecting activities of various types and intensities. Perform the workout and estimate the number of calories expended (burned) in the workout using an online activity calculator such as the ACE calorie calculator.

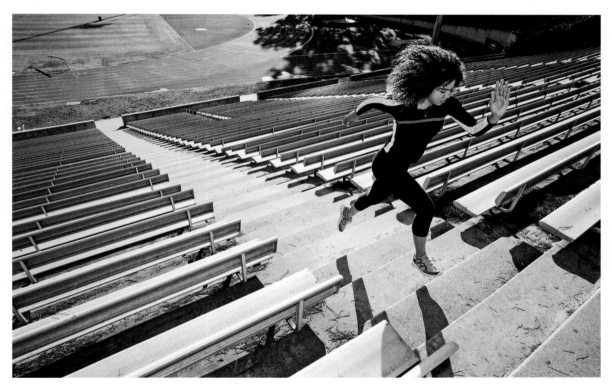

Take action with the Burn It Up workout.

CHAPTER REVIEW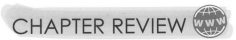

Reviewing Concepts and Vocabulary

Answer items 1 through 5 by correctly completing each sentence with a word or phrase.

1. _____ occurs when you expend as many calories as you consume.

2. Foods that are high in calories but low in nutrients are said to contain _____ calories.

3. _____ are the substances that make up protein.

4. A portion of food is the amount of a specific food on your plate; it differs from a _____, which is the recommended amount of a specific food.

5. The minimum amount of a nutrient necessary to meet health needs is called the Recommended _____.

For items 6 through 10, match each term in column 1 with the appropriate phrase in column 2.

6. carbohydrate   a. major source of energy

7. protein   b. regulates cell activity

8. fiber   c. solid at room temperature

9. saturated fat   d. cannot be digested by the body

10. mineral   e. building block for your body

For items 11 through 15, respond to each statement or question.

11. Describe your body's need for fat and the best types to include in your diet.

12. Describe some common myths about food and explain how they might affect you.

13. Explain how FDA-approved food labels can help you eat well.

14. Describe several guidelines about eating before physical activity.

15. Describe several guidelines for saying no in situations when you might feel pressured to do something you don't want to do.

Thinking Critically

Write a paragraph to answer the following question.

Your friend asks for your advice about her diet. She wonders whether the food choices she makes are important or whether she only needs to count calories. She has also started to increase her physical activity and wonders how that will affect her caloric and nutritional needs. What advice would you give your friend?

Project

You learned about MyPlate in this chapter. MyPlate was preceded by a similar diagram called MyPyramid and, before that, the Food Guide Pyramid. Other diagrams, such as the rainbow-themed Canada's Food Guide, have been developed to help people make sound nutrition decisions. Check out these diagrams, choose the one that you like best, and explain your reasons, or create a new nutrition diagram to help people better understand the types of food in a healthy diet.

Stress Management

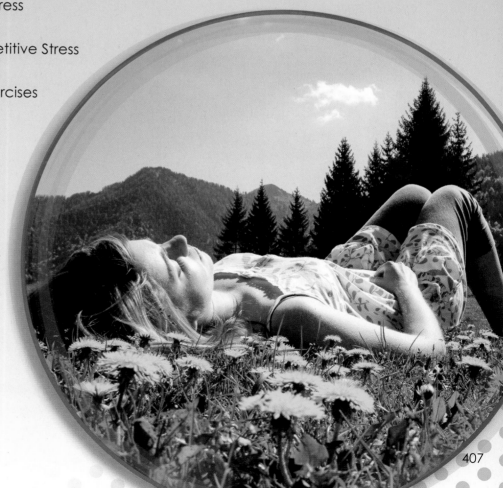

LESSON 17.1
Facts About Stress

Lesson Objectives

After reading this lesson, you should be able to

1. define *stress* and *stressor* and describe the stress responses of general adaptation syndrome;
2. define *distress* and *eustress* and describe some common causes of stress;
3. identify and describe some of the effects of stress; and
4. define *coping skills* and explain why they are important and discuss the value of seeking help when you experience stress.

Lesson Vocabulary

alarm reaction
coping
coping skills
distress
eustress
general adaptation syndrome
stage of exhaustion
stage of resistance
stress
stressor

Have you ever given a performance or speech in front of a lot of people? Did it make you anxious? If so, your heart rate may have increased and your muscles may have gotten tense. Stressful situations can bring these changes about by causing your body to release a chemical called *adrenaline*. The changes are part of what is called the *stress response*—your body's way of preparing you to deal with a demanding situation.

You probably face stressful situations every day that affect you both physically and emotionally. In fact, two-thirds of Americans report feeling "stressed out" at least once a week. In this lesson, you'll read more about stress, how your body responds to it, and stress management. Along with regular physical activity and good nutrition, stress management should be a priority in your healthy lifestyle. This lesson will teach you about the Stress Management Pyramid and its five steps (figure 17.1).

My sister did a bungee jump at the amusement park. She said, "Try it, it's great!" I didn't! It stressed me out. I realized that what was stressful for me was not for her.

Anthony DiGennaro

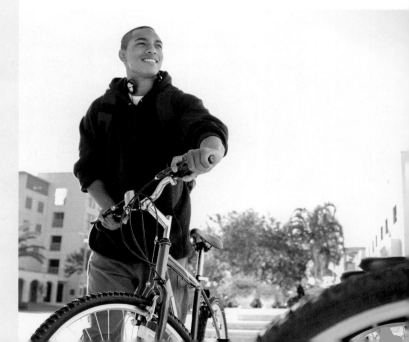

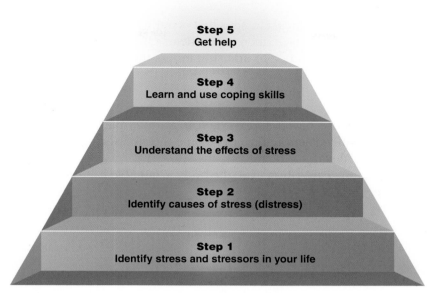

Figure 17.1   The five steps of the Stress Management Pyramid.

Step 1: Identify Stress and Stressors

Stress is the body's reaction to a demanding situation. A **stressor** is something that causes or contributes to stress. As shown in figure 17.1, the first step in managing stress is to identify stress when you have it.

When you're in a highly stressful situation, a series of physical changes takes place automatically. As researcher Hans Selye showed, when people are exposed to stressors, they undergo what is called **general adaptation syndrome**, which includes three stages (see figure 17.2). In responding to a stressor, the body first initiates an **alarm reaction**. Anything that causes you to worry, get excited, or experience other emotional and physical changes can be a stressor and thus can start your body's alarm reaction. For adults, common stressors include bills, vacation plans, work responsibilities, and family conflicts. Common stressors for teenagers include grades and schoolwork, family arguments, peer pressure, moving to a new home, serious illness or death in the family, poor eating habits, lack of physical activity, feelings of loneliness, a

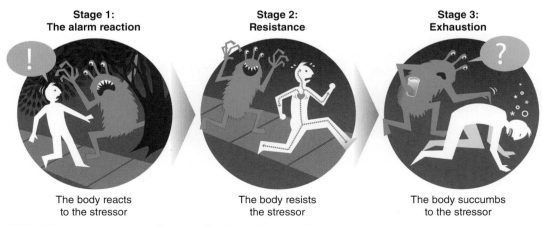

Figure 17.2   The three stages of general adaptation syndrome.

> One person's stress is another's pleasure.
>
> *Ruth Lindsey, fitness author*

change or loss of friends, substance abuse, bullying, and trouble with school or legal authorities.

Some of the physical changes that occur when your body starts its alarm reaction to a stressor, such as an increase in heart rate, are shown in figure 17.3. After your body has had a chance to adjust, it enters the second stage of general adaptation syndrome, the **stage of resistance**, in which your body systems start to resist or fight the stressor. In the case of an illness, antibodies are sent out to fight. In the case of a physical stressor, such as doing heavy exercise, the heart rate increases to supply more blood and oxygen to various parts of your body. In most cases, your resistance is enough to overcome the stressor, and you adapt by returning to your normal state of being.

In extreme cases, however, the body is not able to resist and thus enters the third stage of the syndrome—the **stage of exhaustion**. In this case, medical treatment may be necessary. If the stressor is too great, as in the case of a disease that the body and medicine cannot fight, death can occur.

Step 2: Identify Causes of Stress

To be able to manage stress, you first have to know its causes (see step 2 of figure 17.1). Before learning more about the causes of stress, however, it is important to learn more about it. Not all stressful experiences are harmful. Scientists use the term **eustress** to describe positive stress (figure 17.4). Situations that can produce eustress include riding a roller coaster, successfully competing in an activity, passing a driving test, playing in the school band, and meeting new people. Eustress helps make your life more enjoyable by helping you meet challenges and do your best.

Negative stress is sometimes called **distress**, which is produced by situations that cause worry, sorrow, anger, or pain. A situation that causes eustress for one person can cause distress for another. For example, an outgoing person might look forward to joining extracurricular activities at school or attending social

FIT FACT

The prefix *eu* in the word *eustress* is taken from the word *euphoria*, which means a feeling of well-being.

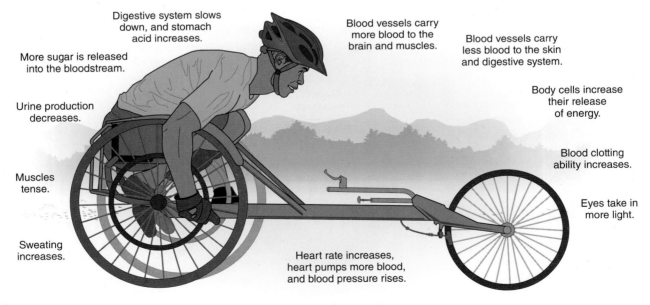

Figure 17.3   The stress response: Your body's way of preparing.

Digestive system slows down, and stomach acid increases.

More sugar is released into the bloodstream.

Urine production decreases.

Muscles tense.

Sweating increases.

Blood vessels carry more blood to the brain and muscles.

Blood vessels carry less blood to the skin and digestive system.

Body cells increase their release of energy.

Blood clotting ability increases.

Eyes take in more light.

Heart rate increases, heart pumps more blood, and blood pressure rises.

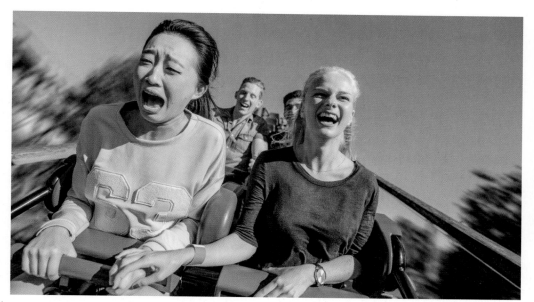

Figure 17.4 Stress can be positive or negative.

events, whereas a shy person might dread the same situations. In addition, the same experience can be eustressful for you at one time (taking a test for which you're well prepared) and distressful at another (taking a test for which you are not prepared). You'll learn more about identifying stressors in your own life in the Self-Assessment feature that follows this lesson.

Distress can negatively affect your total health and fitness (more on this in the next section). To control stress in your life, you need to understand the cause of the stress you're experiencing. Some causes of stress are described in the following sections.

Physical Stressors

Physical stressors are conditions in your body or environment that affect your physical well-being. Examples include thirst, hunger, overexposure to heat or cold, lack of sleep, illness, pollution, noise, accidents, and catastrophes such as a flood or fire. Even excessive exercise can be a stressor, as in the case of athletes who overtrain. However, healthy, fit people are better able to adapt to the changes produced by physical stressors.

Emotional Stressors

Emotions such as fear, anger, grief, depression, worry, and even falling in love are powerful stressors that can strongly affect your physical and emotional well-being. Another cause of emotional stress is overload—taking on more tasks than you can accomplish in the time available. To prevent or correct overload, learn to say no and develop your time management skills.

Social Stressors

Social stressors arise from your relationships with other people. Each day, you have interactions with your family members, friends, teachers, employers, and others, and some may be difficult or unpleasant. As a teenager, you're probably exposed to many social stressors. The coping skills described in this lesson can help you deal with social stressors.

Step 3: Understand the Effects of Stress

Once you understand the causes of stress, you can then better understand the effects of it. High levels or prolonged periods of stress can lead to both physical and emotional changes. Physical effects include increased stomach acid, which can aggravate ulcers, as well as high blood pressure, which can lead to serious cardiovascular diseases and disorders. Prolonged stress can also lower the effectiveness of your body's immune system, making you more susceptible to certain diseases. Other physical signs of stress include the following.

Acne flare-ups	Headache	Neckaches
Allergy flare-ups	Hyperventilation	Perspiring
Backaches	Increased blood pressure	Shortness of breath
Blurred vision	Indigestion	Tightness in throat
Constipation	Irregular heartbeat	Tightness in chest
Diarrhea	Light-headedness	Trembling
Difficulty sleeping	Muscle spasms	Upset stomach
Extreme fatigue	Muscle tension	Vomiting

Many stress-related health problems in the United States require medical attention, which should give us all the motivation we need to deal effectively with stress, especially distress.

Emotional effects of stress include feelings of nervousness; anger, anxiety, or fear; frequent criticism of others; frustration; forgetfulness; difficulty paying attention; difficulty making decisions; irritability; lack of motivation; boredom, depression, or withdrawal; and change in appetite.

FIT FACT
A study indicated that in recent years there has been a 35 percent increase in college students who seek help with mental health issues. One reason for the increase is the rise in rates of anxiety and depression among young adults. The good news, however, is that this increase also reflects a greater availability and use of mental health services.

Steps 4 and 5: Learn Coping Skills and Get Help

Once you've learned about the causes and effects of stress, you can move to step 4 of the pyramid—learning and using coping skills. **Coping** means attempting to deal with problems, and **coping skills** are techniques that you can use to manage stress and address problems. The next lesson describes five types of coping skills.

Coping skills can be very helpful for managing stress, but at times we all need assistance when things are not going well (step 5). As you learned in an earlier chapter, social support is important for a variety of reasons. It is especially helpful when you are experiencing stress. Good sources of support can include parents, other family members, teachers, clergy, and friends. In addition, experts such as school counselors, guidance counselors, nurses, and physicians can provide advice about stress management and dealing with depression. There are also mental health professionals who can help people manage stress. You can find out about such resources by asking a doctor, school counselor, or hospital referral service. Special hotlines are also available for assistance (see the web resource for more information).

SCIENCE IN ACTION: **Depression Among Teens**

Psychologists and public health scientists have done considerable research about depression among teens. As many as one in four teens report feeling sad for as long as two weeks at some point during the high school years. Although feeling sad is something that we all experience from time to time, extended bouts of sadness can be a sign of depression. Other common feelings—such as anxiety, restlessness, guilt, and irritability—can also be signs of depression when experienced in excess. Other, more serious signs of depression include feelings of emptiness and hopelessness. The risk of suicide is higher among teens who are depressed than those who are not. The U.S. National Institute of Mental Health offers the following suggestions for helping a friend who shows signs of depression.

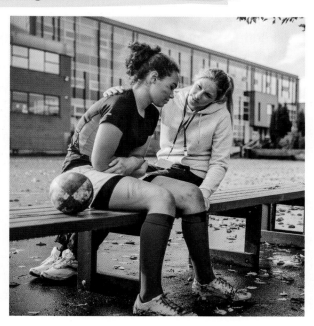

- Encourage your friend to talk to an adult and get evaluated by a doctor.
- Offer emotional support, understanding, patience, and encouragement.
- Talk with your friend—not necessarily about depression—and listen carefully.

- Never discount the feelings your friend expresses, but point out realities and offer hope.
- Never ignore comments about suicide; report them to a trusted adult.

STUDENT ACTIVITY

Interview a school guidance counselor or school nurse. Ask what help your school offers to help reduce stress and depression among teens. Ask what students can do to help. Write a summary of the interview.

LESSON REVIEW

1. How do you define *stress* and *stressor,* and how does your body respond to them?
2. How do you define *distress* and *eustress,* and what are some of the common causes of stress?
3. What are some of the physical and emotional effects of stress?
4. What are coping skills, and why are they important? What is the value of seeking help when you experience stress, and how can you find help?

SELF-ASSESSMENT: **Identifying Signs of Stress**

All people experience some negative stress in their lives, and when you do, your body sends off certain signals. You'll learn to identify some of these signals in this self-assessment.

Table 17.1 lists some common signs of stress. You may notice some of these signs when you are not under excessive stress, but they're often especially apparent in times of great stress.

One way to determine whether an activity is stressful to you is to self-assess for signs of stress before and after the activity. Working with a partner, use the following steps to look for the signs of stress included in table 17.1. Record results as directed by your instructor. Remember that self-assessment information is confidential and shouldn't be shared without the permission of the person being tested.

1. Lie on the floor, close your eyes, and try to relax. Have your partner count your pulse and your breathing rate. Ask your partner to observe you for irregular breathing and unusual mannerisms and evaluate how tense your muscles seem. Report any feeling of butterflies in your stomach or other indicators of stress to your partner. Record your results, then have your partner lie down while you assess them.

2. Next, all members of the class write their names on a piece of paper and place the papers in a hat or box. The teacher will then draw names until only three remain in the container. The students whose names remain will each give a one-minute speech about the effects of stress. During and after the name drawing, observe your partner. Look for signs of stress. Also, notice your own feelings during the drawing. Finally, observe the people who were required to make a speech. Write down your observations about stress symptoms in you, your partner, and other class members. Refer to table 17.1 as needed.

3. Finally, walk or jog for five minutes after your second stress assessment. Then, once again, work with a partner to assess your signs of stress. Notice that the exercise causes your heart rate and breathing rate to increase. At the same time, however, it may help reduce earlier signs of the emotional stress related to the possibility of performing in front of the class. Record your observations.

TABLE 17.1   Signs of Stress

Heart rate	Is it higher than normal?
Muscle tension	Are your muscles tighter than usual? • Arms and shoulders • Back and neck • Legs
Mannerisms	Are unusual mannerisms present? • Frowning or twitching • Hands to face (nail biting)
Nervous feelings	Do you feel different than you normally do? • Feeling of butterflies in stomach • Tense or anxious feelings
Breathing	Is your breathing different than usual? • Irregular • Rapid or shallow

Managing Stress

Lesson Objectives

After reading this lesson, you should be able to

1. describe several types of physical coping techniques;

2. describe several types of emotional coping techniques;

3. describe several types of social and spiritual coping techniques; and

4. describe several types of intellectual coping techniques.

Lesson Vocabulary

competitive stress
mindfulness
rumination
runner's high

What causes you stress? How do you react to stress? Do you have strategies for dealing with your stress? Are they healthy strategies? As you learned in the previous lesson, the first three steps in the Stress Management Pyramid require you to identify stress and its causes and effects in your life. The fourth step refers to learning coping skills that you can use to manage stress. There are four types of coping skills that are discussed in this lesson.

- Physical coping skills, such as exercising, reducing muscle tension, and getting enough sleep

- Emotional coping skills, such as laughing and thinking positively

- Social and spiritual coping skills, such as seeking social or spiritual support or getting professional help

- Intellectual coping skills, such as using problem-solving techniques and managing time

> Taking tests and speaking in public make me nervous. I learned some stress management techniques and now I do better.
>
> *Gail D'Spain*

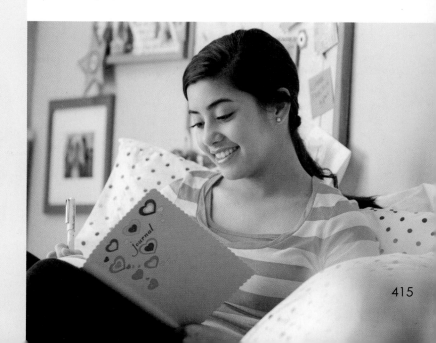

415

Physical Coping

The first type of coping skill involves taking physical steps to deal with stress. Here are some examples of techniques you can use.

- *Do regular physical activity.* Regular physical activity can help you reduce your stress. Noncompetitive physical activity can help you get your mind off of stressful situations. For example, people who jog regularly report experiencing a **runner's high**, or feelings of eustress experienced during or after a run. Similar feelings of eustress are experienced during or after other forms of vigorous aerobic exercise.

- *Reduce your breathing rate.* Sit or lie down quietly. Take a long slow breath, breathing in through your nose for 4 to 6 seconds. Exhale slowly through your mouth, again for 4 to 6 seconds. Repeat several times.

- *Reduce muscle tension.* Relaxing your muscles can help you reduce distress. You'll learn helpful relaxation techniques for reducing muscle tension in this chapter's Taking Action feature.

- *Rest in a quiet place.* Take time out to relax in a quiet place indoors or outdoors. Read. Listen to peaceful music.

- *Eat a nutritious, well-balanced diet.* Good nutrition contributes to good health, which can help you handle stress better. On the other hand, foods or drinks high in caffeine may cause you to be irritable and restless.

- *Get enough sleep.* Lack of sleep can lead to distress—in fact, lack of sleep is itself a stressor. Some problems might be easier to handle when you feel rested. Try to sleep at least 8 hours a night.

- *Pay attention to your body.* Notice how your body reacts in different situations. If you experience physical signs of distress, use some of the stress-management techniques described in this lesson.

- *Do relaxation exercises.* Perform the exercises shown in the following section. Consider yoga, tai chi, stretching exercises, and deep breathing exercises.

Emotional Coping

You can also manage stress by using emotional coping skills. Here are some examples.

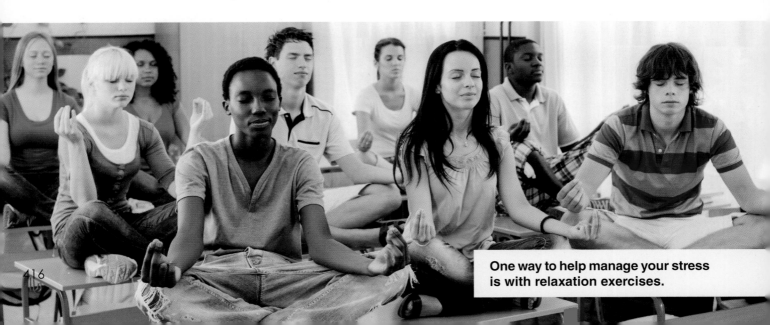

One way to help manage your stress is with relaxation exercises.

SCIENCE IN ACTION: Mindfulness

Mindfulness is a state of being characterized by a focus on the present moment. People in a state of mindfulness can enjoy what is happening right now, shutting out thoughts of past failures and concerns about the future.

Researchers have identified useful methods of mindfulness training that include breathing and relaxation exercises, positive mental imagery, avoiding negative thoughts, and other coping strategies and techniques such as those described in this lesson. A review of studies indicates that mindfulness training can reduce anxiety and depression, reduce harmful thoughts, and promote better social coping. Many schools have implemented programs designed to promote mindfulness with a focus on improving student attention, achievement, and classroom behavior; improving social–emotional skills such as social and empathy skills; and reducing test anxiety. Mindfulness training can also benefit athletes by helping them reduce competitive stress (see Taking Charge feature). Obviously, limiting time on digital devices and designating time free from devices is important if mindfulness training is to be effective.

Mindfulness training can help you if you are overly involved in gaming or using social media. If your school has a mindfulness training program, you may benefit from participating. If not, you can practice the coping skills and other techniques described in this lesson—many of these skills are similar to those used in mindfulness training programs.

STUDENT ACTIVITY

Search the term "mindfulness" to see if you find consistency in the definition of the term. Investigate different mindfulness training programs offered in person or on the web. Which do you think is most likely to be effective?

- *Try not to let little things bother you.* Many events in life are simply not worth stressing over. For example, if you're disappointed, remind yourself that a situation might be better the next time.

- *Think positively.* Positive thoughts can help you reduce distress. For example, try thinking that you *will* get a hit in the softball game instead of worrying about striking out. In softball, and all activities of life, success does not come with every attempt you make. Even the best hitters only get a hit about 30 percent of the time. Making an effort to perceive a stressor as a challenge rather than as a problem can help you think positively.

- *Avoid negative thoughts.* **Rumination** means to repeatedly think about a past—often distressing—event. Rumination can lead to additional distress rather than reducing it. To avoid rumination and negative thoughts, try focusing on positive thoughts, changing your way of thinking, or focusing on something pleasant.

- *Change the way you think.* Not all problems can be solved, but you can still deal with them effectively. For example, suppose you're asked to trim the hedges at home. You do the job, then find that you did it incorrectly. You can't change what you've already done, but you can reduce stress by recognizing that all people make mistakes. You can also learn from your mistake and make sure you understand the directions next time so that you can do a better job.

- *Be flexible.* In stressful situations, be willing to bend a little and adjust to changes as the situation demands.

- *Have fun.* Laughter can help reduce distress. Take time to laugh and do things that are fun for you. Enjoy your life!

FIT FACT
The World Health Organization (WHO) identifies gaming disorder as an official mental disorder, which occurs when "gaming takes precedence over other life interests and daily activities." Similarly, the Addiction Center identifies social media addiction as "devoting so much time and effort to social media that it impairs other important life areas." Many people who are not addicted still spend considerable time gaming or using social media, which can limit their ability to achieve mindfulness.

TECH TRENDS: **Preventing Cyberbullying**

Bullying is a major source of stress among teens. Stopbullying.gov, a U.S. government website, defines bullying as "unwanted, aggressive behavior among school aged children that involves a real or perceived power imbalance. The behavior is repeated, or has the potential to be repeated, over time. Bullying includes actions such as making threats, spreading rumors, attacking someone physically or verbally, and excluding someone from a group on purpose."

Many other websites have also been designed to prevent bullying. In addition to defining bullying, these websites discuss who is at risk of bullying, how to prevent bullying, methods of responding to bullies, and how to get help regarding bullying. Teens more likely to be targeted for bullying include those who are perceived as different from their peers, as weak or unable to defend themselves, or as having few friends. However, all teens can be subjected to bullying at one time or another. Others who face higher risk for bullying include teens who are lesbian, gay, bisexual, or transgender, as well as those with a disability.

Many of the websites discuss cyberbullying—bullying that occurs over social media, text messages, and chatrooms. Cyberbullying is different from other forms of bullying because it can be done 24-7, it often reaches teens when they are alone and without social support, and anonymous messages can be posted and distributed to many people very quickly. Technology also makes it relatively easy to take, post, and spread embarrassing photos to be used in cyberbullying.

Some of these websites, including those described on the web resource, offer content designed to help schools assess bullying and create effective anti-bullying rules and policies.

USING TECHNOLOGY

Investigate your school to see if it has anti-bullying policies. Assess the extent of bullying and cyberbullying in your school. Assessment tools are available on anti-bullying websites.

▌Social and Spiritual Coping

You can also manage stress by using social and spiritual coping skills. The following list gives some examples, all of which relate to getting help—the top step in the Stress Management Pyramid.

- *Seek help from friends and family.* When you feel down, don't keep it to yourself. Talk to family members and friends you trust. Just talking about problems can often help reduce distress.

- *Seek spiritual guidance.* Again, just talking to others often helps reduce stress, and trusted spiritual advisors may be able to offer additional help.

- *Seek professional help.* Sometimes it's necessary to seek professional help from a school official (such as a guidance counselor) or, after consulting a parent or guardian, an outside professional (such as a counselor or psychiatrist).

Adopting the right attitude can convert a negative stress into a positive one.

Hans Selye, stress researcher

▌Intellectual Coping

The final type of coping skill, intellectual coping, involves using your thought processes to manage stress. Here are some examples of techniques you can use.

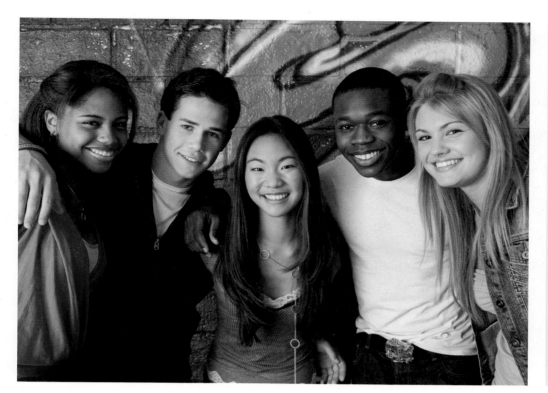

- *Use problem solving.* Rather than worrying about a problem, use the scientific method to solve problems that cause stress. Consider several solutions and the likely results of each, choose the best one, and carry it out.
- *Establish your priorities and tackle one thing at a time.* If several problems pile up, ask yourself which is most important and which can wait.
- *Manage your time effectively.* Prioritize your activities so that you have time for the most important things. Learn to say no to new responsibilities and activities if you can't give them the time required.
- *Use mental imagery.* In stressful situations, imagining pleasant circumstances can help you relax. Try imagining a pleasant outdoor scene before a test or when you have thoughts that make you feel anxious. Some athletes listen to relaxing music before a competition to help reduce mental activity.

LESSON REVIEW

1. What are some examples of physical coping techniques?
2. What are some examples of emotional coping techniques?
3. What are some examples of social and spiritual coping techniques?
4. What are some examples of intellectual coping techniques?

TAKING CHARGE: **Managing Competitive Stress**

A little stress can give you more energy and help you meet a challenge. However, the effects of too much stress can interfere with your performance, especially during a competition. To do your best, you need to recognize the symptoms of **competitive stress** and know how to manage them. Here's an example.

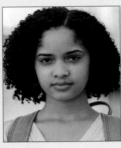
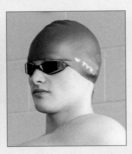

Shelly watched from the bottom row of the bleachers as Willie shook his shoulders and arms. Shelly knew that swimmers do that to help them stay relaxed.

"You're the best, Willie! You're going to win!" Shelly had to yell so that Willie would hear her because the crowd was cheering so loudly.

Willie thought to himself, *I'm not so sure.* He shook his shoulders and legs again.

"You can do it!" Shelly screamed. "You're faster than anyone! We're all behind you!" She wasn't sure whether Willie heard her.

Willie had heard, and he thought, *That's exactly the problem! The whole school is watching! My parents, too! If I don't get at least second place, our team might not make it to the regionals. The way my stomach feels, these people are more likely to see me throw up than win the 200.*

Willie knew it was just stress. He'd felt the same way at the last meet. And Shelly had told him she felt the same kind of stress during a debate last week. The debate coach had shown her how to slow down her breathing to help her relax, and she had shown Willie how to do it.

Shelly stood up and took a deep breath. Willie saw her and did the same thing, and then he grinned to let her know he felt better. Willie was ready.

FOR DISCUSSION

How were Willie's muscles affected by the stress he felt? What were his other symptoms? How was Willie's stress similar to the stress Shelly had felt before her debate? What advice would you give Willie and Shelly (or anyone who is in a similar situation)? Consider the guidelines in the following Self-Management feature as you answer these discussion questions.

SELF-MANAGEMENT: **Skills for Managing Competitive Stress**

In the second lesson of this chapter, you learned that doing regular, noncompetitive physical activity can help you reduce stress. On the other hand, stress can be caused or increased by competitive sports and other competitive activities, such as performing a music solo or giving a speech. Factors that can make these activities stressful include being evaluated by others, performing in front of a crowd, and feeling that the outcome is important. If you get involved in situations that cause competitive stress, use the following guidelines to help you manage your stress.

- *Learn to identify signs of stress.* You can learn this skill by using the self-assessment included in this chapter.

- *Use muscle relaxation techniques.* Use the muscle relaxation techniques presented in this chapter's Taking Action feature.

- *Get experience.* Remember that most people feel stressed the first few times they compete or perform in public. With experience, competing and performing become easier.

- *Practice and prepare.* Practice and preparation help you experience eustress when competing and performing, thus helping you achieve your full potential. When you practice, try to simulate the real event. Practices with an audience can help you prepare.
- *Use mental imagery.* Some people do well in practice but not in actual competition. One method used by experienced competitors to address this issue is mental imagery. During the real event, they imagine themselves as they are in practice—relaxed and confident.
- *Use a routine.* For example, golfers find a regular putting routine very helpful. Following a routine before and during a competitive event can help you stay focused and avoid being affected by factors around you.
- *Take a deep breath and slow your breathing.* For example, take a deep breath before shooting a free throw or performing a solo. If you find yourself becoming tense, slow down your breathing—it can help.
- *Use other effective methods of managing stress.* Use the ways of managing stress discussed earlier in this lesson.

ACADEMIC CONNECTION: Literacy

As you know, *literacy* refers to being educated or cultured. In addition to physical literacy, it includes literacy in language (ability to read, write, and speak effectively), mathematics, science, humanities (including art and music), health, and technology. But how can you find reliable sources of information to increase your understanding in these areas and other topics such as stress management? People who have studied library and information science (LIS) can assist you; your school librarian is one such person.

If you're like most teens today, you probably use the Internet to search for information, but you need make sure the information you find is from a reliable source. (See chapter 19 for more on this subject.) Even with easily accessible information on the Internet, it's still important for you to know how to find information in print resources as well. One indicator of college and career readiness is the ability to integrate information from a variety of print and digital resources to answer questions. School libraries have print materials (books, magazines, journals, and other documents) and extensive digital materials (online journals, documents, and resources) to help you in your studies. Explore your school library and consult with the school librarian to learn about the best methods for gathering information.

Taking Action: Performing Relaxation Exercises

Did your self-assessment indicate that you have a high level of stress? Even if it didn't, you will have to deal with stressful situations from time to time. One way to manage the effects of stress on your body is to perform relaxation exercises, such as deep breathing, meditation, guided imagery exercises, and simple stretching techniques. Relaxation exercises may feel unfamiliar or even uncomfortable the first time you try them, but as with any skill, you can learn to use them effectively if you practice them properly and regularly. **Take action** by trying the muscle relaxation exercises on the following pages.

RELAXATION EXERCISES FOR STRESS MANAGEMENT

Did your self-assessment indicate that you have a high level of stress? In this activity, you will get the opportunity to perform several exercises that are useful in reducing stress. You will also get the opportunity to practice a muscle relaxation procedure called contract-relax.

You can do exercises at almost any time and place. You might do them when you are sitting and studying or while you are riding or waiting for a bus. You can do most of them lying down or from a sitting position. You can even adapt some of these exercises to do them while standing.

Rag Doll

1. Stand or sit in a chair with your feet apart. Stretch your arms and trunk upward as you inhale.

2. Exhale and drop your body forward. Let your trunk, head, and arms dangle between your legs. Keep your neck and trunk muscles relaxed. Remain relaxed like a rag doll for 10 to 15 seconds.

3. Slowly roll up, one vertebra at a time. Repeat the stretch and drop.

Neck Roll

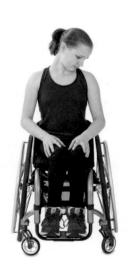

1. Sit in a chair or on the floor with your legs crossed.

2. Keeping your head and chin tucked, inhale as you slowly rotate your head to the left as far as possible. Exhale and slowly return your head to the center.

3. Repeat the movement to the right.

4. Rotate three times in each direction, trying to rotate farther each time so that you feel a stretch in the neck.

5. Now drop your chin to your chest. Inhale as you slowly roll your head in a half circle to the left shoulder, and then exhale as you roll it back to the center. Repeat the movement to the right shoulder.

   Caution: Do not roll your head backward or in a full circle.

Body Board

1. Lie on your right side. Hold your arms over your head.
2. Inhale and stiffen your body as if you were a wooden board. Then exhale as you relax your muscles and collapse completely.
3. Let your body fall without controlling whether you tip forward or backward.
4. Lie still as you continue letting the tension go out of your muscles for 10 seconds. Then repeat the exercise on your left side.

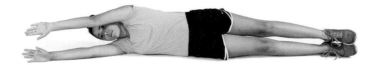

Jaw Stretch

1. Sit in a chair or on the floor with your head erect and your arms and shoulders relaxed.
2. Open your mouth as wide as possible and inhale. (This may make you yawn.) Relax and exhale slowly.
3. Open your mouth and shift your jaw to the right as far as possible; hold for 3 counts.
4. Repeat the movement to the left. Repeat it on both sides 10 times.

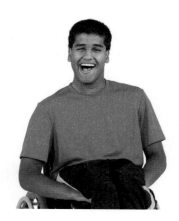

Contract-Relax Method of Muscle Relaxation

Lie on your back with a rolled-up towel placed under your knees. Contract your muscles according to the following instructions. Hold each contraction for 3 counts, then relax for 10 counts. Each time you contract, inhale; each time you relax, exhale.

Do each exercise twice. Try this routine at home for a few weeks. With practice, you should eventually progress to a combination of muscle groups and gradually eliminate the contracting phase of the program.

1. Hand and forearm: Contract your right hand, making a fist. Relax and continue relaxing. Repeat the exercise with your left hand. Repeat it with both hands simultaneously.
2. Biceps: Bend both elbows and contract the muscles on the front of your upper arms. Relax and continue relaxing. Repeat the exercise.
3. Triceps: Bend both elbows, keeping your palms up. Straighten both elbows and contract the muscles on the back of the arm by pushing the back of your hand into the floor. Relax.
4. Hands, forearms, and upper arms: Concentrate on relaxing these body parts all together.
5. Forehead: Make a frown and wrinkle your forehead. Relax and continue relaxing. Repeat the exercise.

6. Jaws: Clench your teeth. Relax. Repeat the exercise.

7. Lips and tongue: With your teeth apart, press your lips together and press your tongue to the roof of your mouth. Relax. Repeat the exercise.

8. Neck and throat: Push your head backward while tucking your chin. Relax. Repeat the exercise.

9. Relax your forehead, jaws, lips, tongue, neck, and throat. Relax your hands, forearms, and upper arms. Keep relaxing all of these muscles.

10. Shoulders and upper back: Hunch your shoulders to your ears. Relax. Repeat the exercise.

11. Relax your lips, tongue, neck, throat, shoulders, and upper back. Keep relaxing these muscles all together.

12. Abdomen: Suck in your abdomen, flattening your lower back to the floor. Relax. Repeat the exercise.

13. Lower back: Contract and arch your lower back. Relax. Repeat the exercise.

14. Thighs and buttocks: Squeeze your buttocks together and push your heels into the floor. Relax. Repeat the exercise.

15. Relax your shoulders, upper back, abdomen, lower back, thighs, and buttocks. Keep relaxing these muscles all together.

16. Shins: Pull your toes toward your shins. Relax. Repeat the exercise.

17. Toes: Curl your toes. Relax. Repeat the exercise.

18. Relax every muscle in your body all together and keep relaxing.

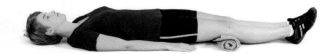

CHAPTER REVIEW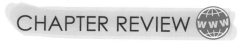

Reviewing Concepts and Vocabulary

Answer items 1 through 5 by correctly completing each sentence with a word or phrase.

1. _____ is the body's reaction to a demanding situation.

2. The first phase of general adaptation syndrome is called the _____.

3. _____ is described as positive stress.

4. Coping that includes exercise and reducing your breathing rate is called _____ coping.

5. Problem solving is a type of _____ coping.

For items 6 through 10, match each term in column 1 with the appropriate phrase in column 2.

6. Stress Management Pyramid step 1   a. identify causes of stress

7. Stress Management Pyramid step 2   b. understand effects of stress

8. Stress Management Pyramid step 3   c. get help

9. Stress Management Pyramid step 4   d. identify signs of stress

10. Stress Management Pyramid step 5   e. learn coping skills

For items 11 through 15, as directed by your teacher, respond to each statement or question.

11. What is the difference between eustress and distress?

12. What are some guidelines for helping a friend who is depressed?

13. How can physical activity help you deal effectively with stress?

14. What is cyberbullying, and why is it a problem?

15. Define mindfulness and explain how it can be achieved, including factors that can limit one's ability to achieve a state of mindfulness.

Thinking Critically

Write a paragraph to answer the following questions.

You've been asked to give a speech to your class. You're concerned that if you refuse the opportunity, you may feel disappointed in yourself. However, you're also afraid that you'll be too nervous to speak in front of a large group. What are the positive and negative consequences of each choice? What decision would you make? How could you manage the stress associated with whichever decision you made?

Project

Keep a journal for one week that documents incidents of stress in your life and observed stress in the lives of friends. Record incidents of bullying and cyberbullying. Use the information from your journal to create a brochure to help teens manage stress or prevent bullying and cyberbullying.

Making Healthy Choices and Planning for Health and Wellness

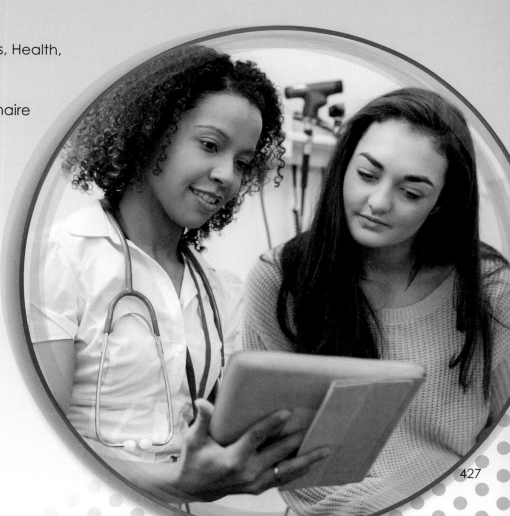

Lifestyle Choices for Fitness, Health, and Wellness

Lesson Objectives

After reading this lesson, you should be able to

1. describe four factors that contribute to early death and differentiate between controllable and uncontrollable risk factors;

2. describe some healthy lifestyle choices other than priority healthy lifestyle choices, and explain how they contribute to fitness, health, and wellness;

3. describe some good safety practices for healthy living; and

4. describe how your physical and social environments affect fitness, health, and wellness.

Lesson Vocabulary

built environment
controllable risk factor
lifestyle
sleep apnea
uncontrollable risk factor

Are you aware of all the things you can do to achieve fitness, health, and wellness? In this lesson, you'll learn about healthy lifestyle choices and how they can help you achieve good fitness, health, and wellness. You'll also learn about environmental and social factors that can influence your fitness, health, and wellness.

Factors Influencing Fitness, Health, and Wellness

As you can see in figure 18.1, four major factors contribute to early death. Most early deaths result from unhealthy lifestyle choices, which means they are preventable. Making healthy lifestyle choices not only reduces the risk of disease and early death but also enhances wellness. For example, not smoking greatly reduces your risk of heart disease and cancer, and you can breathe better, you have a keener sense of smell, and you save the money you would have spent on tobacco and medical care.

> Not all things in life are under my control, but I have learned that there are many things that I can control to help me live a healthy life.
>
> *Savannah Townsend*

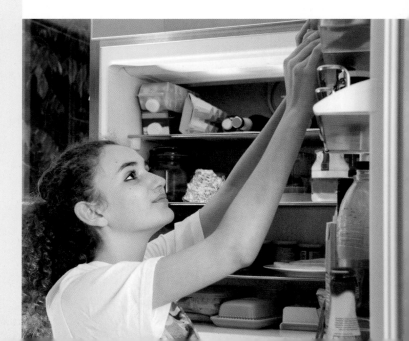

You know by now that a healthy **lifestyle** is a way of living that helps you prevent illness and enhance wellness. Healthy lifestyle choices are ways that you can reduce **controllable risk factors**—the risk factors that you can act upon to change to reduce your risk of many major health problems. For example, one controllable risk factor is sedentary living; simply by being active, you can reduce your health risks.

Other risk factors—such as age and sex—are not in your control and thus are called **uncontrollable risk factors**. Because you cannot do anything about these risk factors, focus instead on those that you can control. This chapter describes several healthy lifestyle choices over which you do have some control.

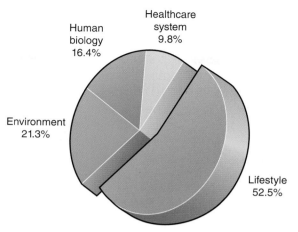

Figure 18.1 Four main factors contributing to early death.

Making Healthy Lifestyle Choices

This book focuses on three priority lifestyle choices—regular physical activity, healthy eating, and stress management—considered to be most important because they can improve the fitness, health, and wellness of virtually all people. However, they are not the only lifestyle choices you can make to promote fitness, health, and wellness. This lesson describes some others.

Adopt Good Personal Health Habits

In elementary school, you most likely learned about personal health habits, such as regular toothbrushing and flossing, good grooming (e.g., hair and fingernail care), handwashing before meals and after bathroom use, and getting a healthy amount of sleep. But how many of these habits have you adopted? Practicing good health habits is one way you can prevent illness and promote optimal quality of life.

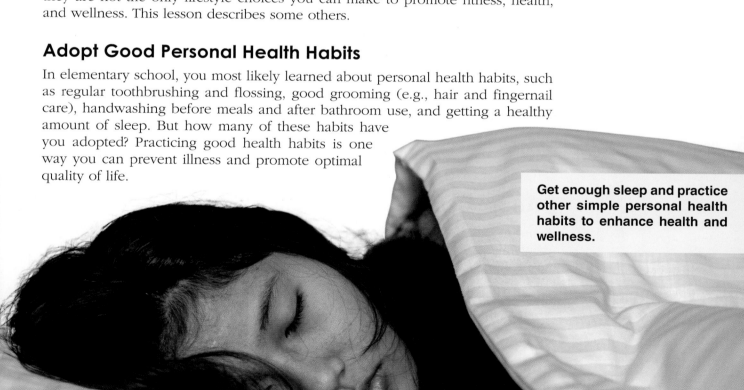

Get enough sleep and practice other simple personal health habits to enhance health and wellness.

TECH TRENDS: Sleep Tracking

Considerable evidence indicates that insufficient sleep can lead to health problems. Most sources indicate that teens need 8 to 10 hours of sleep each night. However, only 25 percent of teens get 8 or more hours of sleep each night. Sleep patterns are also important—people who wake up numerous times or toss and turn frequently during the night are not getting restful sleep.

Sleep apnea is a medical condition that occurs when the muscles in the throat are unable to keep the airway open during sleep, causing interruptions in breathing. Technology is now available to detect sleep apnea and improve the quality of sleep. Physicians can order a sleep study to monitor your patterns of breathing, heart rate, and blood oxygen levels as well as your body movements. Once detected, sleep apnea can be treated by wearing a mask connected to a machine that blows air into the throat to keep the airway open.

Some devices such as activity trackers can be used to determine movement patterns during the night. Sleep tracking devices are most commonly worn on the wrist; however, a ring (Oura Ring) is also available. These devices can be used to screen for sleep problems, but they are not meant to be a method of diagnosing medical problems. If screening with one of these devices indicates restless sleep, consider medical consultation.

Not all high-tech devices are beneficial to sleep. Seven out of 10 teens keep their phone near the bed, 40 percent use their phone within five minutes of going to bed, and one-third of teens wake up at least once a night to check their phone. Keeping a smartphone at the bedside can cause you to wake up when notifications are received. The Kaiser Foundation recommends placing your phone on a charger outside your room so that it will not interrupt your sleep.

USING TECHNOLOGY

Investigate sleep-tracking devices and evaluate their pros and cons. Then analyze your own behavior related to sleep.

Avoid Destructive Habits

Just as healthy habits contribute to good health, destructive habits detract from your fitness, health, and wellness. Examples include (among many others) smoking and other tobacco use, vaping, legal and illegal drug abuse, and alcohol abuse. These destructive habits can impair your ability to perform physical activities and result in various diseases, lowered feelings of well-being, and reduced quality of life.

Adopt Good Safety Practices

FIT FACT

Texting while driving is a major source of automobile accidents—in fact, drivers are 23 times more likely to crash while texting. More generally, driver distraction is the cause of one out of every five fatal accidents in the United States (killing more than 3,000 people each year). A recent survey indicates that 63 percent of teens indicate that they text while driving.

Some of the most common causes of death and injury include motor vehicle accidents, falls, poisonings, drownings, fires, bicycle accidents, and accidents in and around the home. The good news is that many of these injuries and deaths can be prevented by following simple safety rules. One national health goal in the United States is to reduce the number of deaths and injuries resulting from accidents.

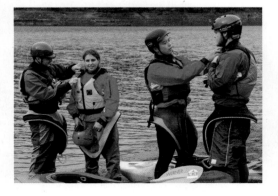

CONSUMER CORNER: **Vaping and E-Cigarettes**

Electronic cigarettes have many names, including e-cigarettes, e-cigs, vape pens, vapes, and mods. They are available in many forms but most have a battery, a heating element, and a place to hold a liquid that usually contains nicotine, flavoring, and other chemicals. The liquid is heated to produce an aerosol (fine spray) that is inhaled into the lungs (vaping). Vaping has been around for decades, but the modern e-cigarette was introduced in the United States in the mid 2000s and since then use has increased dramatically. Although they are promoted as an alternative to smoking and a way to stop smoking, many nonsmokers have begun using e-cigs, creating concerns among health experts. The long-term dangers of vaping are not fully understood, but evidence is accumulating to indicate that it can put your health at risk. In 2019 an epidemic of lung-related illnesses and deaths were associated with vaping.

Of special concern to health and medical experts is the fact that the contents of the liquid in e-cigarettes is often unknown—especially for e-cigs bought on the street. Figure 18.2 shows examples of substances contained in some e-cigs that can be especially damaging to the lungs. Other dangers of vaping include addiction to nicotine and associated health effects (harm to brain development in teens, danger to pregnant women and their babies, fires and explosions from defective batteries, and poisoning from swallowing e-cigarette liquid).

Cigarette use by teens has decreased dramatically over the past 20 years as social norms have changed and smoking has become less fashionable. In addition, public policies now often limit or prohibit smoking in public places, limit tobacco advertisements, and tax tobacco purchases. However, vaping has increased significantly, especially among teens. Experts attribute factors such as marketing campaigns that target teens and use of flavored products as two of the many reasons for this increase. This has prompted health officials to begin implementing policies similar to antismoking policies to reduce the health risks created by vaping.

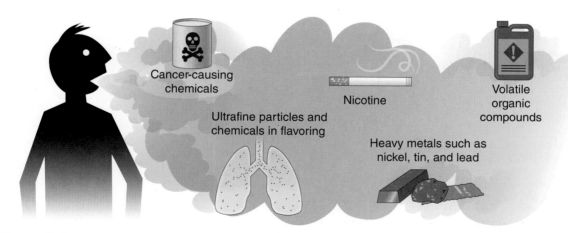

Figure 18.2   Dangerous substances in e-cigarettes.

STUDENT ACTIVITY

Search the CDC website for the terms "vaping" and "e-cigarettes." Prepare a written statement on your findings and share it with your class.

There are a number of healthy lifestyle choices to reduce your risk of accidents, including wearing a seat belt, wearing a helmet when riding a bike or doing inline skating, making sure that poisons are properly labeled, installing and maintaining smoke detectors, practicing water safety, and keeping your home in good repair. And remember—being physically fit can also help you prevent accidents.

Learn Cardiopulmonary Resuscitation (CPR)

Cardiopulmonary resuscitation (CPR) is a first aid procedure that saves many lives each year. When a person's heart or breathing has stopped, CPR uses chest compressions to keep blood flowing, preventing brain damage and death until expert medical help arrives. CPR training is strongly recommended, and many schools and national organizations offer CPR classes and certification. According to the National Institutes of Health, "Even if you haven't had training, you can do 'hands-only' CPR for a teen or an adult whose heart has stopped." However, hands-only CPR is *not* recommended for use with children.

The American Heart Association recommends "two steps to staying alive": First, call 911 or direct someone else to call 911. Second, start chest compressions using the technique shown in figure 18.3. When two people are available, both mouth-to-mouth breathing and chest compression can be used.

CPR techniques and procedures are often revised based on new research and findings. For this reason, a regular check of the National Institutes of Health website for the latest information is recommended.

Learn the Heimlich Maneuver (Abdominal Thrusts)

The Heimlich maneuver (also called *abdominal thrusts*) is performed when an object blocks a person's airway. As shown in figure 18.4, the person administering the maneuver stands behind the person who is choking with their arms around the person's waist. The fist of one hand is placed just above the choking person's navel, with the thumb side of the fist against the body. The other hand is held over the fist. Pulling upward and inward causes pressure to force the object from the windpipe. As with all first aid procedures, training in the Heimlich maneuver is highly recommended.

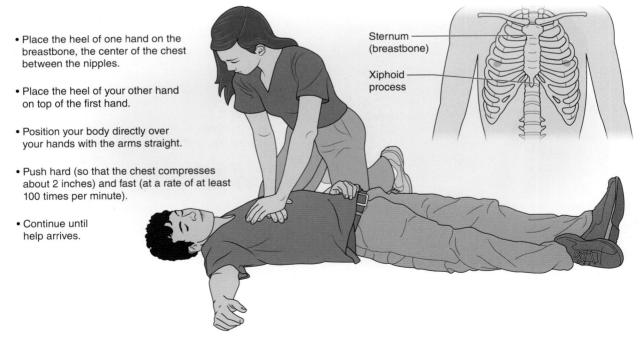

- Place the heel of one hand on the breastbone, the center of the chest between the nipples.

- Place the heel of your other hand on top of the first hand.

- Position your body directly over your hands with the arms straight.

- Push hard (so that the chest compresses about 2 inches) and fast (at a rate of at least 100 times per minute).

- Continue until help arrives.

Sternum (breastbone)

Xiphoid process

Figure 18.3 Technique for performing hands-only CPR.

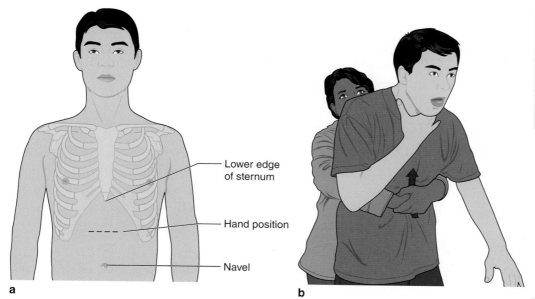

Figure 18.4 The Heimlich maneuver: *(a)* hand placement; *(b)* action—pull upward and inward.

Learn Other First Aid Procedures

Because even people who make healthy lifestyle choices and adopt good safety practices can have accidents, everyone should maintain a first aid kit and know how to administer first aid. In addition to learning how to perform CPR and the Heimlich maneuver, you should also learn how to apply pressure to prevent bleeding, how to clean and treat cuts and open wounds, how to use the RICE formula (rest, ice, compression, and elevation) to treat sprains and strains, and how to use other accepted first aid techniques.

Seek and Follow Appropriate Medical Advice

Even if you make healthy lifestyle choices, you may occasionally become ill. In those cases, seek and follow appropriate medical advice. In fact, for best results,

SCIENCE IN ACTION: The Evolution of CPR

Mouth-to-mouth resuscitation was first used in France in the 1700s, and medical doctors used chest compression to revive people in the late 1800s. Later, "artificial respiration" was modified to use a back-pressure arm-lift method, which in turn was replaced by chest compression and mouth-to-mouth breathing in the 1960s. Later, one-person CPR alternated chest compression with mouth-to-mouth breathing.

Doctors started using these procedures before they were recommended to the general public.

In recent years, CPR has continued to evolve considerably. As shown in figure 18.3, the hands-only method (chest compression) is now used for helping adults and teens in distress. This procedure is easier to do, and experts feel that it will be used more often as a result.

STUDENT ACTIVITY

Do a web search to determine which local organizations offer CPR classes. If possible, take a class and get certified.

get regular medical and dental checkups to help prevent problems before they start. Consult your physician and dentist to determine how often you should be seen. Some people avoid seeking medical help, but as noted in the Fit Fact, this practice can be dangerous because early detection of health problems is often important for an ultimate cure.

The Environment and Fitness, Health, and Wellness

The second leading contributor to early death is an unhealthy environment. It can also cause health problems or detract from personal wellness. Your physical and social environments are both important to your health and wellness.

Physical Environment

The physical environment refers to the air, land, water, plants, and other physical things that exist around you. We know that certain physical environments can be very harmful to your health. For example, people who live in polluted cities are at greater risk of developing health problems than those who live in the countryside, where the air is often cleaner. Your work (or vocational) environment can also have serious consequences for your health. For example, people who work where there is potential exposure to chemicals, fumes, or gases and people who frequent places where smoking is allowed have a higher risk of illness than those who work in less polluted areas. If your job requires you to sit all day without breaks that allow you to get up and move around, you will also have higher health risks.

You may not be able to change all of your physical environment factors; however, you can take action to improve your environment. For example, you can avoid or minimize exposure to smoke-filled places, excessive sun exposure, and exposure to pollutants, such as weed killers and insecticides. To avoid excessive air pollution, exercise away from heavily traveled streets. You can also take certain steps to improve the physical environment—for example, recycling household materials and conserving water and electricity. You can also help people in your community who are making efforts to improve the **built environment**—the physical characteristics of our neighborhoods. Improvements in the built environment, such as adding sidewalks and

Recycling is something everyone can do to aid the environment.

bike paths and improving street lighting and street crossings, have been shown to increase healthy physical activity such as walking and biking in neighborhoods.

Social Environment

Your social environment refers to the settings in which your social interactions take place, including your contacts, conversations, and activities with friends, teachers, work colleagues, and others in leisure-time situations.

Researchers have shown that teens whose friends make unhealthy lifestyle choices are more likely to try risky behavior such as abusing tobacco, drugs, or alcohol. In contrast, teens whose friends and family members make healthy lifestyle choices are more likely to practice healthy behaviors such as being physically active and eating well. With this in mind, choosing supportive friends is important to your health and wellness.

Even if you make good choices, you, like most people, will probably be exposed to unhealthy social environments at some point in your life. If this does happen to you, consider using some of the self-management skills described in this book to help you make good choices in the heat of the moment. For example, practice ways to say no and learn relapse prevention strategies. You do not need to be embarrassed or apologize for practicing healthy behaviors.

> Earth provides enough to satisfy every [person's] need, but not every [person's] greed.
>
> *Mahatma Gandhi, human rights leader*

LESSON REVIEW

1. What are the four factors that contribute to early death, and how do you differentiate between controllable and uncontrollable risk factors?
2. What are some healthy lifestyle choices other than priority healthy lifestyle choices, and how do they contribute to fitness, health, and wellness?
3. What are some good safety practices for healthy living?
4. How do physical and social environments affect fitness, health, and wellness?

SELF-ASSESSMENT: **Healthy Lifestyle Questionnaire**

As you know, wellness is the positive component of good health. The five components of wellness include physical, emotional–mental, social, intellectual, and spiritual wellness. Complete the following questionnaire to assess your current wellness.

1. Read each wellness statement and decide whether you strongly agree, agree, disagree, or strongly disagree.
2. Calculate your score for each wellness component by adding your results for the three questions in that component.
3. Add all five component scores to get your overall wellness score.
4. Use table 18.1 to determine your rating for each component and your overall score. Record your results.

Healthy Lifestyle Questionnaire

Wellness statement	Strongly agree	Agree	Disagree	Strongly disagree
1. I am physically fit.	4	3	2	1
2. I can do the physical tasks needed in my work.	4	3	2	1
3. I have the energy to be active in my free time.	4	3	2	1
Physical wellness score = _____				
4. I am happy most of the time.	4	3	2	1
5. I do not get stressed often.	4	3	2	1
6. I like myself the way I am.	4	3	2	1
Emotional–mental wellness score = _____				
7. I have many friends.	4	3	2	1
8. I am confident in social situations.	4	3	2	1
9. I am close to my family.	4	3	2	1
Social wellness score = _____				
10. I am an informed consumer.	4	3	2	1
11. I check facts before making health decisions.	4	3	2	1
12. I consult experts when I'm not sure of health facts.	4	3	2	1
Intellectual wellness score = _____				
13. I feel a sense of purpose in my life.	4	3	2	1
14. I feel fulfilled spiritually.	4	3	2	1
15. I feel strong connections to the world around me.	4	3	2	1
Spiritual wellness score = _____				
Total wellness score = _____				

Adapted from C.B. Corbin et al., *Concepts of Fitness and Wellness*, 10th ed. (St. Louis, MO: McGraw-Hill, 2013).

TABLE 18.1   Rating Chart: Wellness

Wellness rating	Three-item score	Total wellness score
Good	10–12	≥50
Marginal	8–9	40–49
Low	≤7	≤39

Healthy Lifestyle Planning

Lesson Objectives

After reading this lesson, you should be able to

1. prepare a list of personal needs for healthy lifestyle planning;
2. prepare a list of options for healthy lifestyle planning;
3. prepare a list of goals for healthy lifestyle planning; and
4. prepare a written healthy lifestyle plan and explain how you can evaluate it.

Lesson Vocabulary

consumer community

In other chapters of this book, you've learned the steps of program planning and had the opportunity to prepare several types of physical activity plans. It's also important to plan for the healthy lifestyle choices discussed in this chapter.

The same five steps you've used to plan your physical activity can also be used to prepare plans for eating better, reducing stress in your life, and adopting other healthy behaviors. Jeff was already implementing his physical activity plan but also wanted to make some other lifestyle changes. To plan these changes, he used the five-step approach.

Step 1: Determine Your Personal Needs

As part of learning about SMART goals, Jeff learned that it's important to make goals attainable. If he was going to be successful, he knew he shouldn't try to make too many changes at once. He reviewed some of the healthy lifestyle

> I have made several New Year's resolutions but I didn't stay with them until last year when I made a very specific plan. It helped me to keep my resolution to eat breakfast every day.
>
> *Jeff Weaver*

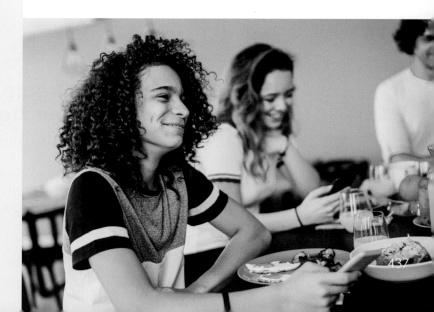

Don't dig your grave with your own knife and fork.

English proverb

choices described in this chapter's first lesson, then decided to start by choosing one area in which he needed improvement. As indicated by the checkmark in the following list, he chose to eat better.

Check one or more areas of personal need in which you want to plan a change.

✓	Eat better	_____	Adopt safety habits
_____	Reduce stress	_____	Seek and follow medical advice
_____	Adopt personal health habits	_____	Learn first aid
_____	Avoid destructive behaviors	_____	Learn CPR

When studying nutrition, Jeff did a self-assessment of his eating habits and found that he could improve in several areas. Specifically, his diet included too much fat, he ate more calories than he should, and he didn't eat the recommended amount of fruits and vegetables.

Step 2: Consider Your Program Options

Based on his needs and nutrition assessments, Jeff's options included changing his eating habits to be healthier.

- Cut the fat in his diet
- Eat more fruits
- Eat more vegetables
- Consume fewer calories

Step 3: Set Goals

To help him eat better, Jeff set some SMART goals.

- Goal 1: Eat at least two servings of vegetables every day for two weeks.
- Goal 2: Eat at least two servings of fruits every day for two weeks.
- Goal 3: Eat at least five total servings of fruits and vegetables every day for two weeks.
- Goal 4: Drink two glasses of skim milk rather than whole milk each day.

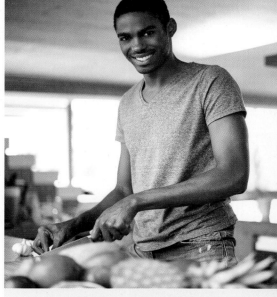

Dietary planning can help you eat more healthfully.

Steps 4 and 5: Create a Written Program and Evaluate Your Progress

Jeff prepared a written plan (see table 18.2) that included each of his SMART goals and a calendar showing each day of the week. He posted the chart on the refrigerator (for the second week, he posted a clean copy of the same chart).

Jeff used checkmarks on his written plan to track his daily goals. He found that he did meet his goal for fruits and his goal for vegetables on all of the days, but

A goal without a plan is just a wish.

Antoine de Saint-Exupéry, writer

CONSUMER CORNER: School-Based Consumer Communities

How do you get good consumer information? One way is to consult a book like *Fitness for Life*. You can also consult experts at your school or high-quality websites such as those described in this book. Another is to establish a school-based **consumer community** for finding and disseminating good information. These communities review scientific information and answer student questions related to fitness, health, and wellness. Some consumer communities provide a newsletter or contribute articles to the school newspaper. Others use the web or the school's intranet (local network) to provide information. Consumer communities with web access may also offer a website featuring articles by students, sources of good consumer information, and answers to student questions. Some high school consumer communities also use social media to share information.

Just as the work of scientists has to be reviewed by peers before it can be published, consumer communities must review their information to make sure that it is accurate and responsibly reported. They typically have older members who assume leadership roles and guide information review. A consumer community provides a great opportunity to learn and serve for teens who are interested in a career in fitness, health, and wellness.

STUDENT ACTIVITY

Check to see if your school has a consumer community. If so, consider participating. If not, consult with a teacher or activities director about starting a consumer community in your school.

on two days he did not eat five fruits and vegetables combined. He met his goal of drinking two glasses of skim milk on five of the seven days. During the second week, he was able to meet all of his goals on every day of the week.

When the two-week period ended, Jeff evaluated his results. He thought he had done pretty well. He was eating more fruits and veggies and had reduced the fat in his diet by drinking skim rather than whole milk. He decided to renew the plan for two more weeks just to be sure he kept on track. After that, he would consider making other healthy lifestyle changes.

In the Taking Action feature, you'll have the opportunity to prepare your own healthy lifestyle plan using the same steps as Jeff. You can also use the planning steps to make lifestyle changes later in life.

TABLE 18.2   **Jeff's Weekly Plan and Log**

Goal	Mon.	Tues.	Wed.	Thurs.	Fri.	Sat.	Sun.
Eat at least 2 daily servings of vegetables.	✓	✓	✓	✓	✓	✓	✓
Eat at least 2 daily servings of fruit.	✓	✓	✓	✓	✓	✓	✓
Eat at least 5 total daily servings of vegetables and fruit.	✓	✓		✓		✓	✓
Drink 2 daily glasses of skim milk rather than whole milk.	✓	✓		✓		✓	✓

LESSON REVIEW

1. How do you prepare a list of personal needs for healthy lifestyle planning?
2. How do you prepare a list of options for healthy lifestyle planning?
3. How do you prepare a list of goals for healthy lifestyle planning?
4. How do you prepare a written healthy lifestyle plan, and how do you evaluate it?

TAKING CHARGE: **Thinking Success**

An optimist is a person who expects a good or favorable outcome when performing a specific activity or task. This optimistic outlook is called "thinking success." A person who thinks success, or has positive thoughts, will succeed more often than a person who has negative thoughts. Here's an example.

Aaron loves baseball. For two years, he played on a team that won most of its regular season games. The team even played in the league's championship game. During that time, Aaron played well at second base and hit a few home runs.

This year, Aaron moved up to a new team. Most of the players at the new level were older, bigger, and stronger than Aaron. During the first game, he was hit by a pitch once and struck out in his other at bats. In fact, he

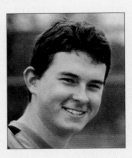

didn't get the bat on the ball even one time.

Aaron's coach noticed that he was no longer swinging with confidence. Luckily, he also knew that Aaron had the physical strength and skills needed to hit the ball. He knew Aaron just needed to change the way he was thinking. He wouldn't hit the ball until he thought he could. The coach had Aaron do some practice drills that he could successfully complete. He taught Aaron to visualize himself hitting the ball and to say "yes, yes, yes" as he stood waiting for the pitch.

The coach also taught Aaron not to obsessively think about the times he'd struck out or failed to make a play. "After all," the coach said, "even the best professionals only get a hit about one out of every three tries. The next play is the one to think about." As Aaron regained his confidence, he improved his hitting.

FOR DISCUSSION

How did Aaron's negative feelings affect the way he played baseball with the new team? How was he able to change his attitude to think about success? What are some other ways a person can change negative thoughts into positive ones? Consider the guidelines in the following Self-Management feature as you answer these discussion questions.

SELF-MANAGEMENT: **Skills for Thinking Success**

One reason that some people fail to stick with a healthy lifestyle program is that they don't believe in themselves. Many people make New Year's resolutions, but not all accomplish their goals. Use the following guidelines to help you succeed.

- Assess your feelings about success. Complete the worksheet provided by your teacher, and then use your answers to see where you might change in order to improve your chances of being successful.

- Set attainable goals and use self-monitoring to reinforce your successes.
- Use self-assessments to help you set goals and evaluate your progress.
- Choose activities that you enjoy and that match your abilities.
- Practice to improve your performance skills.
- Find friends with similar interests who support you.
- Take steps to avoid relapse and say no to things you don't want to do.

- Learn how to overcome the barriers to success.
- Work to build healthy self-perceptions and self-confidence.
- Practice relaxation techniques that can help you overcome competitive stress.
- Learn the steps in planning for healthy lifestyle change.
- Become an informed consumer.
- Avoid unhealthy physical and social environments.

Taking Action: **Your Healthy Lifestyle Plan**

In the second lesson of this chapter, you read about Jeff's plan for adopting a healthy lifestyle. **Take action** by selecting at least one of the healthy lifestyle choices presented at the beginning of this lesson and preparing a plan to make a positive change in this area. You won't be able to carry out your plan in class; it will be something that you do on your own.

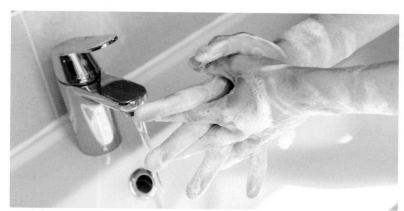

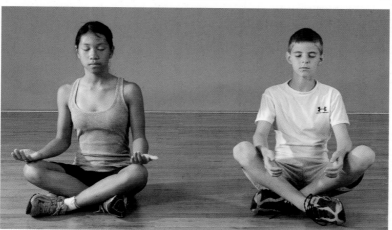

Take action by making a positive lifestyle change, such as adopting personal health practices.

CHAPTER REVIEW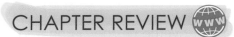

Reviewing Concepts and Vocabulary

Answer items 1 through 5 by correctly completing each sentence with a word or phrase.

1. Risk factors that you can change are referred to as _____ risk factors.

2. _____ is another name for mouth-to-mouth breathing and chest compression.

3. A technique to prevent choking is called _____.

4. Changing the physical environment to make it easier to walk or ride a bicycle is referred to as changing the _____ environment.

5. Groups of students who band together to improve health are called school-based _____.

For items 6 through 10, match each term in column 1 with the appropriate word or phrase in column 2.

6. e-cigarette   a. abdominal thrusts

7. sleep apnea   b. age

8. uncontrollable risk factor   c. vaping

9. chest compression   d. CPR

10. Heimlich maneuver   e. sleep disorder characterized by interruptions in breathing

For items 11 through 15, as directed by your teacher, respond to each statement or question.

11. Describe several healthy lifestyle changes that can improve a person's fitness, health, and wellness.

12. Explain the difference between controllable and uncontrollable risk factors. Give examples.

13. Identify one healthy lifestyle choice and describe how it contributes to fitness, health, and wellness.

14. Explain how a person's environment relates to personal wellness.

15. Describe the five steps in program planning for healthy lifestyles.

Thinking Critically

Write a paragraph to answer the following question.

Choose one destructive behavior identified in this chapter and investigate the harmful effects of the behavior. What actions that can be taken to reduce the behavior in our society, especially among teens?

Project

Many schools have a wellness committee that includes students, teachers, parents, and school staff. Wellness committees often schedule special events such as wellness weeks, during which a schoolwide effort is made to promote fitness, health, and wellness. If your school has a committee, attend a meeting and prepare a report of its activities, indicating how students can become involved. If your school doesn't have a committee, explore ways for getting one created.

UNIT VII

Moving Through Life

Healthy People 2030 Goals and Objectives

Overarching Goals

- Attain healthy, thriving lives and well-being, free of preventable disease, disability, injury, and premature death.
- Eliminate health disparities, achieve health equity, and attain health literacy to improve the health and well-being of all.

Objectives

- Increase the proportion of people who can access electronic health information.
- Increase health literacy of the population.
- Reduce the proportion of people who do no physical activity in their free time.
- Increase the proportion of adolescents and adults who do enough aerobic and muscle building physical activity for health benefits.
- Increase the proportion of teens who play sports and walk or bike to get places.
- Increase the proportion of teens who limit screen time.
- Reduce the proportion of teens with obesity.
- Increase the percentage of worksites that offer physical activity, health promotion, and nutrition programs.
- Increase the proportion of people who get social support.
- Promote healthy development, healthy behaviors, and well-being across all life stages.
- Create social, physical, and economic environments that promote attaining full potential for health and well-being for all.

Self-Assessment Features in This Unit

- Assessing Your Posture
- Analyzing Basic Skills
- Opportunities for Physical Activity Participation Questionnaire

Taking Charge and Self-Management Features in This Unit

- Learning to Think Critically
- Positive Self-Talk
- Choosing Good Activities

Taking Action Features in This Unit

- Your Health and Fitness Club
- Applying Principles
- Taking Advantage of Opportunities

Making Good Consumer Choices

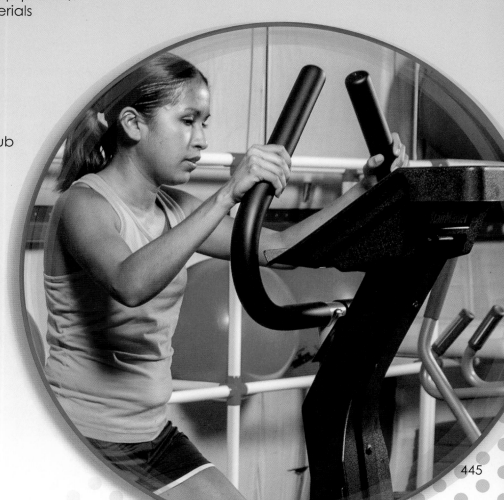

Health and Fitness Quackery

Lesson Objectives

After reading this lesson, you should be able to

1. explain the difference between quackery and fraud;

2. identify and describe some of the ways that you can detect quackery and fraud;

3. identify and describe some of the guidelines for avoiding being a victim of quackery or fraud; and

4. describe some examples of health and fitness misconceptions and quackery.

Lesson Vocabulary

con artist
dehydration
fraud
passive exercise
quack
quackery
scam

You've probably come across ads for health and fitness products and services in newspapers and magazines and on radio, television, and the web. Is a product or service effective simply because it is advertised? Would you buy the product advertised in figure 19.1? In this lesson, you'll learn how to become a wise consumer of health and fitness products.

What Is Quackery? What Is Fraud?

Often, people who want quick results decide to purchase useless health or fitness products or services. In other words, they become victims of **quackery**—a method of advertising that uses false claims to lure people into buying products that are worthless or even harmful. A person who practices quackery is sometimes referred to as a **quack**.

> A woman at the local gym was wearing a plastic suit. I asked, "why?" She said the salesperson told her that it would help her lose weight. I'm not an expert, but I knew that she'd wasted her money and that it could be dangerous.
>
> *Vittoria Russo*

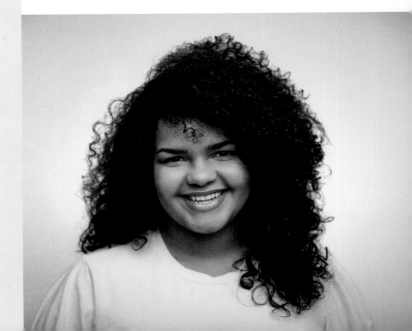

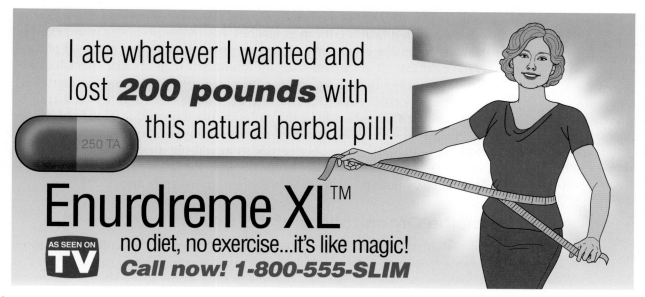

Figure 19.1   Some advertisements make false claims about fitness products and supplements.

Some people who practice quackery actually believe their products work; they may have good intentions but still do harm. Others are guilty of **fraud**. People who practice fraud try to deceive you to get you to buy products or services that they *know* are ineffective or harmful. A person who practices fraud is called a **con artist**. Their actions, sometimes called a **scam**, are designed to take advantage of people. Con artists and scammers are good at making you believe they're offering you a good deal, but deals that seem exceptionally good are often not as good as the con artist makes them seem. Remember, if it seems too good to be true, it probably isn't true. Because fraud and scams are illegal, con artists and scammers may be convicted of a crime.

> Modern health quacks are super salespeople. They play on fear. They cater to hope. And once they have you, they'll keep you coming back for more . . . and more . . . and more.
>
> *Stephen Barrett and William T. Jarvis, consumer fraud experts*

Detecting Quackery and Fraud

People who commit quackery and fraud use a variety of deceptive practices to get you to buy their products or services or use products they endorse. Separating fact from fiction can be difficult. Use the guidelines presented in the following sections to help you spot health and fitness quackery and fraud.

Check Credentials

Be sure that the person you think is an expert really is an expert. A con artist might claim to be a doctor or to have a college or university degree. However, the degree might be in a subject unrelated to health and physical fitness. It might also come from a nonaccredited school; it might even be falsified. You can verify credentials by checking with your local or state health authorities or with professional organizations.

If you have questions about health or fitness, ask a real expert's advice. For example, physical education teachers have a college degree that requires them to study all branches of kinesiology. Some other fitness leaders are certified by a group such as the American College of Sports Medicine. For medical advice, talk to a physician (MD or DO) or a registered nurse (RN). For questions about general health, ask a certified health education teacher. For questions about using exercise to rehabilitate from injury, consult a registered physical therapist (RPT). All of these experts have college degrees and relevant training in their area of specialization.

For questions about diet, food, and nutrition, consult a registered dietitian (RD). Be aware that a person who uses the title of "nutritionist" is not necessarily an expert. Similarly, staff members in health clubs are often not required to hold college degrees. Practitioners certified by a well-respected organization are more qualified than those without certification, but certification without a degree is not adequate to be considered an expert. Neither nutritionists nor health club employees are reliable sources of health or fitness information unless they are an RD.

Check the Organizations of the Experts You Consult

Quacks, con artists, and scammers try to get you to believe that they know more than experts from well-known organizations such as those listed in the Consumer Corner feature. Be wary of people who claim they know more than well-known experts or who try to discredit respected organizations.

Quacks and con artists also often use initials or important-sounding names for fake organizations that are similar to the names of well-known organizations. But anyone can form an organization and use it to try to impress you. Check the background of anyone who claims to be a member of an organization whose name you've never heard.

As a consumer, you need to be informed about the products and services you use. Do not assume that every advertised product is safe and effective. Make complaints to the FTC if you discover a consumer scam. Based on complaints from consumers, the FTC has restrained companies from making false claims and has required them to make refunds to millions of consumers. For example, the FTC has required Reebok and Skechers to make refunds to their customers because of unsupported

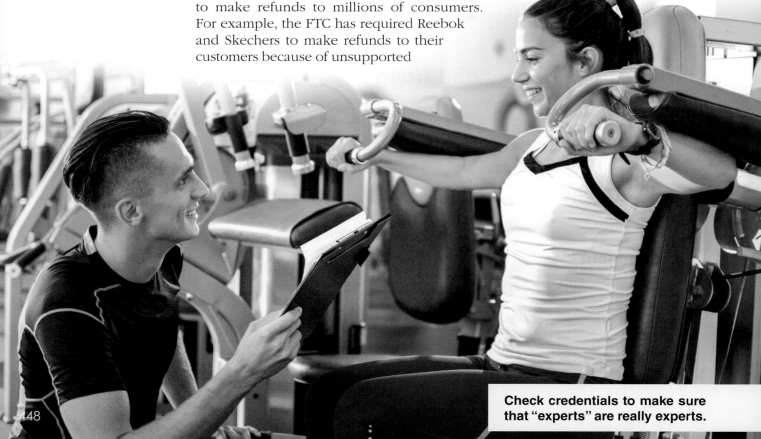

Check credentials to make sure that "experts" are really experts.

CONSUMER CORNER: Reliable Consumer Groups

Many organizations work to protect consumers from misleading advertising and quackery. U.S. governmental agencies that do this type of work include the Centers for Disease Control and Prevention (CDC), the Consumer Product Safety Commission (CPSC), the Federal Trade Commission (FTC), the Food and Drug Administration (FDA), the Department of Agriculture (USDA), and the U.S. Postal Service (USPS). Some reputable private organizations include the Society of Health and Physical Educators (SHAPE America), the American College of Sports Medicine (ACSM), the American Medical Association (AMA), the American Dental Association (ADA), the Academy of Nutrition and Dietetics (AND), the Better Business Bureau (BBB), Consumer Reports, the Cooper Institute, and the Mayo Clinic.

Agencies such as these can provide accurate information, but they do not police all products. Other popular websites may provide unreliable information. *You* make the final decision about buying a product or service, and being informed can help you stay safe and avoid spending money on worthless products.

STUDENT ACTIVITY

Search one or more of the recommended agencies for consumer information about fitness and health products. Prepare a report of the most useful information that you found.

---

claims for "toning" and "shape up" shoes. Herbalife, a manufacturer of supplements, has also been required to refund money to consumers and stop making false claims for their products.

Guidelines for Preventing Quackery and Fraud

Consider the following guidelines before purchasing a product or service.

Be Wary of Salespeople

People who sell products make money by selling them, and salespeople often have little training in health, fitness, and wellness. People who sell exercise equipment or food supplements may know even less about their products than their customers and often stretch the truth. Ask salespeople about their credentials. Before you buy, consult a true expert.

Be Suspicious of Ads Featuring Athlete and Movie Star Testimonials

Athletes and movie stars often do ads endorsing products. They are usually paid for making positive statements but often provide deceptive information. Sports teams sometimes endorse products as well. For example, sports drink may be called the "official drink" of a sports team. Like movie stars and athletes, teams are typically paid for their endorsement. Be skeptical of these types of endorsements.

Be Suspicious of Sales Pitches That Promise Results Too Good to Be True

Look for words and phrases such as *miracle*, *secret remedy*, and *scientific breakthrough*. A quack or con artist is likely to use these or similar terms in a sales pitch

> **FIT FACT**
> A study by the American Council on Exercise (ACE) found so-called "hologram bracelets," worn by many famous athletes, to be ineffective. The bracelets' maker falsely claimed that they improved fitness in areas such as strength, flexibility, and balance.

for an item that is useless. Be suspicious if a salesperson promises immediate, effortless, or guaranteed results.

Be Cautious About Mail-Order and Internet Sales

Because you cannot examine mail-order and Internet products before buying them, you may receive something different than advertised. Before buying from any source, know the company's return policy. Money-back guarantees may seem to protect you, but a guarantee is only as good as the company that backs it. Some have staff members to help you with returns and questions, but many do not. Some may require you to pay return mail costs. Internet-based companies are usually rated for reliability and quality of service, and you should check a company's rating and reviews before buying from it.

Be Wary of Product Claims

A favorite trick of some con artists is to claim that a product is "brand new" or "available in the United States for the first time" to make you think that you're getting something special. Quacks and con artists may also try to get you to believe their product is popular in Europe, Asia, or some other location. This technique is an attempt to impress you, but it does not provide any useful information.

Be Wary of Untested Products

Quacks do not subject their products to thorough scientific testing. Their products are often rushed to market in order to make money as quickly as possible. One way to tell whether a product or service is a good one is to see if information about it has been published in a respected journal. If so, the study was conducted by a qualified expert.

Health and Fitness Quackery

The market is flooded with health and fitness products, many of which are useless. Although some of these products may not be harmful, false claims give people unrealistic expectations about the benefits they can provide. Indeed, many advertisers promote myths about health and fitness. In the section that follows, some products and practices often associated with quackery or fraud are discussed.

Food Supplements

A food supplement is a product that is not part of the typical diet, usually sold in health food stores or online. Supplements are often produced as syrups, powders, or tablets (figure 19.2). Common supplements include protein (amino acids), vitamins, minerals, and herbs. Packaged food—such as canned goods, boxed goods, and frozen foods—must carry a label that informs you of the product's ingredients, but such labels are not required on food supplements.

As you know, manufacturers do not have to prove that a supplement works before they sell it, and the law does not regulate the contents of supplements. Many people have suffered illness and even death as the result of taking supplements marketed as causing fat loss or enhancing performance.

Although food supplements are not regulated, the FDA will investigate if enough complaints are received for a specific supplement. The supplement ephedra, for

FIT FACT

Cellulite is a term often used for fat that causes the skin to look rippled or bumpy. Con artists would have you believe that cellulite is a special kind of fat that can be eliminated with creams or other special products. In fact, cellulite occurs when fat cells become enlarged and is best reduced by expending more calories than you consume.

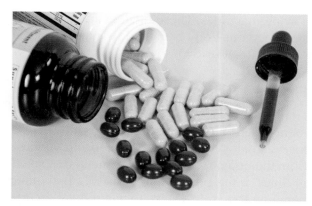

Figure 19.2 Food supplements are not regulated by the government.

example, was banned by the U.S. Food and Drug Administration after being implicated in several deaths. The problem, however, is that new supplements are often sold before the public becomes aware of health problems associated with the product. Taking a supplement about which little is known can be dangerous. For example, as this book went to press, the plant extract kratom is being sold legally in most states. In recent years more than 40 deaths have been linked to kratom use, and despite a report from the National Institute on Drug Abuse (NIDA) that it can cause addiction, withdrawal symptoms, and numerous side effects, kratom use by teens has increased.

Some other supplements are not harmful but simply do not provide the benefits promised by those who sell them. Since being deregulated in 1994, the sale of supplements has increased dramatically, meaning many people are wasting money on products that don't work.

Some supplements can be beneficial if used according to a physician's recommendation. For example, a vitamin B_{12} supplement is recommended for strict vegetarians and vegans, and a folic acid supplement is recommended for expectant mothers. But even vitamins can be dangerous in large amounts. Before you take any supplement, consult a parent or guardian and your family physician.

Sport Supplements

One fad involves the use of sport supplements or sport vitamins intended to enhance athletic performance (also called *ergogenic aids*). Many supplements sold as ergogenic aids are actually quack products that are useless or even harmful to your health. For example, products sold as protein bars are often very high in sugar and calories. As noted earlier in this book, the American Academy of Pediatrics recommends against the use of sports and energy drinks by teens because of the high sugar and caffeine content. Additional information about supplements and ergogenic aids is provided in chapter 11.

Fad Diets

"Lose pounds a day on the ice cream diet!" "The rice diet works wonders!" "Fruit diet dissolves fat!" How many similar weight loss claims have you seen? Each of these claims is an example of a fad diet. Although fad diets are popular because they usually promise fast results, nearly all are nutritionally unbalanced. They often restrict eating to only one or two food groups, or even one specific food. As you've learned, the only safe and effective way to reduce body fatness and lose weight is to combine physical activity with eating fewer calories. Eating healthy, low-calorie foods can help you control your calorie intake.

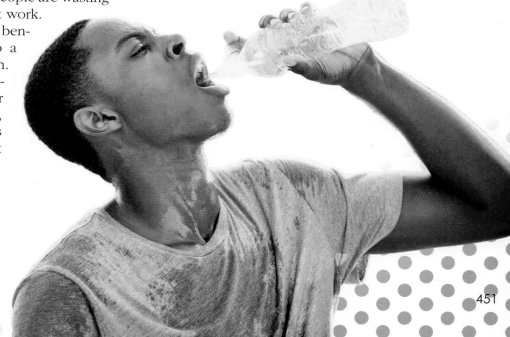

Dehydration

Restricting fluid intake, taking products that cause water loss, and wearing garments that do not allow sweat to evaporate and cool the body (e.g., rubber or plastic clothing) can lead to **dehydration**. Dehydration can cause heat-related conditions such as heat exhaustion and heatstroke and other physical problems such as headache, fatigue, lack of concentration, and mood changes. Drinking water helps you stay hydrated and is important to good health. Unfortunately, some people think that restricting fluids is an acceptable way to lose weight. It is not! Weight loss as a result of water loss is temporary. When fluids are replaced, body weight returns to normal.

Passive Exercise Machines

Passive exercise refers to the use of machines or devices that move your body for you and supposedly promote fat reduction and weight loss. Examples include machines that roll along your hips or legs, vibrating machines that shake certain body areas and are said to "break up" fat cells, and motorized belts, cycles, tables, and rowing machines. These devices are ineffective because your body is moved by outside forces rather than your own muscles.

Figure Wraps

Figure wraps are bandages or nonporous garments used to compress body parts, advertised for weight loss or as a method of losing "inches" from the body. The wraps are sometimes soaked in fluid, or the person may soak in a bath after being wrapped. In reality, they are not effective for either fat loss or size reduction. They can, however, cause overheating and dehydration and can be extremely dangerous to your health.

Spot Reduction

An unqualified fitness instructor might recommend that you perform "spot" fat loss exercises. Those who promote spot fat loss claim that fat can be removed from specific areas in the body by performing exercises that target a specific location. Research shows, however, that no type of exercise causes fat loss at one specific location.

TECH TRENDS: Quack Machines

You've learned in other chapters about many technological innovations that can promote fitness, health, and wellness. However, not all technological devices are safe and effective. Some unscrupulous people sell devices that not only are ineffective but also can be quite dangerous.

One example is the ab stimulator, a device with electrodes that are placed on the abdominal muscles. Electrical current is sent through the electrodes, thus stimulating the muscles. People who advertise these devices claim that you can use them to build strong abdominal muscles without doing any regular abdominal exercises, such as crunches or curl-ups. But studies show that these devices do not build fitness, and the electrodes can cause the heart to beat irregularly and result in serious health problems.

Physical therapists and athletic trainers do use muscle stimulators to help restore normal muscle function in people who have been injured or who are recovering from illness, which can be effective when used by experts for very specific therapeutic purposes. They are not the same as muscle stimulators sold with claims of building abdominal muscle. Be wary of sellers who promise fitness without exercise.

USING TECHNOLOGY

Ask a physical therapist to explain how a muscle stimulator works to help people with injury or illness. Ask for more information about the dangers of using an abdominal muscle stimulator.

LESSON REVIEW

1. What are quackery and fraud, and how do they differ?
2. What are some ways of detecting quackery and fraud?
3. What are some of the guidelines for avoiding being a victim of quackery or fraud?
4. What are some examples of health and fitness misconceptions and quackery?

SELF-ASSESSMENT: **Assessing Your Posture**

Assessing your posture can help you achieve and maintain good posture and prevent problems that could make you susceptible to quackery. You can use the following self-assessment to determine whether your posture is as good as it should be. If you find that improvements are needed, you can work at applying proper biomechanics when sitting, standing, and walking.

For this self-assessment, wear exercise clothing or a swimsuit. Work with a partner to determine each other's scores. Record your results as directed by your instructor.

1. Stand sideways next to a string hanging from a point at least 12 inches (30 centimeters) above your head. The string should be weighted at the bottom so that it hangs straight and reaches nearly to the floor. Position yourself so that the string aligns with the side of your ankle bone.

   - Head: Is the ear in front of the line?
   - Shoulders: Are the shoulders rounded? Are the tips of the shoulders in front of the chest?
   - Upper back: Does the upper back stick out in a hump?
   - Lower back: Does the lower back have excessive arch?
   - Abdomen: Does the abdomen protrude beyond the pelvic bone?
   - Knees: Do the knees appear to be locked or bent backward?

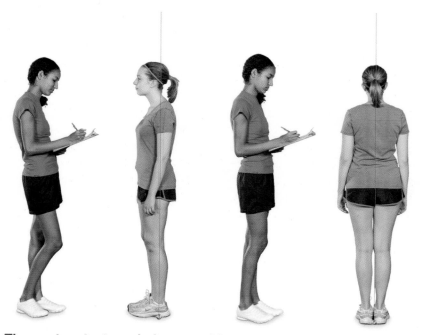

The posture test can help you achieve and maintain good posture.

2. Now stand with your back to the string so that the string is aligned with the middle of your back.
   - Head: Is more than half of the head on one side of the string?
   - Shoulders: Is one shoulder higher than the other?
   - Hips: Is one hip higher than the other?

3. Give yourself 1 point for each question you answered "yes." Add points to get a total score. Then determine your rating in table 19.1.

TABLE 19.1   Rating Chart: Posture Test

Score	Rating
0–1	Good posture
2–4	Can use some improvement
≥5	Needs considerable improvement

Evaluating Health Clubs, Equipment, Media, and Internet Materials

Lesson Objectives

After reading this lesson, you should be able to

1. describe guidelines for evaluating health and fitness clubs;

2. describe guidelines for evaluating exercise equipment;

3. describe guidelines for evaluating websites for fitness, health, and wellness information; and

4. describe guidelines for evaluating exercise videos and magazine articles about fitness.

Lesson Vocabulary

spa
web extension

Where do you get your health, fitness, and wellness information? Have you ever considered how that information is created? People are more interested than ever in health and fitness, and they look to many sources for information. Unfortunately, not all of it is accurate. In this lesson, you'll learn how to evaluate printed material and web resources. First, however, you will learn how to evaluate health and fitness clubs, as well as exercise clothing and equipment.

Evaluating Health and Fitness Clubs

You do not need to join a health club, spa, or gym to attain or maintain fitness. They do offer some advantages: Health clubs offer their members special equipment and personnel, and modern **spas** offer saunas, whirlpool baths, and

My friend was using a supplement. Then he found out that his favorite baseball player was suspended for using a supplement that contained a banned substance. That got his attention, and mine too.

Dontrell Washington

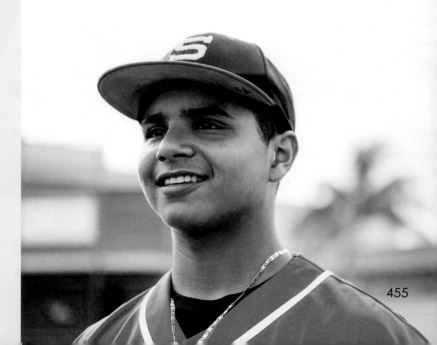

455

other services such as massage and hair and skin care. In addition, some people find that joining a club helps motivate them to exercise and remain physically active. But these services can be expensive, and well-educated people can save money and still get the benefits of regular exercise by designing their own fitness and activity programs without using special facilities or equipment.

Many low-cost programs are offered through community centers, universities, churches, and other groups. In addition, your school may be among the many that have built their own fitness centers, sometimes called *wellness centers*. Such programs can give you the same benefits and motivation as more expensive clubs. Still, if you feel that it would help you stay active, you may be interested in joining a commercial club, spa, or gym at some point. Use the following guidelines when deciding whether to join a health club.

• *If possible, join on a pay-as-you-go basis.* If you sign a contract, make it a short-term one. Read the fine print carefully before signing. Too

often, people pay a lot for a long-term contract, then stop using the facility. It's best to pay for a short membership until you're sure that you'll stick with it. The fine print may contain special clauses that will cost you money. For example, do you still have to pay if you move away? Often, the salesperson pressures you to sign a contract on your first visit, but it's best to think about it for a while before signing.

• *Choose a well-established club.* Such a club is less likely to go out of business. Make sure the facility employs qualified fitness experts and be alert for signs of fitness quackery. If you see them, consider choosing a different club.

• *Make a trial visit to the club.* Visit at a time when you would normally use the club. Make sure you feel comfortable with the employees and other patrons and that the equipment and facilities are available for you to use at that time.

• *Choose a club that meets your personal needs.* For example, a person with joint pain might prefer to avoid activities that stress the joints in favor of swimming for cardiorespiratory

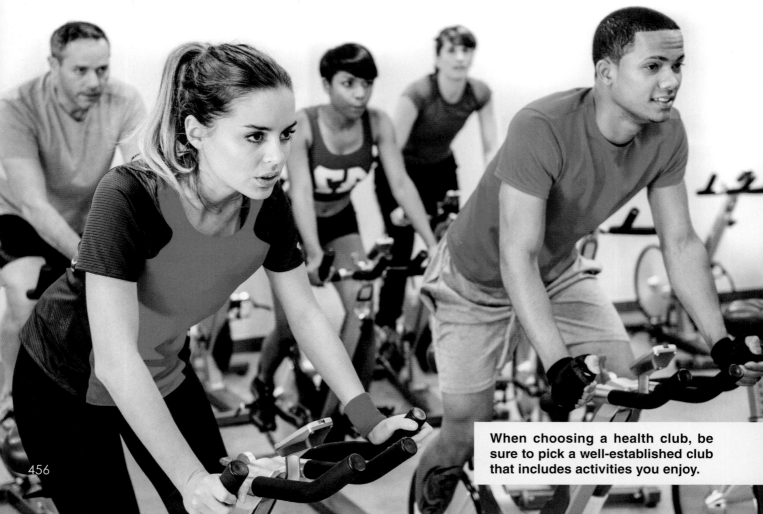

When choosing a health club, be sure to pick a well-established club that includes activities you enjoy.

endurance. Of course, this person should choose a facility that includes a swimming pool.

• *Avoid clubs that cater primarily to bodybuilding for adults.* Research shows that clubs frequented mostly by adults interested in bodybuilding are more likely to sell unproven supplements and even illegal products. Some people who frequent these places subscribe to their own theories and reject scientific evidence developed by experts. Furthermore, practices that may be acceptable for adults are often not appropriate for teens. Find a club that is appropriate for families and teens and employs qualified experts on its staff.

• *Consider any medical needs.* If weight loss is your primary goal, consider joining a program recommended by your physician or sponsored by a hospital rather than joining a health club. If you have a special medical need, you may need the help of a physical therapist.

> Spending money is easy. Spending money wisely is another thing altogether.
>
> *U.S. Federal Trade Commission*

Evaluating Exercise Equipment

Some people choose not to join a club but to buy home exercise equipment instead. If you're considering home exercise equipment, use the following guidelines.

• *Consider inexpensive home equipment.* For resistance exercise, you can use homemade weights, bicycle inner tubes, or rubber or latex bands. To build cardiorespiratory endurance, you can use jump ropes, stepping benches, or stairs. If you're interested in fitness for health and wellness, this equipment may be all you need.

• *Consider your personal needs before buying equipment.* For building muscle fitness, you can use free weights and home exercise machines. For cardiorespiratory endurance, you can use machines such as treadmills, bicycles, and stair steppers. A regular bicycle is also a good choice if you have a safe place to ride. Exercise equipment is often quite expensive, so it's important to choose well. Rather than depending on the advice of a salesperson, consult an expert, the ACSM website, or *Consumer Reports.* Buy from a well-established company that honors the warranty, services the product, and sells replacement parts.

• *Be sure before you buy.* See if you can try equipment owned by a friend or by your school before deciding to buy the product. Avoid investing money in exercise equipment until you're sure you'll use it. Many people buy equipment, then don't use it after the first few months. You can see evidence of this behavior in the many ads for slightly used equipment. Some of the high-tech equipment described in this book, such as pedometers and heart rate watches, can be useful; however, it can be quite expensive, and you may find that you won't use it regularly. In addition, some high-tech products simply are not worth the cost. For example, expensive electrical devices for measuring body fat level are not worth the personal investment when an inexpensive caliper can give you accurate fat measurements.

• *Make sure you have enough space for the equipment.* One of the main reasons people fail to use the exercise equipment they buy is that they don't have a good place to keep it. If you have to get out equipment each time you use it or move it from place to place, you're less likely to use it than if you have an area where you can set it up permanently.

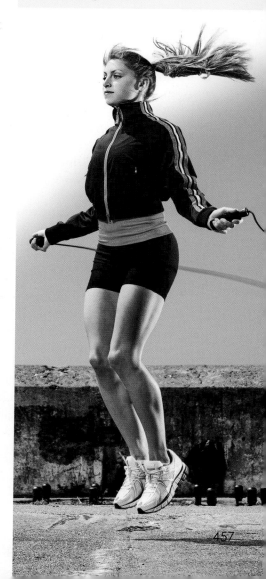

Equipment does not need to be expensive to be effective in promoting fitness.

Evaluating Internet Resources

We depend on the web more than any other source for health and fitness information. Yet research shows that many web sources provide incorrect information. If you use the web to locate information about health, fitness, and wellness, ask yourself the following questions.

• *Who developed the website?* Websites with the best information are often those developed by government agencies, professional organizations, and educational institutions. Governmental health agencies' web addresses end with .gov, professional organizations' web addresses often end with .org, and education institutions' web addresses end with .edu. Choose websites presented by well-known agencies, organizations, and institutions such as those listed in the Consumer Corner feature in the first lesson of this chapter or the web resource. Remember, however, that any organization can now obtain a .org web address, so that alone does not guarantee that the information on the site is reliable. At the same time, some websites with an address ending in .com or .net do provide good information.

• *Did you reach the website you intended to reach?* The Internet Corporation for Assigned Names and Numbers is charged with creating **web extensions** (web address endings). The most common ones are .net, .org, and .com, but there are many, many more (e.g., .book, .movie, and .app). The many web extensions make it difficult to know which websites offer good information. An unscrupulous company may use the same web address as a legitimate company but with a different extension, posing as the real thing (for example, if www.fitnessforlife.org were the website for Fitness for Life, but another organization set up a site at www.fitnessforlife.xyz). Some con artists also use websites with names very similar to legitimate ones in hopes that some people will reach them by accident if they type the intended web address incorrectly. Make sure that you avoid errors when typing web addresses. For more information about good web sources for health and fitness, visit the web resource.

• *Is this web article an advertisement?* Be aware that websites that sell products are more likely to provide false information than those that are authentic web sources. Be aware that Internet searches often lead you to websites that pay to appear at the top of the search list. The FTC requires companies to "clearly and prominently" indicate that an advertisement is an ad. Look beyond the links at the top of the search list and look for "ad" or "advertisement" in front of the URL before clicking on a website. You may also want to check the FTC website for names of companies that have been caught breaking the rules.

Evaluating Exercise Videos and Magazine Articles

Exercise videos and magazine articles, when well done, can be useful to help you stay active and fit. Unfortunately, many contain incorrect information. Guidelines for evaluating exercise videos and articles are provided in the sections that follow.

Evaluating Exercise Videos

Many exercise videos are now available online in addition to traditional formats. One advantage is that many are free; the disadvantage is that anyone can shoot a video and put it online, even if they are not qualified to do so. Before you choose an exercise video, consider the following guidelines.

• *Check the credentials of the creator.* The creator is the person who prepares the exercises, which may then be performed by someone other than the creator. Check whether the creator has a degree or certification from a reputable institution or organization.

• *Choose an exercise program that includes appropriate warm-up and cool-down exercises.* The warm-up and cool-down should be consistent with guidelines provided in this book.

• *Make sure the program contains only safe exercises.* Check to see that the person performing the exercises is doing them properly. This book provides you with information about safe exercises, as well as risky exercises to avoid.

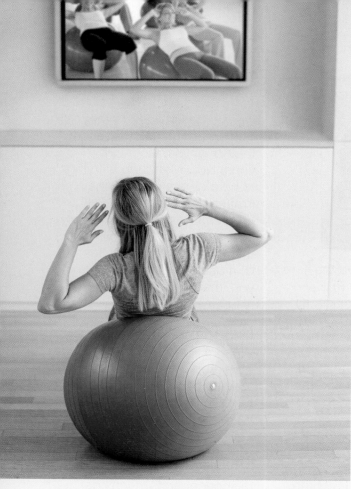

Video exercise routines should be appropriate for your skill and fitness level.

• *Make sure the exercises start gradually and progress in intensity.* If the first part of the exercise program is moderate in intensity, it may serve as the warm-up.

• *Choose a program that is interesting and fun.* Check to see if it includes exercises that you would enjoy doing on a regular basis.

• *Choose a program that is consistent with the information and guidelines included in this book.* If most of the content is good, but some is not, you can modify the exercises in the program or change the order of the routine to make it better.

• *Be aware that free online videos may have unseen costs.* Some online videos are advertised as free, but to make money the website may show ads or require you to register, allowing your personal data to be accessed or sold. A check of the website's privacy policy is recommended.

Evaluating Magazine Articles

Print circulation for teen magazines has decreased in recent years, but millions still read them. Almost all teen magazines also have online editions and some are online only. These magazines, whether print or online, often include articles on exercise. Unfortunately, health and fitness information presented through the media is often misleading or incorrect. How can you evaluate health and fitness information that you read, view, or hear? You can use the guidelines for exercise videos presented in the previous section to evaluate magazine articles as well. If an article promises big results in a short time or promises other benefits that seem too good to be true, find another program.

• *Choose a program that rotates muscle groups and addresses all parts of fitness.* If it claims to be a total fitness program, make sure it includes activities for all parts of fitness and rotates them appropriately.

• *Choose a program that is appropriate for you.* Make sure that the exercises are appropriate for your fitness level. For example, if it says it is for beginners, are the exercises really for beginners?

LESSON REVIEW

1. What are some guidelines for evaluating health and fitness clubs?
2. What are some guidelines for evaluating exercise equipment?
3. What are some guidelines for evaluating websites for fitness, health, and wellness information?
4. What are some guidelines for evaluating exercise videos and magazine articles about fitness?

TAKING CHARGE: **Learning to Think Critically**

A misconception is a belief based on incorrect or misunderstood information or a lack of facts. The best way to counter a misconception is to increase your knowledge so that you can recognize and interpret facts correctly. Here's an example.

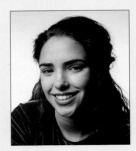

Mary Lou had tried several exercise programs but had not found one that they felt would help them meet their goal of developing muscle fitness. They had never even considered progressive resistance exercise (PRE) because they believed it would cause them to develop big, bulky muscles.

One day, Mary Lou's physical education teacher took her class to the fitness room. There, the teacher explained how to use the free weights and resistance machines. Over the next several weeks, the class practiced the correct use of the PRE equipment. As a class assignment, Mary Lou's teacher had each member of the class find one news article about PRE and write a report on it. In doing the report, Mary Lou learned that muscles do not become bulky if weight training is done properly.

With this new knowledge, Mary Lou realized that the correct PRE program would give them exactly what they were looking for and began working out three days a week. The knowledge they gained about PRE dispelled their original misconceptions. Now Mary Lou is trying to help others change their irrational beliefs about PRE. When friends ask why Mary Lou is trying to build big muscles, Mary Lou replies, "If muscle fitness is what you're after, you should give resistance training a try."

FOR DISCUSSION

What misconception did Mary Lou have? How were they able to build knowledge to dispel a misconception? What are some other misconceptions people have about physical activity? Why do you think people have these misconceptions? Consider the guidelines in the following Self-Management feature as you answer these discussion questions.

SELF-MANAGEMENT: **Skills for Thinking Critically**

Thinking critically means using a problem-solving process before making important decisions, similar to the scientific method. The steps are listed here with examples for using each one to help you select exercise equipment. You can use the same steps to solve problems and make decisions about other important topics.

- *Step 1: Identify the problem to be solved or clarify the decision that must be made.* If you know that you want to improve your muscle fitness but are not sure how to do it, you have to define the problem more clearly. Do you want to improve your health, improve your appearance, or get fit for sport performance? Do you want to

do your exercises at school, join a health and fitness club, buy exercise equipment, or use inexpensive equipment? For this discussion, let's assume that you want to decide what equipment to use in order to build your muscle fitness for good health. Thus the problem has been clearly defined.

- *Step 2: Collect information and investigate.* One way to collect information relevant to the defined problem is to perform self-assessments for muscle fitness. Knowing your current status will help you select exercises to meet your specific needs. You can also consult experts and explore reliable websites, such as those described in this chapter's Consumer Corner feature or in the web resource. In this example, you may also try out several equipment options, perhaps by using the school exercise room, visiting local health and fitness clubs, or trying out machines on display at a sporting goods store. You could also try several of the inexpensive equipment options you've learned about in this book. Focus on finding information that will help you solve the problem you've identified in step 1.

- *Step 3: Develop a plan of action.* Use the information gained from your investigation to formulate a plan. For example, your results from step 2 might indicate that the school exercise room is not open when you are free to use it, and perhaps the health and fitness club is too far from your home and costs too much. In addition, home exercise equipment can be quite expensive. After rejecting these options, then, you might decide to do elastic band

exercises. The equipment is inexpensive, and you can do all the exercises necessary to meet your needs. You could choose several of the exercises described in this book, then make a written plan specifying a schedule and how many sets and reps you'll do each day.

- *Step 4: Put your plan into action.* For a plan to be effective, you must use it. The sooner you begin to act after preparing your plan, the more likely you are to change your behavior. In this example, you would use the plan developed in step 3 to get started with the elastic band exercises.

- *Step 5: Evaluate the effectiveness of your plan.* Use self-assessments and keep a log to chart your progress. As you go forward, you can continue using the five critical thinking steps presented here to solve problems that arise and make effective decisions about your health, fitness, and wellness.

ACADEMIC CONNECTION: **Critical Thinking Skills**

Preparing for a career or for college requires critical thinking skills. Education experts have described learning standards for the English language arts that help you prepare. Following are some of the skills needed for success in the workplace and in college:

- *Demonstrating independence.* In addition to being able to understand ideas presented by others, independence requires you to build on others' ideas and express your own thoughts and views.

- *Building strong knowledge of subject matter.* Research and study are required to develop knowledge in different subject matter areas, including health and physical education. This requires extensive reading and attentive listening.

- *Comprehending as well as knowing facts.* Knowing refers to possessing information

or facts. Comprehending refers to grasping the significance of information or facts.

- *Valuing evidence.* One step in the scientific method is collecting data (tangible evidence). This evidence can be used to help make decisions or solve problems.

- *Using technology capably.* Modern technology makes a considerable amount of information available in an instant. Capable use of technology requires the ability to evaluate the quality of information acquired from the Internet and other technical sources and the thoughtful use of that information.

Practice the self-management skills in this chapter to help you meet these important standards.

Taking Action: **Your Health and Fitness Club**

By now you've learned how to plan a personal physical activity program and are performing it regularly on your own. But you may also enjoy being active with others. Using school facilities and equipment, you can create your own health and fitness club for use during class time. Work with the other students in class to survey the types of activity that class members enjoy.

When putting together a workout for others, consider their current fitness, their skill levels, and their interests. Prepare several exercise stations with a variety of activities and equipment that address all the parts of health-related fitness. Have a class member act as fitness instructor and describe the purpose of each exercise station to the rest of the class. **Take action** by having all class members use the health and fitness club to perform a physical activity workout that meets their personal goals. Evaluate the effectiveness of your health and fitness club.

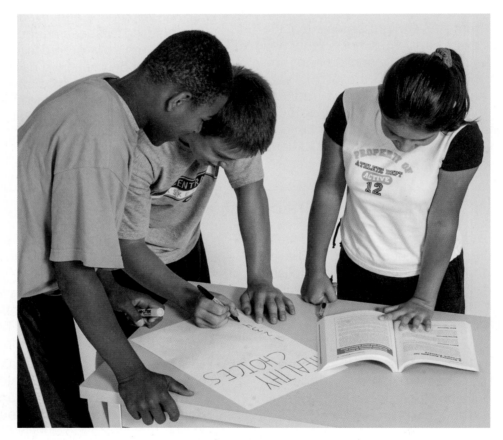

Take action by creating your own health and fitness club.

CHAPTER REVIEW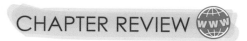

Reviewing Concepts and Vocabulary

Answer items 1 through 5 by correctly completing each sentence with a word or phrase.

1. A method of advertising or selling a health product or service that uses false claims is called _____.

2. Selling a health product you know to be worthless is called _____.

3. A _____ is a product added to the diet rather than being part of the regular diet.

4. _____ exercise uses machines or outside forces to move your muscles.

5. The extension .gov indicates that a website is associated with _____.

For items 6 through 10, as directed by your teacher, match each term in column 1 with the *best* phrase in column 2.

6. physician   a. may not be an expert

7. certified health education teacher   b. provides medical advice

8. registered physical therapist   c. person with a degree in nutrition

9. dietitian   d. provides information about exercise

10. nutritionist   e. provides general health information

For items 11 through 15, respond to each statement or question.

11. Describe three ways to recognize quackery.

12. Describe the posture test and why it is important.

13. Describe three guidelines for selecting a fitness or health club.

14. Describe three guidelines for finding good health information on the web.

15. Describe the five steps for critical thinking that you can use to solve problems and make decisions about physical activity and good health.

Thinking Critically

Write a paragraph to answer the following question.

Your friend Lee visited a health food store and got interested in taking a supplement. He says that he can make his own decision because the products must be safe and effective or they wouldn't be on store shelves. What advice would you give your friend? Explain your reasons.

Project

Visit a local health club, choose an article about exercise from a popular magazine, view an exercise video, or visit a health or fitness website. Use the guidelines presented in this chapter to evaluate its quality and write a brief report of your evaluation.

The Science of Active Living

20

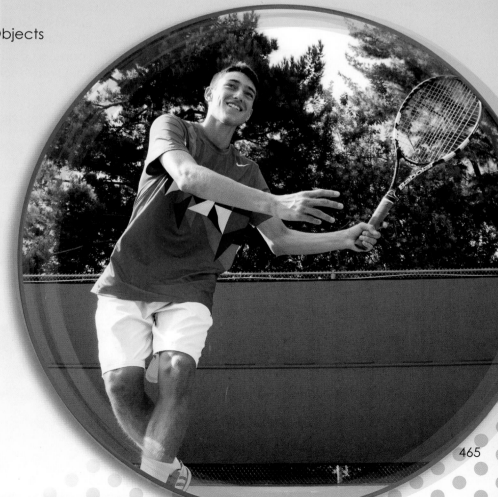

Moving Your Body

Lesson Objectives

After reading this lesson, you should be able to

1. describe how one person (Gretchen) stayed active throughout life;
2. describe nine key biomechanical principles of motor skill learning;
3. describe the two stances commonly used in physical activity; and
4. describe several forms of locomotion and lifting.

Lesson Vocabulary

acceleration
aerodynamics
biomechanical principles
center of gravity
deceleration
force
hydrodynamics
locomotion
resistance
stance
velocity

Throughout this book, you've learned several principles of biomechanics and motor learning and how you can apply them in various situations. In this chapter, you'll review some of these principles and learn about others that can help you move efficiently throughout your life.

When performing activities from the Physical Activity Pyramid, you use motor skills, which range from simple to complex. Successful performance of motor skills requires you to apply principles of human movement. Experts in biomechanics study human movement and help us understand and apply the biomechanical principles in all types of activity.

Learning Skills for Life

When Gretchen was a teen she played softball and basketball. During her 20s and 30s, her job and home responsibilities kept her from playing these team sports, but she stayed active by doing aerobic dance and muscle fitness and flexibility exercises at the local fitness club. During her 40s, Gretchen had more time to get back into sports, so she joined a slowpitch softball league with some friends at work. She also kept up her

> I never thought that I would learn about science in PE. Learning about biomechanical principles helped in science class and with learning skills in sports.
>
> *Rylee Kaczmarek*

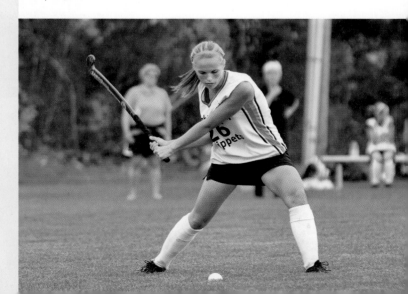

regular exercises at the gym. In her 50s, she decided to try tennis at the urging of a friend who needed a doubles partner. Today, at 74, she walks, does her muscle fitness and flexibility exercises, and plays doubles tennis in a local league. Although her activities have changed over the years, she's never been inactive, and along the way she's developed some great friendships and had a lot of fun.

Early in life, Gretchen was fortunate to have a physical education teacher and coach who taught her the principles of movement. As her life changed, her activities also changed, but she could apply those principles to them. In addition, knowing some movement basics enabled her to have fun participating in activities with friends. In this chapter you will learn principles that helped Gretchen to continue to learn new skills throughout life.

> Excellence is the gradual result of always striving to do better.
>
> *Pat Riley, basketball coach*

Biomechanics and Skill Learning

Biomechanics is a branch of kinesiology that uses principles of physics to help us understand the human body in motion. Physical education teachers and other exercise professionals typically take at least one class in biomechanics and use the information to aid them in teaching motor skills. You can also benefit from learning **biomechanical principles** and applying them to the performance of skills in sports and other activities. In the paragraphs that follow, biomechanical principles in nine different areas are described. These principles relate directly to the motor skills described in this chapter; however, there are many others as well.

1. Stability

Stability of the body, at rest or in movement, is related to the location of the body's **center of gravity** and the base of the body's support. Stability while standing is increased by a wide base of support and a low center of gravity, which is important for activities such as gymnastics and paddleboarding. Staying stable at rest and while moving requires balance, a part of skill-related fitness.

2. Force

To make a body or object move or to stop a moving body or object, **force** must be applied. Many forces are involved, but the contraction of muscles provides the primary force. Applying force in one direction results in the production of force in the opposite direction (for every action there is an equal and opposite reaction).

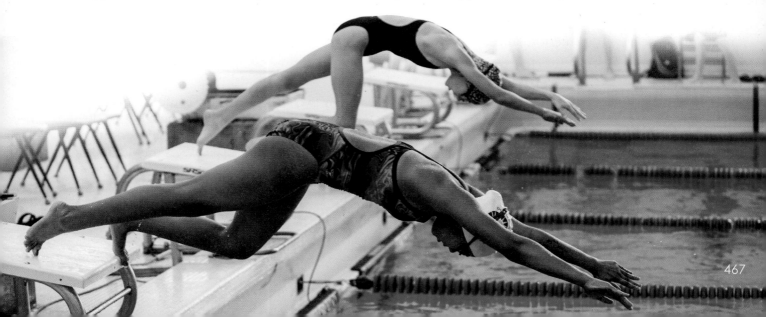

3. Acceleration, Deceleration, and Velocity

Velocity is speed of movement. **Acceleration** (increase in velocity) occurs when a force is applied to a body or object—the bigger the object's mass, the more force must be applied to cause acceleration. **Deceleration** (decrease in velocity) occurs when resistance is applied to an object.

4. Accumulation of Forces

Greater force can be applied to an object or body if each new force is added sequentially. For example, when a person throws a ball effectively, the lower body moves first, the trunk moves second, the upper body moves third, and then finally the arm and hand move (see the Self-Assessment later in this chapter). Force production is greatest if each movement is added after the previous movement has reached its greatest acceleration. The application of force is important in all physical activities.

5. Resistance

Resistance is opposition to a force or movement. Sources of resistance include friction (a force caused by one surface rubbing against another), air (including wind), water, and gravity. Resistance can also be applied by an opposing force such as another player pushing you in football or by a weight on a barbell in progressive resistance training.

6. Levers

A lever is a very basic machine—a bar or stiff, straight object that can be used to lift weight or increase force. Levers can be used to increase force for producing movement. In your body, bones act as levers, and muscle contractions create the force that moves the levers (overcomes a resistance). The body has three types of lever: first, second, and third class (see figure 20.1).

The fulcrum for a first-class lever is located between the resistance and the force applied. The toe raise provides an example for a first-class lever that uses force from muscles to overcome resistance of the body weight (see figure 20.1*a*). A second-class lever has the fulcrum and the force application at each end of the lever with the resistance in the middle (see figure 20.1*b*). The push-up provides an example. A third-class lever has the fulcrum and the resistance at each end of the lever with the force application in the middle (see figure 20.1*c*). The biceps curl provides an example. Third-class levers are the most common for human performance.

7. Angles

An *angle* is defined as a figure formed by two lines originating in the same place. The size of an angle is measured in degrees—for example, a right angle is a 90-degree angle. Understanding angles is important for successful physical performance. For example, when you throw a ball, the angle of release affects the distance and direction it travels. The ground is one line in the angle, and the trajectory of the ball is the other line. In hockey, angles are important for playing the puck off of the wall and passing to teammates.

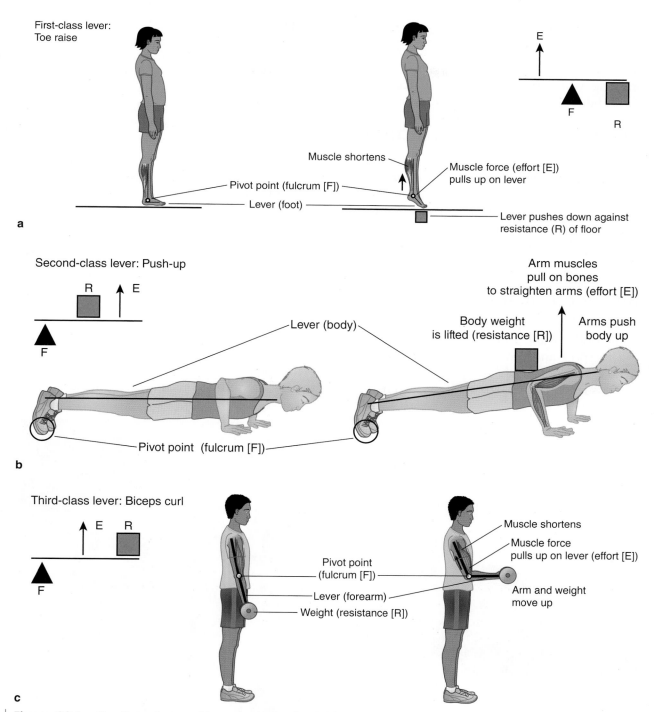

Figure 20.1 The three types of lever in the body: *(a)* first-class lever (toe raise), *(b)* second-class lever (push-up), *(c)* third-class lever (biceps curl).

8. Aerodynamics

In physics, the study of dynamics addresses motion, including factors that cause changes in motion. **Aerodynamics** includes the study of motion in the air (represented in the term by *aero*). Performance is influenced by various aerodynamic factors, including spin (e.g., on a ball), wind (e.g., air resistance in running), and other factors (e.g., turbulence, humidity, and altitude).

9. Hydrodynamics

Hydrodynamics refers to the study of motion in fluids. Factors that affect movement in water include water resistance, turbulence (water movement patterns), and temperature.

▌Fundamental Skills: Stances

Fundamental skills are those that are common to many activities. If you apply the principles of biomechanics when performing fundamental skills, you can use them to help you learn new skills. Virtually all skills are affected in some way by every one of the nine biomechanical principles described previously.

Balanced Stance

The most basic **stance**—the ready position—is with good posture and stability. When performing in sport and other physical activities, you need to use a stance that prepares you for action. For this reason, the balanced stance, sometimes called the *ready stance* or *athletic stance*, is basic to many sport and other physical activities. This stance, shown in figure 20.2, allows you to be stable when standing and prepares you to move in any direction. Some of its characteristics include a wide base (feet shoulder-width apart or slightly more), lowered center of gravity (knees bent), and centered (body is not leaning backward, forward, or to either side).

Variations of the balanced stance are used, for example, by baseball and softball players in the field, basketball players on defense, tennis players when getting ready to receive a serve, and many other participants in a wide variety of physical activity situations. Balance and stability are needed in these cases because the performer doesn't know in which direction they will need to move.

Unbalanced Stance

The unbalanced stance (figure 20.3) is used when a performer anticipates moving in a certain

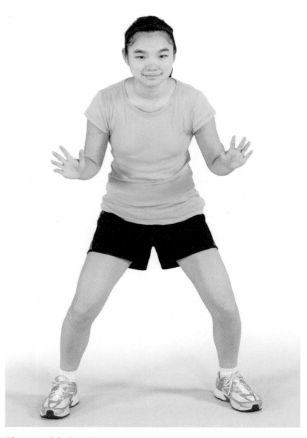

Figure 20.2   The balanced stance.

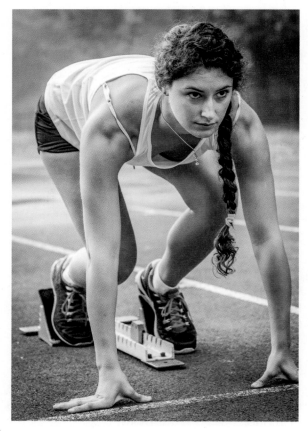

Figure 20.3   The unbalanced stance.

direction. This stance is used, for example, by sprinters and swimmers at the start of a race and by football players lined up for the start of a play. Rather than being stable, a performer using an unbalanced stance leans in the direction of anticipated movement, thus allowing the body to get moving more quickly.

Fundamental Skills: Locomotion and Lifting

Locomotion refers to moving the body from place to place. A *locomotor skill* is a skill that involves movement. In the following paragraphs some basic locomotor skills are described.

Locomotion: Walking, Running, and Sprinting

The most basic forms of locomotion are walking and running. In walking, one foot or the other is in contact with the ground at all times. In running (or jogging), both feet are off the ground for a short time during each stride. The biomechanical principles are especially important to apply when walking, running, and performing other locomotor skills. Sprinting, or fast running, is used for events such as the 100-meter dash and in sports such as soccer.

Locomotion: Jumping and Leaping

Two other common forms of locomotion in sport and other physical activities are jumping and leaping. When jumping, a person pushes off the ground with and lands on two feet (see figure 20.4). A jump can be forward, as in the standing long jump, or upward, as in the vertical jump (figure 20.4). Both of these jumps are used as tests of leg power.

When leaping, a person leaves the ground on one foot and lands on the opposite foot (see figure 20.5). Leaps are common in dance and gymnastics. (Leaping is different from hopping, in which the takeoff and landing is on the same foot).

FIT FACT
It takes 30 times as much force to lift an object as to push it. Pushing is also more efficient than pulling.

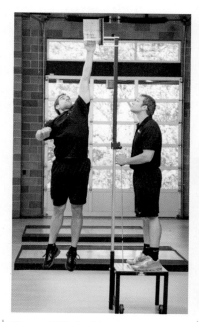

Figure 20.4   Vertical jump.

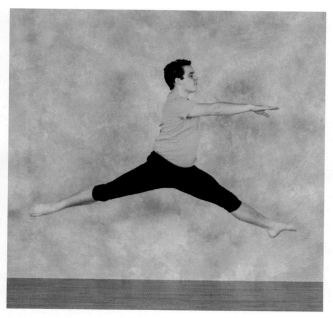

Figure 20.5   Leap.

Elements of jumping and leaping are often combined in physical activities. For example, in the running long jump, the performer leaves the ground on one foot and lands on two feet (see figure 20.6). Although this type of movement is a combined movement, it is commonly referred to as a jump. Plyometrics uses jumping and leaping to build power and muscle fitness.

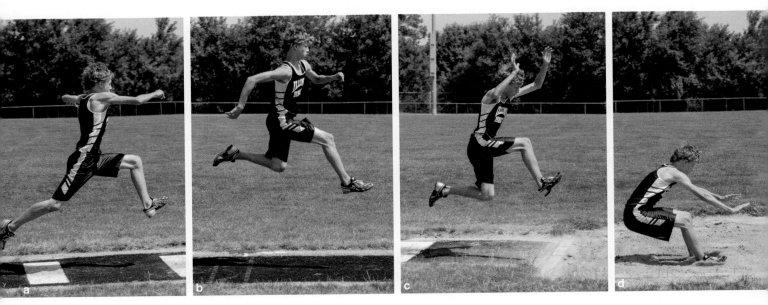

Figure 20.6   Running long jump.

Other Locomotor Movements

Space constraints do not allow for discussion of all forms of locomotor movement. Some examples of other forms are skipping, hopping, galloping, and skating. Crossover running and shuffling are also common in many sports, and there are many variations of moving in water.

Lifting

Lifting is a motor skill used in resistance training and in sports such as weightlifting, powerlifting, and wrestling. The first seven biomechanical principles described earlier are particularly relevant in lifting.

LESSON REVIEW

1. How did Gretchen adapt to stay active throughout life?
2. What are the nine key biomechanical principles of motor skill learning?
3. How do you perform the two types of stances commonly used in physical activity?
4. What are some forms of locomotion, and how do you perform them properly?

SELF-ASSESSMENT: **Analyzing Basic Skills**

In the first lesson of this chapter, you learned about a variety of motor skills, including walking, running, and jumping. In the next lesson, you'll learn about throwing, striking, kicking, and other fundamental skills. In this self-assessment, you'll work with two partners to analyze the fundamental skill of overhand throwing. Use the following steps. Remember that self-assessment information is confidential and shouldn't be shared without the permission of the person being tested.

1. Using a baseball or softball, perform an overhand throw to a partner standing 30 feet (9 meters) away. Your target is the glove or mitt of the person to whom you are throwing. Repeat the throw several times.

2. Have a second partner watch your throws and rate each element using table 20.1. This partner should record the results. Figure 20.7 in the next lesson may be useful as you make your assessment.

3. Rotate your duties so that each member of your team gets a chance to throw and rate.

4. When your ratings are done, use the information you gained to practice throwing properly. You can use peer teaching to help each other improve where needed.

TABLE 20.1   Rating Chart: Overhand Throwing

Throwing mechanics	Needs improvement	Good mechanics
Preparation phase: Stands with the side pointing in the direction of the throw		
Force production phase 1: Reaches backward with the throwing arm and hand; the elbow is at shoulder height or above		
Force production phase 2: Makes a long step forward with the foot opposite of the throwing arm		
Force production phase 3: Turns the lower body toward the target; the upper body lags behind		
Force production phase 4: The shoulders turn toward the target; the upper arm lags behind		
Force production phase 5: The upper arm moves forward; the elbow remains high		
Force production phase 6: The wrist flexes prior to follow-through		
Critical instant: The ball is released at an angle that is appropriate for reaching the target		
Recovery phase: The throwing arm follows through across the body after ball release		

Moving Implements and Objects

Lesson Objectives

After reading this lesson, you should be able to

1. describe several methods (and the related principles) of moving objects with body parts and implements;

2. describe the biomechanics of catching;

3. define aerodynamics and hydrodynamics and explain how each is important to human movement; and

4. describe some factors that help you learn motor skills.

Lesson Vocabulary

complex skill
implement
tracking

What causes an object to move? In many things we do, whether work or play, we use an **implement**—a device or tool that helps us perform a task. For example, we use a rake to clean up leaves in the yard, a shovel to dig holes, and a hammer to pound nails. We also use implements in sport—for example, bats, rackets, clubs, and paddles to hit balls and birdies; oars to propel boats and canoes; sticks to play pool. Of course, we can also use a hand, arm, foot, or leg to kick footballs and soccer balls, throw baseballs and softballs, and strike volleyballs. In all of these examples, we are producing force to move an object.

Skills That Move Objects

Too many skills involve moving objects for us to consider them all here. However, the sections that follow describe some of the more basic skills that use body parts or implements to move objects (for example, throwing, kicking, batting). The descriptions also identify the principles related to performing each skill.

Throwing was easy for me, but I wasn't sure how to help my brother learn to throw. Learning about biomechanics helped me and my brother.

Jorg Dastrup

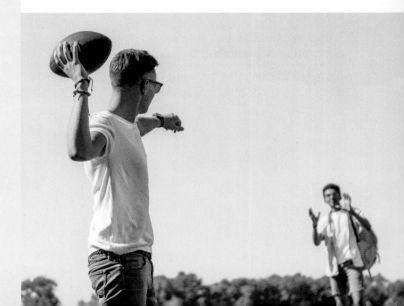

Throwing

The word *throw* means to propel an object through the air using a forward motion of the arm and hand. A throw can be underhand (as in bowling and softball pitching), sidearm (as in some baseball pitches), or overhand (as in most baseball pitches). The focus in throwing is sometimes on accuracy and sometimes on speed or velocity (how hard or fast you throw).

As you know, you move through three stages of learning as you develop a skill such as throwing. In the cognitive stage, you have to think about what you're doing and thus may have to sacrifice speed for accuracy (this is sometimes called the *speed–accuracy trade-off*). As you move through the associative stage, you can move more quickly and still be accurate as you begin to associate your knowledge about throwing with the physical skill itself. In the autonomous stage, you can automatically throw with both speed and accuracy.

Figure 20.7 shows the three stages of an overhand throw: *(a)* force production (levers moved by muscles to produce force in proper sequence), *(b)* ball release (at the critical instant and at the appropriate angle), and *(c)* follow-through (during the recovery phase).

Striking With a Hand or Arm

Striking involves delivering a blow or making contact forcefully. It can be done with a body part, as in using a hand to spike a volleyball or deliver a karate blow, or with an implement, as discussed in a later section. Like throwing, striking can be done at many arm angles, and contact can be made with the hand (open hand, fist, heel of the hand) or the forearms (as in a volleyball dig). Figure 20.8 shows a volleyball serve, which uses a motion very similar to the standard throwing motion. The photos show *(a)* force production (levers moved by muscles to produce force in proper sequence), *(b)* ball strike (at the critical instant and at the appropriate angle), and *(c)* follow-through (during the recovery phase). The strike can be done from a standing jump or a running jump. In this example, the focus is on the mechanics of striking the ball with the arm and hand.

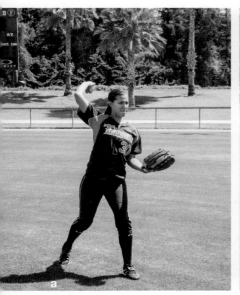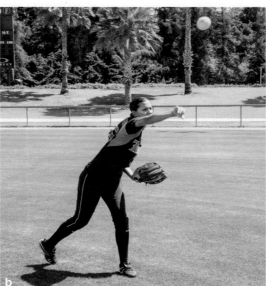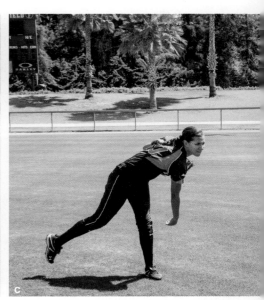

Figure 20.7   Overhand throwing.

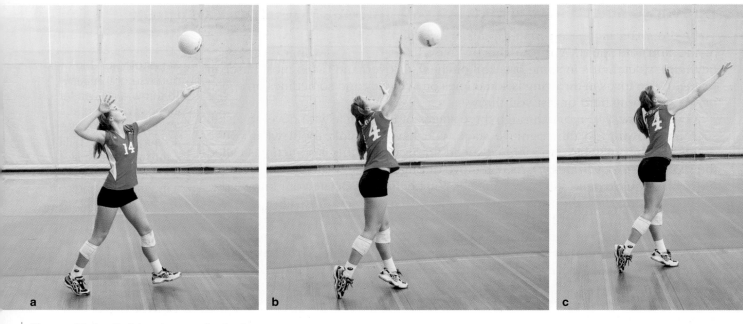

Figure 20.8   Striking for a volleyball serve.

Kicking (Striking With a Foot or Leg)

Kicking, which involves striking with a foot or leg, is used in various sports, including football, soccer, and martial arts. Kicking often involves contact, as when a foot hits the ball in soccer or strikes an object in karate, but some kicks are performed without striking (as in dancing). Kicked objects may be still or moving at the time of contact. Kicking is often preceded by running (as in a football kickoff), and the performer sometimes alternates kicking and running (as in soccer dribbling). Figure 20.9 shows a soccer kick.

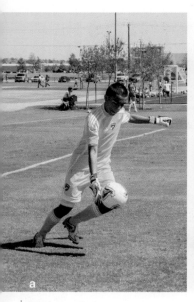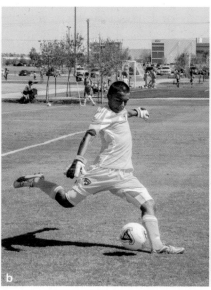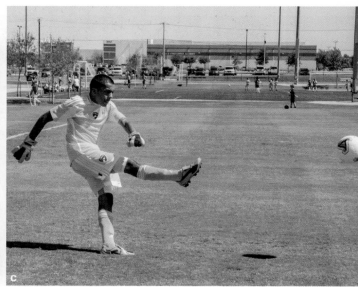

Figure 20.9   Kicking.

Striking With an Implement

As you may recall, an implement is a tool used to accomplish a specific task; examples of sports implements include tennis rackets and baseball bats. Implements are typically used as levers to create a force greater than could be created by the body alone. For example, the most powerful major league pitchers can throw a baseball about 100 miles (160 kilometers) per hour, whereas the most powerful tennis players can serve a ball more than 150 miles (240 kilometers) per hour. Because a tennis racket provides greater leverage (longer lever), it creates greater ball speed.

The process of striking is typically referred to as the *swing*. Some implements are used to strike a moving object, as in tennis, whereas others are used to strike a still object, as in golf. Both kinds of striking are complex skills, but striking a moving object requires the ability to track it—and, in some cases, to toss it so that it can be struck properly, as in a tennis serve. Objects are struck at different angles depending on the sport. For example, a tennis serve goes from high to low, a golf swing from low to high, and a softball swing from front to back.

Catching and Complex Skills

Once an object has been put in motion, it often has to be caught. In many activities you also must perform complex skills that involve using several skills at once. In the paragraphs that follow, catching and complex skills are discussed.

Catching

In sport and other physical activities, *catch* means to grasp and hold onto an object, such as a ball. You can catch with one hand, two hands, or an implement. Catches can be performed either bare-handed or with the assistance of a glove. Sometimes a two-hand catch also requires the use of the arms, such as a football player catching a punt or kickoff. Several kinds of catches are shown in figure 20.10. Some sports require you to use an implement to catch an object; for example, a lacrosse stick is used to catch and throw a ball.

Certain steps are typical regardless of the type of catching. Before you can catch an object, you

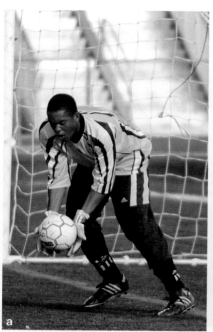
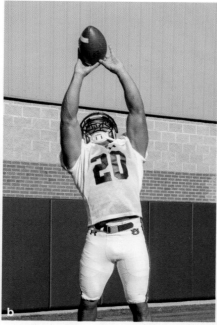
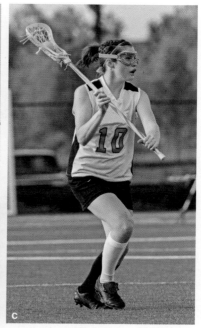

Figure 20.10 Examples of different kinds of catching: *(a)* two hands, below the waist; *(b)* two hands, above the waist; *(c)* with an implement.

TECH TRENDS: **Movement Analysis Apps**

In chapter 13 you learned how coaches and athletes use motion analysis systems to study sport performance and identify areas for improvement. If no software is available, you can use a smartphone to analyze your performance. A softball pitcher, for example, could use the video to study pitching mechanics to see if changes are needed. Similarly, a batter could use video to compare performance when not hitting well to performance when hitting well. Free or low-cost apps are available for use with a smartphone or tablet.

USING TECHNOLOGY

Search the web for sports analysis apps. If possible, download a free app and use a tablet or smartphone to analyze a sport performance. If a download is not possible, read about an app. Prepare a brief report.

must locate it and track it. **Tracking** involves keeping your eye on the object to be caught from the time it is thrown or projected until it gets close enough to catch.

After tracking the ball, you must move your hands, arms, glove, or other catching implement to a location that makes the object easy to receive. The exact positioning of your hands or implement depends on where you will receive the object (see figure 20.11).

In many types of catching, the object is moving very fast. As a result, you should "give" with the blow to absorb the force by allowing the object to continue moving a bit before totally stopping it. For this reason, people who are good at catching are said to have "soft" hands.

Complex Skills

The basic skills described in this chapter, such as walking and running, are the most frequent skills used in sport and physical activity. Many activities, however, require **complex skills**. Some complex skills require the use of several

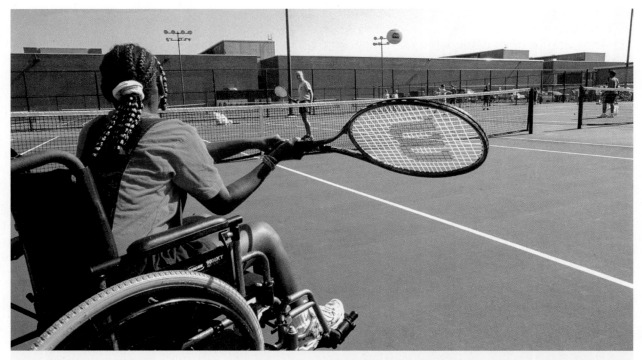

Tennis is an example of a complex skill that requires tracking a ball, moving to it, and striking it.

basic skills in sequence, such as running, catching, and quickly throwing a softball. Dance involves a wide range of intricate sequential steps, including ballet movements, Latin dance moves, and complex hip-hop maneuvers. Other complex skills require the coordination of several different movements—for example, swimming uses virtually all body parts at the same time, and the levers of the upper and lower body must be used in the proper sequence. Even the trunk must move to produce optimal movement through the water.

Aerodynamics and Hydrodynamics

Aerodynamics and hydrodynamics were briefly described in lesson 1. Additional information about both is provided in the sections that follow.

Aerodynamics

Aerodynamics refers to the study of motion in the air. When you use skills at work or play, air can affect your performance. Spin, for example, affects the motion of an object such as a disc in Ultimate. Here are some examples from softball pitching.

- Forward spin (topspin) causes the ball to drop faster than normal.
- Backward spin (backspin) creates lift so that the ball appears to rise (does not drop as fast as normal).
- Sidespin causes the ball to "break" or curve from its normal path.

Spin can also be created by an implement. For example, tennis players swing from low to high to create topspin, which allows them to hit the ball hard and still keep it in bounds because the spin causes the ball to come down faster than normal. As with a pitched softball, sidespin causes a tennis ball to curve. Spin on a football causes it to spiral and stay stable in the air. Spin on a pool or billiard ball causes it to curve or even jump.

Wind can also exaggerate the effect of spin on a ball. For example, if a ball is curving because of spin, the wind may either cause more spin or cause resistance to the curving caused by the spin. In sailing, the wind is essential to the boat's movement, and skilled sailors can use it to move a boat in all directions. Wind can cause resistance in other ways—a headwind, for example, slows a runner.

Moving objects, including your body, can also be affected by humidity, temperature, and altitude. Dry air, for example, provides less resistance than humid air. Very cold air cools an object, which may limit the distance it travels when struck or kicked. The air at high altitude is thinner and therefore provides less resistance than air at lower altitudes.

Hydrodynamics

Hydrodynamics refers to the study of motion in fluid. It's especially important to swimmers, as well as surfers, boaters, kayakers, and rowers. In fact, pushing against the resistance of water is what propels you forward when swimming or using an oar. Water itself moves because of various forces, including

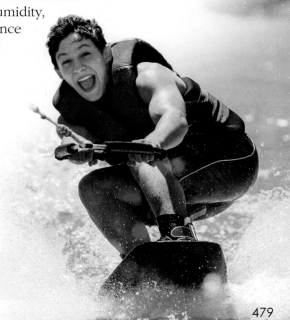

Water resistance affects a variety of water activities.

wind and gravitational pull, which can cause waves. Swimmers' movements also cause the water to move, as does splashing of water against the side of a pool. Waves and other water movements affect performance in these activities.

Motor Learning

Motor learning involves practicing movements in order to improve motor skills. Most movements involved in motor skills are voluntary. When you perform a voluntary movement, such as throwing a ball, your brain signals your nerves, which signal your muscles to contract. The contraction of your muscles then moves your bones (in throwing, the bones or levers of your arm). The movement of the levers provides the force to throw the ball. Some principles of motor learning are described in this section.

There are no shortcuts to success.

*Annika Sorenstam,
Hall of Fame golfer*

Practice

With good practice, you can improve your motor skills. You can get the most out of your practice by getting specific feedback from an instructor or using a video that teaches you about specific mechanics to practice.

Skill Transfer

Once you learn the basics of a motor skill, you can transfer it—that is, use it when learning a similar skill. For example, if you practice to become good at throwing a baseball, it will be easier for you to learn to throw a football and even to strike a volleyball.

Skill Change

If you try to change your technique after learning a skill, it will take some time before you see improvement. For example, if you learn to bowl using a straight ball, then decide to change your delivery to a hook, you may not see immediate improvement. It took a lot of practice for you to learn the first delivery, and it will take time and practice to "forget" it and learn the new one. It's also advisable to avoid making big changes in the way you perform a skill right before you compete or have a test of performance. Allow yourself time to learn the new delivery.

Mental Practice

Mental practice involves rehearsing a skill in your mind without moving the relevant body parts. It is useful for rehearsing the biomechanics of a movement and has been shown to help people learn skills.

LESSON REVIEW

1. What are some methods (and the related principles) of moving objects with body parts and implements?
2. What are the steps for properly catching a ball?
3. How are aerodynamics and hydrodynamics important to human movement?
4. What are some of the factors that help you learn motor skills?

TAKING CHARGE: **Positive Self-Talk**

Alexis liked to play golf. She thought about trying out for the school team, but she wasn't sure that she was good enough. When she played with her family, she did well, but when she played with people she didn't know, she didn't do as well. Sometimes she talked to herself while playing, saying things like, "Why did you do that, dummy?" or "Oh, no—I'm starting to play badly again." Sometimes she even talked to herself out loud, saying things like, "I got a 7 on that hole? Now I don't even have a chance for a good score!"

After one particular round in which she didn't play as well as she would have liked, Alexis asked her mother,

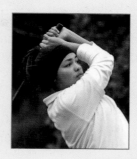

"Why do things always go wrong when I play with people I don't know?" Her mother said that she had read a book by a sport psychologist who recommended avoiding negative self-talk (saying negative things to yourself, which affects your self-confidence and leads to poor play). The key is to replace the negative self-talk with positive self-talk. As Alexis' mom said, "If you expect bad things to

happen, they probably will. Next time you play, try to cut the negative talk and focus on positives. If you have a bad hole, say to yourself, 'It's just one hole—I'm going to do better on the next one.'"

FOR DISCUSSION

What are some examples of negative self-talk common in sport and other activities? What are some examples of positive self-talk that can be used to replace negative self-talk? What other suggestions do you have for Alexis and other people who use negative self-talk? Consider the guidelines in the following Self-Management feature as you answer these discussion questions.

SELF-MANAGEMENT: **Skills for Positive Self-Talk**

Some people are optimists who believe good things are going to happen, and others are pessimists who think bad things are sure to come. Experts in exercise and sport psychology have found that with practice, you can develop "learned optimism." Specifically, you can replace negative thoughts and self-talk with positive thoughts and self-talk. Follow these guidelines to use positivity to improve your performance.

- *Learn the ABCs (adversity, beliefs, consequences).* Learn to recognize when you're facing adversity, which can lead to negative thoughts and negative self-talk. Learn to recognize negative beliefs—if you believe that you're going to do poorly when you face adversity, you probably will. Finally, learn to recognize your feelings about the consequences of adversity. A pessimist might say, "If I do poorly on

one hole in golf, I have no chance to get a reasonable score." Learning to be more realistic about consequences can help you become more optimistic.

- *Accept adversity as a challenge rather than a sure cause of failure.* Adversity causes negative self-talk only if you let it.

- *Alter your beliefs about adversity.* If you accept adversity as a challenge, you can tell yourself to avoid negative thoughts and replace them with positive ones. Experts suggest that replacing negative comments (such as "That was a dumb decision!") with positive ones (such as "I know I can do it!") leads to better performance. So when you're faced with adversity, respond with positive self-talk. Tell yourself, "I believe I can do this!"

>continued

>continued

- *Don't overdramatize the consequences of adversity.* Ask yourself if your view of the potential consequences of a bad performance is pessimistic. If so, replace it with a more realistic or even positive view.

- *Put the past behind you.* Failing at a task or doing less well than you'd like doesn't necessarily mean you'll fail next time. You can't change the past—only the future. Worrying about the past leads to negative thoughts when you play again. Playing badly creates adversity, but positive thinking and positive self-talk can turn the last bad performance into the next good one.

- *Practice creating a cycle of positivity.* A pessimist thinks negatively when faced with adversity. Negative beliefs lead to poor performance, which contributes to more negative thoughts, thus creating a negative cycle. Work instead to create a cycle of positivity. Every time you face adversity, remember the ABCs and practice them. Recognize adversity when it arises and establish positive beliefs ("I know I can do this"). This can lead to positive consequences (improved performance).

- *Be realistic.* You've learned that being realistic is important to setting effective goals. Setting unrealistically high goals can lead to feelings of failure even when you're doing quite well. Remember that practice is necessary for success.

ACADEMIC CONNECTION: Multiple Meanings

Meeting standards for English language arts requires an understanding of the multiple meanings of words. For example, the word *force* has many meanings, including military force (troops and ships), violent force (a physical attack), and mechanical force (energy exerted). In this chapter, *force* refers to energy exerted by the muscles to cause tension or to cause the body or an object to move. Force can also be used to stop a body or object from moving (resistance force). The following fitness-related definition is included in the glossary.

force—Energy exerted by the muscles to cause movement or resist movement.

STUDENT ACTIVITY

Identify other words used in this book that have multiple meanings. An example is the word *power*, which refers to a part of health-related fitness (strength × speed) in this book. But *power* can also refer to possession of influence or control (political power) or a source of energy (electric or solar power). You may want to use the glossary to assist you.

Taking Action: **Applying Principles**

In this chapter, you've learned about several biomechanical principles that are important for performing motor skills in a variety of work and play situations. **Take action** by trying several different skills and describing the principles that apply to the performance of each one.

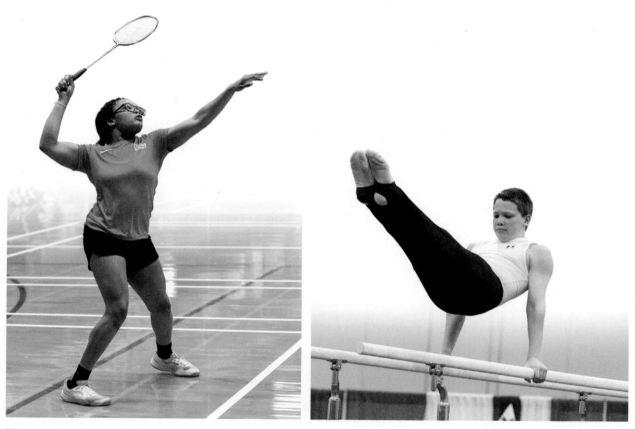

Take action by applying biomechanical principles as you perform different skills.

CHAPTER REVIEW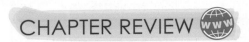

Reviewing Concepts and Vocabulary

Answer items 1 through 5 by correctly completing each sentence with a word or phrase.

1. A _____ refers to a way of standing.

2. Moving your body from place to place is called _____.

3. _____ is the study of motion in fluids.

4. Delivering a blow or making contact forcefully is called _____.

5. When you perform the skill of _____, you must track the object before receiving it.

For items 6 through 10, match each term in column 1 with the appropriate phrase in column 2.

6. transfer   a. study of motion in the air

7. mental practice   b. using one skill to perform another

8. motor learning   c. practicing to improve a skill

9. aerodynamics   d. rehearsing a skill in your mind

10. kicking   e. striking with the foot

For items 11 through 15, respond to each statement or question.

11. Describe three different principles of biomechanics.

12. Describe biomechanical analysis and how it uses technology.

13. Give examples of striking a ball with an implement.

14. What are some aerodynamic factors that influence the flight of a ball?

15. What are some guidelines for eliminating negative self-talk?

Thinking Critically

Write a paragraph to answer the following question.

A friend has been selected to kick a 15-yard field goal at your school's next home football game. If she succeeds, she wins a prize. When she was younger she played soccer, but she has not played in a while. Now she would like your help to improve her kicking. How would you help her win the prize?

Project

To improve academic performance, many schools perform three- to five-minute exercise breaks in the classroom. The breaks include exercises that can be performed in a small space next to desks and often include dance steps. Plan an exercise break for one of your classes. You can use video or music or just lead the group in an exercise. Show it to one of your teachers and ask to present it to the class or have your family members perform it at home.

21

Taking Advantage of Opportunities

In This Chapter

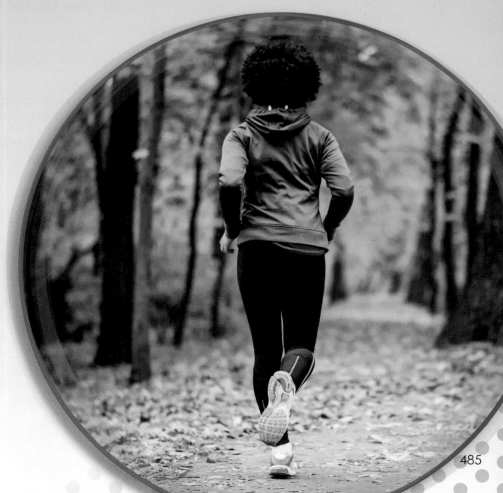

Active Living Opportunities

Lesson Objectives

After reading this lesson, you should be able to

1. define *autonomy* and explain how it relates to decision making about lifelong physical activity participation;

2. describe several sources of information about opportunities for physical activity;

3. explain guidelines for organizing for participation in physical activity and define *extrinsic motivation* and *intrinsic motivation*; and

4. describe some opportunities for helping others be physically active.

Lesson Vocabulary

extrinsic motivation
intrinsic motivation
optimal challenge
self-reward system

In this book you have learned about the health benefits of physical activity and how to plan your own personal physical activity program. If you are to successfully stay active throughout life, you will need to make a commitment to take time to be active. You will also need to take advantage of opportunities available in your community. Some of these opportunities are described in this lesson.

Staying Active After High School

Two years after graduating from high school, a group of friends gathered at Hal's house. He was now married and worked full-time. He'd gained a few pounds since high school and wasn't as active as he had been when he played football. His wife, Fatima, had been a cheerleader but was also less active now that she worked full-time. Hal and Fatima stayed in touch with their friends, but some were off at college, and others were busy working.

> I enjoyed sports in high school but now I realize that I have to make my own opportunities to participate now that I am nearing the end of high school.
>
> *Kelvin O'Neil*

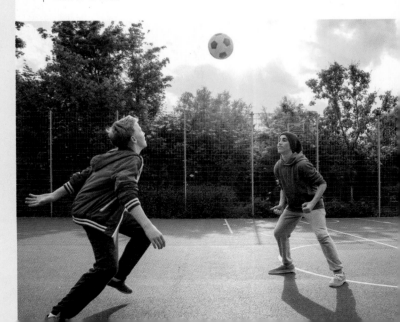

Other people attending the party included Kris, who had also played on the football team. He was now attending a local community college and working part-time. Like Hal, he knew he was less active than he should be. Malia was attending the local university, where she played on the soccer team. She was very active but missed interacting with her friends. Will was also attending the university, where he played some intramurals and worked out at the campus recreation center. Coretta and Jamal had not gone to school with the others but were now neighbors of Hal and Fatima. Jamal played slowpitch softball, and Coretta used some home exercise videos.

The friends decided that it would be good if they could all be more active and spend more time together socially. They decided to do some type of physical activity together to help them be more active and have fun at the same time. The rest of this lesson describes some of the steps that the friends used to investigate opportunities.

Self-determination theory is one theory of human motivation that is often applied to sports and physical activity. The theory places high importance on autonomy—self-direction, or the ability to make decisions for yourself. One goal of this book is to help teens move from having others make decisions for them (dependence) to making decision for themselves (independence). In elementary and middle school, many decisions had been made for Hal, Fatima, and their friends. Even in high school, they were somewhat dependent on parents, teachers, and coaches for many things. Now, however, they have the autonomy to make their own decisions.

The friends used some self-management skills they had learned in high school to search for active opportunities in their community. For example, they had learned how to find social support from friends, but they did have some barriers to overcome. To be active together, they would have to find activities that they were all interested in, times when they would all be available, and locations convenient for everyone. To address these issues, they used critical thinking skills and elements of the scientific method. Like Hal, Fatima, and their friends, you can use the skills you've learned to become more autonomous in making decisions about healthy lifestyles.

Finding Opportunities to Participate

One of the first steps in finding ways to be active is to find out what's available. Options include government agencies, community organizations, worksite programs, commercial options, and places of worship.

Taking Advantage of Opportunities

Once you are aware of opportunities, you'll need to organize and plan to take advantage of them. Some ideas for taking advantage of physical activity opportunities are described in the paragraphs that follow.

Organizing for Participation

After investigating opportunities, Hal and his friends decided to join a co-rec volleyball league sponsored by their community's parks and recreation department. They needed at least 10 people because a team requires 6 participants and they knew that not everyone would be able to make every game due to their busy schedules. They also needed their group to be evenly split between men and women because three of each had to be on the court during every game. The group elected Hal as captain and coach and recruited another couple (Nancy and Cole) who lived nearby. Jennifer also asked her friend Jasmine to join, which brought their total to 10—5 women and 5 men.

Not all people have such a ready-made social group. Here are some good guidelines for finding or forming a group for physical activity participation.

- *Consider nonleague participation as a start.* Joining a club or league can be quite intimidating for some people. If you're just learning an activity, you may first want to join in recreational sessions or take a class at a local club. For example, Coretta had not played much volleyball, so she joined with others in the group to practice at the park before the league started. Will went to the rec center at his university and played in some pickup volleyball games to get some practice.

- *Check with friends at school or work.* Start with a few people, then each can recruit others with similar interests to participate. You might want to start with noncompetitive games before moving on to league play.
- *Check out your work wellness program or school recreation center.* See if there are people interested in the same activity that you can recruit to join you. There might even be an existing club or exercise group that you can join. Club members often get to know each other and then form teams for leagues after starting with recreational play.
- *Check with the organizations listed in table 21.1.* See if they have opportunities for individuals or small groups to join larger teams.

Daring to Try

Sometimes one of the hardest things to do is simply dare to try, especially when you're starting something new and don't have others to do it with. Coretta had friends to support her, so joining them on a volleyball team was not as threatening as it might have been. Still, she lacked confidence, so before the volleyball league began she joined with others to practice. She was initially motivated by her desire to please her friends in the group—she didn't want to let them down.

Coretta's initial motivation for playing is called **extrinsic motivation**, or motivation that comes from outside the individual (for example, pressure from others, external rewards). In this case, Coretta wanted to be on the team not because she particularly enjoyed volleyball but because the team needed another player. Even after trying recreational volleyball, she felt very nervous when she first played on the competitive team. As she got better, however, she started to look forward to the

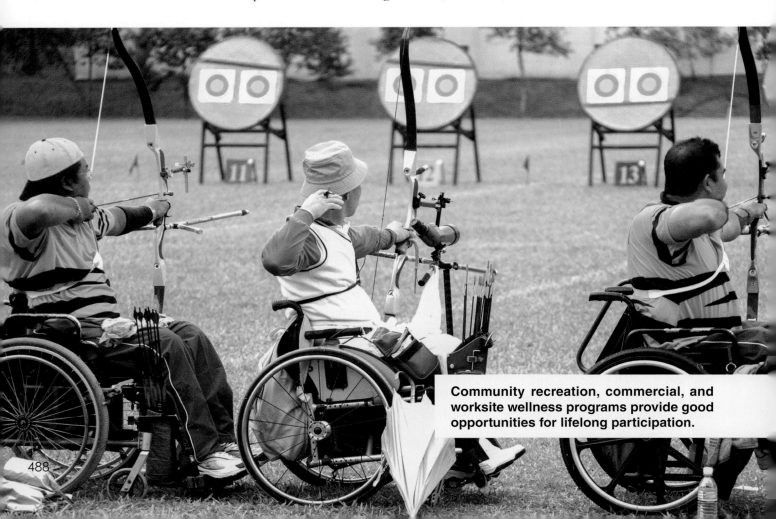

Community recreation, commercial, and worksite wellness programs provide good opportunities for lifelong participation.

TABLE 21.1 **Finding Opportunities for Physical Activity in the Community**

Type	Examples	How to contact
• Government agencies • Youth programs • Sport leagues • Facilities (tennis courts, bike trails, golf courses, hiking trails, parks) • Community centers • Zoos and cultural centers • Museums	• Local parks and recreation department • State parks and recreation department • Local public school programs	Do a web search to locate the agency. Search for a specific department or facility.
National sport organizations	• U.S. Olympic Committee (Team USA) • United States Tennis Association • Amateur Softball Association of America • National Senior Games Association • Special Olympics • U.S. Paralympics	Do a web search to locate the organization. For sites such as TeamUSA.org, use the pull-down menu to find specific sport pages.
Community organizations	• YMCA and YWCA • Boys & Girls Clubs of America • Activity-specific clubs (for example, walking, jogging, and tennis clubs) • Sport organizations (e.g., Little League baseball)	Do a web search for the organization name and your town or city name (for example, "YMCA Los Angeles"). Contact the organization by phone or in person.
Worksite programs	• Company wellness programs • Company fitness centers • Company sport leagues and teams	Check with your human resources office to see what's available.
Commercial options	• Health and fitness clubs and spas • Private sport facilities (sport fields, ice rinks, skating rinks or parks, golf courses, leagues) • Dance and yoga studios • Martial arts studios • Youth activity centers • Physical therapy centers	Do a web search for the activity and your town or city name (for example, "yoga studios Detroit"). Contact the facility by phone or in person.
Places of worship (for example, church, synagogue, mosque)	• Sport leagues • Exercise groups • Social groups	Check with your religious organization's office or look for listings in the bulletin or newsletter.

> You can motivate by fear, and you can motivate by reward. But both those methods are only temporary. The only lasting thing is self-motivation.
>
> *Homer Rice, football coach*

games. She was no longer playing to please someone else (extrinsic motivation); she was now playing because she enjoyed it (**intrinsic motivation**). Intrinsic motivation is personal and comes from within the individual (for example, fun, joy of participation).

In school, Coretta had learned about **optimal challenge** (see figure 21.1). In her practice group, she tried to do things that were neither too easy nor too hard. Because the challenge was reasonable, she found success rather than failure. In turn, this success encouraged her to keep trying. Gradually, she started to enjoy herself, and that made her want to keep participating.

Coretta also learned to reward herself for her performance rather than rely on praise from others. If she had gone right into the volleyball league without practicing first, she might have become frustrated and quit trying.

Kris had a very different experience. He became bored with the volleyball team. Although he liked being with his friends, his volleyball skills were better than his friends' skills, and he lost interest in the games. It took encouragement and even pleading from his friends (extrinsic motivation) to keep him coming. Ultimately, he dropped out of the league, and the team finished with nine players.

Sometimes you need a little external motivation to get you going. But researchers have shown that people who have intrinsic motivation (such as Coretta) are more likely to stick with participation long-term than people who are extrinsically motivated (such as Kris). One way to come up with your own intrinsic motivation is having a **self-reward system**, or finding ways to reward yourself for your efforts rather than expecting others to reward you.

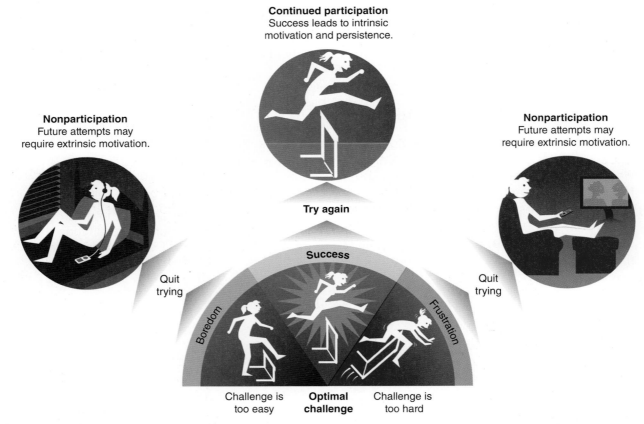

Continued participation
Success leads to intrinsic motivation and persistence.

Nonparticipation
Future attempts may require extrinsic motivation.

Nonparticipation
Future attempts may require extrinsic motivation.

Try again

Success

Quit trying

Quit trying

Boredom

Frustration

Challenge is too easy

Optimal challenge

Challenge is too hard

| **Figure 21.1**   Finding an optimal challenge helps you achieve success and intrinsic motivation.

Helping Others in Physical Activity

In the years ahead, you'll find that having active people around you helps you be more active. You'll also have the opportunity to help others be physically active. A few of these opportunities are described in the following list.

• *Family activities.* As the saying goes, "families that play together stay together." You can use the skills you've learned in this class to help family members be active. Examples include family outings (such as camping, fishing, and biking trips), family exercise sessions (such as walks and hikes), and family activity nights (such as bowling or skating night). Although not all family members will always like the same activities, you can also support each other's activities—for example, watching a family member's team play or praising the jogger in the family for sticking with it over time.

• *Coaching.* When you were younger, you may have played a sport such as soccer or tee ball. If so, someone coached your team. You can give back by volunteering to coach children in your neighborhood or your own children. Training for volunteer coaches is provided by many organizations.

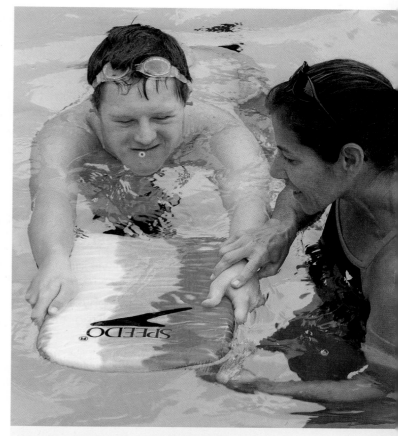

Helping others learn skills can be very rewarding.

TECH TRENDS: Finding Support for Active Living

Social support is important in helping people adopt and stick with healthy lifestyle changes. Research indicates that people who have friends who are active are more likely to be active themselves. Modern technology makes it easier than ever for friends to support each other in activity through the web and social media. For example, Hal and his friends could use e-mails, text messages, phone calls, or tweets to encourage each other to come to practice and games.

However, messages from others can also be harmful if not done properly. Autonomy is important—we all want to make decisions for ourselves. Messages that encourage a person to stick with their plan encourage autonomy. On the other hand, messages or comments that treat a person as if you're trying to control their behavior do not. For example, if a person misses a practice, a good message of support might be, "Missed you at practice—hope to see you next time." A not-so-good message might be, "If you keep missing, you will never get better." This message suggests that the person should attend to please someone else.

Appropriately supportive personal messages have been shown to help people who are trying to stop smoking, maintain a healthy weight, or be active for health and fitness.

USING TECHNOLOGY

Work with a group of friends to form a support network. Outline ways in which the group will use technology to support each other in meeting their goals.

LESSON REVIEW

1. How does autonomy relate to decision making about lifelong participation in physical activity?
2. What are some sources of information about opportunities for physical activity?
3. What are some guidelines for organizing participation in physical activity, and how do you define *extrinsic motivation* and *intrinsic motivation*?
4. How can you help others to be physically active?

SELF-ASSESSMENT: Opportunities for Physical Activity Participation Questionnaire

In this self-assessment you will identify opportunities for physical activity available to you in your school and community. Use the portfolio sheet provided to record your results.

1. In table 21.2, list the five physical activities that you are most likely to perform that require a facility or other specialized area outside the home.

TABLE 21.2   Preferred Activities Requiring a Special Facility

	Name of Activity
1.	
2.	
3.	
4.	
5.	

2. In table 21.3, place a checkmark by five different facilities that could be used to perform the activities listed in table 21.2. For these five facilities, record a number from 1 to 5 to indicate how important it would be to have the facility or activity area near where you live (1 = least important and 5 = most important). For those activities that you rate as 3 or higher, list the name of the nearest facility where you can do the activity.

TABLE 21.3   Facility Location Importance

Type of facility	✓	1	2	3	4	5	Facility or activity area
Biking trails							
Boating area							
Climbing area or facility							
Dance studio							
Golf course							
Gym							
Hiking trail							
Ice skating rink							
Indoor sports courts							
Martial arts school							
Open play area (park)							
Outdoor sport courts							
Running track							
Skate park							
Ski slope							
Sports field							
Swimming pool							
Trail (hiking)							
Other							

3. Choose one facility from the list in table 21.3. In table 21.4, record the name of the facility and check the reasons why you will use it.

TABLE 21.4   Reasons for Choosing Facility

Facility name:							
Low cost	Convenient location	Fun activity	Easy to use	Equipment or space available	Safety	No membership required	Other

Physical Education and Career Opportunities

Lesson Objectives

After reading this lesson, you should be able to

1. name and describe the seven characteristics of physical literacy and the five characteristics of health literacy;

2. describe the benefits of high-quality physical education;

3. describe several options for elective physical education; and

4. describe some career opportunities in fitness, health, and wellness.

Lesson Vocabulary

adventure education
cooperative game
dance education
fitness education
outdoor education
professionals
sport education

You are now reading the last lesson in this book. This means that you are about to complete this physical education class. A major goal of this book, as well as the class you are taking, is to help you to be active and adopt other healthy lifestyles throughout life. In this lesson you will learn about physical literacy, the benefits of participating in a high-quality physical education program, physical education elective opportunities, and career opportunities in fitness, health, and wellness.

Physical and Health Literacy

In the first chapter of this book you learned about definitions of literacy, including physical literacy and health literacy. The characteristics of physical literacy described in chapter 1 are shown again in figure 21.2.

> I never played on a sports team in high school, but I have found activities that I enjoy such as yoga and rock climbing. I do them because I like them, not to compete with others.
>
> *Astrid Borgen*

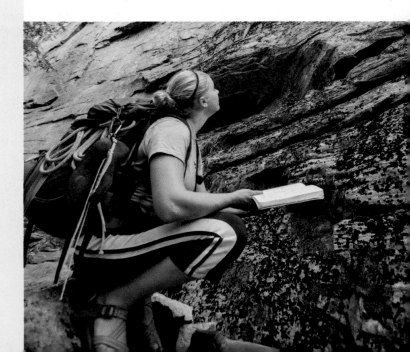

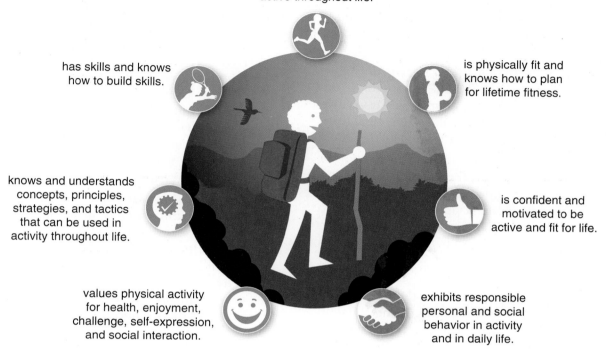

A physically literate person...

is physically active and knows how to stay active throughout life.

has skills and knows how to build skills.

is physically fit and knows how to plan for lifetime fitness.

knows and understands concepts, principles, strategies, and tactics that can be used in activity throughout life.

is confident and motivated to be active and fit for life.

values physical activity for health, enjoyment, challenge, self-expression, and social interaction.

exhibits responsible personal and social behavior in activity and in daily life.

Figure 21.2   The characteristics of physical literacy.

The overarching goal of physical literacy is to help you to be active and fit throughout life. Using the information and self-management skills that you have learned in this book can help you build physical literacy and meet the goal of lifelong active living.

Just as physical literacy is important to lifelong health and wellness, so is health literacy—the capacity to make sound health decisions that lead to adopting healthy lifestyles now and later in life. Knowing how to obtain good health information, how to process it, how to understand it, and how to use it to identify and choose health services prepares you to make appropriate health decisions throughout life. The characteristics of health literacy illustrated in chapter 1 are shown again in figure 21.3.

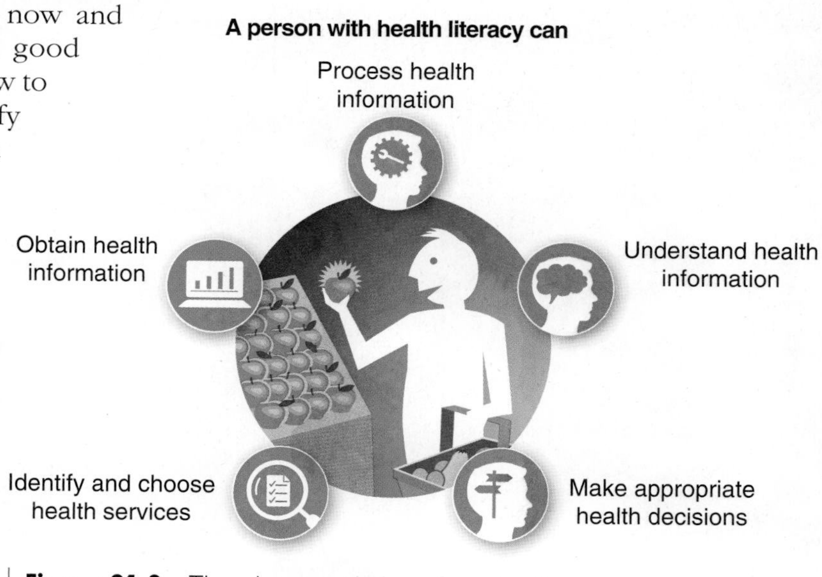

Benefits of High-Quality Physical Education

Kinesiology experts have identified 10 research-based benefits of high-quality physical education (HQPE). In addition

A person with health literacy can

Process health information

Obtain health information

Understand health information

Identify and choose health services

Make appropriate health decisions

Figure 21.3   The characteristics of health literacy.

to helping students to become physically literate, the following are important benefits of HQPE.

1. *Regular physical activity helps prevent disease.* Regular physical activity reduces the risk of hypokinetic diseases, including heart disease, cancer, diabetes, and osteoporosis.

2. *Regular physical activity promotes lifelong wellness.* Health involves more than freedom from disease. Being regularly active improves wellness, including quality of life and sense of well-being.

3. *HQPE provides unique opportunities for activity.* Physical education, including dance education, is the primary subject that provides an opportunity to be active during school hours. Teens who do physical education meet national activity goals more often than those who do not.

4. *HQPE helps fight obesity.* About one-third of youth and two-thirds of adults are overweight or obese. Being active in physical education classes and at other times during the school day helps expend calories to reduce the risk of overweight and obesity.

5. *HQPE helps promote lifelong physical fitness.* Regular physical activity using the FIT formula for each type of physical activity helps build all parts of health-related physical fitness. This enhances health and increases your ability to function effectively in work and play.

6. *HQPE teaches self-management and motor skills.* Teens who have learned self-management skills are more likely to be active after they graduate from school. They know how to plan personal activity programs and avoid quackery. Students who learn a variety of motor skills are more active later in life.

7. *HQPE and regular physical activity promote learning in other academic areas.* Teens who are active and fit score better on academic tests than those who are inactive. Evidence shows that physical activity is necessary for the brain to function optimally. Active students are less likely to miss school or have discipline problems.

8. *HQPE and regular physical activity make good economic sense.* The annual cost of inactive living in the United States is

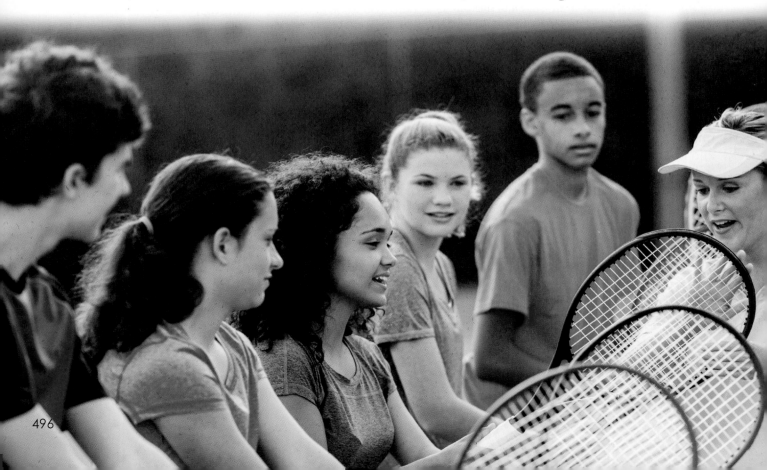

almost $28 billion. A study in the *Journal of the American Heart Association* indicates that the average cost per person is $2,500 a year. Worksite wellness programs enable many companies to save money, reduce absenteeism, and increase job satisfaction. High-quality physical education promotes the same benefits.

9. *HQPE is widely endorsed.* More than 50 organizations in the United States support the value of HQPE in schools, including the American Academy of Pediatrics (AAP), the American College of Sports Medicine (ACSM), the American Heart Association (AHA), the U.S. Centers for Disease Control and Prevention (CDC), and the President's Council on Fitness, Sports, and Nutrition.

10. *HQPE helps educate the total person.* As President John F. Kennedy said, "physical fitness is the basis of all the activities in our society. And if our bodies grow soft and inactive, if we fail to encourage physical development and prowess, we will undermine our capacity for thought, for work, and for the use of those skills vital to an expanding and complex America."

Adapted from G. Le Masurier and C.B. Corbin, "Top 10 Reasons for Quality Physical Education," *Journal of Physical Education, Recreation & Dance*, 77, no. 6 (2006): 44-53.

> **FIT FACT**
> A survey from the Harvard School of Public Health found that more than 90 percent of parents believe schools should provide physical education, particularly for fighting obesity.

Physical Education Elective Opportunities

There are a variety of types of quality physical education programs that can help you become physically literate. Some may be elective classes. You can also use what you have learned in this class to help you choose an elective class in physical education. Some of these are listed in the section that follows.

Conceptual Physical Education

Conceptual physical education refers to physical education classes or units that focus on learning concepts and principles of physical activity and other healthy behaviors. Conceptual physical education also emphasizes self-management skills. The class that you are finishing is an example of a conceptual physical education class. A goal of conceptual physical education is to promote all aspects of physical and health literacy.

Fitness Education

Fitness education refers to physical education classes or units that focus on learning fitness, physical activity, and related health and wellness concepts and principles. The class that you are finishing can be considered to be both a conceptual physical education and a fitness education class.

Advanced Conceptual Physical Education and Fitness Education Classes

Some schools offer advanced conceptual physical education and fitness education classes. You may want to consider one of these classes, if available.

Advanced Skills and Activity Classes

Choosing an elective class in physical education can help you further develop your skills and abilities to stay active after the school years. One option is an advanced skills or advanced activity class. Classes may include all types of activities from the Physical Activity Pyramid. Check to see what classes are offered at your school and which ones have special interest to you. The guidelines in the Self-Management feature at the end of this lesson can also help you make an activity choice.

Sport Education

Sport education is an approach to teaching physical education that is designed to make playing sports fun, interesting, and authentic. In sport education, as in the sporting world itself, the year is divided into several "seasons" (for example, baseball season or soccer season). Early in each season, the class is split into three to five teams, and members remain with the same team throughout the season. Teams practice together to learn skills and compete against other teams in various sport, recreational, and fitness activities. Games are modified to accommodate team size, equipment, and rules, and teams are balanced to make competition fair.

In sport education, team members develop a sense of belonging or team affiliation. Over the course of a season, members play different roles such as coach, fitness trainer, statistician, publicist, equipment manager, scout, scorekeeper, or referee. Game results are posted and standings are updated regularly. Each season concludes with postseason playoffs and an award ceremony. A key aspect of sport education is that team members provide leadership and assume responsibility for activities conducted during each season.

Some schools use the sport education approach when teaching advanced skills and activity classes and some may have specially designed sport education classes.

Adventure Education

Adventure education typically focuses on challenging recreational activities such as rock climbing, orienteering, boating, rafting, and ropes courses. Adventure education units are sometimes taught as part of physical education and sometimes used in camp settings, recreational programs, and even programs designed to train business executives. Among the principal goals of adventure education are trust building, problem solving, and enhancement of self-confidence. This approach often emphasizes placing trust in team members and working together to overcome risks. Although adventure education is often conducted in outdoor and wilderness settings, it can also be conducted indoors using trust-building activities and cooperative games.

Outdoor Education

Like adventure education, **outdoor education** uses activities such as camping, fishing, and hiking to develop physical literacy. Some schools conduct camps where students participate for several days and learn in outdoor settings.

Cooperative Games

Like sport education, **cooperative games** use teams to help students learn teamwork, have fun, and overcome challenges; however, the focus is on working together rather than competing or winning. Some physical education programs include units focused on cooperative games; as previously mentioned, cooperative games are also sometimes part of adventure education. Cooperative games are sometimes used to help people get to know each other (through "icebreakers") as well as build trust.

Trust-building activities can be part of the adventure education curriculum.

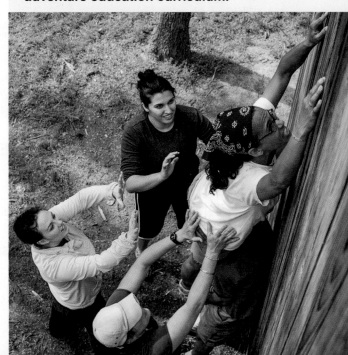

Dance Education

Dance education can be part of a physical education program or a separate program that includes classes or units focused on various forms of dance, including ballet, contemporary, ballroom dance (waltz, foxtrot, and quickstep), Latin (samba, cha-cha, and rumba), hip-hop, jazz, line dance, and swing. Dance education often includes cultural dances as well, such as square dance, Irish dance, and African dance. Aerobic dance and other types of fitness dance such as Zumba may be included as part of dance education or a fitness education unit.

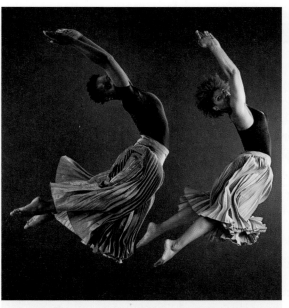

Dance can be part of physical education units or separate dance education classes.

I do not try to dance better than anyone else. I only try to dance better than myself.

Mikhail Baryshnikov, professional dancer

Careers in Fitness, Health, and Wellness

In this book, you've learned about scientists who do research related to fitness, health, and wellness. Scientists typically are experts in one area of science and often have specialties within their area. In many ways, what scientists do is like finding pieces of a puzzle. But new research is not of much value unless it is made available to the general public. This is where professionals come in. **Professionals** are experts in their field who deliver and apply the research developed by scientists. They make sense of the pieces of the puzzle and help people use scientific information to learn and improve themselves. Professionals go through an extended education, typically a bachelor's degree or higher, and often they must also be certified by a professional organization or governmental agency.

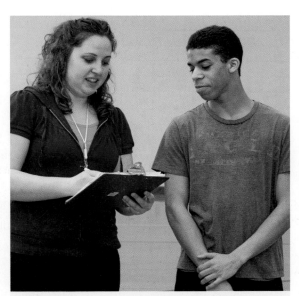

Qualified professionals are a good source of fitness, health, and wellness information.

Now that you're nearing completion of this course, you may want to consider a career in fitness, health, and wellness. Table 21.5 lists some of these possible careers and their descriptions.

TABLE 21.5   **Selected Careers in Fitness, Health, and Wellness**

Specialty	Professional career	Description
Kinesiology		
Biomechanics	Physical education teacher	Teaches physical education
Exercise anatomy	Coach	Coaches sport teams
Exercise physiology	Fitness management	Manages corporate and commercial fitness
Exercise sociology	Fitness leader	Leads exercises at clubs and worksites
Motor learning/control	Personal trainer	Teaches exercise in one-on-one settings
Sport/exercise psychology	Sport management	Applies business principles in sport settings
Sport pedagogy	Sport psychologist	Helps athletes achieve optimal performance
	Athletic trainer	Provides health care for athletes
	Physical therapist	Provides preventive and rehabilitative health care related to musculoskeletal problems
	Occupational therapist	Provides rehabilitative health care related to musculoskeletal problems; helps people with tasks of daily life
	Strength coach	Helps athletes and exercisers build muscle fitness
	Dance teacher	Teaches dance in schools, studios, and other settings
	Recreation leader/therapist	Organizes programs and treats problems through recreation
Nutrition science		
Food science	Clinical dietitian	Works in hospitals and nursing facilities
Food services	Community dietitian	Works with organizations
Food technology	Management dietitian	Works in schools, health care facilities, and institutions such as prisons
Sport nutrition		
Health science		
Environmental health	Health educator	Teaches health concepts in schools
Epidemiology	School health	Provides health care to students
Health statistics	Public health	Works in public health agency
Public health	Worksite wellness	Conducts wellness programs in businesses
Medical and life sciences		
Genetics	Medical doctor	Provides health care (diagnoses and treats)
Immunology	Nurse	Provides health care as part of health care team
Medical technology	Dentist	Provides dental health care
Microbiology	Veterinarian	Provides animal health care
Pathology	Medical technician	Performs laboratory analysis
Virology	Physician's assistant	Helps physicians provide health care
	Chiropractor	Provides health care focused on musculoskeletal system

LESSON REVIEW

1. What are the five characteristics of a physically educated person?
2. What are some of the benefits of high-quality physical education?
3. What are several options for elective physical education?
4. What are some career opportunities in fitness, health, and wellness?

TAKING CHARGE: **Choosing Good Activities**

You can help yourself be active by choosing activities you're likely to do both now and throughout your life. One way to evaluate an activity is to find out the number of people who participate and how long they tend to stay involved. Here's an example.

At a recent high school reunion, the alumni enjoyed seeing their former classmates again. Everyone remembered Norma as an athlete. She had played soccer, basketball, and softball. What a surprise when her classmates discovered that 10 years later Norma was doing very little physical activity! The closest she got to participating in any sport was to watch her son's tee ball games. According to Norma, "It was just too hard

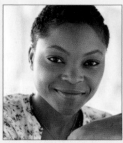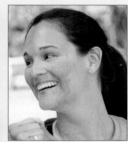

to find people who wanted to play the team sports I used to enjoy."

Kim Lea was just the opposite. In high school, she had always gone to the games to cheer for the team, but she had never dreamed of taking part in a sport. In fact, she would have been the first to admit that she was sedentary. Now, Kim Lea was biking with her two children and organizing her neighborhood aerobics class. She described it this way: "Every Tuesday and Thursday morning, we all get

together and talk while we work out. No one cares how we dress or how good we are. We all just seem to be energized as we go on to our next activities."

FOR DISCUSSION

Why did Norma feel that it was no longer feasible to continue participating in the sports she played in high school? What might help her get involved in physical activity again? Why do you think Kim Lea started to participate in activities? What advice would you have for other people who want to get active later in life? Consider the guidelines in the Self-Management feature that follows as you answer these discussion questions.

SELF-MANAGEMENT: **Skills for Choosing Good Activities**

Research shows that the most active people in society are those who have identified specific activities that they enjoy. For example, many people love tennis, golf, or running and participate in these activities on a regular basis. These people might not have become so active if they were not doing activities that they

especially enjoy. Use the following guidelines to help you find a physical activity (or activities) especially good for you.

- *Consider your physical fitness.* How well you do in an activity depends on your fitness. Choose activities that match your

>continued

>*continued*

abilities in both health- and skill-related fitness, and consider activities that help you build health-related fitness.

- *Consider your interests.* Finding an activity that is fun is very important. Don't be afraid to try an activity that you really enjoy or have always wanted to do just because it doesn't match your fitness profile. The fun new activity might take a while to learn, but it will be worth the time and effort.

- *Consider an activity that you can do with others.* Try to find others of your own ability so that they can support you if you don't learn the activity as quickly as you'd like.

- *Consider the activity's benefits.* If you want to get optimal fitness, health, and wellness benefits, select activities from each area of the Physical Activity Pyramid.

- *Practice, practice, practice.* Becoming skilled in a sport or activity increases your enjoyment. If you choose an activity that is new to you, there is no substitute for practice. To make your practice more productive, consider taking lessons.

- *Consider activities that do not require high levels of skill.* Compared to other activities in the Physical Activity Pyramid, sports require a relatively high level of both sport skill and skill-related fitness in order to play. They also require a lot of practice in order to perform them well. With some exceptions, moderate activities, vigorous aerobic activities, and recreational activities do not require a high level. You might want to consider one of these activities if you're not willing to put in the necessary time to learn a more complicated one.

Taking Action: **Taking Advantage of Opportunities**

In this chapter you learned guidelines for choosing activities that meet your personal needs and interests. Use the guidelines to choose an activity that you enjoy. **Take action** by performing it for at least 30 minutes a day for several days during the upcoming week.

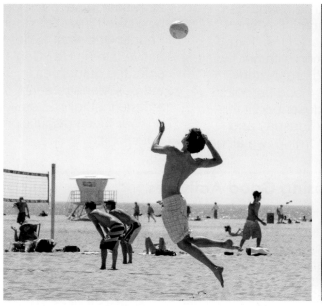 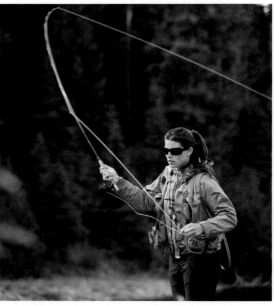

Take action by choosing activities that meet your needs and interests.

CHAPTER REVIEW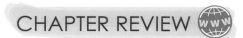

Reviewing Concepts and Vocabulary

Answer items 1 through 5 by correctly completing each sentence with a word or phrase.

1. _____ refers to self-direction, or the ability to make decisions for yourself.

2. Rewarding yourself for your effort in order to build intrinsic motivation is called a _____ system.

3. People who need an external reward to do a behavior have _____ motivation.

4. _____ refers to the capacity to make sound health decisions.

5. _____ education includes challenging recreational activities such as rock climbing.

For items 6 through 10, as directed by your teacher, match each term in column 1 with the appropriate phrase in column 2.

6. self-determination theory   a. places importance on autonomy

7. cooperative game   b. expert

8. optimal challenge   c. emphasizes team building and problem solving

9. professional   d. motivation that comes from within

10. intrinsic motivation   e. ensures success with reasonable difficulty

For items 11 through 15, respond to each statement or question.

11. List and describe some of the benefits of high-quality physical education.

12. List and describe several physical education elective opportunities.

13. List and describe the seven characteristics of physical literacy.

14. Describe the guidelines for choosing activities that can be used for a lifetime.

15. Describe at least one career opportunity from each area of science: kinesiology, nutrition science, health science, and medical and life sciences.

Thinking Critically

Write a paragraph to answer the following question.

You've been asked to form an intramural team for a school league. What steps would you take to organize a team?

Project

Working alone or with a group, develop a directory of physical activity for your community. Include a list of agencies and businesses offering various kinds of physical activity. Consider the following categories and list the activities they provide: local government agencies, community sport organizations, worksite activity programs, local businesses, and places of worship. Use table 21.1 for ideas.

Glossary

absolute strength—Strength measured by how much weight or resistance you can overcome regardless of body size.

acceleration—Increase in velocity.

accelerometer—Device that measures movement; frequently used to measure steps, intensity of movement, and duration of physical activity.

acronym—Specific kind of mnemonic in which the first letters of each word in a phrase are combined to form an easy-to-remember word (for example, FIT—frequency, intensity, and time).

active stretch—Stretch caused by contraction of your own antagonist muscles.

activity neurosis—Condition in which a person feels overly concerned about getting enough exercise and becomes upset if they miss a regular workout.

Adequate Intake (AI)—Dietary reference intake (DRI) used when there is insufficient evidence to establish a Recommended Dietary Allowance (RDA).

adventure education—Physical education approach focused on challenging recreational activities, such as rock climbing, orienteering, and rafting.

aerobic—Term meaning "with oxygen"; often used to describe moderate to vigorous physical activity that can be sustained for a long time because the body can supply adequate oxygen to continue activity.

aerobic capacity—The ability of the cardiorespiratory system to provide and use oxygen during very hard exertion over a specific amount of time, measured by the maximal oxygen uptake test.

aerobic physical activity—Activity that is steady enough to allow your heart to supply all the oxygen your muscles need.

aerodynamics—Study of motion in the air.

agility—Ability to control your body's movements and change body position quickly.

air quality index—Scale used to rate air pollution levels, ranging from good to hazardous.

alarm reaction—First stage of general adaptation syndrome; occurs when your body reacts to a stressor.

amino acid—Building block of protein.

anabolic steroid—Risky synthetic drug that resembles the male hormone testosterone and produces lean body mass, weight gain, and bone maturation.

anaerobic—Term meaning "without oxygen"; often used to describe activities for which the body can't supply enough oxygen to keep going for long periods of time.

anaerobic capacity—The ability of the body to perform all-out exercise using the body's high energy fuel sources (ATP-PC and glycolytic systems); commonly measured using the Wingate Test.

anaerobic physical activity—Activity so intense that your body cannot supply adequate oxygen to sustain it for a long time.

androgen—Hormones primarily associated with male physical characteristics.

androstenedione—A steroid precursor that is converted into anabolic steroids such as testosterone after it enters the body; also called *andro*.

anorexia athletica—Disorder marked by obsessive exercise; most common among athletes involved in sports in which low body weight is desirable (such as gymnastics and wrestling).

anorexia nervosa—Eating disorder in which a person severely restricts the amount of food eaten in an attempt to be exceptionally low in body fat.

antagonist—Muscle or muscle group having the opposite function of another muscle or muscle group.

atherosclerosis—Disease caused by clogging of the arteries.

ATP-PC system—System that uses high-energy fuels called adenosine triphosphate (ATP) and phosphocreatine (PC) to provide energy for very vigorous short bouts of physical activity (15 seconds or less).

attitude—Your feelings about something.

autonomy—Self-direction; ability to make decisions for yourself.

balance—Ability to maintain an upright posture while standing still or moving.

ballistic stretching—Series of gentle bouncing or bobbing motions that are not held for a long time.

basal metabolism—Amount of energy your body uses just to keep you living.

bioelectrical impedance analysis (BIA)—A type of lab assessment that requires a special machine that measures the speed that electrical current moves through the body to measure body composition.

biomechanical principles—Basic laws of physics that help people perform physical tasks efficiently and effectively.

biomechanics—Branch of kinesiology that uses principles of physics to help us understand the human body in motion.

blood pressure—Force of blood against your artery walls.

bodybuilding—A competitive sport in which participants are judged primarily on the appearance of their muscles rather than how much they can lift.

body composition—The proportion of body tissues, including muscle, bone, body fat, and other tissues, that make up your body.

body fat level—Percentage of body weight that is made up of fat.

built environment—Physical characteristics of a neighborhood.

bulimia—Eating disorder in which a person binges, or eats very large amounts of food within a short time, followed by purging.

bullying—Unwanted, aggressive behavior that involves a real or perceived power imbalance.

calisthenics—Exercises done using all or part of the body weight as resistance.

calorie—Unit of energy or heat that describes the amount of energy in a food (the true term is *kilocalorie*).

calorie expenditure—Calories (energy) used in physical activity.

calorie intake—Calories (energy) ingested.

calorimeter—Apparatus used to determine the amount of heat generated by a chemical reaction; also can determine the number of calories in food.

carbohydrate—Type of nutrient that provides you with your main source of energy.

cardiac muscle—Muscle located in the walls of the heart.

cardiorespiratory endurance—Ability to exercise your entire body for a long time without stopping.

cardiovascular disease (CVD)—A physical illness that affects the heart, blood vessels, or blood, such as heart attack and stroke; currently the leading cause of death in the United States.

center of gravity—The location of the center or midpoint of the total body weight.

cholesterol—Waxy, fatlike substance found in meat, dairy products, and egg yolk; a high amount in the blood is implicated in various types of heart disease.

cognitive skills—Abilities that help you gain knowledge from information; examples include being able to concentrate and focusing your attention.

competence—The capability of carrying out a specific task or responsibility.

competitive stress—The body's reaction to participation in a sport or other activity in a competitive environment; may cause distress or eustress.

complete protein—Protein containing all nine essential amino acids; derived from animal sources, such as meat, milk products, and fish.

complex skill—Task that involves complicated movement sequences (for example, serving a tennis ball, hip-hop dancing) or integrating several movements at the same time (for example, stroking, kicking, and breathing in swimming).

con artist—Person who practices fraud.

concentric—A shortening isotonic muscle contraction.

consumer community—A school group or club that reviews scientific information and answers student questions related to fitness, health, and wellness.

controllable risk factor—Risk factor that you can act upon to change.

cool-down—Activity performed after a workout to help you recover.

cooperative game—Game in which teams work together rather than compete.

coordination—Ability to use your senses together with your body parts or to use two or more body parts together.

coping—Dealing with or attempting to overcome a problem.

coping skill—Technique that you can use to manage stress or deal with a problem.

CRAC—Contract-relax-antagonist-contract; a type of PNF stretch that first requires the muscle or muscles to contract and then relax before being stretched by the contraction of the opposing muscle or muscles.

creatine—Natural substance manufactured in the body by meat-eating animals including humans and needed in order for the body to perform anaerobic exercise, including many types of progressive resistance exercise.

criterion-referenced health standards—Fitness ratings used to determine how much fitness is needed to prevent health problems and to achieve wellness.

dance education—An approach to physical education (or a separate program) that focuses on teaching various forms of dance, both in and out of school.

deceleration—Decrease in velocity.

dehydration—A physical condition that occurs when your body does not have enough fluids to function effectively.

dependence—Relying on others to make decisions for you.

determinant—Factor affecting your fitness, health, and wellness.

diabetes—Disease in which a person's body is unable to regulate sugar levels, leading to an excessively high blood sugar level.

diastolic blood pressure—Pressure in your arteries just before the next beat of your heart.

Dietary Reference Intake (DRI)—Amount of a given micronutrient that you should consume daily.

dietitian—Expert in nutrition who helps people apply principles of nutrition in daily life; has a college degree and certification by a reputable national organization.

distress—Negative stress from situations that cause worry, sorrow, anger, or pain.

diversity—The inclusion of different types of people in society regardless of race, ethnicity, age, disability, culture, socioeconomic status, sex, or gender identity.

double progressive system—The most common method of applying the principle of progression for improving muscle fitness—first by increasing reps, and then by increasing resistance or weight.

dynamic movement exercises—Exercises such as jumping, skipping, and calisthenics that are often used in a warm-up for activities requiring strength, power, and speed.

dynamic stretching—Slow movement exercises designed to lengthen the muscles.

dynamic warm-up—Dynamic movement exercises that increase body temperature and get muscles ready for more vigorous exercise; can serve as all or part of the general warm-up.

dynamometer—Device that measures the amount of force produced by a muscle or group of muscles.

eating disorder—Condition that involves dangerous eating habits and often excessive activity to expend calories for fat loss.

eccentric—A lengthening isotonic muscle contraction.

electrolytes—Minerals in your blood and body fluids that are important for normal body functioning and prevention of water loss during exercise.

empathy—The ability to understand and be sensitive to the feelings of others.

empty calories—Calories that provide energy but contain few if any other nutrients.

energy balance—Balance between calorie intake and calorie expenditure.

equity—The personal quality of being fair and impartial (free of bias or favoritism).

ergogenic aid—Anything done to help you generate work or to increase your ability to do work, including performing vigorous exercise.

ergolytic—Term referring to substances that negatively affect performance (*ergo* meaning work, and *lytic* meaning destruction).

e-sports—Organized competitive video gaming.

essential body fat—The minimum amount of body fat that a person needs to maintain health.

etiquette—Typical or expected behavior of a social group.

eustress—Positive stress.

exercise—Form of physical activity specifically designed to improve your fitness.

exercise anatomy—Study of how muscles work together with bones, ligaments, and tendons to produce human movement.

exercise physiology—Branch of kinesiology focused on how physical activity affects body systems.

exercise psychology—Study of human behavior in all types of physical activity, including exercise for fitness and sport.

exercise sociology—Study of social relationships and interactions in physical activity, including sport.

exergaming—Digital games that involve using the large muscles of the body to perform physical activity that improves health-related physical fitness.

extension—A movement that increases the angle between the bones at a joint.

extrinsic motivation—Reason for doing something that comes from an outside source (for example, prizes).

fast-twitch muscle fiber—Muscle fiber that contracts quickly and generates more force than slow-twitch muscle fiber; important for strength activities.

fat—Nutrient that provides energy, helps growth and repair of cells, and dissolves and carries certain vitamins to cells.

feedback—Information you receive about your performance, including suggestions for making changes in order to perform better.

fiber—Type of complex carbohydrate that your body cannot digest.

fibrin—Substance involved in blood clotting.

fitness education—Classes or units in physical education focused on learning fitness and activity concepts and self-management skills that can help you be active throughout your life.

fitness profile—Brief summary of your fitness self-assessment results.

fitness target zone—Optimal range of physical activity for promoting fitness and achieving health and wellness.

FITT formula—Formula to determine the appropriate frequency, intensity, time, and type of physical activity.

flexibility—Ability to use your joints fully through a wide range of motion without injury.

flexion—A movement that reduces the angle between the bones at a joint.

food label—Nutritional information that appears on food packaging.

food supplement—Product taken as an addition to a person's basic diet (for example, vitamins, minerals, and herbs); also called a *dietary supplement*.

force—Energy exerted by the muscles to cause movement or resist movement.

fraud—Intentional use of deception to get you to buy products or services known to be ineffective or harmful.

free time—Time left over after work, school, and other commitments have been accounted for.

frequency—How often a task is performed; in the FITT formula, it refers to how often physical activity is performed.

functional fitness—Capacity to function effectively when performing normal daily tasks.

general adaptation syndrome—Body's reaction to stress in three phases: alarm reaction, stage of resistance, and stage of exhaustion.

general warm-up—Five to 10 minutes of light- to moderate-intensity physical activity that prepares your body for more intense exercise.

glycolytic system—System that uses glucose stored in the muscles and liver as glycogen to provide energy for activities that last between 11 seconds and about 90 seconds.

goal setting—Process of establishing objectives to accomplish; the objectives for lifetime fitness are to achieve good fitness, health, and wellness and to adopt a healthy lifestyle.

graded exercise test—Test used to detect potential heart problems by exercising on a treadmill while your heart is monitored by an electrocardiogram.

group cohesiveness—Working together toward a common goal.

health—Freedom from disease and a state of optimal physical, emotional–mental, social, intellectual, and spiritual well-being (wellness).

health literacy—The capacity to make sound health decisions that lead to adopting healthy lifestyles now and later in life.

health-related physical fitness—Parts of physical fitness that help a person stay healthy; includes cardiorespiratory endurance, flexibility, muscular endurance, strength, power, and body composition.

health science—Area of study that focuses on preventing and treating illness and promoting wellness.

heart attack—Condition in which the blood supply within the heart is severely reduced or cut off, which can cause an area of the heart muscle to die.

heart rate reserve (HRR)—Difference between the number of times that your heart beats per minute at rest and during maximal exercise.

heat index—Scale that rates the safety of the environment for exercise based on temperature and humidity.

hemoglobin—A protein in red blood that picks up oxygen for delivery to the cells via the arteries.

high-density lipoprotein (HDL)—Lipoprotein often referred to as *good cholesterol* because it carries excess cholesterol out of your bloodstream and into your liver for elimination from your body.

human growth hormone (HGH)—Illegal drug that is exceptionally dangerous, especially for teens; causes premature closure of bones and can have deforming and even life-threatening effects.

humidity—Relative amount of moisture in the air.

hydrodynamics—Study of motion in fluids.

hyperkinetic condition—Health problem caused by doing too much physical activity.

hypermobility—Unusually large range of motion in the joints; sometimes erroneously referred to as *double-jointedness*.

hypertension—Condition in which blood pressure is consistently higher than normal.

hyperthermia—Exceptionally high body temperature often associated with exposure to hot or humid environments.

hypertrophy—Increase in muscle fiber size.

hypokinetic condition—Health problem caused partly by lack of physical activity.

hypothermia—Abnormally low body temperature often associated with exposure to cold and windy environments.

implement—Device or tool used to perform a task.

inactive—Refers to a person who fails to meet national physical activity guidelines.

inclusion—Including all people, especially those who have previously been excluded.

incomplete protein—Protein that contains some, but not all, essential amino acids.

independence—Making decisions on your own; autonomy.

intensity—Magnitude or vigorousness of a task; in the FITT formula, it refers to how hard you perform a physical activity.

intermediate muscle fiber—Fiber with characteristics of both slow- and fast-twitch fibers.

interval training—Type of training that uses bouts of high-intensity exercise followed by rest periods.

intrinsic motivation—Reason for doing something that comes from within (for example, enjoyment, desire to be more fit).

isokinetic exercise—Type of isotonic exercise in which movement velocity is kept constant through the full range of motion.

isometric exercise—Exercise involving isometric contractions in which body parts do not move.

isotonic exercise—Exercise involving isotonic contractions in which body parts move.

kinesiology—Study of human movement.

kyphosis—Posture problem characterized by rounded back and shoulders.

laws of motion—Rules of physics that help us understand human movements.

leadership—Ability to motivate and help people in a group work toward a common goal.

lean body tissue—All tissue in the body other than fat.

leisure time—Time free from work and other commitments; also called *discretionary time*.

lifestyle—The way you live.

lifestyle physical activity—Activity done as part of daily life (such as walking to school or doing yardwork).

lifetime sport—Sport in which you're likely to participate throughout your life.

ligament—Tough tissue that holds bones together.

locomotion—Movement of the body from place to place.

long-term goal—Goal that takes months or even years to accomplish.

lordosis—Posture problem characterized by too much arch in the lower back; also called *swayback*.

low-density lipoprotein (LDL)—Type of lipoprotein often referred to as *bad cholesterol* because it is most likely to stay in your body and contribute to atherosclerosis.

macronutrient—Nutrient that supplies the energy your body needs to perform daily tasks; comes in three types—carbohydrate, protein, and fat.

maturation—Process of becoming fully grown and developed.

maximal heart rate—Number of times your heart beats per minute during very vigorous activity; the highest your heart rate can go.

maximal oxygen uptake test—Lab measure considered to be the best for assessing fitness of the cardiovascular and respiratory systems; see also *aerobic capacity*.

medical science—Science that provides medical practitioners with research evidence for medicine and medical procedures.

metabolic equivalent (MET)—Measure that refers to metabolism (the use of energy to sustain life), with 1 MET representing the energy you expend while resting; multiples are used to describe the intensity of all types of physical activity.

metabolic syndrome—Condition in which a person has high body fat, large girth, and other health risks, such as high blood pressure, high blood fat, and high blood sugar.

MET minute—Unit of measure calculated to determine energy expended when you know the MET value of the activity and the amount of time spent doing it.

micronutrient—Nutrient (vitamin or mineral) that your body needs in smaller amounts than it needs carbohydrate, protein, and fat.

microtrauma—Invisible injury, caused by repeated use or misuse of a body part, that may not result in immediate pain, soreness, or symptoms.

mindfulness—State of being characterized by a focus on the present moment.

mixed fitness activities—Activities that combine several different activities, such as vigorous aerobics, anaerobics, and muscle fitness exercises, in a single workout.

mnemonic—A term that is useful to help remember specific information, such as an acronym (for example, FIT).

moderate physical activity—Activity that requires energy expenditure four to seven times greater than that required by being sedentary (that is, 4 to 7 METs).

motor learning—Process of acquiring a motor skill; also an area of study within kinesiology that relates to acquiring motor skills.

motor skill—The learned ability to use the muscles and nerves together to perform a physical task (for example, throwing, running).

motor unit—A group of nerves and muscle fibers that work together to cause movement.

muscle bound—Having tight, bulky muscles that inhibit free movement.

muscle contraction—Activation of muscle fibers; also called muscle action.

muscle dysmorphia—Condition in which a person is obsessed with building muscle.

muscle–tendon unit (MTU)—Skeletal muscles and the tendons that attach them to bones.

muscular endurance—Ability to use your muscles many times without tiring.

neuromotor exercise—A method of training that involves balance, coordination, and agility as well as resistance and flexibility exercise.

nutrition science—Study of the processes by which a plant or animal uses food to grow and sustain life.

obesity—Condition of being especially overweight or high in body fat.

object—An item used in sport and physical activity (for example, a ball or hockey puck).

Olympic weightlifting—Sport involving free weights in which athletes try to lift a maximum load; includes two lifts (the snatch and the clean and jerk).

one-repetition maximum (1RM)—Test of muscle strength in which you determine how much weight you can lift (or how much resistance you can overcome) in one repetition.

optimal challenge—Activity that is neither too hard nor too easy, which allows success and encourages continued participation.

osteoporosis—Condition in which bone structure deteriorates and bones become weak.

outdoor education—An approach to physical education that occurs in an outdoor classroom.

overexercising—Doing so much exercise that you increase your risk of injury or soreness.

overuse injury—Injury resulting from repeated movement that causes wear and tear in your body.

overweight—Condition of weighing more than the healthy range.

oxidative system—System that uses both glucose and glycogen stored in the body to produce energy.

passive exercise—Use of a machine or device that moves your body for you; ineffective at building fitness.

passive stretch—Stretch requiring an assist from an external source (gravity, a partner, or some other source).

peak bone mass—Highest bone density achieved during life; typically occurs in late adolescence or early adulthood.

PED—Performance-enhancing drugs.

pedometer—Small battery-powered device that can be worn on your belt to count your steps.

personal needs profile—Chart listing self-assessment scores and corresponding ratings.

personal program—Written individualized plan designed to change behavior (the way you live) to improve fitness, health, and wellness.

physical activity—Movement using the large muscles; includes sport, dance, recreational activity, and activities of daily living.

physical activity compendium—List of physical activity that tells you the intensity of various activities.

Physical Activity Pyramid—Model that describes the various types of physical activity that produce good fitness, health, and wellness.

Physical Activity Readiness Questionnaire for Everyone (PAR-Q+)—Seven-question assessment of medical and physical readiness that should be taken before beginning a regular physical activity program for health and wellness.

physical fitness—Capacity of your body systems to work together efficiently to allow you to be healthy and effectively perform activities of daily living.

physical literacy—Being physically educated; a physically literate person does regular activity, is fit, has skills, values activity, and knows the implications and benefits of physical activity.

Pilates—Form of training designed to build core muscle fitness; named for Joseph Pilates, who described core exercises and developed special exercise machines for building core muscles.

plyometrics—Type of training designed to increase athletic performance using jumping, hopping, and other exercises to cause lengthening of a muscle followed by a shortening contraction.

PNF stretching—Flexibility exercise using proprioceptive neuromuscular facilitation; a variation of static stretching that involves contracting a muscle before stretching it.

power—Capacity to use strength quickly; involves both strength and speed.

powerlifting—Competitive sport using free weights and involving only three exercises: bench press, squat, and deadlift.

principle of overload—The most basic law of physical activity, which states that the only way to produce fitness and health benefits through physical activity is to require your body to do more than it normally does.

principle of progression—Principle stating that the amount and intensity of your exercise should be increased gradually.

principle of rest and recovery—Principle stating that you need to give your muscles time to rest and recover after a workout.

principle of specificity—Principle stating that the type of exercise you perform determines the type of benefit you receive.

priority healthy lifestyle choice—Key lifestyle choice (regular physical activity, sound nutrition, and stress management) that helps you prevent disease, get and stay fit, and enjoy a good quality of life.

process goal—Goal relating to what you do rather than the product resulting from what you do.

product goal—Goal relating to what you get as a result of what you do.

professional—Highly educated person who delivers information and helps people apply it to improve their lives.

progressive resistance exercise (PRE)—Exercise that increases resistance (overload) until you have the amount of muscle fitness you want; also called *progressive resistance training* (PRT).

prohormones—Nonsteroid substance that leads to the formation of a steroid.

protein—Group of nutrients used for building, repairing, and maintaining your body cells.

ptosis—Posture problem characterized by protruding abdomen.

quack—Person who practices quackery.

quackery—Method of advertising or selling that uses false claims to lure people into buying products that are worthless or even harmful.

quality of life—Satisfaction with your current life status.

range of motion (ROM)—The amount of movement in a specific joint that is considered to be healthy (neither too much nor too little).

range-of-motion (ROM) exercise—Exercise that requires a joint to move through a full range of motion either using your own muscles or with the assistance of a partner or therapist.

ratings of perceived exertion (RPE)—Method of estimating exercise intensity using self-estimates.

reaction time—Amount of time it takes to move once you recognize the need to act.

Recommended Dietary Allowance (RDA)—Minimum amount of a nutrient necessary to meet the health needs of most people.

recreation—Something you do during your free time.

relative strength—Strength adjusted for your body size.

reps—Short for *repetitions*, the number of consecutive times you do an exercise.

resting metabolism—Number of calories expended by your body for basic functions and typical light activities done during the day.

rhabdomyolysis—Condition in which muscle fibers break down and are absorbed into the bloodstream.

RICE—Formula in which each letter represents a step in the treatment of a minor injury: R = rest; I = ice; C = compression; E = elevation.

risk factor—Any action or condition that increases your chances of developing a disease or health condition.

rule—Guideline or requirement for conduct or action.

rumination—Repeatedly thinking about the past or a past—often distressing—event.

runner's high—The eustress people feel when they run or do exercise that they enjoy.

saturated fat—Fat that is solid at room temperature and is derived mostly from animal products, such as lard, butter, milk, and meat.

scam—Actions designed to take advantage of people, often motivated by potential financial gain.

scoliosis—A posture problem that occurs when the spine has too much sideways curve.

sedentary—Not engaging in regular physical activity from any of the steps of the Physical Activity Pyramid.

self-management skill—Skill that helps you adopt a healthy lifestyle now and throughout your life.

self-reward system—System of rewarding yourself for your efforts to build motivation rather than expecting others to reward you.

sensitivity—In this book it refers to paying attention to the feelings and concerns of others.

set—One group of repetitions.

short-term goal—Goal that can be reached in a short time, such as a few days or weeks.

side stitch—Pain in the side of the lower abdomen that people often experience during sport activity, especially running.

skeletal muscle—Muscles that you consciously control that produce movement involved in physical activity.

skill—Ability to perform a specific task effectively that results from knowledge and practice.

skill-related physical fitness—Parts of fitness that help a person perform well in sports and activities requiring certain skills; the parts include agility, balance, coordination, reaction time, and speed.

skill warm-up—Performing the skills to be used in an activity to prepare the body for the activity.

skinfold—Fold of fat and skin used to estimate total body fat level.

sleep apnea—Disorder that results in poor sleep or inability to sleep, characterized by pauses in breathing or shallow breathing during sleep.

slow-twitch muscle fiber—Muscle fiber that contracts at a slow rate, is usually red because it has a lot of blood vessels delivering oxygen, and generates less force than fast-twitch muscle fiber but is able to resist fatigue.

SMART goal—Goal that is specific, measurable, attainable, realistic, and timely.

smooth muscle—Muscles found in various body organs such as the walls of blood vessels and the lungs, eyes, and intestines.

social–emotional learning—A type of learning that focuses on interpersonal skills, self-control, and self-awareness.

social justice—A concept in which equity or justice is achieved in every aspect of society rather than in only some aspects or for some people.

spa—Facility offering saunas, whirlpool baths, and other services such as massage and hair or skin care.

speed—Ability to perform a movement or cover a distance in a short time.

sport—Physical activity that is competitive and has well-established rules.

sport education—Approach that seeks to make physical education both fun and interesting by dividing the year into seasons similar to those found in the sport world.

sport pedagogy—Art and science of teaching physical activity; includes applying motor learning principles to help people learn motor skills and studying the best ways to teach and learn the principles of physical activity derived from the sciences.

sportspersonship—Having respect for people on opposing teams; being a good winner and not being a poor loser.

sprain—Injury to a ligament.

stage of exhaustion—Third stage of general adaptation syndrome; occurs when the body is not able to resist a stressor well enough.

stage of resistance—Second stage of general adaptation syndrome; occurs when the immune system starts to resist or fight the stressor.

stance—Way of standing.

state of being—Overall condition of a person.

static stretch—Stretch performed slowly as far as you can without pain, until you feel a sense of pulling or tension.

strain—Injury to a tendon or muscle.

strategy—Master plan for achieving a goal or set of goals.

strength—Maximal amount of force your muscles can produce.

stress—Body's reaction to a demanding situation.

stressor—Something that causes or contributes to stress.

stretching warm-up—A way of preparing for physical activity using flexibility exercises performed after several minutes of general exercise.

stroke—Condition in which the supply of oxygen to the brain is severely reduced or cut off.

systolic blood pressure—Pressure in your arteries immediately after your heart beats.

tactic—Specific method for carrying out a strategy.

tai chi—Ancient form of exercise that originated in China and whose basic movements have been shown to increase flexibility and reduce symptoms of arthritis in some people.

target ceiling—Your upper recommended limit of activity for optimally promoting fitness and achieving health and wellness.

T-booster—Supplements that often falsely promise a variety of benefits, including (but not limited to) increased energy, increased muscle mass, and improved sexual function.

teamwork—Cooperative effort of all team members to strive for a common goal in the most effective way.

tendon—Tissue that connects muscle to bone.

test battery—A group of several fitness tests.

threshold of training—Minimum amount of overload you need in order to build physical fitness.

time—Length of a task; in the FITT formula (first *T*), it refers to the optimal length of an activity session designed to improve fitness and promote health and wellness.

Tolerable Upper Intake Level (UL)—Maximum amount of a vitamin or mineral that can be consumed without posing a health risk.

tracking—Using vision to follow the path of an object, such as a thrown ball.

trans-fatty acid—Product made from unsaturated fat by means of a process that renders it solid at room temperature (for example, solid margarine); also known as trans fat. It has been banned from food by the FDA.

trust—Belief that others are honest and reliable.

type—The specific kind of task; in the FITT formula (second *T*), it refers to the specific kind of physical activity that is performed.

uncontrollable risk factor—Risk factor that you cannot do anything to change.

underweight—Condition of weighing less than the healthy range.

unsaturated fat—Fat that is liquid at room temperature; derived mostly from plants, such as sunflower, corn, soybean, olive, almond, and peanut.

velocity—Speed of movement.

vigorous aerobic activity—Aerobic activity intense enough to elevate your heart rate above your threshold of training and into your target zone for cardiorespiratory endurance.

vigorous recreation—Activity done during your free time that is fun and typically noncompetitive, but intense enough to elevate your heart rate above your threshold of training and into your target zone for cardiorespiratory endurance.

vigorous sport—Sport activity that elevates your heart rate above your threshold of training and into your target zone for cardiorespiratory endurance.

warm-up—A series of activities that prepares the body for more vigorous exercise.

web extension—Ending of a web address, such as .gov, .org, and .com.

wellness—Positive component of health that involves having a good quality of life and a good sense of well-being.

windchill factor—Index used to determine when dangerously low temperatures and unsafe wind conditions exist.

workout—The part of the physical activity program during which a person does activities to improve fitness.

yoga—Activity that originated in India and includes exercises and breathing techniques, as well as occasional meditation.

Index

Photo Credits

About the Authors

Charles B. ("Chuck") Corbin, PhD, is a professor emeritus in the College of Health Solutions at Arizona State University. He has published more than 200 journal articles and has authored or coauthored more than 100 books, including *Fitness for Life, Fitness for Life: Middle School, Fitness for Life: Elementary School*, and *Concepts of Fitness and Wellness*, all of which earned the Text and Academic Authors Association's Texty award for excellence demonstrated over time. Dr. Corbin is internationally recognized as an expert in physical activity, health, and wellness promotion and youth physical fitness. He has presented keynote addresses at more than 40 state conventions, made major addresses in more than 15 countries, and presented numerous named lectures. He is a past president and emeritus fellow of the National Academy of Kinesiology; a fellow of the American College of Sports Medicine (ACSM), National Association for Kinesiology in

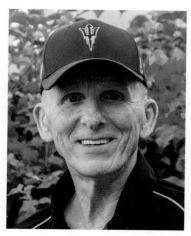

Higher Education (NAKHE), and the North American Society of Health, Physical Education, Recreation and Dance Professionals; and an honorary fellow of SHAPE America. His awards include the Lifetime Achievement Award and the Healthy American Fitness Leaders Award from the President's Council on Sports, Fitness and Nutrition (PCSFN); the Luther Halsey Gulick Award, Physical Fitness Council Honor Award, Margie R. Hanson Award, and Scholar Award from SHAPE America; and the Hetherington Award, the highest honor of the National Academy of Kinesiology. He received distinguished alumnus awards from the University of New Mexico and the University of Illinois. He was selected to the SHAPE America Hall of Fame. He served for more than 20 years as a member of the advisory board of FitnessGram and was the first chair of the science board of PCFSN.

Darla M. Castelli, PhD, is a professor in the department of kinesiology and health education at the University of Texas at Austin. Her work examines the effects of physical activity and metabolic risk factors on cognitive health. Dr. Castelli strives to understand how physical activity can reverse the effects of health risk. She has been working with school-age youth in physical activity settings for more than 25 years, leading several physical activity interventions (e.g., Kinetic Kidz, FITKids1, FITKids2, Active + Healthy = Forever Fit, and Fitness 4 Everyone). Dr. Castelli has received teaching awards in both the public school setting (e.g., Maine Physical Education Teacher of the Year) and in higher education (e.g., University of Illinois Teaching Excellence Award and University of Texas at Austin Kinesiology and Health Education Graduate Teaching Award). She is an active fellow in the National Academy of Kinesiology. As a fellow in the SHAPE

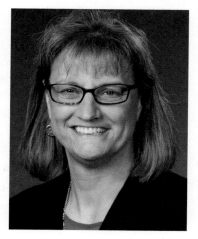

America Research Council and a past Young Scholar Award recipient from the National Association for Kinesiology and Physical Education in Higher Education (NAKPEHE) and the International Association for Physical Education in Higher Education (AEISEP), her research has been funded by the National Institutes of Health, the Robert Wood Johnson Foundation, the American Dietetic Foundation, and the U.S. Department of Education. She has presented her work at U.S. Congress and Senate briefings in Washington, D.C., in support of the FIT Kids Act. Dr. Castelli has been a member of two Institute of Medicine committees, one on fitness measures and health outcomes in youth physical activity and one on physical education in the school environment. She received a BS from Plymouth State University, an MS from Northern Illinois University, and a PhD from the University of South Carolina.

Benjamin A. Sibley, PhD, is a professor in the department of recreation management and physical education at Appalachian State University. Dr. Sibley received a BS in exercise science from Wake Forest University, an MAT in physical education from the University of South Carolina, and a PhD in sport and exercise psychology from Arizona State University. He is designated as a Certified Strength and Conditioning Specialist (CSCS) by NSCA, is certified as a CrossFit Trainer (CF-L3), and has served as a NASPE Physical Best Instructor. He has been a member of SHAPE America since 2003, currently serves on the SHAPE America Professional Preparation Council, and has served on the editorial board for the *Journal of Physical Education, Recreation and Dance* (JOPERD). Dr. Sibley has published and presented numerous papers on physical activity among children and adults, in particular addressing motivation for physical activity and the relationship between physical activity and cognitive performance. In his leisure time, Dr. Sibley enjoys exercising, outdoor activities, cooking, and spending time with his wife and two children.

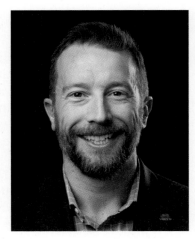

Guy C. Le Masurier, PhD, is a professor of sport, health, and physical education at Vancouver Island University in British Columbia, Canada. Dr. Le Masurier has published numerous articles related to youth physical activity and physical education, and he has given more than 50 research and professional presentations at national and regional meetings. He is the lead author of *Fitness for Life Canada* and coauthor of *Fitness for Life, Seventh Edition*; *Health Opportunities Through Physical Education*; *Fitness for Life: Middle School*; and *Fitness for Life: Elementary School*. Dr. Le Masurier has served as an editorial board member for *Research Quarterly for Exercise and Sport* and the *International Journal of Physical Education*, and he reviews research for numerous professional journals. Dr. Le Masurier is a research fellow of SHAPE America. He serves his island community as a volunteer firefighter and loves to grow vegetables.

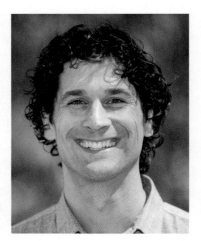